PEDIATRIC ONCOLOGY

W. Archie Bleyer
Ronald D. Barr
(Eds.)

Cancer in Adolescents and Young Adults

With 199 Figures and 90 Tables

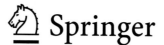

Library of Congress
Control Number: 2007930206
ISBN 978-3-540-40842-0
Springer Berlin Heidelberg New York
ISSN 1613-5318

W. Archie Bleyer
St. Charles Medical Center
Bend, Oregon, USA
Email: ableyer@scmc.org

Ronald D. Barr
McMaster University
Hamilton, Ontario, Canada
Email: rbarr@mcmaster.ca

Springer is part of Springer Science+Business Media.

Springer.com

© Springer-Verlag Berlin Heidelberg 2007

Medical Editor: Dr. Ute Heilmann, Heidelberg, Germany
Desk Editor: Meike Stoeck, Heidelberg, Germany
Cover design: Erich Kirchner, Heidelberg, Germany
Layout: Bernd Wieland, Heidelberg, Germany
Production: LE-TEX Jelonek, Schmidt & Vöckler GbR, Leipzig
Reproduktion and Typesetting: Arnold & Domnick, Leipzig

24/3100/YL – 5 4 3 2 1 0
Printed on acid-free paper

Letter from the Chair of the Children's Oncology Group

Supported by the National Cancer Institute, the Children's Oncology Group designs and conducts clinical trials, correlative laboratory research, and epidemiological studies of cancer in infants, children, and adolescents. More than 200 member institutions in the United States, Canada, Europe, Australia, and New Zealand participate in these clinical trials, as we strive to improve survival rates and lessen the late effects of cancer treatment in this population. Older adolescent and young adult participation in clinical trials is significantly lower than that of younger patients, and parallels the relatively worse treatment outcomes for each cancer type in this population.

The Adolescent and Young Adult Committee of the Children's Oncology Group was formed to focus research attention on this population, develop treatment protocols, increase participation in clinical trials, and ultimately improve survival rates for adolescents and young adults.

The following chapters highlight the initial efforts of this Committee in addressing the scope of the problem of adolescent and young adult underrepresentation in clinical trials and offer evidence that such a discrepancy may partially explain outcome differences. In addition, these chapters present information about biologic differences between specific cancer subtypes most common in younger children and those exhibited by the same cancers in adolescents and young adults, and offer plausible explanations for outcome differences as well as potential treatment strategies.

This textbook is the first comprehensive resource on cancer in adolescents and young adults. The presenting symptoms and signs, diagnosis, staging, treatment, and late effects are reviewed for each of the common malignancies in the age group, together with the epidemiology (incidence, mortality, survival, and their trends) and risk factors published earlier this year (Bleyer WA, O'Leary M, Barr R, Ries LAG (eds) (2006) Cancer Epidemiology in Older Adolescents and Young Adults 15 to 29 Years of Age, including SEER Incidence and Survival, 1975–2000. National Cancer Institute, NIH Pub. No. 06-5767, Bethesda MD; also available at www.seer.cancer.gov/publications/aya). The principles and practices of care for the adolescent and young adult patient with cancer are then discussed, with separate chapters covering specialized units, adherence/compliance, psychological support and issues, quality of life outcomes, rehabilitation and exercise, late effects, ethical issues, access to care after therapy, future health, resources for survivors, and financial considerations. There are also chapters on access to care before and during therapy, clinical trials, future challenges and opportunities, and international perspectives.

The epidemiology portions use both the International Classification of Childhood Cancer and the International Classification of Diseases-Oncology because cancers occurring in this age group span the pediatric-to-adult spectrum of diseases. I believe this textbook will help educate medical providers and the public about cancer incidence and survival in this age group, and provide the impetus for further research to improve the survival and the quality of life of these young people.

Gregory H. Reaman, MD

Letter from the Chair
of the Eastern Cooperative
Oncology Group and
President of the Coalition
of Cancer Cooperative Groups

Adolescents and young adults 15–29 years of age are making the transition from childhood to adulthood, not only physically and psychologically, but also financially and educationally. When the burden of cancer is added, it becomes part of this extraordinary and challenging time in their growth and development. They are also unique in the types of cancers that they develop and present problems that neither pediatric nor adult-treating oncologists are fully comfortable in managing. It is no surprise, therefore, that 15- to 29-year-olds are often lost in a healthcare system that concentrates on pediatric and adult cancers, with the resultant limited participation of the intermediate age group in clinical trials.

Until recently, little attention and few resources were devoted to studying the incidence, biology, and treatment outcomes in this age group. With the ability to gather data specific to this age group, the National Cancer Institute (NCI) Surveillance Epidemiology and End-Results (SEER) program allows us to estimate that, in the year 2000, there were nearly 68,000 new cases of cancer among 15- to 39-year-olds in the United States. In 15- to 29-year-olds, the focus of this textbook the estimate is 21,500 new cases. Compared to the estimated 9,200 cases diagnosed in children younger than 15 years of age, the cancer incidence rate in 15- to 29-year-olds was nearly 2.5-fold greater. Among 15- to 39-year-olds, it was nearly 7.5-fold greater.

With the establishment of the Adolescent and Young Adult Committee of the NCI-funded Children's Oncology Group and with support from the AFLAC Insurance Company, an organized program in research and education for and about young people with cancer has recently been initiated. I first heard of this initiative in 1996 when I was Chair of the Cooperative Group Chairs. It has taken a decade to reach this point, but the wait has been worthwhile.

This year the NCI is conducting a 1-year-long evaluation of the issues facing older adolescents and young adults with cancer. Known as a Progress Review Group, this effort is being cosponsored by the NCI and the Lance Armstrong Foundation. Its mission is to identify and prioritize the scientific, medical, and psychosocial barriers facing adolescent and young adult cancer patients and to develop strategies to improve their outcomes. I have had the privilege to co-Chair, along with Drs. Barry Anderson and Archie Bleyer, the Clinical Trials/Research Subcommittee of the Progress Review Group and expect the initiative to succeed in its goal to increase the participation of young adults and older adolescents in clinical trials.

This textbook, the first comprehensive treatise on cancer in adolescents and young adults, should help enable the mission of the Progress Review Group. It reviews the presenting symptoms and signs, diagnosis, staging, treatment, and late effects for each of the common malignancies in the age group. It supplements a monograph published earlier this year on the epidemiology (incidence, mortality, survival, and their trends) and risk factors of cancer in 15- to 29-year-olds (Bleyer WA, O'Leary M, Barr R, Ries LAG (eds) (2006) Cancer Epidemiology in Older Adolescents and Young Adults

15 to 29 Years of Age, including SEER Incidence and Survival, 1975–2000. National Cancer Institute, NIH Pub. No. 06-5767, Bethesda MD; also available at www.seer.cancer.gov/publications/aya). It would not have been possible without the support of the cooperative group enterprise in the United States, or without the extensive data collection efforts of the NCI's SEER program.

I congratulate the authors and look forward to a successful impact of the book and national initiative.

Robert Comis, MD

Contents

9   Non-Hodgkin Lymphoma

Catherine Patte, W. Archie Bleyer, and
Mitchell S. Cairo

10   Central Nervous System Tumors in Adolescents and Young Adults

David A. Walker, Anne Bendel, Charles Stiller,
Paul Byrne, and Michael Soka

11   Soft-Tissue Sarcomas

Karen H. Albritton, Andrea Ferrari,
and Michela Casanova

12   Bone Sarcomas

Michael S. Isakoff, Michael J. Harris,
Mark C. Gebhardt, and Holcombe E. Grier

13   Malignancies of the Ovary

Jubilee Brown, Thomas Olson, and Susan Sencer

22 Drug Compliance by Adolescent and Young Adult Cancer Patients: Challenges for the Physician

Benjamin Gesundheit, Mark L. Greenberg,
Reuven Or, and Gideon Koren

23 Psychological Support for Adolescents and Young Adults

Christine Eiser and Aura Kuperberg

24 Psychosocial Support

Brad J. Zebrack, Mark A. Chesler,
and Anthony Penn

25   Health-Related Quality of Life

Ernest R. Katz, Tasha Burwinkle, James W. Varni,
and Ronald D. Barr

26   Rehabilitation and Exercise

Marilyn J. Wright

27   Adolescent and Young Adult Cancer Survivors: Late Effects of Treatment

Smita Bhatia, Wendy Landier, Andrew A. Toogood,
and Michael Hawkins

28   Ethical Issues for the Adolescent and Young Adult Cancer Patient: Assent and End-of-Life Care

Susan Shurin and Eric Kodish

Contributors

Karen H. Albritton, M.D.
Dana Farber Cancer Institute
44 Binney Street, Boston, MA 02115, USA

Banu Arun M.D.
The University of Texas
MD Anderson Cancer Center,
1515 Holcomer Blrd., Houston, TX 77030, USA

Mary Baron Nelson, M.S.
Children's Hospital Los Angeles,
4650 Sunset Boulevard, Los Angeles, CA 90027, USA

Ronald D. Barr, M.B. ChB, M.D.
McMaster University
1280 Main Street West, Hamilton, Ontario,
L8S 4J9 Canada

Anne Bendel, M.D.
Department of Hematology/Oncology
Children's Hospital and Clinics of Minnesota
2525 Chicago Ave. S,
MS 32-4150, Minneapolis, MN 55404, USA

Smita Bhatia, M.D.
City of Hope Medical Center,
1500 East Duarte Road
Duarte, CA 91010-3000, USA

Jillian M. Birch, Ph.D.
Cancer Research UK
Paediatric and Familial Cancer Research Group
University of Manchester and Royal Manchester
Children's Hospital, Stancliffe, Hospital Road,
Manchester M27 4HA, UK

W. Archie Bleyer, M.D.
St. Charles Medical Center
Bend, 2500 NE Neff Road OR, 97701, USA

Jubilee Brown, M.D.
The University of Texas MD Anderson Cancer
Center, 1515 Holcombe Blvd.
Houston, Tx 77030, USA

Tasha Burwinkle, Ph.D.
Department of Pediatrics
Texas A and M College of Medicine
Temple, TX 76508, USA

Paul Byrne
Queen's Medical Centre, University Hospital,
NHS Trust
Derby Road, Nottingham NG7 2UH,
UK

Troy Budd
Cancer Therapy Evaluation Program
Division of Cancer Treatment and Diagnosis
National Cancer Institute,
Executive Plaza North, Bethesda, MD, 20892, USA

Mitchell S. Cairo, M.D.
Department of Pediatrics
Children's Hospital of NewYork-Presbyterian
Columbia University, 180 Fort Washington
New York, NY, 10032, USA

Michela Casanova, M.D.
Pediatric Oncology Unit
Istituto Nazionale Tumori,
Via Venezian 1, 20133 Milano, Italy

Mark A. Chesler, Ph.D.
University of Michigan
Ann Arbor, MI 48109-1882, USA

Louis S. Constine, M.D.
University of Rochester Medical Center, Departments
of Radiation Oncology and Pediatrics
601 Elmwood Are, Rochester, NY 14642, USA

Ursula Creutzig, M.D.
Universitats-Kinderklinik
Albert-Schweitzer Str. 33, 48149 Munster,
Germany

John W. Cullen, M.D.
Children's Hematology-Oncology Associates,
Denver, Co 80210, USA

Tim Eden, M.B. BS, M.D.
Academic Unit Paediatric Oncology
Christie Hospital, NHS Trust
Wilmslow Road, Manchester,
M20 4Bx, United Kingdom

Christine Eiser, Ph.D.
University of Sheffield, Western Bank
Sheffield S10 2TP, UK

Robert Fallon, M.D., Ph.D.
University of Indiana, Dept. of Hermatology/
Oncology
702 Barnhill Dr., Indianapolis, IN 46202, USA

Andrea Ferrari, M.D.
Pediatric Oncology Unit
Istituto Nazionale Tumori
Via Venezian 1, 20133 Milano, Italy

David R. Freyer, D.O.
DeVos Children's Hospital
Grand Rapids, Michigan State University College of
Human Medicine
JO Michigan Street N.E., East Lansing,
MI 48823, USA

Wayne L. Furman, M.D.
Department of Hematology/Oncology, St. Jude
Children's Research Hospital
University of Tennessee
332 N. Lauderdale, Memphis, TN 38101, USA

Mark C. Gebhardt, M.D.
Dana Farber Cancer Institute
44 Binney Street, Boston, MA 02115, USA

Benjamin Gesundheit M.D.
Hadassah Hebrew University Medical Center
Jerusalem, Israel

Mark L. Greenberg, M.B. ChB
The Hospital for Sick
Children, 555 University Arenne
Toronto, ON M5G 1x8, Canada

Holcombe E. Grier, M.D.
Dana Farber Cancer Institute
44 Binney Street, Boston, MA 02115, USA

Michael J. Harris, M.D.
Hackensack University Medical Center,
30 Porspect Are, Hackensack, NJ 07601, USA

Michael Hawkins, MSc
University of Birmingham
Queen Elizabeth Hospital, Birmingham, B15 2TT, UK

Cynthia E. Herzog, M.D.
The University of Texas MD Anderson Cancer
Center, Division of Pediatrics
1515 Holcombe Boulevard, Houston, Tx 77030,
USA

D. Ashley Hill, M.D.
Washington University Medical Center
660 S Euclid Ave, St Louis, MO 63110, USA

Melissa M. Hudson, M.D.
St. Jude Children's Research Hospital, 332 North Lauderdale
University of Tennessee, College of Medicine
332 North Landerdele, Memphis, TN 38105, USA

Michael S. Isakoff, M.D.
Dana Farber Cancer Institute
44 Binney Street, Boston, MA 02115, USA

Ernest R. Katz, Ph.D.
Children's Hospital Los Angeles and the Keck School of Medicine, University of Southern California,
4650 Sunset Boulevard, Los Angeles,
CA 90027, USA

Karen E. Kinahan, M.S.
Robert H. Lurie Comprehensive Cancer Center of Northwestern University,
Northwestern Medical Faculty Foundation
Chicago, Il 60611, USA

Eric Kodish Ph.D.
Department of Bioethics
The Cleveland Clinic Foundation
9500 Euclid Avenue, NA1-05, Cleveland,
OH 44195, USA

Gideon Koren, M.D.
Division of Clinical Pharmacology and Toxicology,
The Hospital for Sick Children
555 University Avenue, Toronto, Ontario M5G 1X8,
Canada

Aura Kuperberg, Ph.D.
University of Southern California
Children's Center for Cancer and Blood Diseases,
Children's Hospital of Los Angeles, 4656 Sunset
Boulevard, Los Angeles, CA 90027, USA

Wendy Landier, RN
City of Hope Medical Center
1500 East Duarte Road, Duarte, CA 91010-3000, USA

Michael LaQuaglia, M.D.
Memorial Sloan Kettering Cancer Center,
1275 York Ave, New York, NY 10021, USA

Michael Leahy, M.B. B.S., Ph.D.
Department of Medical Oncology
Christie Hospital NHS Trust
Wilmslow Road, Manchester M20 4BX,
UK

Ian Lewis, M.D.
Department of Paediatric and Adolescent Oncology,
St James University Hospital
Beckett Street, LS 9 7TF, UK

Marcio H. Malogolowkin, M.D.
Keck School Of Medicine of USC
Dept. of Hematology/Oncology
4650 Sunset Blvd., Los Angeles, CA 90027, USA

Giuseppe Masera, M.D.
University of Milano-Bicocca
Hospital San Gerardo
Via Perigolesi 33, 20052 Monza, Italy

Leonard J. Mattano, M.D.
Michigan State University/Kalamazoo Center for Medical Studies,
1000 Oakland Drive, Kalamazoo, MI 49008, USA

Michael Montello, M.D.
Cancer Therapy Evaluation Program, Division of Cancer Treatment and Diagnosis,
National Cancer Institute
Executive Plaza North, Bethesda, MD 20892, USA

Sue Morgan, RN
Department of Paediatric and Adolescent Oncology,
St James University Hospital
Beckett St, Leeds LS9 7TF
UK

Alexis Mottl, BA
University of Rochester Medical Center
601 Elmwood Are, Rochester, NY 14642, USA

James Nachman, M.D.
Wyler Children's Hospital
University of Chicago Medical Center,
5841 South Maryland Ave, Chicago, IL 60637, USA

Odile Oberlin M.D.
Institut Gustave Roussy
Pediatric Department, Villejuif 94800, France

Kevin C. Oeffinger, M.D.
Department of Pediatrics
Memorial Sloan Kettering Cancer Centre
1275, York Ave, New York, NY 10021, USA

Thomas Olson, M.D.
Division of Pediatric Hematology/Oncology
Childrens Healthcare of Atlantiat Egleston
2015 Uppergate Drive
Atlanta, GA 3022, USA

Reuven Or, M.D.
Hadassah Hebrew University Medical Center, PO Box
12000 Jerusalem, 91120 Israel

Alberto S. Pappo, M.D.
Texas Children's Cancer Center
6621 Fannin St., MC 3–3320
Houston, TX 77030, USA

Catherine Patte, M.D.
Department of Pediatrics
Institut Gustave Roussy, Villejuif 94800, France

Anthony Penn, M.B., ChB
Bristol Royal Hospital for Children
Bristol, BS 16 1CE, UK

Marianne Phillips, M.B., ChB
Department of Oncology
Princess Margaret Hospital for Children
Roberts Road, Perth, Western Australia 6006,
Australia

Jack Plaschkes, M.D.
University Children's Hospital, Dept. of
Pediatric Sugery
Bern, Switzerland

Lynn A.G. Ries, MS
Surveillance, Epidemiology and End Results Program,
National Cancer Institute
Bethesda, Maryland, USA

Beverly Ryan, M.D.
Department of Pediatric Oncology
Tomorrows Children's Institute
Hackensack University Medical Center
177 Summit Ave, Hackensack, NJ 07601, USA

Susan Sencer, M.D.
Children's Hospitals and Clinics of Minnesota
2525 Chicago Ave. S
Minneapolis, MN 55404, USA

Susan Shurin, M.D.
National Heart, Lung, and Blood Institute, National
Institutes of Health
Bethesda, MD 20892, USA

Stuart Siegel, M.D.
University of Southern California
Keck School of Medicine,
Los Angeles, CA 90089-9034, USA

Michael Soka
Nottingham Children's Brain Tumour Research
Centre, Nottingham City Hospital
Nottingham, NG7 24H, UK

Charles Stiller, Ph.D.
University of Oxford, Childhood Cancer Research
Group
Woodtsock Road, Oxford, OX2 6HJ, UK

Cameron K. Tebbi, M.D.
Pediatric Hematology Oncology
Tampa Children's Hospital
3001 W. ML King Boulevard
Tampa, Florida 33607, USA

Andrew A. Toogood, M.B. B.S.
University of Birmingham
Queen Elizabeth Hospital,
Birmingham, B15 2TI, UK

Tanya M. Trippett, M.D.
Memorial Sloan-Kettering
Cancer Center, Pediatric Hematology/Oncology
1275 York Ave, New York, NY 10021, USA

James W. Varni, Ph.D.
Texas A&M University
College Station, TX 77843-3137, USA

Steven G. Waguespack, M.D.
Department of Endocrine Neoplasia
and Hormonal Disorders
The University of Texas MD Anderson Cancer Center
1515 Holcombe Boulevard,
Houston, TX 77030, USA

David A. Walker, M.B. B.S.
Medical School of Nottingham QMC
Nottingham, NG72UH, UK

Samuel A. Wells, M.D.
Duke University, Medical Centre
Durham NC 27710, USA

William G. Woods, M.D.
Children's Hospital of Atlanta
Emory University,
2015 Uppergate Drive, GA 30322, Atlanta, USA

Marilyn J. Wright, BScPT
McMaster Children's Hospital
Box 2000, Hamilton, Ontario, Canada, L8N 3Z5

Brad J. Zebrack, Ph. D.
University of Southern California
669 West 34th St, Los Angeles, CA 90089-0411, USA

Arthur Zimmermann, M.D.
University of Bern
Murtenstraße 31, 3010 Bern
Switzerland

Introduction

Archie Bleyer • Karen H. Albritton •
Lynn A.G. Ries • Ronald Barr

1.1 Introduction

This is the first textbook of its type, a comprehensive treatise on cancer in adolescents and young adults who are 15 to 29 years of age when diagnosed. The impetus for this book is the lack of attention that has been paid to this age group, scientifically, therapeutically, psychosocially, and economically. During the past half-century, children (younger than 15 years of age) with cancer have been a singular focus of treatment and research. The advances among children with cancer have been among the most dramatic in the history of medicine, and the cooperative infrastructure that has supported this success has been among the most organized in the history of science. In 1971, the US National Cancer Act led to another highly organized effort that has significantly improved the outcome of adults with cancer, in whom the median age was at that time in the 60s. Meanwhile, substantially less attention has been given to the age group of cancer patients in between. Yet, cancer develops in 2.7 times more people in the 15 to 29 year age group than in those younger than 15 years of age, and the incidence of cancer has increased more rapidly in this older age group than in the younger population. Moreover, the relative improvement in the survival rate in young adults has not kept pace with that achieved in younger patients.

Reasons for this lack of progress certainly include issues specific to this age group: some inherent in the disease or the patient (differences in biology or intolerance of therapy), some inherent in the system (treatment by physicians less familiar with the disease, delay in recognition of malignancy, lack of available clinical trials, or failure to enroll patients on available trials),

Table 1.1 Incidence of invasive cancer in the period 1996–2001 reported according to age. Modified from Bleyer et al. [1]. *SEER* Surveillance, Epidemiology, and End Results

Age at diagnosis (years)	<5	5–9	10–14	15–19	20–24	25–29	30–34	35–39	40–44
United States population, year 2000 census, in millions	19.175	20.549	20.528	20.219	18.964	19.381	20.510	22.706	22.441
Incidence of invasive cancer, 1996–2001, per million, SEER	206	111	125	203	352	547	843	1289	2094
No. of persons diagnosed with invasive cancer, year 2000, U.S.	3,954	2,281	2,566	4,105	6,675	10,602	17,085	29,269	46,993

and some influenced by the psychosocial milieu of the patient (unwillingness to participate in clinical trials, delays in seeking medical attention with symptoms of cancer, poor compliance with treatment). A further consideration is that the physical, emotional, and social challenges posed by cancer in adolescence and early adult life are often unique and especially difficult for patients, families, and healthcare providers alike.

In contradistinction to younger and older patients with cancer, until recently adolescents and young adults with cancer have had no national program to address their special problems. This review describes these issues relevant and specific to adolescents and young adults with cancer and their caregivers. The ultimate goal is to heighten awareness of a relatively neglected group of patients who, during the current half-century, deserve better.

A recently published monograph from the Survaillance, Epidemiology, and End Results (SEER) program of the National Cancer Institute (NCI) and the Children's Oncology Group of the United States describes the epidemiology of cancer between 15 and 30 years of age [1]. Previously, a brief summary of the epidemiology of cancer among 15- to 19-year-olds in the United States appeared in a monograph in 1999 [2], but neither monograph includes diagnostic or therapeutic considerations. The data reported in the more recent monograph are included in the epidemiology sections of this treatise, as provided by the SEER and the United States government [3], and are analyzed with the methods described in the monograph [4].

Each disease-based chapter follows a standard outline, beginning with the epidemiology of the disease including incidence, mortality, and survival rates, and risk factors/etiology, and continuing summaries of diagnosis, treatment, and outcome. Each of the disease-based chapters is authored by at least one pediatric oncologist and at least one academic oncologist who is an expert in the investigation of adult patients with cancer (medical oncologist, surgical oncologist, or radiation oncologist). Each chapter has been reviewed before publication by a member of our editorial staff and epidemilology sections were reviewed by an epidemiologist.

1.2 Epidemiology

1.2.1 Classification System

Invasive cancer refers to any malignancy except non-melanoma skin cancer (squamous and basal cell carcinoma), in situ cancer of the breast or uterine cervix, or ovarian cancers of borderline significance. It does include low-grade brain tumors (e.g., "benign astrocytoma" and juvenile pilocytic astrocytoma) with low metastatic potential since these tumors can be fatal because of local growth. There are two basic systems of classification: the International Classification of Diseases for Oncology (ICD-O) and the International Classification of Childhood Cancers (ICCC). The ICD evolved first, and has been through several iterations

[5]. The ICCC was developed later [6] to better characterize the pediatric cancers than did the ICD. The ICD was based primarily on the site in the body where cancer arises (e.g., gastrointestinal tract, genitourinary system, respiratory system, and the breast), which is relatively easy to determine in the adult patient in part because most adult cancer at the time of diagnosis is localized. The vast majority of pediatric cancers are usually disseminated when they are diagnosed and only the tissue of origin can be determined. The ICD is therefore topographic and the ICCC is primarily histology-based. A proposal that synthesizes the ICCC and ICD systems for adolescents and young adults has been published [7]. More information on classification and how the epidemiology data were tabulated may be found in the monograph cited previously [1].

1.2.2 Incidence

In the United States, as in most economically advantaged countries of the world, 2% of all invasive cancer occurs in the 15-year interval between the ages of 15 and 30 years. This compares with cancer before age 15 years, which accounts for 0.75% of all cancers. There are 2.7 times more patients diagnosed during the second 15 years of life than during the first 15 years. At the turn of the millennium, in the year 2000, nearly 21,400 persons in the United State of 15 to 29 years of age were diagnosed to have invasive cancer (Table 1.1). Since the incidence of cancer increases exponentially as a function of age between 10 and 80 years of age (Fig. 1.1), approximately half of these patients are 25 to 29 years of age.

1.2.2.1 Age-Specific Incidence

Figure 1.1 shows the incidence of all invasive cancer in the United States from 1975 to 2000 as a function of 5-year age intervals from birth to 85+ years. The straight line in Fig. 1.1B, which is presented on a logarithmic scale, indicates that the incidence increases exponentially with age from 10 to 55 years, and throughout the adolescent and young adult years, which suggests that a common age-dependent oncogenic process is active, such as telomerase shortening, or that the mutation-to-malignancy rate constantly increases with age.

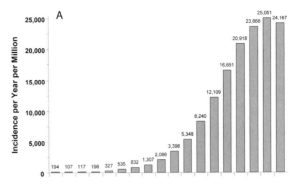

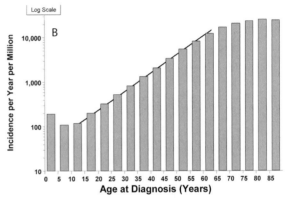

Figure 1.1

Incidence of all invasive cancer in the United States from 1975 to 2000 as a function of 5-year age intervals from birth to 85+ years. The ordinate is linear in A and logarithmic in B. The *straight line* in B indicates that the incidence is exponentially correlated with age from 10 to 55 years, and throughout the adolescent and young adult years. Surveillance, Epidemiology and End Results (SEER), 1975–2000

1.2.2.2 Gender-Specific Incidence

Figure 1.2 shows the incidence of all invasive cancer in the United States from 1975 to 2000 as a function of 5-year age intervals from birth to 85+ years separately for females (Fig. 1.2A) and males (Fig. 1.2B). Females demonstrate the exponential risk pattern from age 10 to 50 years. Males have a third peak that appears during the young adult age range, at approximately

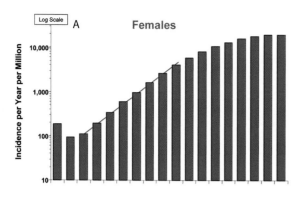

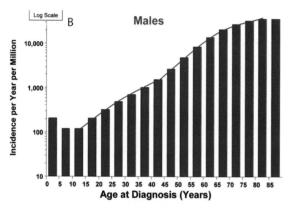

Figure 1.2

Incidence of all invasive cancer in the United States from 1975 to 2000 as a function of 5-year age intervals from birth to 85+ years among females (A) and males (B), each expressed on semi-logarithmic coordinates. SEER, 1975–2000

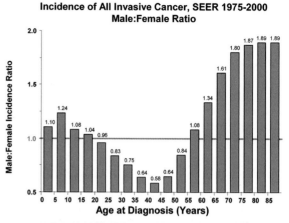

Figure 1.3

The relative risk of developing cancer in males versus females: dependence on age. SEER, 1975–2000

likely than girls to develop cancer, and older adult males are much more likely than the opposite sex to suffer a malignancy. The switchover from a male predominance in childhood to a female predominance occurs in the 15 to19 year age group. Between the ages of 10 and 40 years, the male:female ratio declines linearly to the 40- to 45-year nadir.

1.2.2.3 Ethnicity-Specific Incidence

The dependence of cancer incidence on race and ethnicity as a function of age is shown in Figs. 1.4 and 1.5. The non-Hispanic white population has had the highest incidence during the first 40 years of life. Over the age of 40 years, African Americans have been at the highest risk. Americans of Hispanic/Latino, Asian, and Pacific Islander descent are the next most likely. American Indians and Native Alaskans have had the lowest incidence at all ages. Males and females each follow the race/ethnicity incidence patterns described above, with males demonstrating more marked differences (Fig. 1.6).

1.2.2.4 Types of Cancer

The common types of cancer and their relative proportion of all invasive cancers that occurred in 51,479 15-

25 years of age. This intermediate peak may have occurred in males as a result of Kaposi sarcoma and HIV-related lymphoma during the AIDS epidemic of the 1980s and early 1990s. Alternatively, another age-dependent oncogenic mechanism may occur in young adult males that may also contribute to their risk.

Figure 1.3 demonstrates the dependence on age of the relative risk of developing cancer in males versus females. The male:female ratio has a nadir between the ages of 40 and 45 years, during which females are almost twice as likely to develop invasive cancer. At both ends of the age spectrum, in children and older adults, the ratio is reversed. Boys are 10 to 25% more

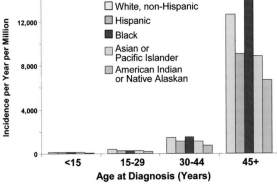

Figure 1.4

The incidence of all invasive cancer according to race/ethnicity as a function of age from birth to +45 years. SEER, 1990–1999

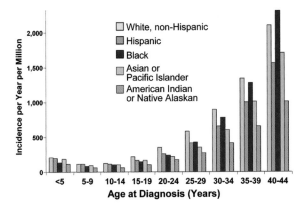

Figure 1.5

The incidence of all invasive cancer according to race/ethnicity as a function of 5-year age intervals from birth to 44 years. SEER, 1990–1999

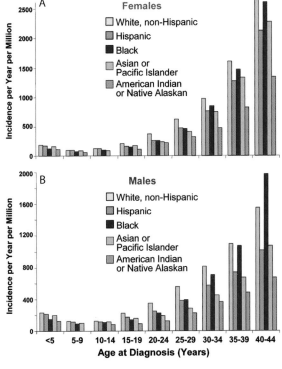

Figure 1.6

The incidence of all invasive cancer according to race/ethnicity as a function of 5-year age intervals from birth to 44 years among females (A) and males (B). SEER, 1990–1999

tumors (6%), breast cancer (5%), bone sarcomas (3%, predominantly osteosarcoma and Ewing tumor), and extragonadal germ cell tumors like teratocarcinoma and dysgerminoma (2%).

The distribution of the most frequent cancers within 5-year age intervals within the 15- to 29-year age range is shown in Figs. 1.8–1.10. The most dramatic changes in the types of cancer as a function of age between 15 and 29 years of age are melanoma (from 9th most frequent in the 15- to 19-year age group to 1st most frequent in the 25- to 29-year age group), leukemia (from 2nd most frequent to 11th), female genital tract malignancies (from 10th to 2nd most frequent), testicular carcinoma (8th to 3rd), and bone sarcomas (5th to 12th).

to 29-year-old Americans registered by SEER during the period 1975–2000 is shown in Fig. 1.7. Lymphoma accounted for the largest proportion, 19% of all cases, with Hodgkin lymphoma the most frequent, accounting for 12% of all cases by itself. Second in frequency was melanoma (11%) and testis cancer (11%), followed in rank order by female genital tract malignancies (10%, predominantly carcinoma of the uterine cervix and ovary), thyroid cancer (10%), soft-tissue sarcomas (8%), leukemia (6%), brain and spinal cord

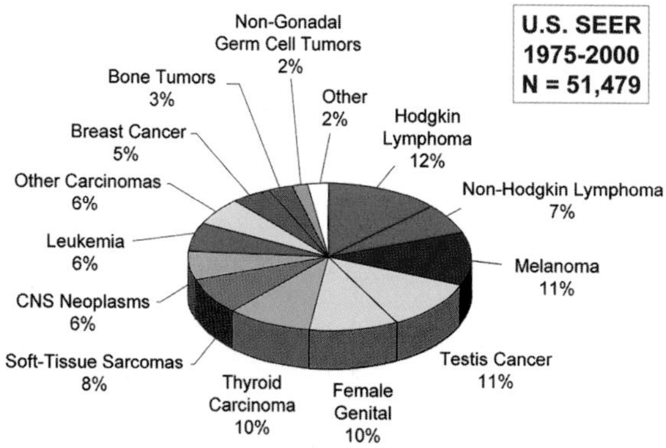

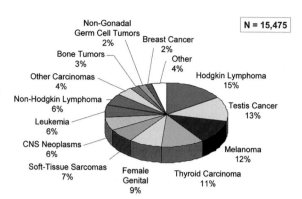

Figure 1.7

The common types of cancer and their relative proportion of all invasive cancers that occurred in 51,479 15- to 29-year-old Americans registered by SEER during the period 1975–2000

Figure 1.9

The distribution of the most frequent cancers within 5-year age intervals and within the 20- to 24-year age range. The total number of patients available for analysis was 15,475. SEER, 1975–2000

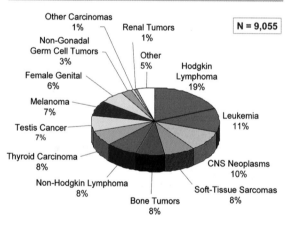

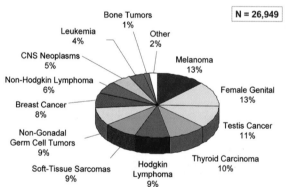

Figure 1.8

The distribution of the most frequent cancers within 5-year age intervals within the 15- to 19-year age range. The total number of patients available for analysis was 9,055. SEER, 1975–2000

Figure 1.10

The distribution of the most frequent cancers within 5-year age intervals within the 25- to 29-year age range is shown in Figs. The total number of patients available for analysis was 26,949. SEER, 1975–2000

1.2.2.5 Trends in Incidence

Between 1975 and 2000, cancer increased in incidence in all age levels below 45 years of age (Fig. 1.11). Most of the increase in incidence in 25- to 44-year-olds occurred in males (Fig. 1.12), in large part due to increases in soft-tissue sarcoma (notably Kaposi sarcoma), non-Hodgkin lymphoma, and testicular carcinoma (Fig. 1.13). Among females less than 45 years of age, the greatest increases occurred in germ cell tumors (Fig. 1.14).

There is evidence that the increase in incidence has declined among 15- to 29-year-olds, with a leveling off

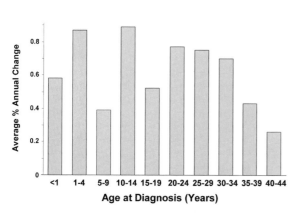

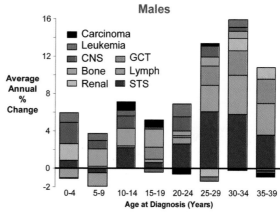

Figure 1.11

Change in the incidence of all invasive cancer between 1975 and 2001. SEER, 1975–2001

Figure 1.13

Increase in the incidence of cancer among males between 1975 and 1998, compiled from SEER data

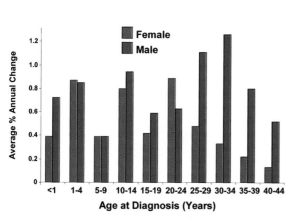

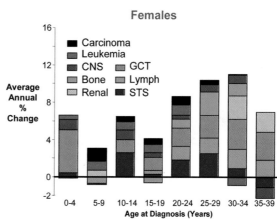

Figure 1.12

Change in the incidence of all invasive cancer between 1975 and 2001 according to gender. SEER, 1975–2001

Figure 1.14

Increase in the incidence of cancer among females between 1975 and 1998, compiled from SEER data

of the incidence rate among 15- to 24-year-olds and a decrease after a peak in the late 1980s and early 1990s in 25- to 29-year-olds (Fig. 1.15). The latter is primarily due to cancers related to the HIV epidemic that occurred during the years before the rise in cancer incidence during the early 1980s in this age group.

1.2.3 Mortality and Survival

1.2.3.1 Age- and Gender-Specific Mortality

The national mortality rate of all invasive cancer as a function of age at death in shown in Fig. 1.16. Largely,

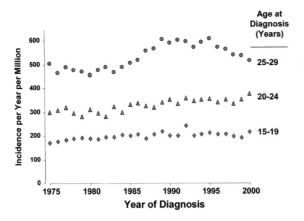

Figure 1.15

Change in the incidence of invasive cancer in three different age groups (15 to 19 years, 20 to 24 years, and 25 to 29 years) as a function of the year of diagnosis. SEER, 1975–2000

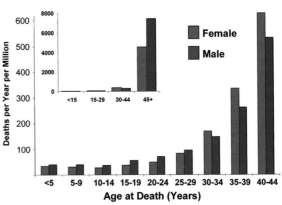

Figure 1.16

The national mortality rate of all invasive cancer as a function of age at death in the period 1975–2000

the age-dependent cancer mortality rate reflects the incidence profile (Fig. 1.6). More males die of cancer above age 45 years (Fig. 1.16, inset). From 30 to 45 years of age, deaths among females predominate. In younger patients, the mortality rate is higher among males (Fig. 1.16). Figure 1.17 shows the gender-specific ratio of the mortality rate to the incidence rate for the era 1975–2000. When the mortality rate is considered relative to the variation in incidence, it can be seen that, among all age groups from age 10 to 45 years of age, more men than women have died of cancer. This suggests that the cancers that occurred in adolescent and young adult males during 1975–2000 were more lethal than those in women, or that the treatment was less effective or efficacious.

1.2.3.2 Ethnicity-Specific Mortality

Figures 1.18 and 1.19 present the mortality rate for all invasive cancer according to ethnicity and age of death up to 45 years. The mortality rate generally reflects the incidence rate (Figs. 1.4 and 1.5), with the exception of the population of 15- to 44-year-old African-Americans, who had a higher mortality rate relative to their incidence than any of the other races/ethnicities evaluated.

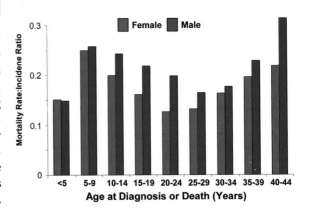

Figure 1.17

Ratio of national mortality rate to SEER incidence for all invasive cancer among males and females in the period 1975–2000

1.2.3.3 Trends in Mortality

The mortality rate from invasive cancer declined during the period 1975–2000 in all age groups below age 45 years, but the least improvement occurred in the 20- to 44-year-olds (Fig. 1.20). This pattern – less progress among young adults than among children and young adolescents – is true for both genders (Fig. 1.21)

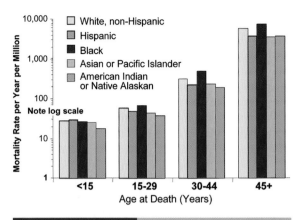

Figure 1.18

National mortality rate of all invasive cancer in the United States according to race, including American Indians/Alaskan natives, in the period 1990–2000, as a function of age from birth to 45+ years

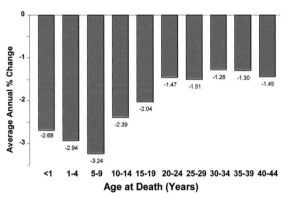

Figure 1.20

Change in the national mortality rate of all invasive cancer in the United States during the period 1975–2000

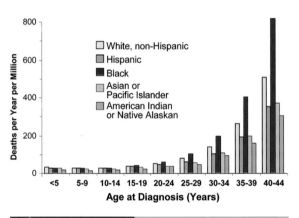

Figure 1.19

National mortality rate of all invasive cancer in the United States according to race, including American Indians/Alaskan natives, in the period 1990–2000, as a function of 5-year age intervals from birth to 44 years

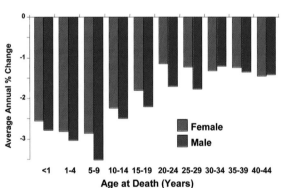

Figure 1.21

Change in the national mortality rate of all invasive cancer in the United States during the period 1975–2000, as a function of gender

and for whites and African Americans (Fig. 1.22). Among African Americans, however, the rate of progress in reducing cancer mortality was considerably lower, particularly among the 15- to 24-years olds (Fig. 1.22).

1.2.4 Survival

In the United States, cancer and suicide are the leading causes of nonaccidental death among adolescents and young adults. Among 20- to 39-year-olds, cancer causes more deaths than heart disease, HIV infection,

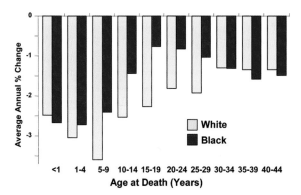

Figure 1.22

Change in the national mortality rate of all invasive cancer in the United States during the period 1975–2000, as a function of race

diabetes mellitus, chronic liver disease (including cirrhosis), cerebrovascular disease, and congenital anomalies (Table 1.2) [8]. In females, deaths caused by cancer occur at more than twice the frequency of the second leading cause of death caused by disease (Table 1.2).

Rates of survival up to 20 years after a diagnosis of invasive cancer is shown in Fig. 1.23 for all patients followed by SEER during the period 1975–1999, and in Figs. 1.24 and 1.25 for the females and males during

this era, respectively. Among 15- to 29-year-olds and females 30 to 44 years of age, survival after an invasive cancer diagnosis was comparable to that in persons who were younger than age 15 years when diagnosed. In males older than 30 years, survival was worse. Above age 45 years, survival was considerably worse, and comparable in men and women, in large part due to death from causes other than cancer.

Survival as a function of race/ethnicity among 15- to 29-year-olds with cancer is shown in Fig. 1.26; the era is more recent (and the follow-up shorter), 1992–1999, since race/ethnicity data for other than whites and African Americans were not available until the 1990 census. American Indians and Native Alaskans have had the worst survival, with more than 35% of the patients dying within 2 years, nearly twice the death rate observed among other races/ethnicities. African Americans have had the second worst survival outcome.

Figures 1.27–1.29 display the average annual percent change (AAPC) in 5-year relative survival of patients diagnosed between 1975 and 1997, inclusive, as a function of age at diagnosis, in 5-year age increments [9]. Relative survival refers to adjustment of the observed survival relative to the survival expected from population norms of the same age, and thereby partially corrects for deaths due to causes other than cancer. The average annual percent change in survival

Table 1.2 Top eight causes of death due to disease in those aged 20 to 39 years in the United States in 2002 (accidents and homicides excluded). Modified from Jemal et al. (2005) [8]. *HIV* Human immunodeficiency virus, *Dis.* disease, *Cong.* congenital, *Cerebrovasc.* cerebrovascular

	Male & Female	Deaths		Males	Deaths		Females	Deaths
1	Suicide	10,684	1	Suicide	8,771	1	Cancer	5,403
2	Cancer	10,029	2	Heart diseases	5,590	2	Heart diseases	2,640
3	Heart diseases	8,230	3	Cancer	4,626	3	Suicide	1,913
4	HIV disease	4,597	4	HIV disease	3,206	4	HIV disease	1,391
5	Diabetes mellitus	1534	5	Diabetes mellitus	905	5	Cerebrovasc. Dis.	740
6	Chronic Liver Dis.	1327	6	Chronic Liver Dis.	852	6	Diabetes mellitus	629
7	Cerebrovasc. Dis.	1482	7	Cerebrovasc. Dis.	742	7	Chronic Liver Dis.	475
8	Cong. Anomalies	983	8	Cong. Anomalies	552	8	Cong. Anomalies	431

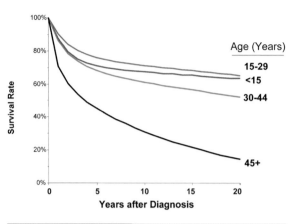

Figure 1.23

Rates of survival up to 20 years after a diagnosis of invasive cancer according to age, in the period 1975–1999 (SEER)

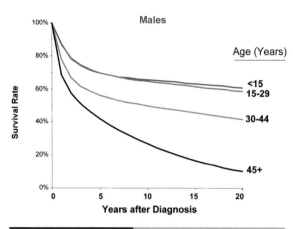

Figure 1.25

Rates of survival among males up to 20 years after a diagnosis of invasive cancer according to age, in the period 1975–1999 (SEER)

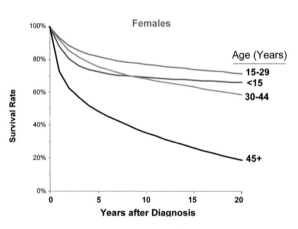

Figure 1.24

Rates of survival among females up to 20 years after a diagnosis of invasive cancer according to age, in the period 1975–1999 (SEER)

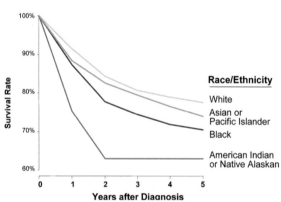

Figure 1.26

Short-term survival as a function of race/ethnicity among 15-to-29-year-olds diagnosed with invasive cancer during the period 1992–1999 (SEER)

for females and males are evaluated separately in Figs. 1.28 and 1.29. An explanation of how SEER applies the AAPC and relative survival parameters is given in Bleyer et al (2006) [10].

Steady progress in improving the 5-year survival rate has occurred among children and older adults. Between 15 and 45 years of age, however, progress in survival improvement has been a fraction of that achieved in younger and older patients, and among patients 25 to 35 years of age, there has been no evidence of an improvement in survival from all invasive cancers considered together since 1975 (Fig. 1.27).

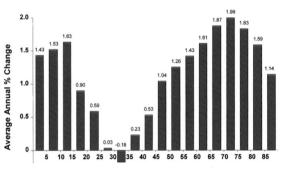

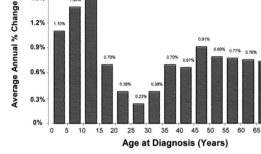

Figure 1.27

Change in the 5-year relative survival rate of all invasive cancer in the period 1975–1997 (SEER) as a function of 5-year age increments

Figure 1.28

Change in the 5-year relative survival rate of females with invasive cancer in the period 1975–1997 (SEER) as a function of 5-year age increments

Most of the older adolescent–young adult deficit has occurred among males (Fig. 1.28), but females have not been spared (Fig. 1.29).

To determine whether the early-adult survival gap was apparent at follow-up time points earlier and later than 1 year, 1- and 10-year relative survival intervals were examined and compared with the 5-year relative survival (Fig. 1.30) [10]. In this analysis, the survival rates during the 1995–1999 era were compared with those of the 1975–1999 era and expressed as the percentage improvement since the earlier era, and individual year-to-year age groups were evaluated instead of the 5-year age groupings. All three survival parameters (1-, 5- and 10-year survival rates) showed the same profile (Fig. 1.30A), with a nadir in progress occurring between the ages of 25 and 40 years (the red zone in Fig. 1.30). The 10-year survival pattern showed an even greater disparity with progress made in other age groups, than either the 1- or 5-year follow-up data. As in the analyses that utilized the average percent change method, young adult males exhibited a more striking deficit than females of the same age group (Fig. 1.30B).

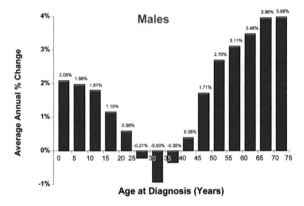

Figure 1.29

Change in the 5-year relative survival rate of males with invasive cancer in the period 1975–1997 (SEER) as a function of 5-year age increments

1.2.4.1 Conditional Survival

Conditional survival expresses change in prognosis for survivors as a function of their time since diagnosis [11]. When applied to cancer, this matrix estimates the risk of dying after an interval of survival and allows survivors and their healthcare providers to know what the risks are at intervals after diagnosis, and to base prognostication and follow-up accordingly [12, 13].

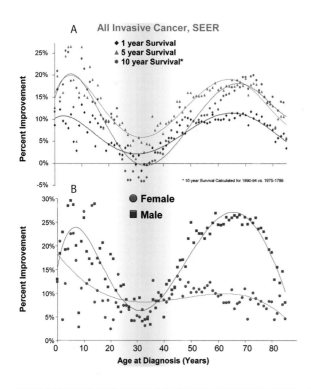

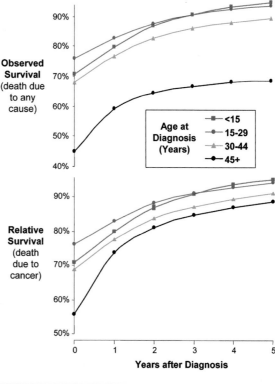

Figure 1.30

A Comparison of the 1-year (*blue diamonds*), 5-year (*red triangles*), and 10-year (*green circles*) survival rates during the period 1995–1999 compared with those of the period 1975–1999, expressed as the percentage improvement since the earlier era, as a function of individual year-to-year age groups (SEER). B Percentage improvement in overall survival among females (*pink*) and males (*blue*) as a function of age at diagnosis during the period 1995–1999. The *red zone* indicates a nadir in progress between the ages of 25 and 40 years

Figure 1.31

Improvement in 5-year conditional survival (freedom from death of any cause) for four age groups: younger than 15 years, 15–29 years, 30–44 years, and 45 years and older when diagnosed with all invasive cancer, during the first 5 years following diagnosis (SEER, 1975–2000). *Upper panel* Observed survival (freedom from death by any cause); *lower panel* relative survival (freedom from death due to cancer)

The NCI SEER database was used to determine the conditional survival of 15- to 29-year-olds diagnosed with cancer during the period 1975–2000 and to compare their results with younger and older patients diagnosed during the same interval. In Fig. 1.31, the observed conditional survival is shown for four age groups: younger than 15 years, 15 to 29 years, 30 to 44 years, and 45 years and older when diagnosed with cancer. The upper panel shows absolute survival (free-dom from death of any cause) and the lower panel depicts relative survival (freedom from death attributable to having had a diagnosis of cancer). Whereas 15- to 29-year-olds diagnosed with cancer during the past quarter century had a better prognosis at diagnosis (as shown by the values in Fig. 1.31 at time zero), their probability of survival thereafter did not increase as rapidly as it did in younger and older patients, particularly for relative survival.

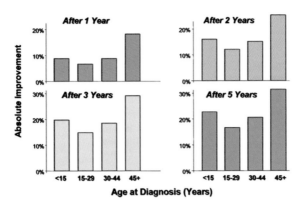

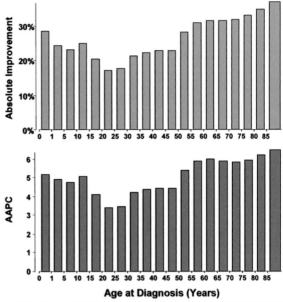

Figure 1.32

Comparison of improvement in 5-year conditional relative survival (freedom from death by cancer) at 1, 2, 3, and 5 years after diagnosis of any invasive cancer as a function of age at diagnosis (SEER, 1975–2000)

Figure 1.33

Improvement in 5-year relative conditional survival (freedom from death due to cancer) 5 years after diagnosis of all invasive cancer as a function of age at diagnosis from birth (<1 year) and then at 5-year age groups to 85+ years (SEER, 1975–2000). *Upper panel* Absolute improvement from 1975 to 2000; *lower panel* Average annual percent change (AAPC) during the period 1975–2000

Conditional survival in all SEER-registered patients with cancer at 1, 2, 3, and 5 years after diagnosis as a funktion of age is shown in Fig. 1.32. A deficit among 15- to 29-year-olds is apparent at the earliest follow-up and continues at the same magnitude throughout the 5-year postdiagnosis period.

The conditional relative survival 5 years after diagnosis is further analyzed in Fig. 1.33 for 5-year age intervals. The upper panel demonstrates the absolute percent improvement in conditional survival from 1975 to 2000. The lower panel shows the AAPC, using the same method as shown for change in survival at diagnosis (Fig. 1.27). In both cases, the 20- to 29-year age group had the least improvement in conditional survival, and those 15 to 19 years of age at diagnosis had the next worst improvement

These profiles may be interpreted to mean that during the past 25 years, young adults with cancer have not enjoyed the improved prognosis with the passage of time since diagnosis to the extent that younger and older patients have. This deficit in progress is in addition to the deficit in survival improvement measured at diagnosis described above and shown in Figs. 1.27–1.30).

The reason for a deficit in conditional survival

among young adults relative to younger and older patients is not known. One explanation is that the kinds of cancer that occur in this age group are distinctly different than those that occur in younger and older persons. It is possible that the mix of sarcomas, lymphomas (both Hodgkin and non-Hodgkin lymphoma), leukemia, thyroid cancer, melanoma, testicular carcinoma, breast cancer, and carcinoma of the uterine cervix that occurs in young adults may not have the same year-to-year improvement as the array of cancers in younger and older patients. It is possible that it may take longer in the young adult age group than 5 years after diagnosis to realize an eventual overall gain that matches younger and older patients. Another possibility is that the therapeutic gains made in younger and older patients have not occurred to the same degree in young adults and older adolescents – an explanation that has been applied to the deficit in survival at the time of diagnosis. Either way, however, survival at diagnosis and conditional survival up to 5 years after diagnosis indicates that young adults and older adolescents deserve a better trend in outcome than that which has occurred during the last quarter century.

1.2.5 Etiology and Risk Factors

As in younger patients, little is known about the causes of cancer in adolescents and young adults. Whereas cancers in infants and young children are likely to be influenced strongly by congenital and prenatal factors, and cancers in the elderly population are most strongly linked with environmental causes, the cancers in young adults and older adolescents may be a combination of both. Very few cancers in this age group have been attributed directly to single environmental or inherited factors. An exception is clear cell adenocarcinoma of the vagina or cervix in adolescent females, with most cases caused by diethylstilbestrol taken prenatally by their mothers in an attempt to prevent spontaneous abortion. Radiation-induced cancer may occur in adolescents and young adults after exposure during early childhood. In fact, many of the adolescent and young adult cancers that have been linked to an identifiable cause are second malignant neoplasms in patients who were treated with chemotherapy and/or radiotherapy for a prior cancer.

Given that the duration of exposure to potential environmental carcinogens is directly proportional to age, it is not surprising that tobacco-, sunlight-, or diet-related cancers are more likely to occur in older adolescents than in younger persons. With the probable exception of melanoma, cancers known to have been related to environmental exposures in older adults have not been implicated with any certainty to environmental agents in 15- to 30-year-olds. In most people, it appears to take considerably longer than one or two decades for these environmentally related cancers to become manifest. The logical hypothesis is that adolescents who develop cancer after a carcinogenic exposure have a predisposing genotype. For example, melanoma is more common among Australian adolescents than among those elsewhere in the world, as described above. The Australia data does suggest that solar exposure may be able to induce skin cancer before the end of the second decade of life, at least in that part of the world.

Besides intense sun exposure, exposure to other environmental carcinogens, including tobacco, recreational drugs, alcohol, and sexually transmitted diseases, begins or intensifies during this age period. Cancer control efforts to reduce teenage exposure to these carcinogens are unlikely to affect rates of cancers in adolescents, but should decrease rates in adults.

Lymphoma, sarcoma, melanoma, and cancer of the breast, thyroid, colon, and liver may also occur at higher frequency during this period of life in persons with inherited conditions (see Chaps. 9, 11, 12, 16–18, and 20). On aggregate, however, these cancers account for only a small proportion of the cancers that occur during adolescence and early adulthood.

1.3 Diagnosis

1.3.1. Signs and Symptoms

With few exceptions, the signs and symptoms of cancer in young adults and older adolescents are similar to those of the same cancer in younger and older patients. Nonetheless, knowing the most common sites of disease in this age group helps in directing the evaluation of the symptoms and in formulating the most appropriate differential diagnosis. The examiner who is not aware of the prominence of sarcomas, thyroid and testicular cancer, and melanoma in this age group may overlook these possibilities when taking the history and performing the physical examination.

Because of the psychological and social factors that affect adolescents and young adults, patients in this age range may be at higher risk for a delay in diagnosis, a factor that may impact their cancer survival. In a study of the interval between symptom onset and diagnosis (lag time) in 2,665 children participating in Pediatric Oncology Group therapeutic protocols between 1982 and 1988, Pollock and colleagues found by multivariate analysis that for all solid tumors except Hodgkin lymphoma, lag time increased as age increased [14]. In addition, data from the University of Texas

MD Anderson Cancer Center indicates, that among 15- to 29-year-olds with newly diagnosed, previously untreated cancer, the lag time to diagnosis was correlated with the quality of health insurance. Those with public or no health insurance had statistically longer lag times in five of the six cancers evaluated [15, 16]. In multivariate analysis, only the type of cancer and quality of health insurance were significantly correlated with lag time. Gender, age subgroup, race/ethnicity, religion, marital status, rural vs. urban residence, and median household income and population density of the zip code of residence were not correlated.

The reasons for delay in seeking medical care and obtaining a diagnosis are multiple:

1. Adolescents and young adults have a strong sense of invincibility. Out of denial, they may delay seeing a physician for symptoms. Even when seen, they may give poor historical information, especially to a physician untrained to "read between the lines" of an adolescent's history. Some of the most advanced disease presentations occur in adolescents. We have had older adolescents with extraordinarily large masses of the breast, testes, abdomen, pelvis, and extremity that they had harbored for months because they were too embarrassed to bring the problem to anyone's attention.

2. Too many young adults are not receiving routine medical care. Young adults and older adolescents have the lowest rate of primary care use of any age group in the United States [17]. Regardless of health insurance status, adolescents and young adults are more likely than younger children to lack a usual source of care. Without a primary physician who knows the patient's baseline heath status, the symptoms of cancer can be missed.

3. Physicians may be poorly trained or unwilling to care for adolescents and young adults.

4. Adolescents and young adults are not "supposed to" have cancer. Clinical suspicion is low, and symptoms are often attributed to physical exertion, fatigue, and stress.

5. Young adults are the most underinsured age group, falling in the gap between parental coverage and programs designed to provide universal health insurance to children (Medicaid and Children's Health Insurance Programs), and the coverage supplied by a full-time secure job. Lifetime uninsured rates for those who present for care peak for females between ages 15 and 17 years (19%) and for males between ages 18 and 21 years (24%). True uninsured rates are likely to be higher, as those who do not present for care may not do so because of lack of insurance [18–21].

Given the lack of routine care, empowering young adults and older adolescents for self-care and detection is important. Certainly, self-examination of the skin and, in females, of the breasts should be encouraged. However, at this age, it may be most difficult to teach the importance of early detection of cancer, because at no other time in life is the sense of invincibility more pervasive. Adolescents should be taught especially to examine themselves for cancers that increase in incidence during this time period. This is particularly true for testicular self-examination, a subject that is obviously difficult to bring up and teach at this age. On the other hand, there is little evidence that testicular self-examination screening is effective. The American Cancer Society encourages self-examination of the skin and breasts, and increasing the awareness of testicular cancer in young men, but routine testicular self-examination is not recommended. Teaching testicular cancer awareness to high school and college students may not be as difficult as it may seem. A preliminary assessment of teaching testicular self-examinations showed that anxiety was no greater in students who were exposed to presentations on testicular cancer and testicular self-examination than in those who did not receive this training [22]. In addition, efforts should be made to educate teenagers about the treatment and cure rates of cancer in children and young adults in order to dispel the fatalistic perception that arises from knowing older individuals (grandparents and others) who have died from cancer.

1.3.2 Radiologic and Pathologic Considerations

A diagnosis in adolescents and young adults may be more favorably facilitated compared to children. Young adults are able to describe and localize signs and symptoms of the malignancy and biopsy specimens are more easily obtained. Knowing the most common sites and histology of malignancies in the age group assists in evaluating symptoms and in selecting the most appropriate imaging and biopsy procedures. Noninvasive imaging without the need for sedation, endoscopy, and minimally invasive surgery are all available for patients in this age group. Although these are used more often in adolescents and young adults than in children because they are easier to obtain, it is possible that they are underused in this group in comparison with older patients, because of a lack of insurance and other economic constraints, difficulty taking time off from work, transportation limitations, and a lack of understanding on the part of the professional staff as to what diagnostic and staging procedures are appropriate.

1.4 Treatment

As is true at any age, treatment depends on the type and stage of the tumor. In general, however, the therapeutic management of cancers in adolescents and young adults differs from that in adults because of physiologic, psychological, and social differences. Although there is a dearth of publications that address these issues, several provide advice on how to manage the cancers that occur in this age group [23–33].

1.4.1 Choice of Treatment Setting and Specialist

A central, complex issue is the appropriate specialist to manage the treatment of the young adult and adolescent – a pediatric oncologist or an adult oncologist (medical, radiation, surgical, or gynecologic oncologist). Leonard and his colleagues surmised that, at least in the United Kingdom, adult oncologists are "untutored in arranging ancillary medical, psychological, and educational supports that are so important to people who are facing dangerous diseases and taxing treatment at a vulnerable time in their lives" and "unpracticed in managing rare sarcomas," and pediatric oncologists "have little to no experience in epithelial tumors or some of the other tumors common in late adolescence" [34]. The (admittedly biased) American Academy of Pediatrics issued a consensus statement in 1997, in

which it indicated that referral to a board-eligible or board-certified pediatric hematologist-oncologist and to pediatric subspecialty consultants was the standard of care for all pediatric and adolescent cancer patients [35]. A wider consensus panel that included adult oncologists, the American Federation of Clinical Oncologic Societies, also concluded that "payors must provide ready access to pediatric oncologists, recognizing that childhood cancers are biologically distinct" and that the "likelihood of successful outcome in children is enhanced when treatment is provided by pediatric cancer specialists" [36]. However, neither of these statements defines an age cutoff for the recommendation.

Currently, the choice of specialist is made haphazardly and probably depends on the decision of the referring physician. Younger children obtain care primarily from pediatricians who refer to pediatric centers and specialists. Young adult and older adolescent patients are seen by a breadth of specialists for their presenting symptoms of cancer. These include internists, family physicians, gynecologists, emergency room physicians, dermatologists, gastroenterologists, neurologists, and other specialists. These physicians may have very different referral patterns [37]. In addition, when a referral of a young adult or adolescent patient is made to an oncologic subspecialist, the latter may be a medical, radiation, surgical, or gynecologic oncologist, or other oncologic specialist.

The switch from predominantly pediatric specialist management to adult management occurs not at age 21 years, or even at age 18 years, as might be expected, but around age 15 years. A cancer registry review in Utah, a state that has only one pediatric oncology treatment facility, showed that only 36% of oncology patients aged 15–19 years were ever seen at the pediatric hospital [38]. A study of the National Cancer Data Base found that, for nearly 20,000 cases of cancer in adolescents aged 15–19 years, only 34% were treated at centers that had NCI pediatric cooperative group affiliation [39]. Research is only now being done to ascertain the reasons for this practice pattern.

The answer to which specialist is most appropriate certainly varies from case to case. Patients at any age who have a "pediatric" tumor, such as rhabdomyosarcoma, Ewing sarcoma, and osteosarcoma, will probably benefit from the expertise of a pediatric oncologist, at least in the form of consultation. Children younger than age 18 years and their parents may benefit from the social and supportive culture of a pediatric hospital regardless of the diagnosis. Individuals between the ages of 16 and 24 years may have varying levels of maturity and independence, and the choice of physician and setting for their care should be determined individually. Pediatric oncologists may be less adept at a nonpaternalistic relationship with the patient (and potentially his or her spouse) and less inclined to consider issues such as sexuality, body image, fertility, and the like. Adult oncologists are more accustomed to dose delays and adjustments, and may be less willing to be aggressive with dosing that can be tolerated by the younger patient.

In the end, the decision should be based in large part on which setting will provide the patient with the best outcome. If these are equivalent, "social" or "supportive" factors should weigh into the decision. Little comparative outcome data are available. Stock and colleagues compared patients between the ages of 16 and 21 years who were registered on either a pediatric (Children's Cancer Group, CCG) or adult (Cancer and Leukemia Group B, CALGB) treatment protocol between 1988 and 1998. The remarkably significant results were a 6-year event-free survival of 64% for those treated on the CCG study and 38% for those treated on the CALGB study [40]. At the University of Texas MD Anderson Cancer Center, results of treatment for acute myeloid leukemia (AML) in adults improved substantively after treatment derived from pediatric trials was introduced into the institution's trials [41]. The analysis of data from the National Cancer Database revealed that adolescents (ages 15–19 years) with non-Hodgkin lymphoma, leukemia, liver cancer, and bone tumors have a survival advantage if treated at an NCI pediatric group institution [23].

The British, although hindered by the limited size of their patient population (only 600 cancer cases per year between the ages of 13 and 20 years), have pioneered the solution of treating young adult and adolescent patients at a unique "adolescent oncology unit" [42]. This provides the adolescent with age-specific nursing care, recreation therapy, and peer companionship. Perhaps it is appropriate to have as a goal, centers and oncologists devoted solely to the care of this group

of patients. This topic has its controversies and is discussed further in Chap. 33.

1.4.2 Surgery

In general, surgery is performed more readily and anesthesia is easier to administer in larger patients. Another advantage is that young adults are generally healthier than older patients. The main disadvantage in fully grown patients relative to children is that the older patients generally have fewer compensatory mechanisms to overcome the deficits and disabilities resulting from the surgical resection of large tumors. Decisions to use sedation and anesthesia commonly employed in younger children (e.g., topical anesthetic for venipunctures) should be individualized to the adolescent/young adult patient, but should not be dismissed as unnecessary just because of the patient's "maturity."

1.4.3 Radiation Therapy

Compared to children, adolescents and young adults are less vulnerable to the adverse effects of ionizing radiation. This is particularly true for the central nervous system, the cardiovascular system, connective tissue, and the musculoskeletal system, each of which may be irradiated to higher doses and/or larger volumes with less long-term morbidity than in younger patients. By analogy, older adolescents who are still maturing may be more vulnerable to radiation toxicities than older persons at those sites and tissues that are still undergoing development such as the breast and gonads. Breast cancer, for example is more likely in women who received radiation for Hodgkin lymphoma if the radiation was administered between the onset of puberty and the age of 30 years [43]. Remarkably little is actually known about the differential normal-tissue effects of radiotherapy in patients between 15 and 30 years of age.

1.4.4 Chemotherapy

The acute and chronic toxicities of chemotherapeutic agents are generally similar in children, adolescents, and young adults. Exceptions are that older patients in this age range may experience a greater degree of anticipatory vomiting, have a somewhat less rapid recovery from myeloablative agents, and have fewer stem cells in the peripheral blood available for autologous rescue. Adolescents and young adults certainly can tolerate more intensive chemotherapeutic regimens than older adults, because of better organ (especially renal) function. This should encourage those treating patients in this age group to push the limits of dose intensification. At the University of Texas MD Anderson Cancer Center, the more rigorous pediatric regimen for acute lymphoblastic leukemia (ALL) was adopted successfully years ago. Subsequently, the center also integrated the more intensive AML regimen used by pediatric oncologists into the adult therapy program for AML. In London, Verrill and his colleagues found the use of pediatric regimens for the treatment of young adults (ages 16 to 48 years) with Ewing sarcoma "rational and feasible" without excessive dose delays or modifications [44].

Adherence to therapeutic regimens, particularly oral chemotherapy, is also much more problematic in teenagers and young adults than in younger and older patients [45–48].

1.4.5 Psychosocial and Supportive Care

The greatest difference in the management of adolescents and young adult patients is in the supportive care, particularly psychosocial care, that they require. These patients have special needs that are not only unique to their age group but also broader in scope and more intense than those at any other time in life.

Young adult and older adolescent patients are on the cusp of autonomy, starting to gain success at independent decision-making, when the diagnosis of cancer renders them "out of control" and often throws them back to a dependent role with parents and authority figures (by circumstance and/or by choice). Sometimes the patient has become distanced from his or her nuclear family but has not yet developed a network of adult support relationships. The young adult or adolescent patient usually has many new roles they are just trying to master when the cancer diagnosis hits: high school student, college student, recent graduate, newlywed, new employee, or new parent. How

can they succeed when, in addition to all of these stresses, cancer intervenes? How can they plan and begin their future when they suddenly realize that they may not have one? What will happen if they cannot graduate, keep their friends, finish their education, get a good job, marry, have children, or be whatever they aspire to be?

Because of the complex issues of dependence, decision-making during cancer therapy is different for the patient, family, and physician of an adolescent/young adult than for either younger patients (which is more paternalistic) or for the older adult (more patient-centered). The young adult patient may wish to make his or her own decisions, but his or her understanding of the illness may be incomplete or flawed [49].

Honing social and interpersonal skills is an important developmental milestone during adolescence. Cancer treatment for these patients must accommodate this important developmental process. We have discharged a patient from the intensive care unit to allow her to attend her senior prom, and readmitted her when the party was over. Yet boundaries must be set, so that treatment effectiveness is not compromised to keep a "social calendar." Certainly, cancer therapy causes practical problems in social arenas. Adolescent and young adult patients, who are developmentally dependent on peer-group approval, often feel isolated from peers by their experience; the cancer patient's issues are illness and death, while their peers are consumed by lipstick and homework. All adolescents agonize over their personal appearance and hate to be singled out or to appear different. In adolescents with cancer, having to be isolated from peers and society by having a disease that makes them different and having to be treated separately is often devastating. In addition, many of the adverse effects of therapy can be overwhelming to an adolescent's or young adult's self-image, which is often tenuous under the best of circumstances. Weight gain, alopecia, acne, stunted growth, and mutilating surgery to the face and extremities are examples of adverse consequences that can be devastating to an adolescent's self-image. In particular, hair loss is cited over and over as a huge blow to the adolescent or young adult (especially the female) with cancer.

Other challenges include the time away from school, work, and community that therapy requires and the financial hardships that occur at an age when economic independence from family is an objective. There may be guilt if not attending to these responsibilities, or stress and fatigue if trying to keep up a semblance of normal activity.

This is a period when sexuality, intimacy, and reproduction are central. A young adult is supposed to attract a mate and reproduce. However, the young adult with cancer may feel or look unattractive, may be uninterested in or unable to have sex, and may be infertile. A feeling of impotence can pervade.

Most patients are in a relationship or hope to be in one. However, the relationship will be tested by the strain of the cancer diagnosis and its therapy. Patients may wonder whether the partner stays in the relationship out of guilt or sympathy. Some significant others may feel ignored by medical staff because they are not formally a "family member." After treatment, commitment to the relationship in the face of fear of relapse or infertility can be difficult for both parties. Those contemplating having children often worry about passing on a genetic predisposition to cancer.

A wide range of financial situations is seen in the young adult population. Some patients are still happily dependent on their parents. Some are just striking out on their own but, without a long-standing job or savings, may have to return to dependence on parents or get public assistance. Others are trying to begin a career, but long work absences threaten their job security or growth. As stated above, this age range is the most medically uninsured. As a result, many young adult patients incur high medical bills, and at a time in life when they may least be able to afford them. Future insurability is certainly a stressful issue for all of these patients.

Medical professionals caring for the adolescents and young adults may be used to the psychosocial problems more common in either younger children or older adults. Extra effort, including patient and family support groups specifically geared to this age bracket, should be made to uncover and address these needs, to increase compliance, reduce stress, and improve the quality of life during cancer therapy. Established theories of developmental behavior should be used to systematically improve our care of these patients. As Christine Eiser states, "only by seeing adolescents with

cancer as adolescents will we ultimately be acceptable as sources of support" [50]. Only by seeing young adults with cancer as young adults will we ultimately be able to optimize their care.

1.4.6 Lack of Participation in Clinical Trials

More than 90% of children with cancer who are younger than 15 years of age are managed at institutions that participate in NCI-sponsored clinical trials, and 55 to 65% of these young patients are entered into clinical trials. In contrast, only 20 to 35% of 15- to 19-year-olds with cancer are seen at such institutions, and only approximately 10% are entered into a clinical trial [51, 52]. Among 20- to 29-year-olds, the participation rate is even lower, with fewer than 10% being seen at member institutions of the cooperative groups, either pediatric or adult, and only approximately 1% of 20- to 29-year-olds entering clinical trials of the pediatric or adult cooperative groups. Among older patients, the trial participation rate is higher, putatively between 3 and 5%. The high proportion of older adolescent and young adults who are not entered into clinical trials is referred to as the "adolescent and young adult gap." This gap has been observed throughout the United States and spares no geographic region or ethnic group [53].

The reasons for the gap are to a large extent unknown and are undoubtedly multifactorial, as explained in Chap. 5. A factor that does not explain the discrepancy is the participation of minority adolescent patients in clinical trials. Although minority patients are known to be underrepresented in visits to physician offices [54], they have equal or higher rates of entry into clinical trials. The participation rate of older adolescent patients is lower than rates of younger patients of corresponding ethnicity and socioeconomic status.

The dramatically lower clinical trial participation rate by young adults may help to explain the lower-than-expected improvement in their outcome relative to younger and older patients. A report on 38,144 young adults with sarcoma diagnosed during the period 1975–1998 and followed by the United States SEER program may provide insight into the relative lack of progress [55]. In this study, the average annual percent change in 5-year survival as a function of patient age was compared with national sarcoma treatment trial data obtained on 3,242 patients entered onto NCI-sponsored trials during 1997–2002. For bone and soft-tissue sarcomas (except Kaposi sarcoma), the least survival improvement occurred between the ages of 15 and 45 years. For Kaposi sarcoma, the pattern was reversed, with the greatest survival increase occurring in 30- to 44-year-olds. The lowest participation rate in NCI-sponsored sarcoma treatment trials was found to be among the 20- to 44-year-olds. For Kaposi sarcoma patients, the highest accrual rate was found among the 35- to 44-year-olds. The age-dependent survival improvement and clinical-trial accrual patterns were directly correlated (soft-tissue sarcomas, $p < 0.005$; bone sarcomas, $p < 0.05$; Kaposi sarcoma, $p = 0.06$), regardless of whether the accrual profile demonstrated a decline or a peak (Kaposi sarcoma) during early adulthood. Thus, the lack of survival prolongation in 15- to 44-year-old Americans with non-Kaposi sarcomas may be a result of their relative lack of participation in clinical trials. If so, reversing the shortfall in survival among young adults with sarcomas, as was accomplished in Kaposi sarcoma patients, should benefit from increased clinical trial availability, access, and participation.

Studies of younger children have certainly shown a survival advantage to children enrolled in clinical trials for ALL [56], non-Hodgkin lymphoma [57], Wilms tumor [58], and medulloblastoma [59]. Similar analyses of data for adolescents are sparse. In the United States and Canada, a comparison of 16- to 21-year-olds with ALL or AML showed that the outcome was superior in patients with either cancer treated on CCG trials than in those not entered [60]. In France, The Netherlands, and North America, older adolescents with ALL treated in pediatric clinical trials have fared considerably better than those treated on adult leukemia treatment trials [61–63]. In Germany, older adolescents with Ewing sarcoma who were treated at pediatric cancer centers had a better outcome than those treated at other centers [64]. In Italy, young adults with rhabdomyosarcoma fared better if they were treated according to pediatric standards of therapy than if treated ad hoc or on an adult sarcoma regimen [65].

On the other hand, a population-based study of 15- to 29-year-olds with acute leukemia in England and Wales showed no difference between patients treated on national clinical trials and those not entered, or between those managed at teaching hospitals as opposed to nonteaching hospitals [66]. This observation appears to be exceptional, however, in that subsequent national AML trials in the United Kingdom have shown some of the best results reported to date [67].

1.4.7 Quality of Survival

The quality of survival, both during and after therapy, is a critical issue for adolescents and young adults. Quality of life is poor during the months and years when most adolescents and young adults with cancer are treated, and the acute and delayed toxicities of cancer therapy are undeniably among the worst associated with the treatment of any chronic disease. The acute toxicities of nausea, vomiting, mucositis, alopecia, weight gain (or excessive loss), acne, bleeding, and infection are generally harder for adolescents to cope with than for either younger or older persons. Delayed complications may be of low concern to patients in this age group during treatment, but after therapy has been completed these complications can be frightening and real. Cardiomyopathies, growth disturbances, and neuropsychological side effects are examples of adverse late effects that are hard to describe in a meaningful way before initiating therapy to an adolescent or young adult. A particularly tragic example of an unanticipated late effect is the development of a second malignancy in a patient cured of their original disease.

Many adolescent and young adult cancer survivors cite fertility as a primary concern that impacts the quality of their life. Most do not recall an adequate discussion of the risks of infertility or methods to decrease the risks with their physician at the initiation of therapy. The risk of infertility for an individual is difficult to predict. Direct radiation exposure of the gonad had been studied more extensively than other chemotherapy exposures. Permanent ovarian damage occurs between 5 and 20 Gy, with higher doses required in younger females [68]. The male germinal epithelium is much more sensitive to radiation-induced damage, with changes to spermatogonia resulting from as little as 0.2 Gy. Testicular doses of less than 0.2 Gy had no significant effect on follicle-stimulating hormone

(FSH) levels or sperm counts, whereas doses between 0.2 and 0.7 Gy caused a transient dose-dependent increase in FSH and a reduction in sperm concentration, with a return to normal values within 12 to 24 months. No radiation dose threshold has been defined above which permanent azoospermia is inevitable; however, doses of 1.2 Gy and above are likely to be associated with a reduced risk of recovery of spermatogenesis. The time to recovery, if it is to occur, is also likely to be dose dependent [69]. Cranial radiation impairs gonadal hormone synthesis and can result in a decreased production of luteinizing and follicle-stimulating hormones. Alkylating chemotherapeutic agents carry a high risk of infertility, but the exact dose required or the rates associated with combination agents are unavailable. Recommendations for preservation, evaluation, and counseling have recently become available [70–73].

The quality-of-life issues that arise during and after cancer therapy have been the focus of studies in children and older adults, but have not received the same attention or study in adolescents and young adults. A few studies have found certain trends that should be tested in future studies. A higher risk-taking behavior has been noted among survivors of Hodgkin lymphoma occurring during childhood and adolescence [74], an observation that does not appear to be limited to this disease. On the other hand, evidence also suggests that adolescent and young adult cancer survivors show better attendance and performance at school and work [75]. Persistent anxiety over relapse, death, or late effects is likely to be higher in adolescents who were cognitively aware of the severity of their illness than in those treated in early childhood (the Damocles syndrome) [76]. The paucity of quality-of-life data in this age group is another manifestation of the general neglect of these patients.

1.5 Summary

Cancer is 2.7 times more likely to develop in a patient at the age of 15 to 30 years than during the first 15 years of life, and yet is uncommon relative to older ages, accounting for 2% of all invasive cancer. Malignant disease in persons 15 to 30 years of age has no age counterpart. It is unique in the distribution of the types that occur, with Hodgkin lymphoma, melanoma, testis cancer, female genital tract malignancies, thyroid cancer, soft-tissue sarcomas, non-Hodgkin lymphoma, leukemia, brain and spinal cord tumors, breast cancer, bone sarcomas, and nongonadal germ cell tumors accounting for 95% of the cancers in the age group. In the mere 15 years of the age span, the frequency distribution of cancer types changes dramatically, such that the pattern at age 15 years does not resemble that at age 30 years. It is unique with regard to the physical nature and emotional needs of the hosts that develop it, and in the current failure to improve survival prolongation or mortality reduction relative to other age groups. Adolescents and young adults with cancer also face unique psychosocial challenges in the arenas of self-image, independence/dependence, finances, and relationships. Fortunately, the incidence increase observed during the past quarter century is declining, and in the older end of the age range appears to be returning to incidence rate of the 1970s.

Males in the age group have been at higher risk of developing cancer, the risk being directly proportional to age in the group. Non-Hispanic white people have had the highest risk of developing cancer during this phase of life, and Asians, American Indians and Native Alaskans the lowest. Males have had a worse prognosis, as have African-American, American Indians, and native Alaskans among the races/ethnicities evaluated.

The most disturbing epidemiologic finding is the lack of progress in survival improvement among older adolescents and young adults relative to all other ages. Whereas the diagnosis of cancer in this age group used to carry a more favorable prognosis, on the average, relative to cancer at other ages, survival improvement trends portend a worse prognosis for young adults diagnosed with cancer today. During the last 25 years, the incidence of cancer in this age range has increased more and the reduction in cancer mortality has been lower than in younger or older patients.

Proposed reasons for this gap in outcome include lack of health insurance and poor participation by older adolescents and young adults with cancer in clinical trials: in the United States, only approximately 1% of 15- to 29-year-olds with cancer are entered onto clinical trials, in contrast to more than 50% of younger patients.

Despite the fact that there are nearly three times as many cases of cancer in individuals who are 15–29 years of age as in those less than 15 years of age. Yet the former has its own organized cooperative oncology group and the latter does not. Adolescent and young adult oncology patients should be viewed as a distinct age group that, like pediatric, adult, and geriatric patients, has unique medical and psychosocial needs. This mindset will help bring the problem into focus and will help those caring for adolescents or young adults to find solutions. A specific discipline for this special population is just beginning to evolve. Meanwhile, resources should be devoted to educating the public, health professionals, insurers, and legislators about the special needs of these patients. The overriding issues to be addressed are the lagging improvements in survival and the special psychosocial needs of this age group.

To address this problem, the United States NCI and the NCI-sponsored pediatric and adult cooperative groups have launched a national initiative to improve the accrual of adolescents and young adults with cancer into clinical trials. In North America and Australia, the newly formed Children's Oncology Group has taken a leadership role in this effort. In conjunction with the NCI and NCI-sponsored adult cooperative groups, four initiatives were identified as priorities for development: (1) improving access to care through understanding barriers to participation; (2) developing a cancer resource network that provides information about clinical trials to patients, families, providers, and the public; (3) enhancing adolescent treatment adherence (compliance with protocol-prescribed therapy); and (4) increasing adolescent accrual and adult participation in sarcoma trials designed specifically for patients in this age group. However, reasons other than poor clinical trial participation, such as undescribed differences in biology, delays in diagnosis, poor compliance or intolerance of therapy, and treatment by physicians less familiar with the disease, may also be contributing to this outcome disparity [77], and need to be studied.

Surviving adolescence and young adulthood is difficult enough, even when all is well and health is not limiting. Cancer makes this phase of life extraordinarily more challenging and demanding. The medical community caring for these patients should pay special attention to the unique transitions faced by adolescents and young adults with cancer at the times of diagnosis, informed consent, initiation of therapy, school and employment reentrance, completion of therapy, posttreatment follow-up, and switching from pediatric to adult care [78, 79]. Ideally, specialized adolescent and young adult cancer units should be developed in the anticipation that the centralization of care and the availability of age-targeted clinical trials will lead to improved treatment, survival, and quality of life.

Thus, cancer during adolescence and early adult life is an underestimated challenge that merits specific resources, solutions and a national focus. Future research should elucidate why the outcomes have lagged behind and identify the efforts, including better clinical trial accrual, that will remedy the disparity. Finally, more scholarly and focused attention on the unique psychosocial needs of this population will improve the quality of their cancer care and the quality of their survival.

References

1. Bleyer WA, O'Leary M, Barr R, Ries LAG (eds) (2006) Cancer Epidemiology in Older Adolescents and Young Adults 15 to 29 Years of Age, Including SEER Incidence and Survival, 1975–2000. National Cancer Institute, NIH Pub. No. 06-5567, Bethesda MD; also available at www.seer.cancer.gov/publications/aya

2. Smith MA, Gurney JG, Ries LAG (1999) Cancer among adolescents 15–19 years old. In: Ries LAG, Smith MA, Gurney JG, Linet M, Tamra T, Young JL, Bunin GR (eds) Cancer Incidence and Survival Among Children and Adolescents: United States SEER Program 1975–1995. NCI, SEER Program NIH Pub No 99-4649 Bethesda, MD

3. Ries LAG, Eisner MP, Kosary CL, et al (eds) SEER Cancer Statistics Review, 1975–2002, National Cancer Institute. Bethesda, MD, http://seer.cancer.gov/csr/1975_2002/, based on November 2004 SEER data submission, posted to the SEER web site 2005

4. Bleyer A, Hag-Alshiekh M, Pollock B, Ries LAG (2006) Methods. In: Bleyer WA, O'Leary M, Barr R, Ries LAG (eds) Cancer Epidemiology in Older Adolescents and Young Adults 15 to 29 Years of Age, Including SEER Incidence and Survival, 1975–2000. National Cancer Institute, NIH Pub. No. 06-5567, Bethesda MD; also available at www.seer.cancer.gov/publications/aya

5. Fritz A, Percy C, Jack A, et al (eds) (2000) International Classification of Diseases for Oncology (3rd edn). World Health Organization, Geneva

6. Steliarova-Foucher E, Stiller C, Lacour B, Kaatsch P (2005) International Classification of Childhood Cancer (3rd edn). Cancer 103:1457–1467

7. Barr RD, Holowaty EJ, Birch JM (2006) Classification schemes for tumors diagnosed in adolescents and young adults. Cancer 106:1425–1430

8. Jemal A, Murray T, Ward E, Samuels A, Tiwari RC, Ghafoor A, Feuer EJ, Thun MJ (2005) Cancer statistics, 2005. CA Cancer J Clin 55:10–30

9. Bleyer A, Viny A, Barr R (2006) Introduction. In: Bleyer WA, O'Leary M, Barr R, Ries LAG (eds) Cancer Epidemiology in Older Adolescents and Young Adults 15 to 29 Years of Age, Including SEER Incidence and Survival, 1975–2000. National Cancer Institute, NIH Pub. No. 06-5767, Bethesda MD; also available at www.seer.cancer.gov/publications/aya

10. Bleyer W, Barr R (2006) Highlights and challenges. In: Bleyer A, O'Leary M, Barr R, Ries LAG (eds) Cancer Epidemiology in Older Adolescents and Young Adults 15 to 29 Years of Age, Including SEER Incidence and Survival, 1975–2000. National Cancer Institute, NIH Pub. No. 06-5767, Bethesda MD; also available at www.seer.cancer.gov/publications/aya.

11. Chambless LE, Diao G (2005) Estimation of time-dependent area under the ROC curve for long-term risk prediction. Stat Med 25:3474–3486

12. Kato I, Severson RK, Schwartz AG (2001) Conditional median survival of patients with advanced carcinoma: surveillance, epidemiology, and end results data. Cancer 92:2211–2219

13. Merrill RM, Henson DE, Barnes M (1999) Conditional survival among patients with carcinoma of the lung. Chest 166:697–703

14. Pollock BH, Krischner JP, Vietti TJ (1991) Interval between symptom onset and diagnosis of pediatric solid tumors. J Pediatr 119:725–732

15. Bleyer A, Ulrich C, Martin S, et al (2005) Status of health insurance predicts time from symptom onset to cancer diagnosis in young adults. Proc Am Soc Clin Oncol 23:547s

16. Martin S, Ulrich C, Munsell M, Lange G, Taylor S, Bleyer A (2005) Time to cancer diagnosis in young Americans depends on type of cancer and health insurance status. Value Health 8:344; The Oncologist (in press)

17. Ziv, A, Boulet JR, Slap GB (1999) Utilization of physician offices by adolescents in the United States. Pediatrics 104:35–42

18. Robert Wood Johnson Foundation (2003) Report by Families USA & The Lewin Group

19. DeNavas-Walt C, Proctor BD, Mills RJ (2004) Income, Poverty, and Health Insurance Coverage in the United States: 2003, U.S. Government Printing Office, Washington, DC, U.S. Census Bureau, Current Population Reports, pp 60–226.

20. Fishman E (2001) Aging out of coverage: young adults with special health needs. Health Affairs 20.6:254–266

21. White PH (2002) Access to health care: health insurance considerations for young adults with special health care needs/disabilities. Pediatrics 110:1328–1335

22. Friman PC, Finney JW, Glasscock SG, et al (1986) Testicular self-examination: validation of a training strategy for early cancer detection. J Appl Behav Anal 19:87–92

23. Albritton K, Bleyer A (2003) The management of cancer in the older adolescent. Eur J Cancer 39:2548–2599

24. Lewis IJ (1996) Cancer in adolescence. Br Med Bull 52:887–897

25. Reaman G, Bonfiglio J, Krailo M, et al (1993) Cancer in adolescents and young adults. Cancer 71:3206–3209

26. Selby P, Bailey C (eds) (1996) Cancer and the Adolescent. BMJ Publishing Group, London, pp 276–283

27. Yarcheski A, Scoloveno MA, Mahon NE (1994) Social support and well-being in adolescents: the mediating role of hopefulness. Nurs Res 43:288–292

28. Manne S, Miller D (1998) Social support, social conflict and adjustment among adolescents with cancer. J Pediatr Psychol 23:121–130

29. Nichols ML (1995) Social support and coping in young adolescents with cancer. Pediatr Nurs 21:235–240

30. Novakovic B, Fears TR, Wexler LH, et al (1996) Experience of cancer in children and adolescents. Cancer Nurs 19:54–59

31. Pelcovitz D, Libov BG, Mandel F, et al (1998) Post-traumatic stress disorder and family functioning in adolescent cancer. J Trauma Stress 11:205–221

32. Blum RW, Garell D, Hodgman CH, et al (1993) Transition from child-centered to adult health care systems for adolescents with chronic conditions: a position paper of the Society for Adolescent Medicine. J Adolesc Health 14:570–576

33. Rait DS, Ostroff J, Smith K, et al (1992) Lives in a balance: perceived family functioning and the psychosocial adjustment of adolescent cancer survivors. Fam Process 4:383–397

34. Leonard RC, Gregor A, Coleman RE, et al (1995) Strategy needed for adolescent patients with cancer. BMJ 311:387

35. American Academy of Pediatrics Section on Hematology/Oncology (1997) Guidelines for the pediatric cancer center and role of such centers in diagnosis and treatment. Pediatrics 99:139–141

36. American Federation of Clinical Oncologic Societies (1998) Consensus statement on access to quality cancer care. J Pediatr Hematol Oncol 20:279–281

37. Goldman S, Stafford C, Lenarsky C, et al (2000) Older adolescents vary greatly from children in their route of referral to the pediatric oncologist and national trials [abstract]. Proc Am Soc Clin Oncol 19:1766

38. Albritton K, Wiggins C (2001) Adolescents with cancer are not referred to Utah's pediatric center [abstract]. Proc Am Soc Clin Oncol 20:990

39. Rauck AM, Fremgen AM, Menck HR, et al (1999) Adolescent cancers in the United States: a National Cancer Data Base (NCDB) report. J Pediatr Hematol Oncol 21:310

40. Stock W, Sather H, Dodge RK, et al (2000) Outcome of adolescents and young adults with ALL: a comparison of Children's Cancer Group (CCG) and Cancer and Leukemia Group B (CALGB) regimens. Blood 96:467a

41. Kantarjian HM, O'Brien S, Smith TL, et al (2000) Results of treatment with hyper-CVAD, a dose-intensive regimen, in adult acute lymphocytic leukemia. J Clin Oncol 18:547–561

42. Lewis IJ (1996) Cancer in adolescence. Br Med Bull 52:887–897

43. Clemons M, Loijens L, Goss P (2000) Breast cancer risk following irradiation for Hodgkin disease. Cancer Treat Rev 26:291–302

44. Verrill MW, Judson IR, Fisher C, et al (1997) The use of paediatric chemotherapy protocols at full dose is both a rational and feasible treatment strategy in adults with Ewing's family tumours. Ann Oncol 8:1099–1105

45. Festa RS, Tamaroff MH, Chasalow F, et al (1992) Therapeutic adherence to oral medication regimens by adolescents with cancer. I. Laboratory assessment. J Pediatr 120:807–811

46. Tamaroff MH, Festa RS, Adesman AR, et al (1992) Therapeutic adherence to oral medication regimens by adolescents with cancer. II. Clinical and psychologic correlates. J Pediatr 120:813–817

47. Tebbi CK (1993) Treatment compliance in childhood and adolescence. Cancer 71:3441–3449

48. Kyngas HA, Kroll T, Duffy ME (2000) Compliance in adolescents with chronic diseases: a review. J Adolesc Med 26:379–388

49. Everhart C (1991) Overcoming childhood cancer misconceptions among long-term survivors. J Pediatr Oncol Nurs 8:46–48

50. Selby P, Bailey C (eds) (1996) Cancer and the Adolescent. BMJ Publishing Group, London, p 274

51. Kyngas HA, Kroll T, Duffy ME (2000) Compliance in adolescents with chronic diseases: a review. J Adolesc Med 26:379–388

52. Everhart C (1991) Overcoming childhood cancer misconceptions among long-term survivors. J Pediatr Oncol Nurs 8:46–48

53. Ross JA, Severson RK, Robison LL, et al (1993) Pediatric cancer in the United States. A preliminary report of a collaborative study of the Children's Cancer Group and the Pediatric Oncology Group. Cancer 71:3415–3421

54. Ziv A, Boulet JR, Slap GB (1999) Utilization of physician offices by adolescents in the United States. Pediatrics 104:35–42

55. Bleyer A, Montello M, Budd T, Saxman S (2005) National survival trends of young adults with sarcoma: lack of progress is associated with lack of clinical trial participation. Cancer 103:1891–1897

56. Meadows AT, Kramer S, Hopson R, et al (1983) Survival in childhood acute lymphocytic leukemia. Effect of protocol and place of treatment. Cancer Invest 1:49–55

57. Wagner HP, Dingeldein-Bettler I, Berchthold W, et al (1995) Childhood NHL in Switzerland: incidence and survival in 120 study and 42 non-study patients. Med Pediatr Oncol 24:281–286

58. Lennox EL, Stiller CA, Morris-Jones PH, Wilson-Kinnier LM (1979) Nephroblastoma: treatment during 1970–3 and the effect on survival of inclusion in the first MRC trial. Br Med J 2:567–569

59. Duffner K, Cohen ME, Flannery JT (1982) Referral patterns of childhood brain tumors in the state of Connecticut. Cancer 50:1636–1640

60. Nachman J, Sather HN, Buckley JD, et al (1993) Young adults 16–21 years of age at diagnosis entered onto Childrens Cancer Group acute lymphoblastic leukemia and acute myeloblastic leukemia protocols. Results of treatment. Cancer 71:3377–3385

61. Stock W, Sather H, Dodge RK, et al (2000) Outcome of adolescents and young adults with ALL: a comparison of Children's Cancer Group and Cancer and Leukemia Group B Regimens. Blood 96:467a

62. de Bont JM, van der Holt B, Dekker AW, et al (2004) Significant difference in outcome for adolescents with acute lymphoblastic leukemia treated on pediatric versus adult ALL protocols in the Netherlands. Leukemia 18:2032–2053

63. Boissel N, Auclerc MF, Lheritier V, et al (2003) Should adolescents with acute lymphoblastic leukemia be treated as old children or young adults? Comparison of the French FRALLE-93 and LALA-94 trials. J Clin Oncol 21:774–780

64. Paulussen S, Ahrens S, Juergens HF (2003) Cure rates in Ewing tumor patients aged over 15 years are better in pediatric oncology units. Results of GPOH CESS/EICESS studies. Proc Am Soc Clin Oncol 22:816

65. Ferrari A, Dileo P, Casanova M, et al (2003) Rhabdomyosarcoma in adults. A retrospective analysis of 171 patients treated at a single institution. Cancer 98:571–580

66. Stiller CA, Benjamin S, Cartwright RA, et al (1999) Patterns of care and survival for adolescents and young adults with acute leukemia – a population-based study. Br J Cancer 79:658–665

67. Webb DK, Harrison G, Stevens RF, et al (2000) Relationships between age at diagnosis, clinical features, and outcome of therapy in children treated in the Medical Research Council AML 10 and 12 trials for acute myeloid leukemia. Blood 98:1714–1720

68. Lo Presti A, Ruvolo G, Gancitano RA, Cittadini E (2004) Ovarian function following radiation and chemotherapy for cancer. Eur J Obstet Gynecol Reprod Biol 113:S33–40

69. Howell SJ, Shalet SM (2005) Spermatogenesis after cancer treatment: damage and recovery. J Natl Cancer Inst Monogr 34:12–17

70. Lee SJ, Schover LR, Partridge AH, et al (2006) American Society of Clinical Oncology recommendations on fertility preservation in cancer patients. J Clin Oncol 24:2917–2931

71. Roberts JE, Oktay K (2005) Fertility preservation: a comprehensive approach to the young woman with cancer. Natl Cancer Inst Monogr 34:57-59

72. Davis M (2006) Fertility considerations for female adolescent and young adult patients following cancer therapy: a guide for counseling patients and their families. Clin J Oncol Nurs 10:213–219

73. Beerendonk CC, Braat DD (2005) Present and future options for the preservation of fertility in female adolescents with cancer. Endocr Dev 8:166–175

74. Wasserman AL, Thompson EI, Wilmas JA, et al (1987) The psychological status of survivors of childhood/adolescent Hodgkin disease. Am J Dis Child 141:626–631

75. Hays DM, Landsverk J, Sallan SE, et al (1992) Educational, occupational, and insurance status of childhood cancer survivors in their fourth and fifth decades of life. J Clin Oncol 10:1397–1406

76. Koocher GP, O'Malley JE (1981) The Damocles Syndrome. Psychosocial Consequences of Surviving Childhood Cancer. McGraw-Hill, New York

77. Barr RD (1999) On cancer control and the adolescent. Med Pediatr Oncol 32:404–410

78. MacLean WE, Foley GV, Ruccione H, et al (1996) Transitions in the care of adolescent and young adult survivors of childhood cancer. Cancer 78:1340–1345

79. Glasson JE (1995) A descriptive and exploratory pilot study into school re-entrance for adolescents who have received treatment for cancer. J Adv Nurs 22:753–758

History of Adolescent Oncology

Cameron K. Tebbi

Contents

2.1 Introduction

The history of adolescent and young adult oncology, as a distinct entity, is relatively short. Nevertheless, the true chronicle of cancer in the young is centuries old. Such history is inevitably intertwined with that of cancer and medicine. While reports of adolescents and young adults are not specifically recorded, evidence indicates that cancer in adolescents precedes and transcends human written history [1–3]. The types of cancer most prevalent in this age group have been found or reported throughout the ages. One of the earliest cases of cancer was found by Louis Leaky in 1932 in the remains of either a Homo erectus or an Australopithecus and was suggestive of a Burkitt lymphoma. Cancer, including osteosarcoma, which has its peak occurrence in the second decade of life, has been found in Egyptian mummies. A case of possible osteosarcoma was also discovered in the mummified skeletal remains of a Peruvian Inca. In recorded history, a clear description indicating knowledge of cancer dates back to at least 1500 BC. The Edwin Smith Egyptian Papyrus, which was written between 3000 and 1500 BC, describes eight cases of tumors that were treated by cauterization with a tool called the "fire drill" [1]. The writing on the papyrus admits that there is no treatment. Hippocrates (450–370 BC) recognized the disease and theorized that it was caused by the imbalance of four humors, and specifically excess of black bile emanating from the spleen [1]. He recognized the difference between benign and malignant tumors and described cancers of many body sites. It was Hippocrates who coined the terms "carcinos" and "carcinoma," Greek words referring to the shape of a crab. The crab symbol still has currency as a sign of cancer.

The earliest documented cure for cancer is found in Ramayana, the Hindu epic. This recommends arsenic paste to slow down the growth of the tumor. By the second century AD, Leonide of Alexandria used a scalpel for the first time during an operation which, combined with cauterization to prevent hemorrhage, was to destroy the remnants of the cancer. During the same century, Galen, the Greek physician, became the first known oncologist. He considered metastatic cancer to be an incurable disease. By 50 AD, Romans had discovered that some tumors could be resected by surgery and cauterized, but no medicine was effective. Little was added to the ancient knowledge and treatment of cancer up to 1500 AD, when the practice of autopsy, later popularized by Harvey (1628), became widespread. In 1761 Giovanni Morgagni of Padua made autopsy a routine procedure to relate the disease and cause of death. John Hunter, the Scottish surgeon (1728–1793), differentiated resectable from nonresectable tumors and suggested that some cancers can be cured by surgery.

During the same era, causes such as snuff (John Hill 1761) and exposure to soot (Percival Pott 1775) were related to nasal and scrotal cancer, respectively. These represent the earliest recognitions of carcinogenesis. The first cancer hospital was founded in the 18th century in Reims, France, to control the spread of cancer, which was then assumed to be an infectious disease. During the same period, Joseph Recamier described and used the term metastasis to indicate blood-born spread of cancer. Rudolph Virchow (1821–1902), a German pathologist, correlated microscopic pathology with the course of the disease. In 1895, Wilhelm Conrad Roentgen discovered the X-ray and was awarded the first Nobel Prize for his contribution. Three years later, French scientists Pierre and Marie Curie discovered radium. Between 1900 and 1950, radiotherapy was developed as an effective treatment of cancer.

In the more recent era, the search for the etiology of cancer had a major boost when, in 1911, Peyton Rous demonstrated that sarcomas in Plymouth Rock hens can be transferred to normal animals by injection of cell-free filtrates of the tumor [4]. He received the Nobel Prize for his discovery in 1966. The search for other viruses and organisms followed. At one point, cancer was incorrectly attributed to parasitic infections, a "discovery" that erroneously was rewarded with a Nobel Prize to Fibiger in 1926 [5].

In 1958 Sir Dennis Burkitt described a type of lymphoma, which now bears his name, in African children [6]. The geographic distribution and its relation to the Epstein-Barr virus and possibility of cure opened a new era of research. The introduction of the concept of "oncogenes" enhanced the understanding of the control of cell division in normal and transformed cells and their role in cancer [7, 8] and resulted in the presentation of a Nobel Prize to J. Michael Bishop and Harold E. Varmus in 1989.

More recently, revolution in molecular genetic research has resulted in a better understanding of many types of cancer. The advent of microarry technology will undoubtedly expand the field. The potential of genetic technology for therapeutic purposes has now been well demonstrated [9, 10]. The development of a monoclonal antibody production technique by Kohler, Milstein, and Jerne has revolutionized the diagnosis and treatment of cancer [11]. For their discovery in 1975, they were awarded the Nobel Prize in Medicine in 1984.

Colchicine, benzol, and arsenic were the earliest effective chemotherapy agents used for cancer; however, these had severe side effects. During the Second World War it was noted that exposure to mustard gas, a chemical warfare agent, resulted in leukopenia. It was then deduced that this might damage rapidly growing cells in cancer. By the 1940s, intravenous mustard was used in mouse and man, and proved to be temporarily effective in the control of lymphomas [12, 13]. This opened the era of chemotherapy and encouraged the search for other chemotherapeutic agents for the treatment of cancer. In 1947, Sidney Farber of Boston reported temporary remissions in acute leukemia in children by using aminopterin [14]. Two years later, methotrexate was used for "acute leukemia and other forms of incurable cancer" [15]. The same investigator introduced adrenocorticotrophic hormone for the treatment of childhood acute leukemia [16]. The development of a host of other effective agents, including antineoplastic antibiotics, alkylating agents, vinca alkaloids, nitrosoureas, hormones, enzymes, antimetabolites, topoisomerase inhibitors, and biological response modifiers, followed. The utility of each agent and best mode of administration and combination, and development of in vitro and animal models resulted in new hope for the treatment and cure of cancer.

Pediatric oncology took the lead in organizing groups to systematically test the effects of various new cancer chemotherapy compounds and combinations. In 1955, the Acute Leukemia Chemotherapy Group A, later to be called Children's Cancer Group (CCG), was established to conduct research on childhood cancer. Cancer Chemotherapy Group, later renamed Southwest Oncology Group (SWOG) was formed. In 1979, the pediatric division of SWOG separated to become the Pediatric Oncology Group (POG). Likewise, the Cancer and Leukemia Group B was established in 1955 with a pediatric division, which was separated and its institutions amalgamated into POG and CCG in 1980.

Despite the golden opportunities that a combination of adult and pediatric groups had created, no attempts were made to establish adolescent sections or programs in those early days. Over time, the American clinical investigation organizations expanded their membership to include international members from across the globe. Other pediatric clinical trial groups (i.e., National Wilms' Tumor Study Group, NWTS, and Intergroup Rhabdomyosarcoma Study Group, IRSG), were established in 1969 and 1972, respectively. All children's trial groups admitted pediatric, adolescent, and young adult patients to their protocols. Despite these developments, adolescent and young adult patients had fallen through the cracks. The activity of these groups, which was initially limited to the evaluation of chemotherapy agents, eventually expanded to include scientific research in areas such as, for example, tumor biology, molecular genetics, drug resistance, biological responses, immunotherapy, transplantation, nursing, epidemiology, and cancer control.

With the merger of four major national pediatric group organizations (i.e. CCG, POG, NWTS, and IRSG), in the year 2000, into a single national group called Children's Oncology Group (COG), an expanded Adolescent and Young Adult Committee was established to address the needs of these patients.

2.2 Background for Establishment of Adolescent/Young Adult Oncology as an Entity

From time immemorial, adolescents have been criticized for their behavior. Socrates complained that "children today are tyrants; they contradict their parents, gobble their food, and tyrannize their teachers." Homer declared "thou knowst the over-eager vehemence of youth, how quick in temper, and in judgment weak." Shakespeare suggested that teenagers be put into suspended animation until of age [17]. Some characteristics of adolescents, including ambivalence, rebellion, desire for freedom from family, conflicts with parents, reaction with intensity, choice of music, identification with peer group, and sexual activities, have created a negative stereotype for this age group. An imbalanced rate of demands for privileges and acceptance of responsibility, coupled with the desire to be different, has led to labeling adolescents as difficult and unruly. Often the behavior of adolescents is frowned upon with antipathy and dislike, if not abhorrence, not realizing these characteristics may be appropriate for this age group, and likely constitute one of the pillars of human advancements over the ages.

For adolescents, the transition from childhood to adult status is equally difficult and stressful. As such, many experience ambivalence, and physical and emotional turmoil, which threaten their ability to become healthy and productive adults. Cancer, a catastrophic, life-threatening disease, has major physical, functional, psychological, and social implications, which are multiplied in the adolescent and young adult age group. While cancer in this age group is not rare, it poses a unique enough challenge to require specialized services [18]. In the 1970s, when cancer was becoming a more "chronic" disease, and promising reports of successful treatment in types of cancer, which heretofore was deemed incurable, appeared in the literature, physicians began treating their patients with curative rather than palliative intents [19]. At that point, it became apparent that a catastrophic disease with uncertain outcome requiring intensive therapy is difficult to face without a major social support system [20]. It had been recognized for some time that care for adolescent/young adult patients requires an understanding of the process of physical, mental, psychological, and social growth and development [21]. Adolescent services had been in existence in the United States since 1951, when Dr. J. Roswell Gallagher established adolescent medicine and a unit at Boston Children's Hospital [22]. Against this background, the first adolescent oncology unit was established in 1978. Establishment of the unit, where this writer was the director, was by a grant from the National Cancer Institute (NCI). The unit was established through the efforts and support of Dr. James Wallace, then the director of the Division of Cancer Control and Rehabilitation, and endorsement of Dr. Gerald Murphy, then the Institute Director at Roswell Park Memorial Institute. While adolescent medicine as an entity was not new, the idea of a separate unit for adolescent/young adult oncology patients was unique. Establishment of a unit specifically dedicated to cancer was received enthusiastically by patients and their families alike. The reception by medical and surgical subspecialists was far less enthusiastic. There was significant opposition, expressed and implied, by various medical and surgical services. The ten-bed unit, which was located in a separate building and connected to the main hospital, proved to be resented by most departments on several principles. Most medical and surgical staff physicians preferred their patients to be hospitalized on their own floors. Some were unwilling to lose the adolescent population from their services, which was another deterrent to admission to the units. Our much more modern facility for adolescents and young adults than the then older hospital floors was also resented. Only with the strong support of Dr. Gerald Murphy, the devotion and resilience of the unit staff, and demand of patients and their families, has the unit survived and flourished. Dr. Murphy had personal experience with adolescents through his own biological and adopted children, and had significant knowledge of adolescents' desires and behavior.

The physical structure of the unit, which was designed with the patients' input, proved to be a major draw. The unit was painted with bright colors and geometric designs appealing to adolescent and young adult patients. It included a sizeable patient lounge with bright furniture, a large aquarium, and decora-

tions. Patient rooms were designed with adolescent and young adult patients in mind [23]. An arcade-like recreation room with the latest in electronic games then available, foozball, air hockey, bumper pool table, jukebox, stereo system, large TV, and musical instruments, drew the patients' friends to visit them in the hospital. An extensive exercise and arts and crafts room, a classroom, and a library with books and magazines appealing to the age group, were provided. A well-stocked and equipped kitchen with dining room allowed patients or their parents to cook and dine together. There was no dress code. A laundry room was available to patients so that they could wear their own, not the hospital, clothes. A room designated as a quiet room was furnished for patients and their families who wanted to take some time off and not be disturbed by anyone, including medical personnel. A separate parents' lounge and room to stay when their child was critically ill allowed parents to be involved, but not intrusive. Selection of the staff for the unit was based largely on their desire and ability to work with adolescent/young adult patients. Primary nursing care proved to be essential for the operation of the unit. Various programs were designed to promote communication and support emotional stability in crisis situations. A teacher visited patients on a daily basis and through an agreement with a local college, post-secondary education was available. In retrospect, the educational opportunities offered, especially for those less engaged in school prior to the diagnosis of cancer, was an important function of the unit [23]. Among other programs offered were music therapy, group sessions, and career planning. The unit, in those early days, offered a computer for patients' use, which was then unique. With a grant from Poets and Writers Inc., a creative writing program was established. The unit's monthly newsletter, entitled "Now and Then News," often contained excellent articles or poems expressing patients' and staff's feelings and experiences.

Offices of the staff, including the medical director, patient care coordinator, family counselor, and occupational therapist, were in the unit and open to patients and their families and friends. Patients' records were computerized, allowing access, using a series of codes, to the patients' prior admissions and discharge notes. This was probably one of the earliest attempts at computerized medical record keeping. The unit shared a research laboratory, and accepted pre- and postdoctoral trainees.

The rules governing the unit, including visiting hours and visitors' age limit and number, were liberal [17]. A family night was hosted on a monthly basis for the patients and their families to attend. In-patient field trips decreased the monotony of staying in the hospital, which were then, as a rule, lengthier and more frequent than they are today. A home- and terminal-care program was designed for patients who opted to stay at home. An evaluation program periodically examined satisfaction with the various aspects of the unit's operation by the patients, their families and staff [23, 24].

Shortly after the establishment of the unit, it became apparent that information regarding care of the adolescent oncology patients was scanty, if not nonexistent. In a series of investigations, the medical and psychological effects of the diagnosis and treatment of cancer in adolescents were probed. Since nowhere are these effects more exaggerated than with loss of a limb and its effect on body image, physical, psychological, and social functioning of the patient, a major effort was placed on study of this subject. These studies described various aspects of the bone tumors [25–27] and the short- and long-term effects of the amputation on the patients' lives [28, 29]. With some degree of surprise, the research found that, in general, despite all adversities, in the long-term most amputee patients had adjusted to their circumstances and were leading full and productive lives [28, 29]. Other investigations probed the role of social support systems in adolescent/young adult patients [20, 30]. Evaluation of the pattern of religiosity and locus of control revealed that adolescent cancer patients were not significantly more religious than established norms [31]. However, among younger adolescents, the diagnosis and treatment of cancer may have accelerated the development of internality, which is expected to be associated with increased age [31]. Early during the establishment of an adolescent/young adult unit, significant noncompliance with self-administered cancer therapy was noted. This led to a series of studies of patients and parents of adolescent cancer patients, and a means to improve compliance [32–37]. Since the psychological aspects of the disease play an important role in the care of patients,

great emphasis was placed on this aspect of care [24, 38, 39]. Depression had been observed and studied extensively in adult cancer patients, but no systematic evaluation was available for adolescent oncology patients. In a series of studies, the rate of self-reported depression in cancer patients was probed [40]. Issues pertaining to long-term survivors were another venue for early research. With improved survival, the short- and long-term sequelae of cancer and its effects on the vocational achievements of the patients and their function in the workplace were examined [41, 42]. This disclosed a greater degree of functional deficit in unemployed versus employed cancer survivors, and in health, life, and disability insurance issues [41]. Nevertheless, there was no significant relationship between health status and employment. As a whole, former cancer patients had a higher average income compared to a control group, and were competitive members in the workplace [41]. The experiences in establishment of a specialized unit, care, and nutrition for these patients were published [21, 43]. This, along with annual adolescent oncology conferences, attracted a significant number of interested individuals to work and train in the unit. Publication of the first book solely devoted to adolescent oncology [44] increased the awareness of cancer in adolescents and young adults, albeit to a limited extent.

In 1989, when Dr. Gerald Murphy left Roswell Park, the unit, which was then by far the most modern and progressive floor of the hospital, was viewed as an "extravagance" by the new administration. For cost-cutting purposes, it was decided that its resources should be shared with pediatrics. Consequently, in October of 1989, despite the pleas of dedicated staff and patients, the unit was merged with pediatrics and the adolescent/young adult cancer program was effectively closed.

A new chapter in adolescent and young adult oncology commenced when in October 1992, the American Cancer Society (ACS) sponsored a workshop on Adolescents and Young Adults with Cancer [45]. The conference served as a watershed for recognition of the special needs of this group of patients. It was attended by, and had the support of, Dr. Gerald P. Murphy who, after leaving Roswell Park Cancer Institute and State University of New York, had accepted a position as the chief medical officer of the ACS. To organize this conference was a departure from prior attitudes toward the importance of specialized care for adolescent and young adult cancer patients. In fact, before the leadership of Dr. Murphy, when an earlier conference entitled "Advances in Care of the Child with Cancer", was being planned by the ACS in 1985, this writer suggested that the subject of adolescent oncology be included in the agenda. The organizer of that conference indicated that nothing was new or important enough in adolescent oncology to merit a session, and the subject was declined. The 1992 "Adolescent and Young Adult Conference" was attended by many leaders in pediatrics, adolescent medicine, and medical and surgical oncology. Among these were chairs of then major pediatric cancer groups. The workshops included sessions on long-term care and lifetime follow-up [46], insurance and employability [47], psychological and emotional issues, specialized support groups/compliance issues [48], and clinical research implications [49]. The published proceedings of the conference had an important conclusion, which recognized cancer as a significant health problem in the adolescent and young adult population [45]. It observed that the rate of cancer in patients 15 to 19 years of age is equal to that of 0- to 4-year-olds, and 1.6 times that in patients between 5 and 14 years of age [50, 51]. The conclusions also brought attention to the relatively infrequent participation of adolescent and young adults in cooperative group trials and superior outcome of those treated based on a national protocol as compared to Surveillance, Epidemiology, and End Results (SEER) data [50]. This observation has ignited new initiatives to include these individuals in cancer trials [51–54]. The 1992 conference also emphasized the necessity for long-term follow up and psychosocial support, and called attention to discrimination in insurance and employment [50]. The concluding remarks included recommendations to remedy these concerns [50].

Another chapter in the history of adolescent oncology was begun in 1998 when the CCG initiated an "Adolescent Young Adult Committee" under the leadership of Dr. W. Archie Bleyer. When in the year 2000 the COG was formed from the predecessor childhood cancer cooperative groups, the Adolescent and Young Adult Committee was endorsed and expanded.

Intuitively, the genesis of the committee was recognition of the fact that there are currently approximately 37 million individuals between the ages of 10 and 19 years living in the United States. Based on SEER data, the incidence of cancer in the United States among the adolescent and young adult population during the 1990s is 203 new cases per million population [55], which, while higher than the rate reported from the United Kingdom, is similar to those elsewhere [56–58]. The incidence of cancer in 15- to 19-year-olds is on the rise [52, 59–63]. In the United States, this has increased an average of 0.7% per year from 1975 to 1998 [18, 53], yet no age-defined health-care system or providers are generally available to the majority of adolescents [64]. Thus, the healthcare of this group of patients is fragmented and is divided between medical, pediatric and general practitioners, and others [18, 65]. On the other hand, in the United States, the mortality from cancer has decreased at the rate of 3.3% per year for the period 1965–1974 and 2.6% per year for the period 1975–1984, a trend that continues to date. Similar progress is reported in Europe [60, 61, 66].

The importance of the clinical trials strategy group of the COG Adolescent and Young Adult Committee is underscored by the lack of clinical trial participation of older adolescent and young adults with cancer. Compared to children [51, 67], a far lower percentage of adolescents are entered into clinical trials [64, 67–70]. Unlike pediatric oncologists, who treat the majority of their patients according to an established protocol, and often, if not always, belong to a cooperative group, in the United States medical oncologists infrequently enter their patients in group studies [71]. In contrast to patients under age 15 years where, irrespective of race [72], 94% are treated in centers that were members of a cooperative group, less than 21% of those 15 to 19 years of age are treated in such institutions [65, 73, 74]. Likewise, adolescent cancer participation in clinical trials remains poor in pediatric centers (34.8%) and other institutions (12.1%) [70, 75]. The age-adjusted registration rate of patients aged 15–19 years to pediatric cooperative groups is only 24% [76]. In one study of 29,859 subjects under 20 years of age entered onto NCI-sponsored clinical trials between January 1, 1991, and June 30, 1994, pediatric cooperative groups accounted for less than 3% of the clinical entrees in the 15 to 19 years age range [67]. Overall, 5% of 15- to 25-years-olds as compared to 60–65% of younger patients in the United States and Canada enter clinical trials [53].

There is some controversy regarding the differences in the response and survival rate of adolescent patients treated by medical and pediatric oncologists and in oncology centers and elsewhere [18, 56, 71, 77, 78]. However, there is no question that to obtain uniform results and to better understand the biology, course of the disease, and survival, these patients must be treated in an organized fashion. To add to this mix, many adolescent patients are treated by nononcology subspecialists, such as neurosurgeons and other surgical specialists.

The reduction in the mortality rate among adolescent and young adults has lagged behind those of young children [52–54, 79, 80]. While the main reason for such a disparity may have a biological basis, as evidenced by the poorer response of similar patients treated with the same protocol [80], other factors are also to be considered. A uniform, meticulous, systematic approach to the subject is needed. Lack of a separate and identifiable health-care system for adolescent/young adult patients in the United States and elsewhere will probably result in the continued division of adolescent oncology patients among various subspecialties [81].

While the problems and special needs of adolescent oncology patients are well recognized, their priority remains low [81]. The current challenge faced by the general medical and pediatric establishment and the COG remains to assure that adolescents with cancer receive the benefits of treatment in an age-appropriate setting and be included in clinical trials and research [82, 83]. With this background, during its short existence, the COG Adolescent and Young Adult Committee has taken steps to organize a comprehensive program including subcommittees for all major categories of oncological disorders common among adolescent and young adult patients. The Committee now consists of more than 120 members who represent nearly 20 disciplines, and is sustained by funding from the NCI and the health insurance industry. It is organized into three Strategy Groups (disease-specific clinical trials, behavioral oncology and health services research, and

epidemiology research, and awareness) and a sentinel task force on survivorship transition. In addition, the Committee has established task forces on access to clinical trials and care, cancer control and community oncology programs, adolescent treatment adherence, exercise and adventure therapy, and development of an informative website.

Unfortunately, years after the demonstration of the benefits of treatment of adolescent patients in a unit of their own [23, 84, 85], only a handful of specialized adolescent oncology services in the United States and elsewhere are operational. In the United Kingdom, the Teenage Cancer Trust (TCT) is an advocate of these units [85, 86] (see Chapter 21). There are currently eight operational units, and there are plans for the establishment of a TCT unit in every regional cancer center [85, 86]. Adolescent oncology units can provide an environment where the age-appropriate atmosphere and facilities coupled with medical technological and psychosocial expertise can provide specialized care while reducing dropouts of the treatment and short- and long-term side effects of cancer and its therapy. In an inquiry sent to 238 COG institutions in the United States, of the 196 institutions that responded to a questionnaire, only 1 hospital had a formal designated adolescent oncology unit (unpublished observation, Tebbi 2004). In the same inquiry, ten admitted their patients to a general adolescent unit, and only seven had staff who specifically identified with the care of these patients (unpublished data, Tebbi 2004). While adolescents are generally resilient [87, 88], in adult units these patients are frightened by the generation gap, adults disfigured by cancer, and rigid rules imposed upon them while they are hospitalized. Medical oncologists tend to regard 16- to 21-year-olds as adults and do not make a distinction between them and older patients [70]. Furthermore, diagnoses common in older adults are rare in adolescents and young adults [70]. While disputed, at least for some oncological diseases, the treatment of adolescents according to a pediatric protocol has yielded better results than on medical oncology protocols [18, 71, 89]. In a pediatric setting, however, adolescents and young adults are often demeaned by an atmosphere created for very young children and the childlike manner with which they often are dealt, not considering their age and accomplishments. The patients are often bypassed by the pediatric staff, who habitually deal with their parents rather than directly with the patient. Thus, the trend that has already started in the United States [23] and the United Kingdom [85, 86] of establishing adolescent oncology units, is needed to expand and remedy the situation. Designation of a special December 2003 issue of the European Journal of Cancer and an adolescent oncology conference in London in March 2004 are positive steps toward these goals.

2.3 Developments in the Psychosocial and Long-Term Care of Adolescent and Young Adult Oncology Patients

The history of the development of adolescent oncology is incomplete if one is remiss in mentioning the developments in psychosocial and long-term care of the patients [90]. During the period 1975–1984, the survival of adolescent and young adults with cancer had increased to 69%, with improvements in most major categories of cancers [57]. In this period of time, with increased survival, the problems concerning quality of life have gained prominence. Subjects such as "psychological aspects of cancer survivors," "late effects," "long term survivors clinics," "second cancer," and "transition to adult care," which did not exist before, have found their way into the lexicon of oncologists in the United States and elsewhere [80, 82, 91–94]. Likewise, with significant societal changes in the 1970s and 1980s, the subject of death and dying, which once was "taboo," is discussed openly and has become a new area for research and open discussion. Hospice care, initially introduced by physician Dame Cicely Saunders in the UK in the early 1960s and culminating with the opening of the first hospice in 1967, has found its way to the United States and has become a part of end-of-life patient care. The American Academy of Hospice and Palliative Care, originally chartered as the Academy of Hospice Physicians, was established in 1988 [95]. Publication of 500 interviews with dying patients entitled "On Death and Dying" and analysis by Dr. Elisabeth Kubler-Ross [96] catalyzed a more open discussion with dying individuals, including adolescent and young adult patients. The trend continues with most major adult and pediatric cancer study groups establishing committees on end-of-life care.

2.4 Summary

The understanding of cancer in adolescents is perpetually unfinished; the final answers not yet known, if they ever will be. The age-old questions of etiology are still the same today as they have been for millennia. The challenge remains to use today's technology to better understand the exact causes responsible for the development of cancer in the young, which has perplexed those who have come before us, and prevent the disease in those who are yet to come. Until methods for etiology-derived prevention of cancer becomes available, efforts need to be continued to use the latest available tools for early diagnosis and therapy, and to reduce the visible and invisible scars of the disease and its treatment [18, 80].

References

1. Haagensen CD (1933) An exhibit of important books, papers and memorabilia illustrating the evolution of the knowledge of cancer. Am J Cancer 18:42–126
2. Weiss L (2000) Observations on the antiquity of cancer and metastasis. Cancer Metastasis Rev 19:193–204
3. Weiss L (2000) Early concepts of cancer. Cancer Metastasis Rev 19:205–217
4. Rous P (1911) Transmission of a malignant new growth by means of a cell free filtrate. J Am Med Assoc 56:198
5. Fibiger J (1913) Untersuchung uber eine Nematode (Spiroptera sp.) und deren Fahigkeit, papillomatose und carcinomatose Geschwulstbildungen in Magen der Ratte hervorzurfen. Z Krebsforch 13:217
6. Burkett D (1958) A sarcoma involving the jaws in African children. Br J Surg 46:218–223
7. Stehelin D, Varmus HE, Bishop JM, Vogt PK (1976) DNA related to the transforming gene(s) of avian sarcoma viruses is present in normal avian DNA. Nature 260:170–173
8. Sharp PA (1980) Molecular biology of viral oncogenes. Cold Spring Harb Symp Quant Biol 44:1305–1322
9. Anderson WF (2000) Gene therapy scores against cancer. Nature Med 6:862–863
10. Anderson WF, Blaese RM, Culver K (1990) Treatment of severe combined immunodeficiency disease due to adenosine (ADA) deficiency with autologous lymphocytes transduced with human Ada gene. Hum Gene Ther 1:331–362

11. Kohler G, Milstein C (1975) Continuous cultures of fused cells secreting antibody of predefined specificity. Nature 256:495–497

12. Goodman LS, Wintrobe MW, Dameshek W, et al (1946) Nitrogen mustard therapy. Use of methyl-bis (beta-chloroethyl) amine hydrochloride for Hodgkin disease, lymphosarcoma, leukemia and certain allied and miscellaneous disorders. JAMA 132:126–132

13. Gilman A (1963) The initial clinical trial of nitrogen mustard. Am J Surg 105:574–578

14. Farber S, Diamond LK, Mercer RD, et al (1948) Temporary remissions in acute leukemia in children produced by folic acid antagonist, 4-aminopteroylglutamic acid (Aminopterin). N Engl J Med 238:787

15. Farber S (1949) Some observations on the effect of folic acid antagonists on acute leukemia and other forms of incurable cancer. Blood 4:160–167

16. Farber S (1950) The effect of ACTH in acute leukemia in childhood. In: Mote JR (ed) Proceedings of the First Clinical ACTH Conference. Blakiston, New York, pp 328

17. Tebbi CK, Stern M (1984) Burgeoning specialty of adolescent oncology. Cancer Bull 36:265–271

18. McTiernan A (2003) Issues surrounding the participation of adolescents with cancer in clinical trials in the UK. Eur J Cancer Care 12:233–239

19. Tebbi CK (ed) (1982) Preface in Major Topics in Pediatric and Adolescent Oncology. G. K. Hall Medical Publishers, Boston, Massachusetts

20. Tebbi CK, Stern M, Boyle M, et al (1985) The role of social support systems in adolescent cancer amputees. Cancer 56:965–971

21. Tebbi CK (1983) Care for adolescent oncology patients. In: Higby DJ (ed) Supportive Care in Cancer Therapy. Martinus Nijhoff, Boston, Mass, pp 281–309

22. Prescott HM (1998) J. Roswell Gallagher and the origins of adolescent medicine. In: Heather Munro Prescott (ed) A Doctor of Their Own. Harvard University Press, Cambridge, pp 37–47

23. Tebbi CK, Koren BG (1983) A specialized unit for adolescent oncology patients. Is it worth it? J Med 14:161–184

24. Tebbi CK, Tull R, Koren B (1980) Psychological research and evaluation of a unit designed for adolescent patients with oncology problems. Proc ASCO 21:238

25. Tebbi CK, Freeman AI (1984) Osteogenic sarcoma. Pediatr Rev 6:55–62

26. Tebbi CK, Gaeta J (1988) Osteosarcoma. Pediatr Ann 17:285–300

27. Tebbi CK (1993) Osteosarcoma in childhood and adolescence. Hematol Oncol Ann 1:203–228

28. Tebbi CK, Richards ME, Petrilli AS (1989) Adjustment to amputation among adolescent oncology patients. Am J Pediatr Hematol Oncol 11:276–280

29. Boyle M, Tebbi CK, Mindell E, Mettlin CJ (1982) Adolescent adjustment to amputation. Med Pediatr Oncol 10:301–312

30. Rafferty JP, Berjian RA, Tebbi CK (1980) Perceived Psychological Climate of Family Members of an Adolescent With Cancer. Proceedings of the National Forum on Comprehensive Cancer Rehabilitation. Commonwealth University Press, Richmond, VA, pp 16–21

31. Tebbi CK, Mallon JC, Bigler LR (1987) Religiosity and locus of control of adolescent patients. Psychol Rep 1:683–696

32. Tebbi CK, Cummings KM, Zevon MA, et al (1986) Compliance of pediatric and adolescent cancer patients. Cancer 58:1179–1184

33. Tebbi CK, Mallon JC (1986) Compliance with cancer therapy in pediatric and adolescent patients. The Candlelighters Childhood Cancer Foundation Progress Reports VI:9–10

34. Tebbi CK, Richards ME, Cummings KM, et al (1988) The role of parent–adolescent concordance in compliance with cancer chemotherapy. Adolescence 23:599–611

35. Tebbi CK, Richards ME, Cummings KM, Zevon MA (1989) Attributions of responsibilities cancer patients and their parents. J Cancer Educ 4:135–142

36. Tebbi CK, Cummings KM, Zevon MA, et al (1988) Compliance of Pediatric and Adolescent Cancer Patients. In: Oski FA, Stockman JA III (eds) Yearbook of Pediatrics. St. Louis, pp 387–388

37. Tebbi CK (1993) Treatment compliance in childhood and adolescence. Cancer 71:3441–3449

38. Young-Brockoff D, Rafferty JP, Berjian RA, Tebbi CK (1980) The psychological needs of cancer patients, implications for counseling and rehabilitation. Proceedings of the National Forum on Comprehensive Cancer Rehabilitation, Commonwealth University Press, Richmond, VA, pp 16–21

39. Tebbi CK (1988) Psychological consequences of childhood and adolescent cancer survival. In: Oski FA, Stockman JA III (eds) Yearbook of Pediatrics, St. Louis, pp 387–388

40. Tebbi CK, Bromberg C, Mallon J (1988) Self-reported depression in adolescent cancer patients. Am J Pediatr Hematol Oncol 10:185–190

41. Tebbi CK, Bromberg C, Piedmonte M (1989) Long-term vocational adjustment of cancer patients diagnosed during adolescence. Cancer 63:213–218

42. Tebbi CK, Bromberg J, Sills I, Cukierman J, Piedmonte M (1990) Vocational adjustment and general well-being of young adults with IDDM. Diabetes Care 13:98–103

43. Tebbi CK, Erpenbeck A (1996) Cancer. In: Rickett VI (ed) Adolescent Nutrition. Chapman and Hall, New York, pp 479–502

44. Tebbi CK (1987) Major Topics in Adolescent Oncology. Futura, Mount Kisco, New York

45. American Cancer Society (1993) Workshop on Adolescents and Young Adults with Cancer Atlanta, Georgia, October 2–3, 1992. Cancer 7:2410–2412

46. Bleyer WA, Smith RA, Green DM, et al (1993) Workgroup #1: Long-term care and lifetime follow-up. Presented at the American Cancer Society Workshop on Adolescents and Young Adults with Cancer, Atlanta, GA, 1992. Cancer 7:2413

47. McKenna RJ, Black B, Hughes R, et al (1993) Workgroup #2: Insurance and employability. Presented at the American Cancer Society Workshop on Adolescents and Young Adults with Cancer, Atlanta, GA, 1992. Cancer 7:2414

48. Baker LH, Jones J, Stoval A, et al (1993) Workgroup #3: Psychosocial and emotional issues and specialized support groups and compliance issues. Presented at the American Cancer Society Workshop on Adolescents and Young Adults with Cancer, Atlanta, GA, 1992. Cancer 7:2419–2422

49. Hammond GD, Nixon DW, Nachman JB, et al (1993) Workgroup #4: Clinical research implications. Presented at the American Cancer Society Workshop on Adolescents and Young Adults with Cancer, Atlanta, GA, 1992. Cancer 7:2423

50. Reaman GH (1993) Observations and conclusions. Presented at the American Cancer Society Workshop on Adolescents and Young Adults with Cancer, Atlanta, GA, 1992. Cancer 7:2424

51. Bleyer WA (1993) What can be learned about childhood cancer from "Cancer statistics review 1973–1988". Cancer 71:3229–3236

52. Bleyer WA (2002) Cancer in older adolescents and young adults: epidemiology, diagnosis, treatment, survival and importance of clinical trials. Med Pediatr Oncol 38:1–10

53. Bleyer A (2002) Older adolescents with cancer in North America deficits in outcome and research. Pediatr Clin North Am 49:1027–1042

54. Bleyer WA (2001) Adolescents and young adults with cancer: a neglected population. In: Perry MC (ed) ASCO Educational Book, 37th Annual Meeting, Spring 2001, pp 125–132

55. Ries LAG, Eisner MP, Kosary CL, et al (eds) (2000) SEER Cancer Statistics Review, 1973–1997. National Cancer Institute, Bethesda, MD

56. Stiller CA, Eatock EM (1999) Patterns of care and survival for children with acute lymphoblastic leukaemia diagnosed between 1980 and 1994. Arch Dis Child 81:202–208

57. Smith MA, Gurney JG, et al (eds) (1999) Cancer incidence and survival among children and adolescents: United States Seer Program 1975–1995, National Cancer Institute, SEER Program. Bethesda, NIH Pub. No. 99–4649, pp 157–164

58. Cotterill SJ, Parker L, Malcolm AJ, et al (2000) Incidence and survival for cancer in children and young adults in the north of England, 1968–1995: a report from the Northern Region Young Persons' Malignant Disease Registry. Br J Cancer 83:397–403

59. Bleyer WA (1999) Point/Counterpoint, ASCO News, April 1999, p 18

60. Gatta G, Capocaccia R, Coleman MP, Ries LA, Berrino F (2002) Childhood cancer survival in Europe and the United States. Cancer 95:1767–1772

61. Otten J, Philippe N, Suciu S, et al, EORTC Children Leukemia Group (2002) The Children's Leukemia Group: 30 years of research and achievements. Eur J Cancer 38:S44–49

62. Gatta G, Capocaccia R, De Angels R, et al (2003) Cancer survival in European adolescents and young adults. Eur J Cancer 39:2600–2610

63. Barr R (2001) Cancer control in the adolescent and young adult population: special needs. In: Perry MC (ed) ASCO Educational Book, 37th Annual Meeting, Spring 2001, pp 133–137

64. Sateren WB, Trimble EL, Abrams J, et al (2002) How sociodemographics, presence of oncology specialists and hospital cancer programs affect accrual to cancer treatment trials. J Clin Oncol 20:2109–2117

65. Bernstein L, Sullivan-Halley J, Krailo MD, Hammond GD (1993) Trends in patterns of treatment of childhood cancer in Los Angeles County. Cancer 71:3222–3228

66. Whelan J (2003) Where should teenagers with cancer be treated? Eur J Cancer 39:2573–2578

67. Bleyer WA, Tejeda H, Murphy SB, et al (1997) National cancer clinical trials: children have equal access; adolescents do not. J Adolesc Health 21:366–373

68. Rogers AS (1997) Adolescents under enrollment in national clinical research: it is time to ask why. J Adolesc Health 21:374–375

69. Newburger PE, Elfenbein DS, Boxer LA (2002) Adolescents with cancer: access to clinical trials and age-appropriate care. Curr Opin Pediatr 14:1–4

70. Brady AM and Harvey C (1993) The practice patterns of adult oncologists' care of pediatric oncology patients. Cancer 71:3237–3240

71. Jeha S (2003) Who should be treating adolescents and young adults with acute lymphoblastic leukaemia? Eur J Cancer 39:2579–2583

72. Bleyer WA, Tejeda HA, Murphy SB, et al (1997) Equal participation of minority patients in U.S. national pediatric cancer clinical trials. J Pediatr Hematol Oncol 19:423–427

73. Ross JA, Severson RK, Pollock BH, Robison LL (1996) Childhood cancer in the United States. A geographical analysis of cases from the Pediatric Cooperative Clinical Trials groups. Cancer 77:201–207

74. Ross JA, Severson RK, Robison LL, et al (1993) Pediatric cancer in the United States. A preliminary report of a collaborative study of the Childrens Cancer Group and the Pediatric Oncology Group. Cancer 71:3415–3421

75. Shochat SJ, Fremgen AM, Murphy SB, et al (2001) Childhood cancer: patterns of protocol participation in a national survey. CA Cancer J Clin 51:119–130

76. Liu L, Krailo M, Reaman GH, Bernstein L (2003) Surveillance, epidemiology and end results. Childhood Cancer Linkage Group. Cancer 97:1339–1345

77. Stiller CA, Eatock EM (1999) Patterns of care and survival for children with acute lymphoblastic leukaemia diagnosed between 1980 and 1994. Arch Dis Child 81:202–208

78. Rauck AM, Fremgen AM, Hutchison CL, et al (1999) Adolescent cancers in the United States. A National Cancer Data Base (NCDB) report. J Pediatr Hematol Oncol 21:310

79. Irken G, Oren H, Gulen H, et al (2002) Treatment outcome of adolescents with acute lymphoblastic leukemia. Ann Hematol 81:641–645

80. Albritton K, Bleyer WA (2003) The management of cancer in the older adolescent. Eur J Cancer 39:2584–2599

81. Kelly D, Mullhall A, Pearce S (2003) Adolescent cancer – the need to evaluate current service proviso in the UK. Eur J Oncol Nurs 7:53–38

82. Barr RD (1999) On cancer control and the adolescent. Med Pediatr Oncol 32:404–410

83. Keohan ML (2001) Adolescents and young adults with cancer: what will it take to improve care and outcome? In: Perry MC (ed) ASCO Educational Book, 37th Annual Meeting, Spring 2001, pp 138–140

84. Geehan S (2003) The benefits and drawbacks of treatment in a specialist Teenage Unit – a patient's perspective. Eur J Cancer 39:2681–2683

85. SIOP News (2003) Teenage cancer units provide "invaluable" care for the "Lost Tribe". SIOP News, Vol 28

86. Whiteson M (2003) The Teenage Cancer Trust – advocating a model for teenage cancer services. Eur J Cancer 39:2688–2693

87. Woodgate RL (1999) A review of the literature on resilience in the adolescent with cancer: part II. J Pediatr Oncol Nurs 16:78–89

88. Woodgate RL (1999) Conceptual understanding of resilience in the adolescent with cancer. Part I. J Pediatr Oncol Nurs 16:35–43

89. Stock K, Sather H, Dodge RK, et al (2000) Outcome of adolescents and young adults with ALL: A comparison of Children's Cancer Group (CCG) and cancer and Leukemia Group (CALGB) regimens. Blood 96:467a

90. Zeltzer LK (1993) Cancer in adolescents and young adults psychosocial aspects: long-term survivors. Cancer 71:3463–3468

91. Madan-Swain A, Brown RT, Foster MA, et al (2000) Identity in adolescent survivors of childhood cancer. J Pediatr 25:105–115

92. Madan-Swain A, Brown RT, Sexson SB, et al (1994) Adolescent cancer survivors: psychosocial and familial adaptation. Psychosomatics 35:453–459

93. Leonard RC, Gregor A, Coleman RE, et al (1995) Strategy need for adolescent patients with cancer. Br Med J 311:387

94. Rosen DS (1993) Transition to adult health care for adolescents and young adults with cancer. Cancer 71:3411–3414

95. Holman GH, Forman WB (2001) On the 10th anniversary of the Organization of the American Academy of Hospice and Palliative Medicine (AAAPM): the first 10 years. Am J Hosp Palliat Care 18:275–278

96. Kubler-Ross E (1969) On Death and Dying. MacMillan, New York

Epidemiology and Etiology of Cancer in Adolescents and Young Adults

Jillian M. Birch • Archie Bleyer

Contents

3.1 Abstract

The epidemiology of cancer has been studied in children and older adults for nearly half a century. Remarkably little attention has been paid to the cancers in between, especially those that occur between 13 and 30 years of age. Not only are the array of cancers that are diagnosed in this age range unique, recent evidence suggests that they are biologically different and may thereby have different etiologies. Many cancers peak in incidence in older adolescents and young adults. Close scrutiny of overall incidence rates indicate that there is an intermediate peak between the well-known childhood cancer peak and the predominant one that occurs in the elderly. If the cancers that account for the childhood peak are *embryonal/fetal cancers* and those that account for the peak late in life as the *cancers of aging*, the young adult-older adolescent peak may be considered as being due to *cancers of intermediate growth and maturation*. For most of the past quarter century, the incidence of cancers of maturation has been increasing for reasons that have not yet been ascertained. The trends and patterns of incidence do offer certain clues as to cancer causation in older adolescents and young adults. Detailed analyses of incidence patterns by geographic region and demographic factors, together with determination of variations in incidence in time and space, should provide additional insights into etiology and suggest possible lines of investigation.

3.2 Introduction

In the United States and in England, cancer is the leading cause of nonaccidental death among adolescents and young adults [1, 2]. Among 13- to 19-year-olds in the United States, cancer is the fourth leading cause of all deaths, following accidental injuries, suicide, and homicide [1]. Among 20- to 29-year-old Americans, cancer causes more deaths than either suicide, heart disease, human immunodeficiency virus infection, cerebrovascular disease, or cirrhosis. In females, deaths due to cancer occur at more than twice the frequency of deaths due to the second leading disease-related cause of death [1].

Cancer is predominantly a disease of aging, with a dramatic increase from age 10 to 80 years, and an exponential phase from 40 to 80 years of age (Fig. 3.1) [3]. In economically advantaged countries, the median age is between 65 and 70 years. Thus, most of cancer can be considered as cancers of aging. During the first 5 years of life, there is a peak in incidence, with an entirely different group of cancers that appear to have their origin prenatally during embryogenesis and fetal development. These early cancers may be regarded as embryonal/fetal cancers or cancers of early growth. Many of these cancers are small, round blue-cell tumors that are characteristic of pediatric malignancies. A nadir in incidence occurs at age 10 years, followed by a second peak during adolescence and early adulthood, which is most apparent in males (Fig. 3.1). In this phase, there is another set of cancers that are unique to the age group and to organ systems (Fig. 3.2) [4], which as a group do not occur at any other age (Fig. 3.2). This second set of age-dependent cancers may be regarded as cancers of adult growth and maturation, or young adult cancers (Fig. 3.1) [3]. This chapter reviews the epidemiology of cancer in this age group, specifically in 13- to 29-year-olds. After a review of the age-dependent incidence in England and the United States, patterns of incidence are evaluated for clues as to etiologic factors that may account for the malignancies that occur during this phase of life.

Because the types and distribution of malignancies presenting in adolescents and young adults are markedly different compared with those seen in younger or older patients, the development of specialist services

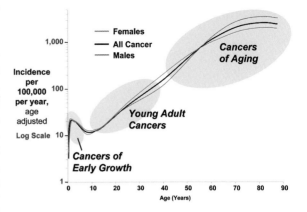

Figure 3.1

Incidence of invasive cancer in the United States as a function of age at diagnosis, overall and by gender, in the period 1975–2001. Rates are age-adjusted to the 2000 United States standard population by 5-year age groups. Data from the United States Surveillance, Epidemiology and End Results (SEER) program [3]

targeted toward adolescent and young adult cancer patients is desirable and necessary to improve all aspects of outcome. In order to develop services that are tailored to the needs of this age group, it is necessary to define the extent and nature of the patient population through precise analyses of relevant population-based data.

3.3 Nosology and Cancer Spectrum

3.3.1 Diagnostic Classification

Two different nosologic systems are used to classify malignancies: one for children and one for adults. The former is known as the International Classification of Childhood Cancer, ICCC, a World Health Organization classification that is based primarily on morphology/histology [5], whereas that for adults is the International Classification of Diseases, ICD system [6–8], which is based primarily on organ site/topography. In general, the ICD system is satisfactory for the majority of cancers occurring in later life, which are mainly carcino-

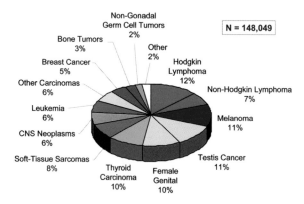

N = 148,049

Non-Gonadal Germ Cell Tumors 2%
Bone Tumors 3%
Breast Cancer 5%
Other Carcinomas 6%
Leukemia 6%
CNS Neoplasms 6%
Soft-Tissue Sarcomas 8%
Thyroid Carcinoma 10%
Female Genital 10%
Testis Cancer 11%
Melanoma 11%
Non-Hodgkin Lymphoma 7%
Hodgkin Lymphoma 12%
Other 2%

Figure 3.2

Types of cancer in 15- to 29-year-olds. Data from the United States SEER program, 1975–1998. *Other Carcinomas* are those that are not carcinomas of the breast, thyroid, or genital systems. The number in the box refers to the total number of cases upon which the array of types is based.

mas, but in young people carcinomas are rare. Therefore, for epidemiological and service planning purposes, data on cancers in young people are best presented mainly in terms of morphology. For the cancers of older adolescents and young adults, the childhood cancer ICCC system, or a modification thereof, has been recommended to be more applicable [9–11]. The rationale for this approach is illustrated in Fig. 3.2, which shows that between two-thirds and three-quarters of 15- to 19-year-old patients and at least half of patients between 20 and 24 years of age have a cancer that a pediatric oncologist would be comfortable and skilful at managing. Nonetheless, although uncommon, many of the cancers of younger and older patients do occur in adolescents [12–15]. Thus, neither histology nor topography provides a completely accurate basis upon which to classify the cancers of adolescents and young adults. One recommendation has been to separate colorectal, salivary, and lung carcinomas from "other carcinomas" within the group of "carcinoma and other epithelial tumors," thereby enumerating the carcinomas that occur at some frequency in younger patients [9]. Breast cancer should also probably be dealt with in this way [16, 17].

A separate nosologic system for cancers that occur in patients 13- to 29-years of age is preferable to a modification of either the ICCC or ICD systems, since this age group is unique in so many ways. Such a classification scheme, specifically tailored to the adolescent and young adult cancer groups, has been published [4]. The scheme is largely based on morphology, and diagnostic groups are specified in terms of the International Classification of Diseases for Oncology (ICD-O) morphology and topography codes [18]. Such a classification scheme can be used in future studies of cancers in adolescents and young adults to achieve a standard format for data presentation to facilitate international comparisons and encourage an interest in research into these cancers.

The scheme was applied to national cancer registration data for England for the years 1979–1997 for patients aged 15 to 24 years [4], and updated data to the year 2000 is presented here. In this age range the main cancers to occur were lymphomas, leukemias, bone tumors, central nervous system (CNS) tumors, germ cell tumors, soft-tissue sarcomas (STS), and carcinomas. In contrast to older age groups in which carcinomas of the lung, breast, large bowel, and prostate account for greater than 50% of all cases [19] at these sites, carcinomas represent only 2% of malignancies in 13- to 24-year-olds. However, certain "adult" cancers are relatively more frequent in this age range. Melanoma and carcinoma of the thyroid represent 8% and 3% of all cancers, respectively, in 15- to 24-year-olds, but across all ages these cancers make up only 2% and 0.4% of the total, respectively [4].

3.4 Incidence

In the United States, nearly 25,000 persons between the ages of 15 and 30 years are diagnosed each year to have cancer (Table 3.1). Data from the United States Surveillance, Epidemiology and End Results (SEER) program indicate that the overall incidence of cancer in 15- to 29-year-olds is twice that in the group of children aged 0 to 14 years (Table 3.1). In the year 2000, 0.6% of all cancer registrations in England were for persons 15 to 24 years of age, inclusive [19]. In the United States, 1.8% of all invasive cancer occurs

Table 3.1 Incidence of invasive cancer in persons less than age 45 years by age group (derived from United States Surveillance, Epidemiology and End Results, SEER, a data; 1975–1999)[a]

Age at diagnosis (years)	<5	5–9	10–14	15–19	20–24	25–29	30–34	35–39	40–44
United States population, year 2000 census (millions)	19.175	20.549	20.528	20.219	18.964	19.381	20.510	22.706	22.441
Average annual increase in invasive cancer, 1975–2000, SEER	1.0%	0.4%	0.9%	0.7%	1.0%	1.9%	1.6%	1.1%	0.4%
Estimated incidence of invasive cancer, year 2000, per 1,000,000 persons	217	113	129	216	365	662	983	1462	2156
No persons diagnosed with invasive cancer, year 2000, United States	4,153	2,314	2,638	4,374	6,928	12,830	20,162	33,197	48,385
					24,132				

[a]Excludes carcinoma in situ (breast and uterine cervix) and nonmelanoma skin cancer

between 15 and 30 years of age (SEER data, 1996–2000). The threefold greater incidence that occurs with just 5 additional years of age is a result of the exponential increase in incidence that occurs between 10 and 55 years of age (Fig. 3.1). From the United States SEER data (Table 3.1), it can be seen that one-half of patients diagnosed at between 15 and 29 years of age are in the 25- to 29-year age range, and one-third are in the 20- to 24-year-old age group.

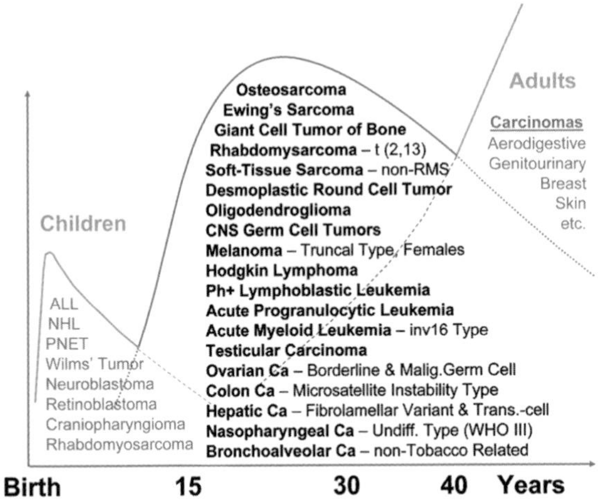

3.4.1 Types of Cancers

The spectrum of cancers in the 15- to 29-year age group (Fig. 3.2) is unique; there is no other age group that has a similar pattern. A variety of cancers ranging from sarcomas to Hodgkin lymphoma to types of carcinomas have their peak in incidence within this age range (Fig. 3.3). For the full 15- to 29-year age span, the order of incidence of the types of cancer is Hodgkin lymphoma, non-Hodgkin lymphoma (NHL), melanoma, testicular carcinoma, female genital tract cancer (primarily cervical and ovarian carcinoma), thyroid

Figure 3.3

Cancers that peak in incidence during childhood (*left peak*), during late adolescence and early adulthood (*middle peak*), and during middle/old age (*right peak*). *Ca* Cancer, *CNS* central nervous system, *ALL* acute lymphoblastic leukemia, *NHL* non-Hodgkin Lymphoma, *PNET* primitive neuroectodermal tumor, *RMS* rhabdomyosarcoma, *Ph+* Philadelphia chromosome-positive, *Malig.* malignant, *Undiff* undifferentiated, *WHO* World Health Organization

Figure 3.4

Types of cancer in 15- to 29-year-olds in 5-year age intervals. Data from the United States SEER program, 1975–1998. Because of the age overlap between the International Classification of Childhood Cancer (ICCC), which is used for pediatric cancers, and the International Classification of Disease, which is used for cancers in adults patients, a combination of both the ICCC and ICD was used to generate the distribution of cancer types.
A Diagnosis between 15 and 19 years, inclusive.
B Diagnosis between 20 and 24 years, inclusive.
C Diagnosis between 25 and 29 years.
The number in the box refers to the total number of cases upon which the array of types in based.

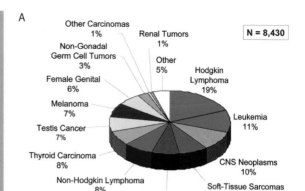

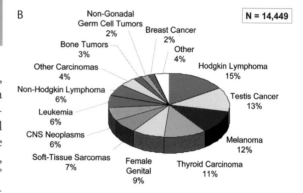

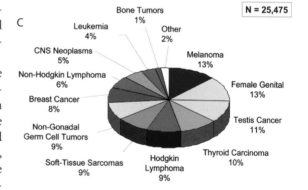

cancer, STS, brain and spinal cord tumors, leukemia, breast cancer, bone sarcomas, and nongonadal germ cell cancer (Fig. 3.2). Most of the common "developmental" malignancies in children (embryonal/fetal cancers of early growth) younger than 5 years of age are virtually absent in 15- to 29-year-olds (Fig. 3.2), including the embryonal malignancies of Wilms' tumor, neuroblastoma, medulloblastoma, ependymoma, hepatoblastoma, and retinoblastoma. In contrast, osteosarcoma, Ewing sarcoma, gonadal germ cell tumors, and Hodgkin lymphoma each peak in incidence during adolescence and young adulthood.

Within the 15-year age span of this age group, the spectrum of cancers also varies dramatically as a function of age (Fig. 3.4). For 15- to 19-year-olds, the ten most frequent cancers, in order of incidence, are Hodgkin lymphoma, leukemia, brain and spinal cord neoplasms, STS, bone sarcomas, thyroid carcinoma, testicular carcinoma, malignant melanoma, and female genital tract malignancies (primarily ovarian carcinoma; Fig. 3.4a). More than 90% of all the cancers in this age group are accounted for by these malignancies. For 20- to 24-year-olds, the ten most frequent cancers, in order of incidence, are Hodgkin lymphoma, testicular cancer, malignant melanoma, thyroid cancer, female genital tract cancer (ovarian and cervical carcinomas), STS, brain and spinal cord tumors, leukemia, NHL, and bone sarcomas (Fig. 3.4b). For 25- to 29-year-olds, the ten most frequent cancers, in order

of incidence, are malignant melanoma, female genital tract tumors (ovarian and cervical carcinomas), testicular cancer, thyroid cancer, Hodgkin lymphoma, STS, breast cancer, NHL, brain and spinal cord tumors, and leukemia (Fig. 3.4c). Nearly 90% of all cancers in both the 20 to 24 and 25 to 29 year age groups are accounted for by the ten most frequent malignancies.

Table 3.2 Registered cases of cancer in 13- to 24-year-olds by age group: Time Period and Main Diagnostic Group, England and Wales, 1979–2000[a]

Age group (years)	1979–1985			1986–1992			1993–2000		
	13–14	15–19	20–24	13–14	15–19	20–24	13–14	15–19	20–24
Tumor type									
Leukemia	249	575	429	191	546	496	241	523	469
Lymphoma	185	1,023	1,258	185	1,007	1,576	256	937	1,506
Malignant brain tumors	189	380	401	152	410	507	203	380	491
Bone tumors	149	360	172	127	310	222	137	386	222
Soft-tissue sarcomas	55	237	269	65	228	300	66	214	279
Germ cell neoplasms	38	297	825	28	332	1,007	63	410	1,215
Malignant melanoma	20	164	405	27	202	664	31	279	752
Carcinoma	75	440	1,141	78	341	1,233	84	448	1,436
Miscellaneous tumors	21	51	54	17	47	67	26	39	48
Unspecified malignant neoplasms NEC	8	48	83	22	155	341	21	87	188
All	989	3,575	5037	892	3,578	6,413	1,128	3,703	6,606
England population (1,000s)	10,309	26,881	25,377	8,106	23,268	26,758	9,670	23,048	24,665

[a]Excludes nonmalignant central nervous system tumors and nonmelanoma skin cancer

Adolescents and young adults rarely develop the cancers that predominate in older adults, such as carcinomas of the aerodigestive and genitourinary tract. Two sarcomas, osteosarcoma and Ewing tumor, account for nearly all of the bone sarcomas in this age group. Both peak between 13 and 19 years of age. Gonadal tumors and Hodgkin lymphoma peak between 20 and 29 years of age.

During the 15-year span from 15 to 30 years of age, malignant melanoma, female genital tract carcinomas (especially cervical carcinoma), and breast cancer undergo a rapid increase in incidence. Concomitantly, leukemia, brain and spinal cord tumors, and bone sarcomas decline sharply in incidence.

The types of STS that occur in 15- to 29-year-olds are also distinct from those seen in younger patients. Specifically, rhabdomyosarcoma predominates among the sarcomas of childhood, accounting for more than 60% of the STS in children less than 5 years of age. In 15- to 19-year-olds, rhabdomyosarcoma accounts for only 25% of the STS in adolescents. Nonrhabdomyosarcoma STS, including synovial sarcoma, liposarcoma, malignant fibrous histiocytoma, and malignant peripheral nerve sheath tumors, account for the rest. Leukemias and lymphomas are also distributed differently in older adolescents than in young children. The incidence of acute lymphoblastic leukemia (ALL) declines steadily with age from the 0- to 5-year age group upwards; it accounts for 30% of all cancers in children younger than 15 years, but only 6% of cancers in adolescents aged 15 to 19 years. Acute myelogenous leukemia (AML) is nearly as common as ALL in 15- to 19-year-olds, and is more common than ALL in 20- to 29-year-olds. The incidence of chronic myelogenous leukemia (CML) increases steadily with age from birth on, but it is not as common as either ALL or AML from 15 to 29 years of age. Juvenile myelomonocytic leukemia is uncommon in all four 5-year age groups before age 20 years, but especially in the 15- to 19-year age group. In 15- to 19-year-olds, NHL is more common

Table 3.3 Cancer incidence rates per 1,000,000 and percentage distribution for main groups of cancers in young persons aged 13–24 years, England and Wales, 1979–2000

	Age group (years)					
	13–14		15–19		20–24	
Tumor type	Rate	% all cancers in group	Rate	% all cancers in group	Rate	% all cancers in group
Leukemia	24.2	22.6	22.5	15.1	18.2	7.7
Lymphoma	22.3	20.8	40.5	27.3	56.5	24.0
Malignant brain tumors	19.4	18.1	16.0	10.8	18.2	7.7
Bone tumors	14.7	13.7	14.4	9.7	8.0	3.4
Soft-tissue sarcoma	6.6	6.2	09.3	6.3	11.0	4.7
Germ cell neoplasms	4.6	4.3	14.2	9.6	39.7	16.9
Malignant melanoma	2.8	2.6	08.8	5.9	23.7	10.1
Carcinoma	8.4	7.9	16.8	11.3	49.6	21.1
Miscellaneous tumors	2.3	2.1	01.9	1.3	2.2	1.0
Unspecified malignant neoplasms	1.8	1.7	04.0	2.7	8.0	3.4
Total	107.1		148.3		235.1	

than ALL. The incidence of NHL increases steadily with age, but the subtype distribution changes from a predominance of lymphoblastic and Burkitt lymphomas during early childhood to a predominance of diffuse large-cell lymphoma during adolescence and early adulthood.

3.4.2 Incidence Rates by Age and Diagnostic Group

The data from England are particularly informative on the incidence rates as a function of age and diagnostic group (Tables 3.2–3.9). Table 3.2 provides the actual number of persons with cancer by age group, cancer type, and era, who were between 13 and 24 years of age, inclusive, and diagnosed between 1975 and 2000. Table 3.3 shows the incidence and percentage distribution of malignant disease among the study population by age group and main diagnostic group. Among 13- to 14-year-olds, the highest rates were seen for leuke-

mias, with lymphomas second highest, then CNS tumors and bone tumors. In this age group, STS, germ cell tumors, melanoma, and carcinomas were relatively uncommon. In comparison with younger adolescents, the most striking difference in the 15- to 19-year-olds was a doubling of the incidence rates for lymphomas, which were the most common malignancies in this age group. Rates for leukemias, CNS tumors, and bone tumors were a little lower than those observed in the 13- to 14-year age group, but increases in rates relative to the younger age group were observed in STS, germ cell tumors, melanoma, and carcinomas. However, rates for these malignancies were still markedly lower than rates for leukemia and lymphoma.

The incidence pattern of cancers in the 20- to 24-year age range was distinctly different in comparison with the younger age group. There was a marked increase in rates of lymphomas, which were the most common malignancies, with a substantial decrease in rates for leukemias. The ratio of lymphomas to leuke-

Table 3.4 Incidence of leukemias and lymphomas per 1,000,000 per year in adolescents and young adults, England and Wales, 1979–2000

Tumor type	Age group (years)		
	13–14	15–19	20–24
Acute lymphoid leukemia	17.0	12.4	6.5
Acute myeloid leukemia	5.7	7.3	8.0
Chronic myeloid leukemia	0.7	1.3	2.3
Other unspecified leukemias	0.8	1.6	1.4
Non-Hodgkin lymphoma	9.1	12.2	15.2
Hodgkin lymphoma	13.2	28.4	41.3

Table 3.5 Incidence of malignant brain tumors per 1,000,000 per year in adolescents and young adults, England and Wales, 1979–2000. *PNET* Primitive neuroectodermal tumor

Tumor type	Age group (years)		
	13–14	15–19	20–24
Astrocytoma	10.4	8.5	9.2
Other glioma	2.7	3.0	4.3
Ependymoma	1.5	1.0	1.1
Medulloblastoma and other PNET	3.0	1.5	1.6
Other and unspecified malignant intracranial and intraspinal neoplasms	1.8	2.0	2.0

Table 3.6 Incidence of bone and soft-tissue sarcomas per 1,000,000 per year in adolescents and young adults, England and Wales, 1979–2000. *STS* Soft-tissue sarcoma

Tumor type	Age group (years)		
	13–14	15–19	20–24
Osteosarcoma	8.4	7.7	3.3
Chondrosarcoma	0.4	0.8	1.0
Ewing tumor	5.2	4.7	2.6
Other bone tumors	0.7	1.1	1.1
Fibromatous neoplasms	1.0	11.7	3.0
Rhabdomyosarcoma	2.8	3.0	1.5
Other and unspecified STS	2.8	4.5	6.6

Table 3.7 Incidence of carcinomas per 1,000,000 per year in adolescents and young adults, England and Wales, 1979–2000. *GU* Genitourinary, *GI* gastrointestinal

Tumor type	Age group (years)		
	13–14	15–19	20–24
Thyroid carcinoma	1.9	4.2	8.6
Other carcinoma head and neck	2.0	2.8	3.6
Carcinoma of trachea, bronchus and lung	0.2	0.4	1.3
Carcinoma of breast	0.0	0.6	5.3
Carcinoma of GU tract	1.5	3.6	20.7
Carcinoma of GI tract	1.8	3.6	7.1
Carcinoma of other and ill-defined sites NEC	1.0	1.7	3.0

Table 3.8 Incidence of germ cell tumors, melanoma and other miscellaneous tumors per 1,000,000 per year in adolescents and young adults, England and Wales, 1979–2000

Tumor type	Age group (years)		
	13–14	15–19	20–24
Germ cell and trophoblastic neoplasms of gonads	3.3	12.5	37.6
Nongonadal germ cell neoplasms	1.3	1.7	2.1
Melanoma	2.8	8.8	23.
Other embryonal tumors NEC	1.6	0.9	0.8
Other specified neoplasms NEC	0.7	1.0	1.4
Unspecified malignant neoplasms NEC	1.8	4.0	8.0

mias was approximately 1:1 in 13- to 14-year olds, but in 20- to 24-year olds this had increased to more than 3:1. However, the most striking differences were in the rates for carcinomas, germ cell tumors, and melanomas, which were the second, third, and fourth most common cancer groups observed in these young adults, respectively. In contrast, bone tumors were much less frequent compared with the younger age groups, but there was an increase in the incidence of STS. The incidence of CNS tumors was fairly similar across all three age groups. The pattern of malignancies that occur in 20- to 24-year-olds overall is therefore very different compared with the younger adolescents. The 15- to 19-year-olds show a transitional pattern. The incidence of all malignancies combined in the 20- to 24-year-age group was more than double that observed in 13- to 14-year-olds.

Table 3.4 shows incidence rates for leukemia subtypes and for NHL and Hodgkin lymphoma. In 13- to 14-year-olds, most leukemias were ALL. Acute myeloid leukemia (AML) accounted for nearly all of the remaining cases. Among 15- to 19-year-olds, there was an increase in rates for AML and a decrease in ALL relative to the younger age group. Among 20- to 25-year-olds, AML was the most frequent subtype, accounting for nearly 50% of the cases. CML was relatively rare at all ages, but showed increasing rates with increasing age. The incidence of CML in 20- to 24-

Table 3.9 Temporal trends in rates of cancer in persons aged 13–24 years, England and Wales, 1979–2000

Tumor type	Average incidence per 1,000,000 per year by time period of diagnosis			
	1979–1985	1986–1992	1993–2000	P for trend
Acute myeloid leukemia	6.7	7.5	7.8	0.03
Non-Hodgkin lymphoma	10.0	14.2	14.7	<0.0001
Hodgkin lymphoma	29.5	32.2	32.1	0.01
Astrocytoma	7.5	9.1	10.9	<0.0001
Ewing's tumor	3.1	3.6	05.1	<0.0001
Germ cell tumor	18.8	22.2	29.0	<0.0001
Melanoma	9.5	14.5	18.3	<0.0001
Thyroid carcinoma	4.5	5.1	7.4	<0.0001
Colorectal carcinoma	2.6	2.3	3.7	0.0007
All cancers	154.1	182.3	198.0	<0.0001

year-olds was more than three times that seen in 13- to 14-year-olds.

In contrast to ALL, rates for NHL increased with increasing age. Only about half of all registered cases were coded to a specific subtype of NHL. The subtypes specified in the dataset are inconsistent with the current international classification of lymphomas, since the classification of NHL has changed substantially during the period covered [20, 21]. However, in summary, nearly 80% of all cases with a specified subtype across the age range 13 to 24 years were classified as diffuse, about 10% as follicular/nodular, and the remainder as other miscellaneous subtypes. The incidence of Hodgkin lymphoma increased markedly with age, and the incidence among 20- to 24-year-olds was more than three times that seen in 13- to 14-year-olds. HD subclassification was consistent across the time period and was based on the Rye Conference scheme [22]. More than two-thirds of the Hodgkin lymphoma cases were coded to a specified subtype. Of these, more than 70% were nodular sclerosing Hodgkin lymphoma, and this proportion did not differ markedly within age groups. Mixed cellularity Hodgkin lymphoma comprised nearly 20% of all specified cases and was somewhat more frequent among 15- to 24-year-olds than in 13- to 14-year-olds. Lymphocyte-predominant Hodg-

kin lymphoma formed less than 10% of all specified cases but was rather more frequent at younger than older ages. Lymphocyte-depleted HD was infrequent across all age groups.

Table 3.5 presents incidence rates of malignant CNS tumors. The most frequent CNS tumor was astrocytoma, and in those with a specified subtype, low-grade astrocytomas were more common than glioblastoma and anaplastic astrocytoma in the 13- to 14-year-olds and 15- to 19-year-olds. However, the difference in rates between low-grade and high-grade astrocytoma was less marked in 15- to 19-year-olds than in the younger age group. In 20- to 24-year-olds, high-grade astrocytomas were more frequent than low-grade variants. Rates for ependymoma did not differ markedly among the age groups, but ependymoma was somewhat more frequent in the youngest group. Medulloblastoma and other primitive neuroectodermal tumors (PNETs) were twice as common in the younger age group as in patients aged 15–24 years. The rates for CNS tumors overall did not differ greatly across age groups. Although rates were only slightly higher in 13- to 14-year-olds than in 20- to 24-year-olds, they constituted 18% of all cases in the younger age group, but less than 8% in the older group (Table 3.2).

Table 3.6 presents the incidence of bone tumors and STS. Rates for bone tumors were higher among patients aged 13 to 19 years than among 20- to 24-year-olds. In all three age groups, osteosarcoma was the most frequent tumor, but the proportion of osteosarcoma was lower in 20- to 24-year-olds, with a relatively higher proportion of chondrosarcoma compared with the younger age groups. Ewing tumor is the second most common type of bone tumor in all three age groups, but rates are higher in 13- to 14-year-olds than at older ages, and the rate in the 20- to 24-year-olds is only half that seen in the youngest group.

STS, although less common than bone tumors, constitute an important group of malignancies in adolescents and young adults. STS represent about 6% of all malignancies in 13- to 14-year-olds. Rates for rhabdomyosarcoma are lower in the 20- to 24-year-olds, but rates for other STS increase with age.

Table 3.7 reports incidence rates for carcinomas. In 13- to 14-year-olds and 15- to 19-year-olds, the head and neck forms the most common primary site group for carcinomas, making up 46% and 41%, respectively, of all carcinomas among these two age groups, but in 20- to 24-year-olds, carcinomas of the head and neck region make up only 25% of all carcinomas. The thyroid is by far the most common primary site for carcinomas in the head and neck, and rates for carcinoma of the thyroid steadily increase across the three age groups. Nasopharyngeal carcinoma (NPC), which is extremely rare in the population in Britain in general, [19] makes up more than 10% of all carcinomas in 13- to 14-year-olds, but represents only 2% among 20- to 24-year-olds, although the rate is similar to that seen in the younger age group.

Carcinomas of the lung, breast, colon, rectum, and bladder constitute nearly 50% of all cancers at all ages [19], but are all uncommon in adolescents and young adults. However, examples of all of these carcinomas are seen, and the rates increase from the 13- to 14-year age group to the 20- to 24-year-olds. The rates for carcinomas of the genitourinary tract show a marked increase across the three age groups. Genitourinary tract carcinomas comprise 18% of all carcinomas in 13- to 14-year olds, but 21% and 42% in the 15- to 19-year-olds and 20- to 24-year-olds, respectively. All sites within the genitourinary tract show increases with age,

but the greatest increases are for invasive carcinoma of the cervix and uterus. The most common sites among carcinomas of the gastrointestinal tract are the colon and rectum in all three age groups. Adrenocortical carcinoma is rare, but is seen across the 13- to 24-year age range.

Table 3.8 includes incidence rates for germ cell tumors, melanoma, and certain tumors that are seen typically in younger children. The most dramatic increase in rates with age among the adolescent and young adult group occurs in the gonadal germ cell tumors, for which the rate increases from 0.33 per 100,000 in 13- to 14-year-olds to 1.25 in 15- to 19-year-olds, and to 3.76 in 20- to 24-year-olds, representing more than an 11-fold increase in rates over the age range. This is entirely due to testicular germ cell tumors. Nongonadal germ cell tumors are much less frequent than gonadal, and although rates increase across the age groups, the trends with age are less dramatic. There is a small decrease in rates with increasing age for intracranial germ cell tumors. Wilms tumor, neuroblastoma, hepatoblastoma, and retinoblastoma have peak incidences in children aged less than 5 years, but a small number of cases have been registered in the adolescent and young adult age range. Cases of pancreatoblastoma and pulmonary blastoma are also present. Collective rates for all of these tumors are shown in the table as "other embryonal tumors NEC." In addition, it is interesting to note that there are several cases of myeloma, which normally occurs in much older patients.

There are also marked differences in the incidences of certain cancers in this age group by gender, ethnicity, and country that are described in more detail elsewhere [23, 24]. Ethnic/racial differences in incidence are particularly apparent between African-American and non-Hispanic white adolescents and young adults. For example, among 15 to 19-year-olds in the United States, the overall incidence of cancer is 50% higher among whites than among blacks. The incidences of specific cancers such as melanoma and Ewing sarcoma are strikingly higher among whites, as is the case for all age groups. ALL, germ cell tumors, and thyroid cancer are also more common among whites than blacks, each by at least twofold. Among the common cancers in this age group, only STS, considered as a group, are more common among blacks than whites. Internationally, the incidence of melanoma varies the most among members of this age group [25], with rates in adolescents up to five times higher in Australia, where the incidence of melanoma is the highest in the world among both adults and children [3, 10].

3.4.3 Incidence by Gender

The incidence of cancer is equal among males and females 15 to 19 years of age, whereas it is 20% higher in boys than girls less than 15 years of age. Individual tumor types have unequal gender distributions in the older adolescent populations, however. The most striking difference is in the incidence of thyroid carcinoma, with females ten times more likely to develop this disease. Females are also 50% more likely to develop melanoma and about 15% more likely to have Hodgkin lymphoma [2]. Alternatively, males are more than twice as likely to be affected with ALL, twice as likely to be diagnosed with NHL or Ewing sarcoma, 50% more likely to develop osteosarcoma, and 20–30% more likely to have a brain tumor [2].

In the British data, examination of the rates of malignancies in males compared with females revealed several statistically significant differences. In ALL overall, the male to female rate ratio was significantly above 1 ($p<0.0001$), and the ratio also increased with increasing age. For AML there was a small excess rate among males ($p = 0.04$), but this did not differ with age. In NHL there was a marked excess rate among males in all age groups ($p<0.0001$), but the male to female ratio fell slightly with increasing age. The pattern of incidence amongst males and females with Hodgkin lymphoma across the three age groups was similar to that seen for NHL, although the male to female ratio was only slightly above 1 ($p=0.013$).

There was a significantly higher incidence of CNS tumors among males than females ($p<0.0001$), a finding which did not differ by age group. Among diagnostic subgroups only, astrocytoma and medulloblastoma/PNET showed significantly higher rates among males ($p<0.01$ and $p<0.0001$, respectively). An interesting pattern was observed among the bone tumors, for which overall there was a significant excess incidence among males ($p<0.0001$), but the ratio of rates in males

and females differed significantly between age groups ($p<0.001$). In osteosarcoma and in Ewing tumor there was a reversal of the ratio of incidence in males to females from an excess rate in females aged 13–14 years, to an excess in males aged 20 to 24 years. The most marked change in incidence rates between males and females with increasing age occurred among the gonadal germ cell tumors. In the 13- to 14-year-olds the ratio of incidence in males to females was less than 0.5, but in 20- to 24-year-olds the male to female ratio had increased to over 17 ($p<0.0001$). Rates for melanoma and carcinoma of the thyroid were markedly higher in females at all ages (in both groups $p<0.0001$). There was an overall significant excess of females with adrenocortical carcinoma ($p = 0.002$). A significant excess incidence rate of NPC and carcinoma of the bladder was seen among males (in both groups $p<0.0001$). Apart from the gender-specific carcinomas (breast, cervix, and uterus) there were no other statistically significant differences in incidence rates among males and females in other main diagnostic groups.

3.4.4 Temporal Trends in Incidence

In the United States, the incidence of cancer among 15- to 29-year-olds has been increasing during the past quarter century (Table 3.1), since the SEER program was first established to track epidemiologic trends. Most of the overall increase in all cancers, however, occurred during the period 1973–1984 (estimated annual increase of 1.6% per year). During the more recent interval of 1985–2000, the increase in incidence was estimated to be only 0.1% per year. This slowing in the increasing incidence in the United States is similar to that observed for younger age groups. NHL and testicular carcinoma have shown the greatest increases in this age group over this interval, each averaging an increase in incidence of over 2% per year for 24 years.

In England, increases in cancer incidence among adolescents and young adults have also been observed (Table 3.9) and they appear to be greater and more sustaining than that noted in the United States (Table 1). Across all diagnostic groups, there was a highly significant increase in incidence rates over time among 13- to 24-year-olds in England (p for trend <0.0001). There was less of a difference during the most recent time interval, similar to the slowing of increase noted in the United States. Rates for leukemias overall remained stable over the study period, but AML showed a small increase (Fig 3.5). NHL showed a highly significant increase with time period, but the increase over time for Hodgkin lymphoma was less marked (*p* for trend <0.0001 and <0.05, respectively) (Fig 3.5). Rates for all CNS tumors increased over time, but among subgroups of brain tumors, only astrocytoma showed a statistically significant increase (*p*<0.0001) (Fig 3.5). Rates for Ewing tumor showed a significant increase, which was particularly marked between the second and third time periods (*p*<0.0001). To what extent this increase in rates for Ewing tumor may be due to changes in diagnostic practice is uncertain, but there were no comparable decreases in rates of other bone tumors. This observation warrants further investigation. Rates for STS overall and for rhabdomyosarcoma also remained unchanged, but rates for fibrosarcoma decreased, while the incidence of other STS increased. This result is probably due to changes in diagnostic criteria and classification following developments in immunohistochemistry and molecular pathology [26], as discussed elsewhere [4].

Marked increases in incidence were also seen for gonadal germ cell tumors (accounted for primarily by testicular tumors), melanoma, and carcinoma of the thyroid (in all cases *p*<0.0001) (Fig 3.6). There was no corresponding significant increase in ovarian germ cell tumors. Colorectal carcinomas showed a significant trend, which was accounted for by an increase between the second and third time periods (*p*<0.001) (Fig 3.6).

3.5 Biological Differences

This topic is covered to a large extent within the individual disease-based chapters in this book and is limited here to a thematic, cross-disease summary. For most cancers that occur throughout the pediatric, adolescent, and young adult age range, the prognosis declines with age. ALL, the most common malignancy in children, is a pertinent example. Between 10 and 35 years of age, the 5-year survival rate plummets from 75–80% to 20–25% (Fig. 3.5) [27–29]. Several studies have attempted to determine whether this decline is

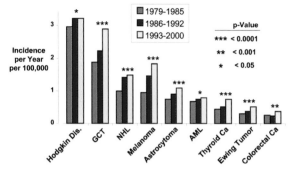

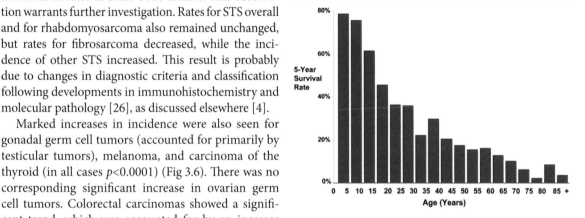

Figure 3.5
Increasing incidence of all common malignancies in England and Wales among 13- to 24-year-olds during the past quarter century

Figure 3.6
Five-year survival rate of patients in the United States SEER program with acute lymphoblastic leukemia by age at diagnosis, 1975–1998 [3]

due to a different biology or to age alone. Compared to children, adolescents and adults with ALL are more likely to have adverse biologic characteristics of their leukemia, such as proT-cell immunophenotype, L2 morphology, Philadelphia chromosome, and other adverse cytogenetics [30, 31]. Alternatively, the Children's Cancer Group (CCG) has shown that, if treatment was risk-stratified based on white blood cell count at diagnosis, FAB (French-American-British) classification and lymphomatous features, older adolescents did nearly as well as those under 15 years [32], and other studies have implicated a treatment effect [33, 34]. Thus far, the impression is that the changes in prognosis based on known biologic predictors do not account for the dramatic decrease in survival.

Observations in Ewing sarcoma suggest a different explanation. In older series, age was felt to be a prognosticator [35, 36]. Indeed, SEER data for all Ewing tumor patients found that between 1985 and 1994, those aged 5–9 years had a 71% 5-year survival, and those aged 10 to 14 years and 15 to 19 years both had a 56% 5-year survival [23]. Unpublished SEER data on adult Ewing sarcoma 1988–1998 had a 45% 5-year survival for those age 20 to 39 years. When presented in aggregate and retrospectively, however, it becomes unclear whether adults were being treated similarly or if more adults had bulky or metastatic disease. In a large analysis of Ewing patients (aged 8 months to 47 years), the age group >15 years had a significantly higher proportion of pelvic primaries and greater tumor volumes [37]. Recently, it has become more common to include adults on Ewing tumor trials. Verrill's group in the United Kingdom treated all Ewing tumor patients from age 16 to 48 years identically with an intensive regimen, and found that age did not influence survival, but volume of tumor did [38]. This was corroborated in the CESS 86 study [39], which intensified treatment for patients with large volume tumors and did not find any impact of age on survival.

On the other hand, in the most recently published CCG/Pediatric Oncology Group study that tested the addition of ifosfamide and etoposide to a standard regimen (doxorubicin, vincristine, dactinomycin, and cyclophosphamide), for nonmetastatic Ewing tumor patients, younger patients again were noted to have a superior outcome (5 year event-free survival 70% for patients <10 years of age, 60% for those 10 to 17 years of age, and 44% for patients 18 to 30 years of age) [40]. This was not explained by any difference in the dose intensity of chemotherapy administered. However, multivariate analysis was not done to determine if the differences in outcome were due to a higher tumor volume, pelvic primary, or male sex, all of which had inferior survival. Interestingly, in this study, the benefit of the addition of ifosfamide and etoposide that was seen in younger patients was not observed in patients older than 17 years, meaning that this may not be the way to overcome the poor prognostic features in older Ewing sarcoma patients.

3.6 Etiology and Pathogenesis

3.6.1 Etiology

As in younger patients, little is known about the causes of cancer in adolescents and young adults. It is likely that environmental agents contribute to the great majority of cancers in older age groups following chronic exposures over many years [41], but in the young there is no opportunity for such long-term exposures. The mechanisms operating between exposure to a risk factor and clinical onset of a cancer in the young may, therefore, be fundamentally different compared with late-onset cancers. In addition, the contributions of the various factors may be proportionally very different and it is likely that genetic susceptibility plays a greater role.

Whereas cancers in infants and young children are likely to be influenced strongly by congenital and prenatal factors, and cancers in the elderly are most strongly linked with environmental causes, the cancers in adolescent and young adult patients may be an interesting combination of both. It has been possible to attribute only very few cancers in this age group directly to single environmental or inherited factors. An exception is clear-cell adenocarcinoma of the vagina or cervix in adolescent females, with most cases caused by diethylstilbestrol taken prenatally by their mothers in an attempt to prevent spontaneous abortion [42]. Radiation-induced cancer may occur in adolescents and young adults after exposure during early childhood; rates of thyroid cancer in children and adolescents have increased in Eastern European and Slavic countries since the Chernobyl accident in 1986 [43]. In fact, many of the adolescent and young adult cancers that have been linked to etiologic factors are second malignant neoplasms in patients who were treated with chemotherapy and/or radiotherapy for a prior cancer.

Given that the duration of exposure to potential environmental carcinogens is proportional to age, it is not surprising that tobacco-, sunlight-, or diet-related cancers are more likely to occur in older adolescents and young adults than in younger persons. Nonetheless, these environmental agents known to be carcinogens in older adults have not been demonstrated to cause cancer with any significant frequency in adolescents. It appears to take considerably longer than one or two decades in most persons for these environmentally related cancers to become manifest. The logical hypothesis is that adolescents who develop cancer after a carcinogenic exposure have a predisposing genotype. For example, melanoma is more common among Australian adolescents than elsewhere in the world, as described above. This suggests that solar exposure may be able to induce skin cancer before the end of the second decade of life, at least in that part of the world. That melanomas during adolescence usually occur in nonexposed areas of the body mitigates against this explanation, and may suggest that the epidemiology of melanoma in Australia is determined more by genetic factors than environmental exposures (cf. Chapter 17).

Besides intense sun exposure, exposure to other environmental carcinogens begins or intensifies during this age period: tobacco use, recreational drug use, alcohol use, and sexually transmitted disease. It is unlikely, however, that cancers resulting from these exposures occur during young adulthood. They are much more likely to occur later in life.

There is accumulating epidemiological evidence that childhood precursor B-cell ALL, which demonstrates a characteristic peak in incidence between the ages of 2 and 6 years, is etiologically linked to delayed exposure to infections in early childhood, resulting in delayed immune stimulation. There is also strong evidence that an initial mutational event occurs in utero and predisposes the child to subsequent development of leukemia in early life [44–48]. Space–time clustering patterns in childhood leukemia also support a role for infections [49]. The decrease in incidence rates in ALL with increasing age following the childhood peak to young adulthood suggests that etiological factors and/or mechanisms may also change with age. Nevertheless, infections may play an important role in the etiology of leukemia in adolescents and young adults, but whereas in young children mainly indirect mechanisms have been proposed, in these

older age groups a directly transforming virus may be more likely [50].

With respect to AML, the increased risk following exposure to certain therapeutic agents used to treat an initial malignancy [51] (i.e., chemical induction of AML) suggests the possibility of a role for environmental chemical exposures in a proportion of cases in young people in general. Higher rates for AML were seen with increasing age among adolescents and young adults, and there was some evidence of an increase in incidence rates over time. The possibility that these patterns of incidence might be due at least in part to postnatal exposures to environmental chemical agents should be given some consideration.

Viruses may also be involved in the etiology of both NHL and Hodgkin lymphoma. An increased risk of NHL has been observed in association with HIV1, HTLV1 and Epstein-Barr virus (EBV). *Helicobacter pylori* infection of the stomach is associated with gastric lymphoma. While these are all relatively rare occurrences and probably account for only a small proportion of total NHL, a role for other viruses and indirect mechanisms involving common infections remain a possibility [52]. EBV infection is linked etiologically to a proportion of Hodgkin lymphoma, particularly the mixed-cellularity subtype. Epidemiological studies have demonstrated that the magnitude of the risk and proportion of cases attributable to EBV infections varies with age, sex, ethnicity, and level of material deprivation. EBV infection is extremely common and other unknown modifying factors are likely to be of importance in the etiology of Hodgkin lymphoma in adolescents and young adults [53, 54].

The decline in the incidence of PNETs, the increase in high-grade astrocytomas, and decrease in low-grade astrocytomas with increasing age may reflect a change in etiological mechanisms in these tumors. A possible role of polyoma viruses, including simian virus 40 (SV40), JC, and BK viruses in CNS tumors has been the subject of much speculation. Viral DNA sequences have been detected in human brain tumors, including PNETs, ependymomas, high- and low-grade astrocytomas, and meningiomas [55–57]. In addition, space–time clustering has been detected in astrocytomas and ependymomas in older children [58]. Presence of space–time clustering is consistent with an infectious etiology. Furthermore, there are similar temporal trends in the incidence of brain tumors in children, adolescents, and young adults [4, 59]. It follows that there may be shared etiological factors for certain brain tumors across these age groups. Hypotheses relating to viral exposures should be investigated.

The increasing ratio of male to female cases across the three age groups 13 to 14 years, 15 to 19 years, and 20 to 24 years suggests that the onset of osteosarcoma and Ewing tumor may be associated with the adolescent growth spurt, which occurs earlier in females than in males. Dietary and hormonal factors may be relevant. The possibility of a viral etiology for osteosarcoma has also been considered, and SV40-like sequences have been detected in osteosarcoma tissue in several studies [60–63]. In the most recent of these studies, the frequency of SV40-like sequences in peripheral blood cells from osteosarcoma patients was compared with that in normal, healthy controls and was found to be substantially increased in the osteosarcoma patients [63]. Space–time clustering has been reported in childhood STS [64]. It would be of considerable interest to determine whether STS in adolescents and young adults exhibit space–time clustering.

The very marked temporal increase in incidence of testicular germ cell tumors in young men has been reported previously. The etiology of testicular germ cell tumors is uncertain, but genetic and hormonal factors, including in utero exposure to estrogen, appear to be implicated [65]. A recent cohort study of young men in Sweden found a positive association between height at 18 years and the incidence of testicular cancer that was not accounted for by gestational age and birthweight. The authors concluded that factors influencing postnatal growth such as diet or growth-related genes might underlie the association [66]. The incidence trends for melanoma of the skin have also been discussed previously. Melanoma of the skin shows associations with socioeconomic factors, skin and hair coloring, certain heritable syndromes, and in particular, patterns of sun exposure [65].

The pattern of carcinomas in adolescents and young adults differs greatly from that seen at older ages. Carcinomas of the head and neck, including thyroid and nasopharynx, make up nearly 30% of carcinomas in the 13- to 24-year age range. The temporal increase in carcinoma of the thyroid in young people has been discussed elsewhere [4]. The highest incidence rates for NPC are found in parts of the Far East where it occurs in association with EBV infection. The rare cases of NPC in young people in Western developed countries may also be associated with EBV, and this should be explored, but it is likely that other cofactors are involved [67]. Carcinoma of the cervix and uterus, although typical of older age groups, is relatively frequent in young adult females and appears to be closely linked with sexually transmitted infections including herpes simplex virus type 2 and human papilloma virus [65]. Other carcinomas seen in adolescents and young adults that occur typically in later life may be strongly associated with genetic predisposition at young ages, as will be discussed below.

3.6.2 Genetic Predisposition and Genetic Susceptibility

In middle to late adult life, cancer occurs as a result of multiple, serially accumulated, genetic changes following decades of exposure to carcinogens like, for example, tobacco smoke. The occurrence of cancer at young ages, when the opportunity for such chronic environmental exposures has not had sufficient time to exist, suggests strongly that individuals are genetically predisposed to develop certain cancers or are genetically susceptible to the carcinogenic effects of environmental agents. In such individuals, the number of genetic changes required to achieve malignant transformation at the cellular level may be reduced and/or metabolic processes modified. In many instances, gene–environment interactions in this age range are more likely to be operative.

Skin cancer, lymphoma, sarcoma, and hepatic cancers also occur at higher frequency in persons with inherited conditions such as neurofibromatosis, ataxia telangiectasia, Li-Fraumeni syndrome, xeroderma pigmentosa, Fanconi pancytopenia, hereditary dysplastic nevus syndrome, nevoid basal cell carcinoma syndrome, multiple endocrine neoplasia syndromes, and Turner syndrome. In the aggregate, however, the cancers that are known to be due to these conditions account thus far for only a small proportion of the cancers that occur during adolescence and early adulthood.

Genetic factors appear to be of etiological importance in CNS tumors in young people. Brain tumors occur in association with several cancer predisposition syndromes that are characterized by germ-line mutations in cancer-associated genes [68]. Of particular relevance to adolescent and young adult cases of high-grade astrocytoma is the possibility that these may arise in patients with germ-line TP53 mutations [69, 70]. Anaplastic astrocytoma shows a peak incidence in the fourth decade of life, and glioblastoma is rare before the age of 30 years [71]. However, in individuals with germ-line TP53 mutations, these tumors tend to arise at much earlier ages [70, 72]. Medulloblastoma, which overall has an incidence peak before 10 years of age, is diagnosed more commonly in older children, adolescents, and young adults with germ-line mutations to the APC (adenomatous polyposis coli) gene [73]. The unusually early age of onset of brain tumors in familial cancer syndromes may represent a combination of genetic susceptibility and environmental exposure. The detection of SV40 viral sequences in tumors from patients with germ-line TP53 mutations is of interest in this context [74]. It appears that genetic factors may be important in the etiology of both osteosarcoma and Ewing tumor. Osteosarcoma is frequently seen in families with germ-line TP53 mutations and cases are usually diagnosed during the teens and twenties [72, 75]. Evidence for genetic susceptibility to Ewing tumor comes from the striking variation in incidence with ethnic origin. Ewing tumor is extremely rare among black Africans and among African Americans [76]. In common with osteosarcoma, STS are a principal component of the cancer predisposition syndrome associated with germ-line TP53 mutations, and in such patients STS are frequently diagnosed at young ages.

Carcinoma of the breast is extremely rare in the adolescent and young adult age range, but is of particular interest since a recent study detected pathogenic alterations in breast cancer susceptibility genes (including BRCA1, BRCA2 and TP53) in 20% of a large series of women with breast cancer diagnosed under the age of 30 years [77]. It is possible that a similarly high rate of mutations in susceptibility genes associated with colorectal carcinoma might also be found among very young patients. Genes of interest in these patients include APC and the mismatch repair genes [78]. The frequency of mutations to relevant genes among these very early onset cases of common carcinomas should be determined.

3.7 Need for an Improved Classification System

Morphology-based classification systems for the analysis and presentation of data on childhood cancers have been in existence for many years [79, 80] and the childhood cancer scheme has been applied to cancer incidence data in adolescents aged 15 to 19 years [23]. Several of the major groups of cancers in children, however (e.g., most embryonal tumors), are so rare as to be irrelevant in adolescents and young adults. Conversely, carcinomas are inappropriately subdivided in the childhood classifications [80]. In an attempt to overcome these problems, one study has used a combination of the childhood classification groups and ICD site groups [82], but this leads to a lack of clarity and coherence in the data. A classification system has been proposed for the adolescent and young adult age range, based primarily on morphology [4]. This classification scheme has now been applied to national data for England and Wales on almost 32,000 cancers in young persons aged 13 to 24 years.

3.8 Conclusions

While a coordinated national approach to the treatment of cancers in younger children was established a half century ago in the United States and a quarter century ago in the United Kingdom, adolescent and young adult cancer patients have not benefited from a similar policy. The adolescent years and early 20s are a crucially important period in terms of educational, social, and career development. Interruption of education, and vocational and professional training following the diagnosis of cancer can have a lasting impact on later life. Furthermore, the potential late effects of cytotoxic treatment can have a greater and more lasting impact in the young, than in the middle-aged and elderly. Loss of fertility, the development of treatment-induced second malignancies, and organ failure are critical considerations in this age group.

Understanding the etiology and biology of cancer in the adolescent and young adult impacts on the management of cancer in this age group, both from a public health cancer-control perspective, and by developing specific therapeutic strategies for a cancer that has a different pathogenesis and biology by virtue of when during life it occurs. Detailed data, as presented above, are of importance in assessing service requirements and in the delivery of services designed to meet the needs of this vulnerable age group. Observation of detailed patterns of incidence can also provide pointers to etiology and identify areas for future research. Classification of cases for analysis that takes into account biological similarities and differences is of critical importance if advances in knowledge and understanding are to be made. Detailed analyses of incidence patterns by geographic region and demographic factors, together with determination of variations in incidence in time and space will provide additional insights into etiology and suggest new lines of investigation, as well as provide a basis for service planning. The chronic occupational and social exposures, including cigarette smoking, which are responsible for the majority of late-onset cancers, are unlikely to be prime causes of cancers in young people. In some circumstances exposure to such environmental agents may be involved in the etiology, but other cofactors, for example genetic susceptibility and hormonal factors, may predominate. The possibility that environmental agents may target different organs and tissues in the growing child leading to different cancers in adolescents and young adults compared with older adults should be considered. In several cancers occurring in young people, the most promising areas for investigation include the role of specific viruses and other infections, dietary factors and their influence on growth and development, and inherited predisposition. Little is known about the etiology of cancer in this fascinating age group and carefully targeted research in this field should produce rewarding results.

Acknowledgements

Data from England presented in this chapter were contributed by the nine regional cancer registries in England and were supplied by the National Cancer Intelligence Centre, London, Director Dr. M.J. Quinn. Statistical analyses were carried out by Dr. R.D. Alston. Data from the United States from the Surveillance, Epidemiology and End Results Program were provided by Lynn Ries.

References

1. Jemal A, Thomas A, Murray T, et al (2002) Cancer Statistics, 2002. CA Cancer J Clin 52:23–47
2. Office for National Statistics; Twentieth Century Mortality. Mortality in England and Wales by age, sex, year and underlying cause: Year 2000 update. London, Office for National Statistics, 2002.
3. Ries LAG, Eisner MP, Kosary CL, et al (eds) (2004) SEER Cancer Statistics Review, 1975–2001, National Cancer Institute. Bethesda, MD, http://seer.cancer.gov/csr/1975_2001/2004
4. Birch JM, Alston RD, Kelsey AM, et al (2002) Classification and incidence of cancers in adolescents and young adults in England 1979–1997. Br J Cancer 87:1267–1274
5. Steliarova-Foucher E, Stiller C, Lacour B, Kaatsch P (2005) International Classification of Childhood Cancer, Third Edition. Cancer 103:1457–1467
6. World Health Organization (1975) International Classification of Diseases, Injuries and Causes of Death. Ninth Revision. World Health Organisation, Geneva
7. World Health Organization (1992) International Statistical Classification of Diseases and Related Health Problems. Tenth Revision. World Health Organisation, Geneva
8. Parkin DM, Whelan SL, Ferlay J, et al (eds) (2002) Cancer Incidence in Five Continents, Vol VIII. IARC, Lyons
9. Fritschi L, Coates M, McCredie M (1995) Incidence of cancer among New South Wales adolescents: which classification scheme describes adolescent cancers better? Int J Cancer 60:355–360
10. Hoff J, Schymura MJ, McCrea Curren MG (1988) Trends in the incidence of childhood and adolescent cancer in Connecticut, 1935–1979. Med Pediatr Oncol 16:78–87
11. Martos MC, Winther JF, Olsen JH (1993) Cancer among teenagers in Denmark, 1943–1979. Int J Cancer 55:57–62

12. Ashikari H, Jun MY, Farrow JH, et al (1977) Breast carcinoma in children and adolescents. Clin Bull 7:55–62

13. Corpron CA, Black CT, Singletary SE, et al (1995) Breast cancer in adolescent females. J Pediatr Surg 30:322–324

14. Franks LM, Bollen A, Seeger RC, et al (1997) Neuroblastoma in adults and adolescents: an indolent course with poor survival. Cancer 79:2038–2035

15. Raney RB, Sinclair L, Uri A, et al (1987) Malignant ovarian tumors in children and adolescents. Cancer 59:1214–1220

16. Ashikari H, Jun MY, Farrow JH, et al (1977) Breast carcinoma in children and adolescents. Clin Bull 7:55–62

17. Corpron CA, Black CT, Singletary SE, et al (1995) Breast cancer in adolescent females. J Pediatr Surg 30:322–324

18. Percy C, Van Holten V, Muir C (eds) (1990) International Classification of Diseases for Oncology (ICD–O). Second edition. World Health Organisation, Geneva

19. Office for National Statistics (2003) Cancer statistics registrations: registrations of cancer diagnosed in 2000, England. Series MB1 no. 31, Office for National Statistics, London

20. Harris NL, Jaffe ES, Diebold J, et al (1999) The World Health Organization Classification of Neoplastic Diseases of the Hematopoietic and Lymphoid Tissues. Report of the Clinical Advisory Committee Meeting, Airlie House, Virginia, Nov 1997. Ann Oncol 10:1419–1432

21. Jaffe ES, Harris NL, Stein H, Vardiman JW (eds) (2001)The World Health Organization Classification of Tumors. Pathology and Genetics of Tumors of Hematopoietic and Lymphoid Tissues. IARC, Lyons

22. Lukes RJ, Craver L, Hall T, et al (1996) Report of the nomenclature committee. Cancer Res 26:1311

23. Smith MA, Gurney JG, Ries LA (1999) Cancer in adolescents 15–19 years old. In: Ries LA, Smith MA, Gurney JG, Linet M, Tamra T, Young JL, Bunin G (eds) SEER Pediatric Monograph, United States SEER Program 1975–1997. National Cancer Institute, Bethesda MD; NIH Pub.No.99–4649

24. Parkin D, Whelan S, Ferlay J, et al (1997) Cancer incidence in five continents. IARC, Lyons, Publications No. 143; volume VII

25. Parkin DM, Kramarova E, Draper GJ, et al (1998) International Incidence of Childhood Cancer Volume II, IARC Scientific Publication #144. International Agency for Research on Cancer, Lyon, France

26. Weiss SW, Goldblum JR (2001) Enzinger and Weiss's Soft Tissue Tumors, 4th edn, St. Louis, Mosby

27. Bleyer A, Montello M, Budd T (2004) Young adults with leukemia in the United States: lack of clinical trial participation and mortality reduction during the last decade. Proc Am Soc Clin Oncol 23:586

28. Rivera GK, Pui CH, Santana VM, et al (1993) Progress in the treatment of adolescents with acute lymphoblastic leukemia. Cancer 71:3400–3405

29. Santana VM, Dodge RK, Crist WM, et al (1990) Presenting features and treatment outcome of adolescents with acute lymphoblastic leukemia. Leukemia 4:87–90

30. Crist W, Pullen J, Boyett J, et al (1988) Acute lymphoid leukemia in adolescents: clinical and biologic features predict a poor prognosis – a Pediatric Oncology Group Study. J Clin Oncol 6:34–43

31. Perentesis JP (1997) Why is age such an important independent prognostic factor in acute lymphoblastic leukemia? Leukemia 4:S4–7

32. Nachman J, Sather HN, Buckley JD, et al (1993) Young adults 16–21 years of age at diagnosis entered on Childrens Cancer Group acute lymphoblastic leukemia and acute myeloblastic leukemia protocols. Results of treatment. Cancer 71:3377–3385

33. Boissel N, Auclerc MF, Lheritier V, et al (2003) Should adolescents (15–20 y) with ALL be treated as old children or young adults? Comparison of the French FRALLE-93 and LALA-94 trials. J Clin Oncol 2:774–780

34. Stock W, Sather H, Dodge RK, et al (2000) Outcome of adolescents and young adults with ALL: a comparison of Children's Cancer Group (CCG) and Cancer and Leukemia Group B (CALGB) regimens (abstracts). Blood 96:467a

35. Rosito P, Mancini AF, Rondelli R, et al (1999) Italian Cooperative Study for the treatment of children and young adults with localized Ewing sarcoma of bone: a preliminary report of 6 years of experience. Cancer 86:421–428

36. Nesbit ME Jr, Gehan EA, Burgert EO Jr, et al (1990) Multimodal therapy for the management of primary, nonmetastatic Ewing's sarcoma of bone: a long-term follow-up of the First Intergroup study. J Clin Oncol 8:1664–1674

37. Cotterill SJ, Ahrens S, Paulussen M, et al (2000) Prognostic factors in Ewing's tumor of bone:analysis of 975 patients from the European Intergroup Cooperative Ewing's Sarcoma Study Group. J Clin Oncol 18:3108–3114

38. Verrill MW, Judson IR, Harmer CL, et al (1997) Ewing's sarcoma and primitive neuroectodermal tumor in adults: are they different from Ewing's sarcoma and primitive neuroectodermal tumor in children? J Clin Oncol 15:2611–2621

39. Paulussen M, Ahrens S, Dunst J, et al (2001) Localized Ewing tumor of bone:final results of the cooperative Ewing's Sarcoma Study CESS 86. J Clin Oncol 19:1818–1829

40. Grier HE, Krailo MD, Tarbell NJ, et al (2003) Addition of ifosfamide and etoposide to standard chemotherapy for Ewing's sarcoma and primitive neuroectodermal tumor of bone. N Engl J Med 348:694–701

41. World Health Organization (2003) The causes of cancer. In: Stewart BW, Kleihues P (eds) World Cancer Report, Chapter 2. IARC, Lyons, pp 22–28

42. Melnick S, Cole P, Anderson D, et al (1987) Rates and risks of diethylstilbesterol-related clear cell adenocarcinoma of the vagina and cervix: an update. N Engl J Med 316:514–519

43. Moysich KB, Menezes RJ, Michalek AM (2002) Chernobyl-related ionising radiation exposure and cancer risk: an epidemiological review. Lancet Oncol 3:269–279

44. Greaves MF (1998) Speculations on the cause of childhood acute lymphoblastic leukemia. Leukemia 2:120–125

45. Kinlen LJ (1995) Epidemiological evidence for an infective basis in childhood leukemia. Br J Cancer 71:1–5

46. Smith MA, Simon R, Strickler HD, et al (1998) Evidence that childhood acute lymphoblastic leukemia is associated with an infectious agent linked to hygiene conditions. Cancer Causes Control 9:285–298

47. Gale KB, Ford AM, Repp R, et al (1997) Backtracking leukemia to birth: identification of clonotypic gene fusion sequences in neonatal blood spots. Proc Natl Acad Sci U S A 94:13950–13954

48. Wiemels JL, Cazzaniga G, Daniotti M, et al (1999) Prenatal origin of acute lymphoblastic leukemia in children. Lancet 354:1499–1503

49. Birch JM, Alexander FE, Blair V, et al (2000) Space–time clustering patterns in childhood leukemia support a role for infection. Br J Cancer 82:1571–1576

50. International Agency for Research on Cancer (1996) Human immunodeficiency viruses and human T-cell lymphotropic viruses: IARC Monographs on the Evaluation of Carcinogenic Risks to Humans, Vol 87. IARC, Lyons

51. Bhatia S, Yasui Y, Robison LL, et al (2003) High risk of subsequent neoplasms continues with extended follow-up of childhood Hodgkin disease: report from the Late Effects Study Group. J Clin Oncol 21:4386–4394

52. Baris D, Zahm SH (2001) Epidemiology of lymphomas. Curr Opin Oncol 12:383–394

53. Glaser SL, Lin RJ, Stewart SL, et al (1997) Epstein-Barr virus-associated Hodgkin disease: epidemiologic characteristics in international data. Int J Cancer 70:375–382

54. Flavell KJ, Biddulph JP, Powell JE, et al (2001) South Asian ethnicity and material deprivation increase the risk of Epstein-Barr virus infection in childhood Hodgkin disease. Br J Cancer 85:350–356

55. Weggen S, Bayer TA, von Deimling A, et al (20001) Low frequency of SV40, JC and BK polyomavirus sequences in human medulloblastomas, meningiomas and ependymomas. Brain Pathol 10:85–92

56. Del Valle L, Gordon J, Assimakopoulou M, et al (2001) Detection of JC virus DNA sequences and expression of the viral regulatory protein T-antigen in tumors of the central nervous system. Cancer Res 61:4287–4293

57. Del Valle L, Gordon J, Enam S, et al (2002) Expression of human neurotropic polyomavirus JCV late gene product agnoprotein in human medullobastoma. J Natl Cancer Inst 94:267–273

58. McNally RJQ, Cairns DP, Eden OB, et al (2002) An infectious etiology for childhood brain tumors? Evidence from space–time clustering and seasonality analyses. Br J Cancer 86:1070–1077

59. McNally RJQ, Kelsey AM, Cairns DP, et al (2001) Temporal increases in the incidence of childhood solid tumors seen in North West England (1954–1998) are likely to be real. Cancer 92:1967–1976

60. Lednicky JA, Stewart AR, Jenkins JJ III, et al (1997) SV40 DNA in human osteosarcomas shows sequence variation among T-antigen genes. Int J Cancer 72:791–800

61. Mendoza SM, Konishi T, Miller CW (1998) Integration of SV40 in human osteosarcoma DNA. Oncogene 17:2457–2462

62. Carbone M, Rizzo P, Procopio A, et al (1996) SV40-like sequences in human bone tumors. Oncogene 13:527–535

63. Yamamoto H, Nakayama T, Murakami H, et al (2000) High Incidence of SV40-like sequences detection in tumor and peripheral blood cells of Japanese osteosarcoma patients. Br J Cancer 82:1677–1681

64. McNally RJQ, Kelsey AM, Eden OB, et al (2003) Space–time clustering patterns in childhood solid tumors other than central nervous system tumors. Int J Cancer 103:253–258

65. Quinn M, Babb P, Brock A, et al (2001) Cancer Trends in England and Wales 1950–1999. Studies on Medical and Population Subjects No.66, London Office for National Statistics

66. Rasmussen F, Gunnell D, Ekbom A, et al (2003) Birth weight, adult height and testicular cancer:cohort study of 337,249 Swedish young men. Cancer Causes Control 14:595–598

67. Griffin BE (2000) Epstein-Barr virus (EBV) and human disease: facts, opinions and problems. Mutat Res 462:395–405

68. Kleihues P, Cavenee WK (eds) World Health Organization, Pathology and Genetics of Tumors of the Nervous System. Chapter 14, Familial tumor syndromes involving the nervous system. IARC, Lyons, pp 215–242

69. Li Y-J, Sanson M, Hoang-Xuan K, et al (1995) Incidence of germ-line p53 mutations in patients with gliomas. Int J Cancer 64:383–387

70. Chen P, Iavarone A, Fick J, et al (1995) Constitutional p53 mutations associated with brain tumors in young adults. Cancer Genet Cytogenet 82:106–115

71. Kleihues P, Cavenee WK (eds) (2000) World Health Organization, Pathology and Genetics of Tumors of the Nervous System. Chapter 1, Astrocytic tumors. IARC, Lyons, pp 9–54

72. Birch JM, Blair V, Kelsey AM, et al (1998) Cancer phenotype correlates with constitutional TP53 genotype in families with the Li-Fraumeni syndrome. Oncogene 17:1061–1068

73. Hamilton SR, Liu B, Parsons RE, et al (1995) The molecular basis of Turcot's Syndrome. N Engl J Med 332:839–847

74. Malkin D, Chilton-MacNeill S, Meister LA, et al (2000) Tissue-specific expression of SV40 in tumors associated with the Li-Fraumeni syndrome. Oncogene 20:4441–4449

75. Birch JM (2003) The Li-Fraumeni syndrome and the role of the TP53 mutations in predisposition to cancer. In: Eeles RA, Easton DF, Eng C, Ponder BA (eds) Genetic Predisposition to Cancer, Second Edition. Edward Arnold, London

76. Parkin DM, Kramárová E, Draper GJ, et al (eds) (1998) International Incidence of Childhood Cancer, Vol II World Health Organisation. IARC Scientific Publications No 144. IARC, Lyons

77. Lalloo F, Varley J, Ellis D, et al (2003) Prediction of pathogenic mutations in patients with early-onset breast cancer by family history. Lancet 361:1101–1102

78. Fearnhead NS, Wilding JL, Bodmer WF (2002) Genetics of colorectal cancer:hereditary aspects and overview of colorectal tumorigenesis. Br Med Bull 64:27–43

79. Birch JM, Marsden HB (1987) A classification scheme for childhood cancer. Int J Cancer 40:624–629

80. Kramárová E, Stiller CA (1996) The International Classification of Childhood Cancer, 1996. Int J Cancer 68:759–765

81. Gatta G, Capocaccia R, De Angelis R, et al and the EUROCARE Working Group (2003) Cancer survival in European adolescents and young adults. Eur J Cancer 39:2600–2610

Access to Care Before and During Therapy

Karen H. Albritton • Tim Eden

Contents

4.1 Introduction

Equitable access to quality healthcare is an ethical tenet that few would question. By access, we mean the timing of treatment, the place of treatment, and the choice of therapy itself. The most important impact of access is in how it affects outcomes. The United States Institute of Medicine Committee on Monitoring Access to Personal Healthcare Services defined access as "the timely use of personal health services to achieve the best possible health outcomes" [1]. We do not expect service or outcomes to be exactly the "same" for various populations, just "equal," which means fair, or equally close to ideal. Adolescents and young adults with cancer should have the same opportunity to achieve their best possible outcome as another older or younger patient.

Are adolescents and young adults really achieving less than their best possible outcome because of how they access their oncologic care? This book and recent editorials have referred to the adolescent oncology patient as a member of a medically "underserved" population. This implies that there is some inequality of services (and therefore outcome) unique to this population.

The question assumes that there is a gold standard, a "best possible health outcome," already defined. In the simplest case, this is long-term cure without significant side effects, and is represented by the chance of achieving that – measured by the event-free survival. The estimates of event-free survival that come from large clinical trials are often held as the "best possible outcome." Population data, on the other hand, tell us not the best possible, but "real world" outcomes.

Different cancers have different biology and, therefore, different event-free survival. Many would also allow that biology within individual tumor diagnoses varies by age and that, therefore, the best possible event-free survival varies by age. Population data (Surveillance, Epidemiology, and End Results, SEER, registry 1986–1995) indeed show that the prognosis of acute lymphoblastic leukemia decreases with age (see Chap. 6), so that the mean 5-year survival of a 15- to 19-year-olds with acute lymphoblastic leukemia is 49%, in comparison to a mean of 81% for a 5- to 9-year-old with the same disease, and 68% for a 10- to 14-year-old. Yet, 15- to 19-year-olds treated on a Children's Cancer Group study had a 5-year survival of 64%, nearly "equal" to that of the 10- to 14-year-olds. If biology alone explained the difference in outcome between children and adolescents, therapy would not be able to overcome this biologic barrier. The concern is that adolescent age, like race, may be a surrogate for other factors that influence survival, and that these factors may not be entirely (or even mostly) biologic, but may in part be related to access to care.

Therefore, the "best possible" goal for 15- to 29-year-olds should probably not be different from that of 10- to 14-year olds; these older patients need easy access to the treatment that can achieve those outcomes. Outcome differentials such as these must make us very concerned with what determines access to different types of therapy. This chapter will examine the little we know of how adolescents and young adults with cancer access health-care services (compared with younger and older cancer patients) and whether their outcomes are influenced by this access.

Such a discussion of access is complicated by two unique issues for this age population. Unlike either children or older adults, adolescents and young adults live in a middle ground where they can access two general healthcare delivery systems: pediatric oncology or medical oncology. Throughout the world, medicine, especially subspecialty medicine, and certainly oncology, is dramatically split into pediatrics (care for children) and internal medicine (care for adults). The problem is the very unclear line between "child" and "adult," with "adolescent" and "young adult"

somewhere in between the two. The American Academy of Pediatrics 1972 revision of its statement on its age purview said the responsibility of pediatrics "usually terminates by 21 years of age" [2]. The current American Academy of Pediatrics mission statement is "to attain optimal physical, mental, and social health and well-being for all infants, children, adolescents, and young adults" [3]. Pediatric hospitals in both the United States and parts of Europe are commonly raising their upper age limits, making the option of care by pediatricians available for individuals into their 20s, but this is not universal. Increasing attention is being paid to the transition of care for adolescents with chronic conditions from child-centered to adult health-care systems, and recommendations made to start considering this transition at age 14 years. What is less apparent is where care should initiate for the adolescent/young adult with a new medical condition, especially one that requires subspecialty care. There are no guidelines that dictate when an adolescent/young adult should seek care with a pediatric specialist or a medical specialist.

Secondly, "best possible outcome" is an ill-defined target in this population. Little outcome data exist that tell us whether there is a differential of care that might dictate the most appropriate site or specialist of care for any specific type of malignancy. Although we know the treatment that achieves the best possible outcome for 15- to 19-year olds with acute lymphoblastic leukemia [4–6], we do not know it for 20- to 24-year-olds, and we certainly do not know it for adolescents and young adults with other cancers. It is also important to acknowledge that survival is not the only outcome of interest; quality of life must be considered too, including late effects. Adolescent and young adult patients should have access to services that provide developmentally appropriate psychosocial support, and minimize side effects and late effects of relevance to the population (e.g., infertility).

4.2 Access to Care Obstacles

Access to care obstacles can be broken down into three categories: strategic/financial factors, provider issues, and personal beliefs, knowledge and behavior [7].

4.2.1 Strategic/Financial Factors

In the United States and other countries without universal healthcare, the financial and insurance status of the patient (and family) may indeed influence access to medical care. Adolescence to young adulthood is an age range with great financial variance. Younger adolescents are usually covered by parental insurance plans. For working class families, there are programs (such as the Children's Health Insurance Plan, CHIP) that provide low-cost insurance for children up to their 19th birthday. For poor adolescents, there is Medicaid. However, there are many adolescents, although eligible, whose parents do not sign up for these programs and therefore remain uninsured – importantly, this means they continue to access services as if they are uninsurable. Furthermore, as children leave their parents' home, they often become uninsured or underinsured. Whilst many colleges provide health services to fully enrolled students, part-time students or students who sporadically attend have limited coverage.

In the United States, young adults are the most under-insured age group, falling in the gap between parental coverage augmented by programs designed to provide universal health insurance to children (Medicaid and CHIP) and the coverage supplied by a full-time secure job [8]. Lifetime uninsured rates for those who present for care peak for females between ages 15 and 17 years (29%) and for males between ages 18 and 21 years (24%) [9]. True uninsured rates are likely to be higher, as those who do not present for care may not do so because of lack of insurance [10]. Recent data found that 33% of males and 27% of females aged 18–24 years are uninsured at a given point in time [11]; another study found 31.4% uninsured for the entire previous year [12].

The hypothesis is that a lack of insurance decreases the therapeutic options for patients (access to second opinions, access to expensive treatments and medication, and choice of specialists). We know that for children under age 15 years with cancer, socioeconomic status appears to have little impact on registration with the Children's Cancer Group, suggesting that low socioeconomic status is not a barrier to access to cooperative group care and clinical trials. However, the reason the majority of 15- to 19-year-olds do not register with the pediatric oncology group is not related to socioeconomic factors, but to age [13].

There is evidence in the United States that there is a delay in the diagnosis of cancer in 15- to 30-year-olds who are under- or uninsured compared with those with private insurance [14]. A study of older adolescent and young adult patients receiving care at the University of Texas MD Anderson Cancer Center found that there was an average difference of 7 weeks in the time from first symptom to diagnosis between those with public insurance and those with private insurance, and on multivariate analysis this was more significant than any other variable (median household income, age, race, urban vs. rural location, etc.) except for tumor type [14].

Other strategic issues for adolescents include the logistics of getting to care. Although adolescents are moving developmentally toward independence from their parents, they rarely have their own stable means of transportation, limiting independent access to care. For example, a sexually active teenager notices a testicular mass. He takes the initiative to see his primary care physician, who orders an ultrasound to be done at the hospital across town. He is unwilling to ask his parents to drive him to the appointment because he is afraid that the mass has something to do with his sexual activity, of which they are not aware, so he does not attend for the planned scan.

In addition, the care that is accessible may not be the most appropriate care. Although there is not a shortage of oncologists in the United States, there are 2.4 medical oncologists for every 15- to 19-year-old cancer patient, but only 0.44 pediatric oncologists. These data were calculated from the number of medical oncologists and pediatric oncologists for 15- to 19-year-old cancer patients in the United States, determined from 2006 Cancer Statistics [15], and the American Board of Internal Medicine (http:\\www.abim.org/resources/dnum.shtm) and American Board of Pediatrics (http://www.abp.org/stats/WRKFRC/Hemo.ppt) board certification data. Furthermore, the pediatric oncologists are not evenly distributed geographically. Ironically, this means that whereas pediatric oncology patients are underserved because of their limited geographic access to care, it means that adolescents might be misserved, by the geographically available, but not necessarily appropriate care. This issue of geography then is complexly tied in with provider services and patient education and choice. The patient may not be aware that traveling further may result in more and perhaps "better" treatment options. Yet when 271 young adult cancer survivors age 14 to 23 years were asked in a United Kingdom survey, 63% reported they would be willing to travel half a day or more for their cancer treatment and 49% would go "any distance or time" to get their cancer care (personal communication, S. Davies, 2005).

4.2.2 Provider Issues

Adolescents and young adults, more than younger children, receive their routine medical care from a heterogeneous population of specialists, and, therefore, have many pathways via which they can access oncologic care. Several recent studies have quantified adolescents' use of health services in the United States [9, 16]. The choice of provider varies with age and gender, with increasing use of family practitioners, internists, and gynecologists and decreasing use of pediatricians as children age. Only 11% of adolescents over the age of 14 years see pediatricians. Regardless of health insurance status, adolescents and young adults are the most likely of any age group to lack a usual source of care [10]. Fifteen- to 24-year olds are the age group with the highest rates of use of the emergency room for any outpatient care: 18.5% of all of their medical visits and 12.6% of all non-injury-related visits are to the emergency room [17]. The lack of a primary physician may be a deterrent to a patient seeking timely attention for early symptoms of cancer, and a physician who is unaware of the patient's baseline medical status may contribute to a failure to recognize the signs of cancer. Clinical suspicion is low (since adolescents and young adults are not "supposed" to get cancer) and symptoms may, and frequently are, attributed to physical exertion, fatigue, and stress.

Although unstudied, the provider whom an adolescent and his/her family chooses to see if there is any suspicion of a malignancy may be different than that chosen for other, more common problems of adolescence. There may be more use of the emergency room and surgical specialists. One pediatric oncology program in Texas examined the difference in the referral source of children under 12 years compared with that of older adolescents (15 to 21 years of age) and found that 15 out of 18 children were referred by primary care doctors (pediatricians, and family practice and emergency room physicians), but that 15 out of 18 older adolescents were referred by adult surgeons or adult oncologists [18]. In a Canadian study of 15- to 19-year olds, 61% contacted a general practitioner with their cancer symptoms during the period 1995–2000. Only 3% saw a pediatrician, compared with 15% of children less than 15 years of age. Twenty-four percent of Canadian adolescents saw an emergency room physician, similar to the 30% of children [19]. It is a logical assumption (currently being studied in the United States) that the type of provider that an adolescent or young adult sees will influence the subsequent referral to oncologic care.

The referral to oncology services is driven largely by physician opinion and preference. A study of adolescent and young adult patients in Britain found that over half of patients had never been given a choice between treatment centers or providers. Although some of the referring decision is certainly based on the diagnostic category (e.g., Wilms tumor vs. cervical cancer), there may be other patient factors involved (age, sex, ethnicity, geographic distance from a pediatric tertiary care center, a patient's insurance status, and perceptions of patient's social situation, or physician characteristics including specialty, years in practice, and location of training). Diagnosis does appear to influence referral; in the Canadian study, 51% of adolescents with leukemia were treated at pediatric centers, but only 11% of those with carcinoma [19]. In the Utah study, 57% of leukemia patients and 11% of carcinoma patients were treated at a pediatric center, but less than 30% of adolescents with brain tumors and lymphoma [20]. In a study of Florida patterns of care, the tumors least likely to be seen at the pediatric centers were Hodgkin lymphoma, "other" tumors, and brain tumors [21]. Some pediatric hospitals have upper age cutoffs that prohibit admissions of older adolescents; in England, most pediatric hospitals do not accept those over age 16 years of age. Anecdotally, few patients are referred to pediatric oncologists after seeing a medical oncologist; a survey of medical oncologists on the subject had a poor response rate (29%) but concluded that medical oncologists believe that they appropriately treated adolescents as adults [22].

To whom should adolescents with cancer be referred for their oncologic care? With the current lack of definitive outcome data, this question remains unanswerable. To start with, it depends on the type and stage of cancer, and the age of the patient. For a patient with a completely resected brain tumor, it may only be a neurosurgeon. For a 19-year-old male with a metastatic malignant melanoma, it may be a medical oncologist.

A compelling reason to choose a site for treatment is because of a proven survival advantage. Such outcome studies are difficult to conduct, as patient numbers with individual tumor types in this age range are small. Several papers have shown a survival advantage to children with cancer treated at specialist pediatric oncology centers [23, 24]. A clinical trial of Ewing sarcoma patients in Germany showed a survival advantage to older adolescents treated at pediatric centers compared with nonpediatric centers, although all patients received the same protocol therapy [25]. Recent data showed a marked survival advantage to older adolescents with acute lymphoblastic leukemia treated on a pediatric oncology group clinical trial compared with those treated on an adult cooperative group clinical trial (cf. Chapter 5) [6, 16]. Data from the National Cancer Data Base indicated that American adolescents aged 15 to 19 years with non-Hodgkin lymphoma, leukemia, liver cancer, and bone tumors had a survival advantage if treated at a National Cancer Institute (NCI) pediatric group institution [26].

The location of treatment may matter the most with regard to how it affects access to and participation in clinical trials. In the United States, 55–65% of children are entered into clinical trials. In contrast, only about 10% of 15- to 19-year-olds with cancer are entered into a clinical trial [13, 27]. Among 20- to 29-year-olds, the participation rate is even lower, with fewer than 10% being seen at member institutions of the cooperative groups, either pediatric or adult, and only about 1% of 20- to 29-year-olds entering clinical trials. This is due largely to the diminishing rate of patients seen at institutions that participate in NCI-sponsored clinical trials. Among older patients, the trial participation rate is

higher, putatively between 3 and 5%, but still much lower than in children. Similarly, in Canada, the TOSS survey found that 21% of adolescents who were referred to pediatric oncology centers were enrolled on clinical trials, but none of those referred to adults centers were on trials [19].

Besides choosing a provider for survival advantage, the patient should choose a provider/center that is comfortable with and skilled in dealing with the psychosocial and developmental issues of the adolescent. Issues such as compliance, importance of a social calendar, different prioritization, and fertility preservation are issues that do not come up as often for younger or older patients, and some providers may not have the experience or communication skills to address them.

In the United States, two leadership bodies have stated that pediatric oncologists are the most appropriate providers for adolescent cancer patients, at least in consultation. A 1997 American Academy of Pediatrics consensus statement considered referral to a board-eligible or board-certified pediatric hematologist-oncologist and pediatric subspecialty consultants as the standard of care for all pediatric and adolescent cancer patients [28]. A wider consensus panel that included adult oncologists, the American Federation of Clinical Oncologic Societies, also concluded that "payors must provide ready access to pediatric oncologists, recognizing that childhood cancers are biologically distinct" and that the "likelihood of successful outcome in children is enhanced when treatment is provided by pediatric cancer specialists" [29]. However, neither of these statements defines an age cutoff for the recommendation. The numbers suggest that, as age increases, there is a steep fall off in observance with this recommendation. A cancer registry review in Utah, a state that has only one pediatric oncology treatment facility, showed that only 36% of oncology patients aged 15 to 19 years were ever seen at a pediatric hospital, compared with 85% of 10- to 14-year-olds and 98% of those younger than age 10 years [20]. A study of the National Cancer Data Base found that for nearly 20,000 cases of cancer in adolescents aged 15–19 years, only 34% were treated at centers that had NCI pediatric cooperative group affiliation [26]. In Canada, 30% of adolescents aged 15–19 years are treated at pediatric oncology centers; 47% of those aged 15–17 years, and 9.6% of those aged 18–19 years [19]. In the United Kingdom, only about 6% of adolescents and young adults 16–24 years of age are recorded on a national registry of all patients treated in the 22 United Kingdom Children's Cancer Study Group pediatric centers.

4.2.3 Personal Belief, Knowledge, Behavior

There are beliefs and behaviors of the adolescent that would impact on their access to oncology care. Adolescents have a strong sense of immortality and invincibility. Out of denial or embarrassment, they may delay seeing a physician for symptoms. Like providers, they rarely suspect cancer. Because no cancers in this age range are targets of screening or self-detection, adolescents are not being programmed to watch for any specific signs or symptoms of cancer. A Canadian study of the time from symptom onset to first healthcare contact showed older adolescents averaged 14 days compared with 9 days for those younger than 15 years [30] Even when seen, they may give a poor history, especially to a physician untrained to "read between the lines" of an adolescent's history. Under therapy, they may struggle to comply with prescribed treatment and appointments. A related issue is the adolescent's prioritization of social calendar over care. Developmentally, they value proximity to friends and social activities and may not be willing to give this up, even if a survival advantage is the trade-off. They also are not trained in self-advocacy, and their parents may not be advocates to the same degree as they would be for younger children. Rather than self-advocate, adolescents tend to "blend in" and not upset the status quo, or question authority. The impact of these patient factors is largely unstudied in adolescent and young adult oncology health services.

It is not known whether adolescents and young adults know they have a "choice" of care between pediatric and medical oncology, tertiary vs. local care, and clinical trial participation. If given a choice, adolescents themselves might choose an adult center over a pediatric center, thinking a pediatric center too juvenile. Finally, adolescents or young adults may impede themselves from getting optimal care because they feel pressure to remain in school or in the workplace (which can be less forgiving environments than for younger children in grade school or older adults in established careers).

4.3 Delay in Diagnosis

Logically, rapid diagnosis and initiation of therapy should identify cancer at early stages, translating into an improved survival rate. This has been proven when screening tests detect early cancers, but it is not clear that it is true for symptomatic cases. In fact, one study of the effect of rapid referral of suspected breast cancer in the United Kingdom found that those with shorter periods were associated with worse prognosis, while another study showed no good evidence that delays in diagnosing colorectal cancer have an impact on staging or health outcomes [31], although delays of 3–6 months in breast cancer patients are associated with reduced survival [32]. In two studies of bone tumors, shorter intervals between onset of symptoms and start of treatment did not improve survival [33, 34].

In younger patients, because of smaller numbers, it is hard to examine a correlation of lag time with survival (for specific diagnoses). In a small study in England, lag time indeed increased with the age of the child, but was not predictive of event-free survival [35]. In a study of the interval between symptom onset and diagnosis in 2,665 children participating in Pediatric Oncology Group therapeutic protocols in the period 1982–1988, Pollock found by multivariate analysis that, for all solid tumors except Hodgkin lymphoma, the lag time increased as age increased [36]. Likewise, the Canadian study found that the time from onset of symptoms to the start of therapy was significantly longer in adolescents of 15–19 years of age than in children (Figure 4.1). Among the adolescents, the delay to treatment was longer when they were treated in an adult center than at a pediatric center (92 vs. 57 days) [19]. The inverse relationship with age appears to be true for some unexpected carcinomas in young people: for both breast cancer and colon cancer, delays in diagnosis increase with age [37], meaning again that young adults may have deleterious delays in diagnosis.

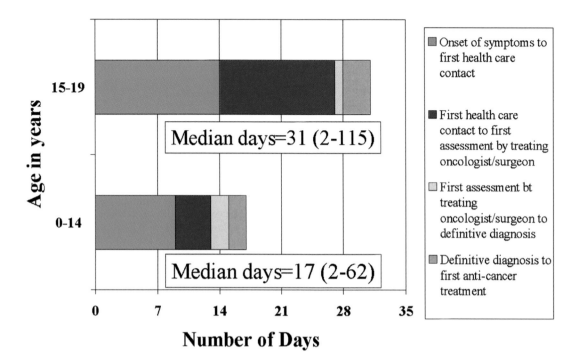

Figure 4.1

The Canadian Childhood Cancer Surveillance and Control Program: diagnosis and initial treatment of cancer in Canadian adolescents 15–19 years of age, 1995–2000 (Ottawa, Canada, 2000)

4.4 Summary

Recommending that adolescents and young adults be treated at pediatric hospitals or by pediatric oncologists has practical constraints. Many pediatric oncologists are uncomfortable caring for older adolescents and young adults. Adult oncologists are often unfamiliar and uncomfortable with the detailed pediatric protocols and older patients cannot be registered on pediatric cooperative trials because of built in upper age limits. Many of the pediatric protocols are written for young children and not for older adolescents. Pediatric hospitals cannot admit patients over a certain age.

The British have pioneered the solution of treating young adult and adolescent patients at a unique "adolescent oncology unit" (see Chap. 21) [38]. This provides the adolescent with age-specific nursing care, recreation therapy, and peer companionship. It is unknown whether this improves survival. One study showed that patient satisfaction was higher in teenage oncology patients treated in a dedicated teenage cancer unit than in adult or pediatric facilities. Several other centers internationally (in Canada, the United States, and Australia) are establishing clinics or programs that seek to establish local "best practice" for adolescents and young adults. Perhaps it is appropriate to have as a goal, centers and oncologists devoted solely to the care of this group of patients. In the meantime, increased cooperation and communication between pediatric and adult oncologists will facilitate the care of this group of patients.

The goal should not be to have all adolescents seen at pediatric cancer centers – the volume would likely overwhelm the system; however, adolescents with cancer should have access to equal services that provide the same outcomes (survival and quality of survival). To fully understand the issue of access we must more fully understand the outcomes. We should worry that only 30% of adolescents are seen at pediatric centers, if more studies clarify that this adversely affects outcomes. There may be patients (such as those with carcinoma) who are better served at adult institutions. The data needs to be looked at in more detail – by diagnosis, age, and treatment – before recommendations can be made.

Outcome studies must not stop at a binary analysis of which provides better survival (pediatric vs. medical oncology), but must characterize the variables that enable better survival (a certain treatment regimen, or level of supportive care or compliance) so that these can be provided equally to all patients.

References

1. Institute of Medicine (U.S.) Committee on Monitoring Access to Personal Health Care Services: Access to Health Care in America (1993). National Academy Press, Washington, DC

2. American Academy of Pediatrics (1972) Council on child health: age limits of pediatrics. Pediatrics 49:463

3. American Academy of Pediatrics: AAP Fact Sheet, http://www.aap.org/visit/facts.htm

4. Boissel N, Auclerc MF, Lheritier V, et al (2003) Should adolescents with acute lymphoblastic leukemia be treated as old children or young adults? Comparison of the French FRALLE-93 and LALA-94 trials. J Clin Oncol 21:774–780

5. de Bont JM, van der Holt B, Dekker AW, et al (2004) Significant difference in outcome for adolescents with acute lymphoblastic leukemia treated on pediatric versus adult ALL protocols in the Netherlands. Leukemia 18:2032–2053

6. Stock W, Sather H, Dodge RK (2000) Outcome of adolescents and young adults with ALL: a comparison of Children's Cancer Group (CCG) and Cancer and Leukemia Group B (CALGB) regimens. Blood 96:467a

7. Facione NC, Facione PA (1997) Equitable access to cancer services in the 21st century. Nurs Outlook 45:118–124

8. Collins SR, Schoen C, Kriss JL, et al (2006) Rite of passage? Why young adults become uninsured and how new policies can help. Issue Brief (Commonw Fund) 20:1–14

9. Ziv A, Boulet JR, Slap GB (1999) Utilization of physician offices by adolescents in the United States. Pediatrics 104:35–42

10. McCormick MC, Kass B, Elixhauser A, et al (2000) Annual report on access to and utilization of health care for children and youth in the United States – 1999. Pediatrics 105:219–230

11. Callahan ST, Cooper WO (2005) Uninsurance and health care access among young adults in the United States. Pediatrics 116:88–95

12. DeNavas-Walt C, Proctor BD, Lee CH (2005) Current Population Reports, P60–229: Income, Poverty, and Health Insurance Coverage in the United States: 2004, in U.S. Department of Commerce. Economics and Statistics Administration. U.S. CENSUS BUREAU (ed), U.S. Government Printing Office, Washington, DC, 2005. http://www.census.gov/prod/2005pubs/p60-229.pdf

13. Bleyer WA, Tejeda H, Murphy SB, et al (1997) National cancer clinical trials: children have equal access; adolescents do not. J Adolesc Health 21:366–373

14. Martin S, Ulrich C, Munsell M, Lange G, Taylor S, Bleyer A: Time to cancer diagnosis in young Americans depends on type of cancer and health insurance status. Value in Health 8 (1):344, 2005; The Oncologist (in press)

15. Jemal A, Siegel R, Ward E, et al (2006) Cancer statistics, 2006. CA Cancer J Clin 56:106–130

16. Ryan SA, Millstein SG, Greene B, Irwin CE Jr (1996) Utilization of ambulatory health services by urban adolescents. J Adolesc Health 18:192–202

17. Burt CW, Schappert SM (2004) Ambulatory care visits to physician offices, hospital outpatient departments, and emergency departments: United States, 1999–2000. National Center for Health Statistics. Vital Health Stat 13:1–70

18. Goldman S, Stafford C, Weinthal J, et al (2000) Older adolescents vary greatly from children in their route of referral to the pediatric oncologist and national trials. Proc Am Soc Clin Oncol 19: (abstr 1766)

19. Klein-Geltink J, Shaw AK, Morrison HI, et al (2005) Use of pediatric versus adult oncology treatment centres by adolescents 15–19 year old: the Canadian Childhood Cancer Surveillance and Control Program. Eur J Cancer 41:404–410

20. Albritton K, Wiggins CL (2001) Adolescents with cancer are not referred to Utah's pediatric center. Proc Am Soc Clin Oncol 19: (abstr 990)

21. Roush SW (1993) Socioeconomic and demographic factors that predict where children receive cancer care in Florida. J Clin Epidemiol 46:535–544

22. Brady AM, Harvey C (1993) The practice patterns of adult oncologists' care of pediatric oncology patients. Cancer 71:3237–3240

23. Stiller CA (1988) Centralisation of treatment and survival rates for cancer. Arch Dis Child 63:23–30

24. Kramer S, Meadows AT, Pastore G, et al (1984) Influence of place of treatment on diagnosis, treatment, and survival in three pediatric solid tumors. J Clin Oncol 2:917–923

25. Paulussen M, Ahrens S, Juergens HF (2003) Cure rates in Ewing tumor patients aged over 15 years are better in pediatric oncology units. Results of GPOH CESS/EICESS studies. Proc Am Soc Clin Oncol 22:(abstr 3279)

26. Rauck AM, Fremgen AM, Hutchison CL, et al (1999) Adolescent cancers in the United States: a national cancer database (NCDB) report. Abstract For The American Society Of Pediatric Hematology/Oncology Twelfth Annual Meeting. J Pediatr Hematol Oncol 21:310

27. Shochat SJ, Fremgen AM, Murphy SB, et al (2001) Childhood cancer: patterns of protocol participation in a national survey. CA Cancer J Clin 51:119–130

28. American Academy of Pediatrics (1997) Guidelines for the pediatric cancer center and role of such centers in diagnosis and treatment. American Academy of Pediatrics Section Statement Section on Hematology/Oncology. Pediatrics 99:139–141

29. American Federation of Clinical Oncologic Societies (1998) Consensus statement on access to quality cancer care. J Pediatr Hematol Oncol 20:279–281

30. Klein-Geltink J, Pogany L, Mery LS, et al (2006) Impact of age and diagnosis on waiting times between important healthcare events among children 0 to 19 years cared for in pediatric units: the Canadian Childhood Cancer Surveillance and Control Program. J Pediatr Hematol Oncol 28:433–439

31. Gonzalez-Hermoso F, Perez-Palma J, Marchena-Gomez J, et al (2004) Can early diagnosis of symptomatic colorectal cancer improve the prognosis? World J Surg 28:716–720

32. Richards MA, Westcombe AM, Love SB, et al (1999) Influence of delay on survival in patients with breast cancer: a systematic review. Lancet 353:1119–1126

33. Goyal S (2004) Symptom interval in young people with bone cancer. Eur J Cancer 40:2280–2286

34. Bacci G (1999) Delayed diagnosis and tumor stage in EWS. Oncol Rep 6:465–466

35. Saha V, Love S, Eden T, et al (1993) Determinants of symptom interval in childhood cancer. Arch Dis Child 68:771–774

36. Pollock BH, Krischer JP, Vietti TJ (1991) Interval between symptom onset and diagnosis of pediatric solid tumors. J Pediatr 119:725–732

37. Sainsbury R, Johnston C, Haward B (1999) Effect on survival of delays in referral of patients with breast cancer symptoms: a retrospective analysis. Lancet 353:1132–1135

38. Lewis IJ (1996) Cancer in adolescence. Br Med Bull 52:887–897

Older Adolescents and Young Adults with Cancer, and Clinical Trials: Lack of Participation and Progress in North America

Archie Bleyer • Troy Budd • Michael Montello

Contents

5.1 Introduction

Whereas the survival longevity benefits of a clinical trial to an individual may be debated [1], there is no question about the value of clinical trials to subsequent generations and to society in general. There is no benefit from the knowledge and experience gained from clinical trials if they are not conducted. In addition, clinical trials are required for new agents to receive federal approval, and for practices to become accepted as standards of care and, after publication, to be disseminated to community practices.

On the side of the personal benefit derived from participation in clinical trials, studies in children have indicated a survival advantage to children enrolled on clinical trials for acute lymphoblastic leukemia (ALL) [2], non-Hodgkin lymphoma [3], Wilms tumor [4], and medulloblastoma [5]. In the United States and Canada, a comparison of 16- to 21-year-olds with ALL or acute myeloblastic leukemia (AML) showed that the outcome was superior in patients treated on CCG trials than in those not entered [6]. Moreover, personal benefit from clinical trial participation may well accrue, especially with regard to quality of life during and after clinical trials.

One example of the benefit of adolescent and young adult participation in clinical trials comes from the recent retrospective comparisons of clinical trials in adolescent and young adult ALL patients. Prior population-based analyses suggest that increasing age was a poor prognostic factor in patients with ALL, but the reason for this correlation is unclear. Three independent groups – in France, the United States and The Netherlands – have extracted retrospectively the data on adolescent and young adult patients who enrolled on either a pediatric or adult clinical trial for ALL. Strikingly similar results were found in all cases: the pediatric regimen resulted in superior outcomes – nearly twice the event-free and overall survival rates – to the adult leukemia trials extant at the time [7–9]. Factors that might contribute to outcome (French-American-British, FAB, classification, presenting white count, cytogenetics) were collected prospectively on the clinical trials and essentially excluded as confounding reasons for decreased survival. Thus, treatment effect has been the favored explanation for the observed differences. In addition, the older adolescents and young adults who participated in the trials were given an opportunity for substantial personal benefit and not just altruism to help succeeding patients of similar age.

This chapter summarizes the evidence for low participation rates of older adolescents and young adults with cancer on clinical trials in the United States. Possible reasons for this are reviewed, and a correlation is described between the lack of clinical trial participation and the relatively worse improvement in survival in adolescent and young adult patients compared with younger and older persons. The overriding premise is that to increase our understanding of cancer in this population and improve outcomes, the rate of clinical trial enrollment of adolescent and young adult cancer patients must be enhanced.

5.2 Deficit in Adolescent and Young Adult Participation in Clinical Trials

As Fig. 5.1 implies, the participation rate of 15- to 19-year-olds in the United States on national cancer treatment trials sponsored by the National Cancer Institute (NCI) during the period 1997–2003 was approximately half that of the corresponding rate in those under 15 years old [10–14]. In 20- to 29-year-olds, it was approximately 15% of the rate in children under 15 years old. With the exception of the most elderly (over 85 years of age), 20- to 29-year-olds are the age group with the lowest clinical trial participation.

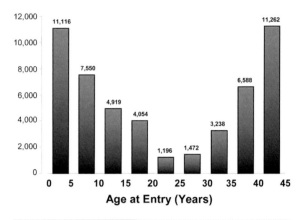

Figure 5.1

Entries of 51,395 patients <45 years of age onto United States National Cooperative Group treatment trials (sponsored by the Cancer Therapy Evaluation Program of the National Cancer Institute Division of Cancer Treatment and Diagnosis) during the period 1997–2003, inclusive. Modified from Bleyer [26]

5.2.1 Race/Ethnicity

A decrease in the participation of minority adolescent patients in clinical trials is not a reason for this deficit in participation, however. In fact, in the United States, minority children and adolescents with cancer show equal or higher rates of entry onto national clinical trials [14]. Figure 5.2 shows the race- and ethnicity-specific accrual for each 5-year age interval from 0 to 40 years of age [12]. The accrual pattern relative to age is similar among all racial and ethnic groups. Specifically, the rate of inclusion of older adolescent patients is lower for non-Hispanic whites, Hispanics, African Americans, Asians, native Indians, Alaskan natives, and Hawaiian and other Pacific Islanders than in the other age groups within their racial or ethnic group. In terms of absolute participation rates as a function of ethnic or racial group, the rate in Hispanic patients is less than one-fifth the rate in white patients, the rate in African-Americans is one-tenth the rate in white patients, and the rate in Asians, native Indians, and Alaskan natives is each about 1% of the rate in white patients (Fig. 5.2) [12]. This suggests that even though the overall nadir pattern is similar across the races and ethnicities evaluated, the relative knowledge gained may well be less in

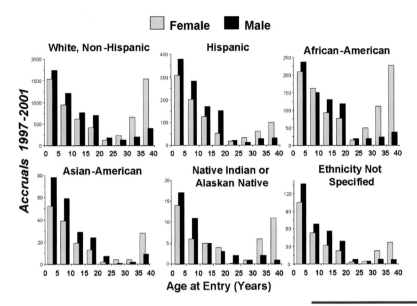

Figure 5.2

Accrual of patients <45 years of age to cooperative group treatment trials by race/ethnicity as a function of age at entry, during the period 1997–2001, inclusive. Modified from Bleyer [26]

the minority populations since there are fewer opportunities to learn about the racial and ethnic differences in the disease and its management.

5.2.2 Gender

The nadir in the clinical trial participation rate at 20–29 years of age is apparent in both females and males, but it is considerably more striking in males (Fig. 5.2). This is the case for all ethnic and racial groups specified above (data not shown).

5.2.3 Residence

Geographically, this gap has been observed throughout the United States and is in striking contrast to the accrual of a majority of patients under 15 years of age to clinical trials in virtually all metropolitan and rural areas across the country [14].

5.2.4 Individual Types of Cancer

Analysis of clinical trial participation broken down by individual types of cancer (i.e., sarcomas [15], leukemia [16], lymphoma [17], brain tumors [18, 19], and breast cancer) showed that participation was once again less in those aged 15 to 29 years than in those in younger or older age groups (Fig. 5.3).

5.3 Current Trends in Clinical Trial Participation by Older Adolescents and Young Adults with Cancer

Unfortunately, a downward trend in the accrual of patients 15–29 years of age onto United States National Cooperative Group treatment trials sponsored by the United States NCI was apparent from 1997 to 2003. The proportion of all patients entered onto the national phase I, II, and III treatment trials declined from 5.5 to 2.5% over this interval. This ominous trend may have been reversed in 2003 as a result, at least in part, of the Children's Oncology Group Initiative described below.

5.4 Reasons for the Lack of Clinical Trial Participation by Older Adolescents and Young Adults with Cancer

The reasons for the gap in the participation of older adolescents and young adults in clinical trials are to a large extent unknown and are undoubtedly multifactorial. The reasons that were identified at an NCI-sponsored workshop on the topic and further developed in subsequent evaluations [20, 21] are summarized in Table 5.1.

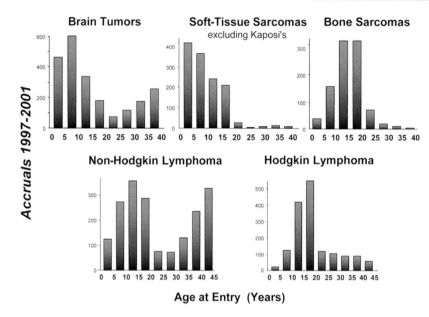

Figure 5.3

Accrual of patients <45 years of age to cooperative group treatment trials by cancer type as a function of age at entry, during the period 1997–2001, inclusive. Modified from Bleyer [26]

A patient between 15 and 29 years of age with newly diagnosed cancer is more likely to be thrust into a state of limbo – both medically and socially – than either a child or an older adult with cancer. Thus, it is no surprise that patients with cancer in this age group are less likely than either younger or older patients to find their way to a clinical trial that could improve their chances of a better outcome. They are less likely than younger patients to find their way to centers that offer clinical trials. Fewer patients in the 15- to 29-year age group are referred to dedicated, comprehensive cancer centers than patients in any other age group, with the possible exception of patients in the most elderly age group (>85 years) [12]. In particular, in the United States, more than 90% of children with cancer who are under 15 years of age are managed at institutions that participate in NCI-sponsored clinical trials. In contrast, only 20–35% of 15- to 19-year-olds with cancer are managed at such institutions [13, 14]. Among 20- to 29-year-olds, the inclusion rate is even lower, with fewer than 10% being treated at institutions that are members of cooperative groups, either pediatric or adult. In adult cancer patients over 40 years of age, the corresponding rate is approximately 20%, including community cancer centers that participate in NCI-sponsored clinical trials (community clinical oncology programs).

The American College of Surgeons (ACoS) has tracked 15- to 19-year-old patients in the ACoS Tumor Registries who were referred to centers that participated in Children's Cancer Group (CCG) or Pediatric Oncology Group (POG) trials. In their National Cancer Database report, those patients 15–19 years of age who were treated at CCG and POG sites with non-Hodgkin lymphoma, liver cancer, ALL, AML, osteosarcoma, or Ewing sarcoma had better 5-year survival rates than those treated elsewhere [22]. However, there were no differences in the 5-year rates for patients with two cancers associated with an excellent outcome, Hodgkin lymphoma and testicular carcinoma, or with brain tumors, one of the cancers associated with the worst prognosis.

Another reason for this deficit is a lack of treatment regimens and clinical trials for young patients. Between 1 and 70 years of age, the age group with the fewest therapeutic cancer trials available to it has been the 15- to 40-year age group (NCI Clinical Therapy Evaluation Program data).

Yet another reason for the deficit in the enrollment of adolescents and young adults with cancer onto clinical trials is that the spectrum of cancers in them differs from that of any other age group. Hence, there is no organized body of research that is dedicated to the spectrum of cancers that affect this age group.

Table 5.1 Potential barriers to participation of older adolescents and young adults in clinical trials

Potential barriers to participation of older adolescents and young adults in clinical trials

Continuity of Care and Philosophy

- Older adolescents and young adults have the lowest rate of primary care use of any age group.
- Adolescents and young adults are more likely than younger children to lack a usual source of care. Without a primary physician whom the patient knows, the patient may be reluctant to trust the medical establishment and the clinical trial enterprise.
- Physicians and other healthcare professionals are either poorly trained or unwilling to care for adolescents.
- Adolescents and young adults aren't "supposed to" have cancer. As a result, clinical suspicion is low, and symptoms are often attributed to physical exertion, fatigue, trauma, and stress.
- Adolescents and young adults have a strong sense of invincibility. Out of denial, they may delay seeing a physician about symptoms. Even when seen, they may give poor historical information, especially to a physician untrained to "read between the lines" of a young person's history.

Economic and Insurance-Based Factors

- In the United States, young adults are the most uninsured and most underinsured age group. Nearly half of all 15- to 19-year-olds lose the healthcare insurance provided by their parents and do not acquire adequate coverage at their next destination in life, whether at an institution of higher learning, through an employer, or by independent means.
- Treating physicians may be reluctant to promote the enrollment of adolescents or young adults onto clinical trials because of the time, cost, and effort involved, not only on their part (and that of their team), but also on the part of the patient and family.
- Health insurance organizations may deter the referral of adolescents and young adults to a cancer center or cooperative group or entry onto clinical trials. Attendees had little direct evidence of this factor, however.

Provider Bias

- Coping with older adolescents and young adults with cancer is difficult in general. The additional burden of clinical trial participation is therefore heavier for adolescents than for younger or older patients.
- Treating physicians may be reluctant to refer adolescent and young adult patients to clinical trials because they perceive these patients as likely to be noncompliant (or nonadherent) with the protocol requirements. These patients are perceived to have enough difficulty complying with the treatment plan and keeping up their lives, without the additional burden of protocol obligations.
- Oncologists (surgeons, radiotherapists, medical oncologists, gynecologists) in private practice may retain these patients rather than refer them to a tertiary-care facility or cooperative group member institution.
- Providers may be biased against clinical trials in adolescents and young adults. Reasons may include the historically better results of standard treatments in adolescents and young adults than in older and younger patients, and the additional effort of entering someone in the age group onto a clinical trial, including having to explain and obtain consent to study entry from both the patient and family.
- Family practitioners, gynecologists, and internists may not regard multimodality therapy as important in older adolescents and young adults as in younger and older patients. Reasons may include the greater use of single-modality therapy in patients in this age range, the additional burden of coordinating multidisciplinary care in the age group, and the historically better results obtained in this age group than in older patients.
- Providers may be unaware of opportunities for clinical trial participation for adolescents and young adults with cancer.

Table 5.1 (continued)

Potential barriers to participation of older adolescents and young adults in clinical trials

Patient/Family Preferences
— Adolescent and young adult patients and/or their parents are more inclined to refuse referral to a cooperative group member institution or to be entered onto a clinical trial.

Provider Age Policies
— The age policies of hospitals may prevent patient access to clinical trials that are under way at the institution. Children's hospitals may have upper age limits that deny the admission of older patients or deny clinical privileges to the treating physician. The reverse may be true for younger patients accessing clinical trials primarily intended for adult patients.
— The clinical trial itself may have age limits that prohibit the entry of an otherwise eligible patient.

Cooperative Group and Cancer Center Limitations
— Pediatric and adult cooperative groups and cancer centers may not allow the enrollment of adolescent and young adults onto clinical trials because of restrictive eligibility criteria.
— A clinical trial may not be available.
— Adult cooperative groups and cancer centers may lack treatment protocols for younger patients.
— Pediatric cooperative groups and hospitals may lack treatment protocols for older patients.
— Clinical trials for the types of cancer that predominate among adolescents and young adults may not be a priority of the cooperative group enterprise.

Adding to this problem is the fact that there is no discipline in medicine devoted to this group. Neither pediatric oncologists nor oncologists who care for adult patients are trained – certainly not optimally – for this set of diseases. Moreover, even those diseases that appear to be the same often have biologic differences. For example, adolescents have different forms of leukemia than either younger or older persons. In particular, the biologic characteristics (and prognosis) of ALL change dramatically in postpubertal patients. Different biologies, likely to respond differently to therapeutics, might best be studied in dedicated and separate clinical trials.

5.5 Survival and Mortality Rates in Adolescents and Young Adults with Cancer

Cancer mortality and survival trends in the United States in 15- to 29-year-olds are behind the gains made in younger and older persons [10–12]. This is particularly true for 20- to 29-year-olds, but it is also apparent for 15- to 19-year-olds [13].

5.5.1 Survival Improvement: From Peak to Nadir

The annual improvement in the 5-year survival rate from 1975 to 1997 averaged 1.5% per year in children under 15 years of age and 1.7% per year in adults 50–85 years of age (Fig. 5.4) [23]. In 15- to 24-year-olds, however, the improvement averaged 0.75% per year, and in 25- to 34-year-olds, there was no perceptible improvement (Fig. 5.4). In the mid 1970s, when national cancer survival rates became available, the 5-year cancer survival rate for Americans was higher in the 15- to 29-year age group than it was in younger or older persons. If the trend of 1975–1997 is projected to 2005, the 5-year survival rate is now lower in the young adult age group than it is in younger and older persons. In a quarter of a century, what was an advantage to be diagnosed with cancer during early adulthood has become a relative disadvantage. To compound matters, the affected population has steadily increased as the "baby boomers" traverse this age range.

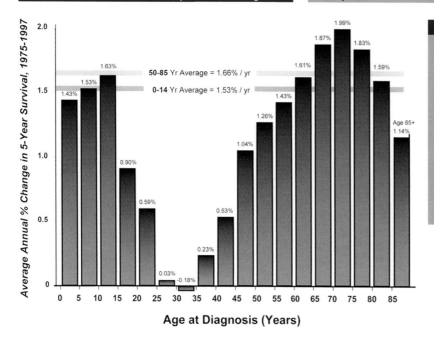

Age at Diagnosis (Years)

Figure 5.4

Average annual percent change in the 5-year survival rate of patients with invasive cancer who were in the United States Surveillance, Epidemiology and End Results (SEER) registry from 1997 to 2001. Data from the National Cancer Institute SEER program, courtesy of Lynn Ries [26]

5.5.2 Survival by Gender and Ethnicity/Race

These ominous trends in survival prolongation among 15- to 29-year-olds are apparent in both males and females, with males showing a greater deficit than females (Fig. 5.5).

5.5.3 Survival by Individual Types of Cancer

These trends have also held true for individual types of cancer, including sarcomas [8], brain tumors (astrocytomas, ependymomas, and other gliomas) [11], leukemia [9], lymphomas [10], and breast cancer. Although 15- to 29- year-olds with leukemia did not have a nadir in outcome improvement, they did have a worse mortality rate relative to their incidence than that of any other age group [9].

5.5.4 Correlation of Survival Improvement and Mortality Reduction

The age-dependent trends in survival improvement are reflected in the age-related trend of reduction in the national cancer mortality rates (Fig. 5.6). For cancer patients younger than age 40 years, the nadirs are

25–29 years and 30–34 years, respectively, with the nadir for mortality reduction expected to be at an older age than that for incidence, since the effect on death would occur later than the effect on survival before death. This correlation also validates the SEER measurements based on a sample of approximately 13% of the United States, whereas the mortality data are for all deaths in the country.

5.6 Why the Lack of Progress in Older Adolescents and Young Adults with Cancer?

Absolute differences in survival between younger patients and adolescent and young adult patients are probably due to a combination of biologic and therapeutic differences, some immutable. However, the marked disparity in survival improvement over time suggests mutable changes disproportionably rendered.

Proposed explanations apply to the patient, healthcare profession, family/community, and society/culture in general [24]. The patient category can be subdivided further into biologic/physical, psychologic/emotional

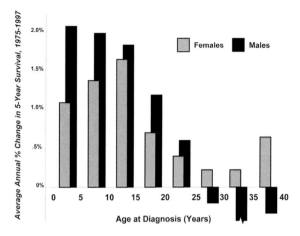

Figure 5.5

Comparison in males and females with invasive cancer of average annual percent change from 1975 to 1997 in the 5-year survival rate (United States SEER program). Modified from Bleyer [26]

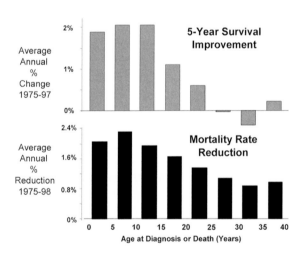

Figure 5.6

Correlation of national cancer mortality rate reduction in the United States as a function of age at death, with the rate of improvement in survival duration as a function of age at diagnosis (data from the United States Census Bureau and United States SEER program)

spiritual, economic/financial, and social factors. Biologic factors include the unique physiologic and pharmacologic characteristics of adolescent and young adult patients and their cancers. The health-care profession explanation includes a lack of awareness by general healthcare providers and of training, knowledge, and experience by oncology specialists. There is no other age during which the time to diagnosis is longer, fewer tumor specimens are available for translational research, or clinical trial participation is lower [11]. The family/community category involves family members and knowledge workers who lack awareness of the problem. Societal issues consist of the challenges societies face in providing for adolescent and young adult healthcare needs. Institutions of higher learning do not have cancer awareness as an essential educational or health evaluation component.

The issue of clinical trial participation seems paramount, since failure to investigate a disease in an age group in which it is prevalent or different is likely to limit the progress that can be made in that group. "No research, no gain" is the explanation. In the United States, the pace of improvement in the 5-year survival rates from sarcoma over the past quarter century has been far less above age 15 years than in younger patients, and this age-dependent pattern is statistically correlated with the rate of clinical trial activity [8]. A report from Australia documented a sharp fall-off in bone sarcoma patients entered onto clinical trials above age 15 years, in association with a drop in survival rate [25].

Although the correlation of outcome improvement with clinical trial participation is not proof of a cause-and-effect relationship, there are reasons to believe that failure to study cancer therapies in specific age subgroups does explain, at least in part, why progress in the age group has fallen behind that achieved in other age groups that have had higher rates of clinical trial participation. The correlation of outcome improvement with clinical trial participation underscores the value of clinical trials in cancer research.

The above considerations suggest several solutions:

1. Societal/cultural: improve awareness of the adolescent and young adult cancer problem.

2. Family/community: improve awareness and health-care insurance to reduce delays in diagnosis and permit participation in clinical trials.
3. Professional: increase awareness and training, and the availability, importance and utilization of clinical trials [15].
4. Personal/patient: overcome invincibility ideation and emphasize importance of health-care and health-care insurance. Another conceptual approach to overcoming the barriers to clinical trial participation faced by adolescent and young adult patients is provided in Table 5.1.

Reversing the trend and allowing older adolescents and young adults to catch up with the progress made in younger and older patients will require a comprehensive effort by multiple organizations, including the federal government, the insurance industry, service groups, the clinical trials cooperative groups, the pediatric academic societies, community agencies, and health-care providers. A multipronged approach to problem solving will be required, beginning with public and professional awareness initiatives such as this report.

In 2000, the Adolescent and Young Adult Initiative of the Children's Oncology Group and the NCI was established as a means to increase the enrollment of adolescents and young adults in cancer clinical trials. This initiative aims to bring advances in cancer education, prevention, and treatment – including educational, social, and emotional development – to this segment of the North American population, and to member sites in Australia, New Zealand, and Europe, whose progress in cancer outcome has fallen behind that achieved in younger and older patients.

The initiative includes several strategies. In all of the pediatric group protocols for malignancies that substantively overlap young adult patients, such as leukemia, Hodgkin lymphoma and the sarcomas, the upper age limit has been raised to 30, 40, or 50 years, depending on the disease. The pediatric group has also opened adult cooperative group trials in melanoma. Reciprocally, an adult cooperative group has opened the pediatric cooperative group trial in Ewing sarcoma. Plans are underway for the pediatric and adult groups to develop and open trials together in other sarcomas.

Other targets for mutual development include ALL, Hodgkin lymphoma, non-Hodgkin lymphoma, and hepatic cancer.

5.7 Summary

Cancer in adolescents and young adults has unique features; this is in addition to the special medical, physical, psychological, and social needs of patients in this age group. The spectrum of malignant diseases in this age group is also different from that in other age groups, and it is strikingly different from that in older persons. At the same time, more young people between 15 and 25 years of age have been diagnosed with cancer than children under 15 years of age, and during the past 25 years, the incidence of cancer in 15- to 29-year-olds has increased faster, and the reduction in cancer mortality has been lower than that in younger or older patients. Whereas it was once a relative advantage to have cancer during the adolescent and young adult years, patients in this age group are now behind patients in other age groups – orphaned in the world of cancer care delivery.

In the United States, older adolescents and young adults with cancer are underrepresented on clinical trials of therapies that could improve their outcome. This pattern is true for both males and females of all ethnic and racial groups. Simultaneously, the survival and mortality rates in these patients have mirrored the clinical trial accrual pattern, with little improvement compared with younger and older patients. This suggests that the relative lack of participation of adolescent and young adult patients in clinical trials has lessened their chances for as good an outcome as those enjoyed by patients in other age groups. The implication is that future progress in the treatment of the cancers among 15- to 29-year-olds will depend largely on increasing their participation in clinical trials. Regardless of whether there is a causal relationship, the impact of low clinical trial activity on furthering our scientific knowledge and management of cancer during adolescence and early adulthood is detrimental.

Thus, the increased availability of and participation in clinical trials is of paramount importance if the current deficits in outcome in young adults and older adolescents are to be eliminated. Eliminating the survival deficit will require a broad initiative to increase clinical trial participation. Ultimately, a new discipline is probably in order to meet the needs of these young patients: adolescent and young adult oncology. These patients deserve trained care providers, specialized clinics and inpatient units, and probably most importantly, dedicated research strategies that are not available through either pediatric or adult care programs.

References

1. Peppercorn JM, Weeks JC, Cook EF, Joffe S (2004) Comparison of outcomes in cancer patients treated within and outside clinical trials: conceptual framework and structured review. Lancet 363:263–270
2. Meadows AT, Kramer S, Hopson R, et al (1983) Survival in childhood acute lymphocytic leukemia. Effect of protocol and place of treatment. Cancer Invest 1:49–55
3. Wagner HP, Dingeldein-Bettler I, Berchthold W, et al for the Swiss Pediatric Oncology Group (SPOG) (1995) Childhood NHL in Switzerland: incidence and survival in 120 study and 42 non-study patients. Med Pediatr Oncol 24:281–286
4. Lennox EL, Stiller CA, Morris-Jones PH, Wilson-Kinnier LM (1979) Nephroblastoma: treatment during 1970–3 and the effect on survival of inclusion in the first MRC trial. BMJ 2:567–569
5. Duffner K, Cohen ME, Flannery JT (1982) Referral patterns of childhood brain tumors in the state of Connecticut. Cancer 50:1636–1640
6. Nachman J, Sather HN, Buckley JD, et al (1993) Young adults 16–21 years of age at diagnosis entered onto Children's Cancer Group acute lymphoblastic leukemia and acute myeloblastic leukemia protocols. Results of treatment. Cancer 71:3377–3385
7. Boissel N, Auclerc MF, Lheritier V, et al (2003) Should adolescents (15–20y) with ALL be treated as old children or young adults? Comparison of the French FRALLE-93 and LALA-94 trials. J Clin Oncol 2:774–780
8. de Bont JM, B. van der Holt B, Dekker AW, et al (2004) Significant difference in outcome for adolescents with acute lymphoblastic leukemia treated on pediatric versus adult ALL protocols in the Netherlands. Leukemia 18:2032–2053
9. Stock W, Sather H, Dodge RK, Bloomfield CD, Larson A, Nachman J (2000) Outcome of adolescents and young adults with ALL:A comparison of Children's Cancer Group (CCG) and Cancer and Leukemia Group B (CALGB) regimens (abstracts). Blood 96:467a
10. Albritton K, Bleyer A (2003) The management of cancer in the older adolescent. Eur J Cancer 39:2548–2599
11. Bleyer A, Budd T, Montello M (2005) Lack of clinical trial participation and of progress in older adolescents and young adults with cancer. Curr Probl Pediatr Adolesc Health Care 35:186–195
12. Bleyer A, Budd T, Montello M (2002) Cancer in older adolescents and young adults. A new frontier. POGO News 9:8–11
13. Bleyer WA (1996) The adolescent gap in cancer treatment. J Registry Manage 23:114–115
14. Bleyer WA, Tejeda H, Murphy SM, et al (1997) National cancer clinical trials: children have equal access; adolescents do not. J Adolesc Health 21:366–373
15. Bleyer A, Montello M, Budd T, Saxman S (2003) Young adults with sarcoma: lack of clinical trial participation and lack of survival prolongation. Proc Am Soc Clin Oncol 21:816
16. Bleyer A, Montello M, Budd T (2004) Young adults with leukemia in the U.S. Lack of clinical trial participation and mortality reduction during the last decade. Proc Am Soc Clin Oncol 22:586
17. Bleyer A, Ries L, Montello M, Budd T (2003) Non-Hodgkin lymphoma: U.S. incidence, outcome and clinical trial participation from birth to age 45. First International Conference on Pediatric Non-Hodgkin Lymphoma, April 10–12, 2003, New York City
18. Bleyer A, Hag-Alshiekh M, Montello M, et al (2004) Older adolescents and young adults with brain tumors in the United States. Lack of clinical trial participation and of survival prolongation and mortality reduction. Proc Intl Symp Pediatr Neurooncol p 52
19. Bleyer A, Montello M, Budd T, Ries L (2003) CNS tumor epidemiology and outcome in the young, 2000–2009. Ten predictions for/from the United States. Neurooncology 5:29 (www.asco.org/ac/1,1003,_12-002489-00_18-002003-00_19-00104011,00.asp)
20. Bleyer A (2002) Older adolescents with cancer in North America. Deficits in outcome and research. Pediatr Clin North Am 49:1027–1042
21. Bleyer A, Albritton K (2003) Special considerations for the young adult and adolescent. In: Kufe DW, Pollock RE, Weichselbaum RR, Bast RC, Holland JF, Frei E (eds) Holland-Frei: Cancer Medicine (6th edition). Decker, Hamilton, Ontario, Canada, pp. 2414–2422
22. Rauck, AM, Fremgen AM, Hutchison CL, et al (1999) Adolescent cancers in the United States: a national cancer data base (NCDB) report. J Pediatr Hematol Oncol 21:310
23. Birch JM (2005) Patterns of cancer incidence in teenagers and young adults: implications for aetiology. In: Eden T, Barr R, Bleyer A, Whiteson M (eds) Cancer and the Adolescent. Blackwell, Malden, Mass, pp 13–31
24. Bleyer A (2005) Cancer in older adolescents and young adults: reasons for lack of progress. Pediatr Blood Cancer 45:376

25. Mitchell AE, Scarcella DL, Rigutto GL, et al (2004) Cancer in adolescents and young adults: treatment and outcome in Victoria. Med J Aust 180:59–62

26. Bleyer A (2005) Lack of participation of young people with cancer in clinical trials: impact on the U.S. In: Eden T, Barr R, Bleyer A, Whiteson M (eds) Cancer and the Adolescent. Blackwell, Malden, Mass, pp 35–42

Acute Lymphoblastic Leukemia

James Nachman • Giuseppe Masera •
W. Archie Bleyer

Contents

6.1 Introduction

Acute lymphoblastic leukemia (ALL) represents approximately 2% of the cancers that occured in 15- to 29-year-olds in the United States during the period 1975–2000 [1]. Their dramatically lower survival rate than in children with ALL, and the recent demonstration that pediatric treatment approaches have been substantively more effective than those used by adult oncologists [2–7], lend emphasis to inclusion of this disease in this textbook of cancer during adolescence and young adulthood.

6.2 Classification System and Methods

In the International Classification of Childhood Cancer (ICCC) (see Chap. 1), ALL is a subgroup of category I(a), lymphoid leukemia. ICCC has two subcategories of lymphoid leukemia, ALL, and non-ALL lymphoid leukemia. ICCC I(b) is labeled "acute leukemia", even though the ALLs are in category I(a). ALL is specified by the ICCC to correspond to the International Classification of Disease – Oncology (ICD-O), Version 3 in Morphology Categories 9828-9837.

Incidence and survival in this chapter are presented for 15- to 29-year-olds, with comparisons to the age groups 0–15 years and 30–44+ years, as appropriate. For some analyses the entire age range from birth to 85+ years is included. The absence of data in any figure or table within this chapter means that too few cases were available for analysis; it does not mean that the rate or change in rate was zero.

6.3 Incidence

6.3.1 Age-Specific Incidence

Figure 6.1 illustrates the strong dependence of ALL incidence on age, with incidence peaks at the ends of the age spectrum and a nadir between 35 and 40 years of age, which is lower than in any other younger or older age group except infants younger than 1 year of age. Table 6.1 lists, for 5-year age intervals less than 40 years of age, the incidence and incidence trends during 1975–2000, and estimates the number of patients with ALL in the United States in the year 2000.

The incidence of ALL as a percentage of all cancers was inversely proportional to age, reflecting the rise in incidence of other cancers beginning at 10 years of age. Within 5-year age groups there was a decrease in incidence in ALL relative to all cancer from 5.8% in 15- to 19-year-olds to 2.0% and 0.3% in 20- to 24-year-olds and 25- to 29-year-olds, respectively. For 15- to 29-year-olds as a group, ALL represented only 2.1% of all cancers.

Figure 6.2 shows the age-dependent incidence of ALL relative to other types of leukemia. ALL decreased in incidence across all age groups, while acute myeloblastic leukemia (AML) and chronic myelogenous leukemia increased in incidence beyond age 5 years. ALL was the most common type in the 15- to 19-year group, occurring at an annual rate of 11.5 per million, twice that of AML. However, over the subsequent two 5-year age groups, ALL and AML incidence curves crossed:

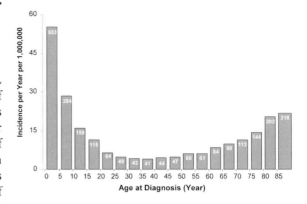

Figure 6.1

Incidence of acute lymphoblastic leukemia (ALL) as a function of age, United States Surveillance, Epidemiology, and End Results (United States SEER) registry, 1975–2000

they were approximately equal in the 20- to 24-year age group, at about 6.6 per million; in the 25- to 29-year age group AML occurred at a rate of 7.5 per million, compared with a rate of 4.9 per million for ALL.

6.3.2 Gender-Specific Incidence

ALL occurred with greater frequency in males of all ages, as shown in Fig. 6.3, with the male predominance greatest in 15- to 29-year-olds at ratios varying from 1.9 to 2.1.

Table 6.1 Incidence, incidence trends and number of patients with acute lymphoblastic leukemia (ALL) in persons younger than 30 years of age, United States (U.S.), 1975–2000

Age at diagnosis (years)	<5	5–9	10–14	15–19	20–24	25–29
U.S. population, year 2000 census (in millions)	19.18	20.55	20.53	20.22	18.96	19.38
ALL						
Average annual incidence per million, 1975–2000, SEER	55.3	28.4	15.9	11.5	6.4	4.9
Average annual % change in incidence, 1975–2000, SEER	0.9%	3.3%	3.8%	2.8%	71.1%	17.6%
Estimated incidence of ALL per million, year 2000, U.S.	60.6	32.8	18.3	12.4	8.5	6.2
Estimated number of persons diagnosed, year 2000, U.S.	1.060	584	375	251	162	120

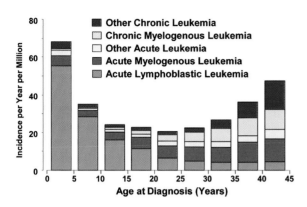

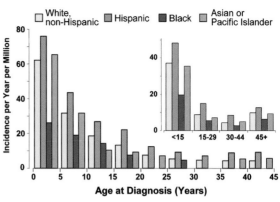

Figure 6.2

Incidence of leukemia by type, age 0–45 years, United States SEER registry, 1975–2000

Figure 6.4

Incidence of ALL by race/ethnicity, United States SEER registry, 1992–2000

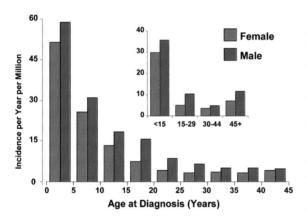

Figure 6.3

Incidence of ALL by gender, United States SEER registry, 1975–1999

6.3.3 Racial/Ethnic Differences in Incidence

The incidence of ALL varied substantively with race/ethnicity (Fig. 6.4). Hispanics experienced the highest rate of ALL at all ages. Among 15- to 29-year-olds, the rate was 14.9 per year per million population, 1.7-fold higher than for non-Hispanic whites, 2.8-fold greater that for African Americans/blacks, and 2.1 times increased over that for Asians/Pacific Islanders. The incidence is lowest in African Americans/blacks in all

age groups. Compared to <15 year-olds, however, in whom the relative absence of ALL among African Americans/blacks was first observed, the disparity among 15- to 29-year olds is not as dramatic (Fig. 6.4 inset).

6.3.4 Incidence Trends

During the period 1975–2000, the incidence of ALL increased significantly among those diagnosed before 30 years of age and after 45 years of age (Fig. 6.5). Among 15- to 29-year-olds, most of the increase was in males, who had the greatest increase in this age group compared with all other ages. Most of the increase in ALL incidence occurred in the 1970s and 1980s. Since 1990, the rates in persons less than 30 years of age have essentially stabilized. In the year 2000, approximately 530 persons 15- to 29-years of age were diagnosed as having ALL (Table 6.1).

6.4 Risk Factors

Numerous risk factors have been investigated as to their potential association with the development of leukemia in children and adolescents, although little is known about such factors for older adolescents and young adults. These have been summarized recently

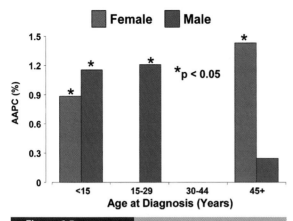

Figure 6.5

Average annual percentage change (AAPC) in the incidence of ALL by gender, United States SEER registry, 1975–2000

into categories based on the degree of certainty of the association, and include demographic, environmental, genetic, and exposure-related factors (Table 6.2). Age, gender, race/ethnicity, socioeconomic status, genetic syndromes, and radiation exposure (in utero and/or therapeutic) are known risk factors for leukemias in younger age groups [8].

Genetic syndromes have been reported in an estimated 2.6% of British children diagnosed with leukemia; 90% of these attributable to Down syndrome (DS, constitutional trisomy 21) [9]. Whereas the pathogenic basis for the 10- to 20-fold increased risk of ALL in individuals with DS has not been elucidated, somatic mutations of the *GATA1* gene are seen in virtually all cases of DS-associated AML and may be implicated in the development of megakaryoblastic AML seen in these patients [10, 11]. Such mutations may also confer enhanced leukemic sensitivity to cytarabine via dysregulation of cytidine deaminase gene expression [12].

Among individuals with neurofibromatosis type 1, homozygous mutations in the neurofibromin tumor-suppressor gene are associated with myeloid leukemias [13]. Characteristic to the chromosome breakage syndromes is DNA instability resulting in aberrant pathways of DNA repair. Mutations associated with leukemic and lymphomatous malignancy have been identified in genes associated with ataxia-telangiecta-

sia, Fanconi anemia (FANC family), and Bloom syndrome [14, 15]. Causative factors in the development of leukemias in those with congenital neutropenia (Kostmann agranulocytosis, Shwachman syndrome) have not been identified. The autosomal dominant form of severe congenital neutropenia is associated with heterozygous mutations in the neutrophil elastase gene (*ELA2*) and consequent alterations in the serine protease neutrophil elastase. Proteolytic regulation of hematopoiesis may be affected [16].

In 1988, Greaves attempted to correlate patterns of infection during infancy with the development of B-precursor ALL in early childhood [17]. Specifically, he hypothesized that exposure to infection during the first year of life purportedly results in immunologic naiveté, a biologically abnormal response to later infection and, rarely, leukemic transformation of a susceptible clone [18, 19]. Support for the hypothesis has been derived mainly from proxy measures of delayed infectious exposure during infancy, including higher socioeconomic status (improved hygiene), social isolation (avoidance of daycare), breast feeding (passive immunity), and birth order (higher rank equated with reduced exposure) [20, 21]. Studies assessing the history of infections during infancy have drawn conflicting conclusions [21, 22].

6.5 Clinical Presentations and Molecular Biology

Data from the Children's Cancer Group (CCG) ALL 1900 studies (conducted during the 1990s) illustrate the differences in molecular biology of ALL between children, young adolescents and older adolescents. Table 6.3 shows the presenting features for patients with B-precursor ALL entered on the CCG 1900 series ALL trials. Older patients had a significantly higher incidence of CALLA common ALL antigen negativity, and significantly higher hemoglobin levels compared to younger patients. Older patients had a significantly lower incidence of lymphomatous features (enlarged liver, spleen, and/or lymph nodes) compared to younger patients. There was no difference in presenting white blood cell count (WBC) for older and younger patients.

Table 6.2 Investigated risk factors for ALL (modified from Bahtia et al. [8])

Degree of Certainty	ALL
Generally accepted risk factors	Males
	Age (2–5 years)
	High socioeconomic status
	Race (whites>blacks)
	In utero x-ray exposure
	Postnatal radiation (therapeutic)
	Down syndrome
	Neurofibromatosis type 1
	Bloom syndrome
	Schwachman syndrome
	Ataxia-telangiectasia
Suggestive of increased risk	Increased birth weight
	Maternal history of fetal loss
Limited evidence	Parental smoking prior to or during pregnancy
	Parental occupational exposures
	Postnatal infections
	Diet
	Vitamin K prophylaxis in newborns
	Maternal alcohol consumption during pregnancy
	Electric and magnetic fields
	Postnatal use of chloramphenicol
Probably not associated	Ultrasound
	Indoor radon

For T-cell ALL, the incidence relative to all ALL was 12.8% in the 1- to 9-year age group, 16.9% in the 10- to 15-year group and 24.7% in the 16- to 21- year age group ($p = 0.0005$; Table 6.4). As for patients with B-lineage ALL, older patients with T-lineage ALL had significantly higher hemoglobin levels and a significantly lower incidence of hepatomegaly and splenomegaly compared to younger patients.

Data from the United Kingdom Medical Research Council showed a higher incidence of Philadelphia-chromosome-positive ALL with increasing age [23].

The Philadelphia chromosome was seen in 1.3% of patients aged 1–9 years, 3.4% of patients aged 10–19 years, and 12.2% of patients aged 20–24 years. On the CCG 1961 trial, 7.5% of patients aged 16–21 years of age with evaluable cytogenetics demonstrated a Philadelphia chromosome [2]. Patients ≥ 10 years of age with B-precursor ALL have a significantly lower rate of the t (12:21) translocation and a lower incidence of high hyperdiploidy compared to younger patients [23, 24]. This may in part be responsible for the worse outcome seen in older patients with ALL.

Table 6.3 Incidence of presenting features in B-lineage ALL by age. WBC White blood cell count, CALLA common ALL antigen

	Age (years)			p value
	1–9	10–15	16+	
WBC > 50 x 10^9/ L	67.7%	67.7%	65.8%	0.50
CALLA Negative	4.2%	8.4%	8.4%	0.0001
Normal liver	46.3%	60.1%	69.4%	0.0000
Normal spleen	49%	54.2%	58.8%	0.05
Normal nodes	48.5%	56.3%	61.7%	0.0007
Hemoglobin > 110 g/ L	8.2%	22.4%	27.3%	0.0000

Table 6.4 Incidence of presenting features in T-Lineage ALL by age

	Age (years)			p value
	1–9	10–15	16+	
WBC > 50 x 10^9/ L	62.4%	50.3%	60%	0.3
CALLA Negative	69.1%	75%	73.8%	0.38
Normal liver	37.3%	48.8%	48.5%	0.06
Normal spleen	29.4%	44.5%	40.0%	0.002
Normal nodes	24.4%	33.7%	31.1%	0.13
Hemoglobin > 110 g/ L	31.1%	51.0%	60.5%	0.0003

Drug sensitivity testing revealed that leukemic cells from older patients demonstrate an increased in vitro drug resistance to prednisone (PDN) and daunomycin (DNR) [25]. Also, ALL in older adolescents may have a different pattern of promoter methylation compared to younger patients [26].

There appears to be no significant difference in presenting features for patients aged 10–15 years and those aged 16–21 years, with the exception that, in the CCG 1961 trial, the percentage of Hispanic patients decreased and the percentage of African American patients increased in the 16- to 21-year age group compared to the 10- to 15-year age group.

6.6 Treatment

Current pediatric protocols are generally based on a model developed by Dr. Riehm for the BFM (Berlin-Frankfurt-Munster) study group. Therapy consists of induction/consolidation, interim maintenance, reinduction/reconsolidation (often referred to as *delayed intensification*), and maintenance phases. Pediatric protocols are characterized by the dose-intensive use of nonmyelosuppressive drugs such as vincristine (VCR), L-asparaginase (L-ASP), corticosteroids; and continuous antimetabolite-based maintenance. CCG-modified BFM therapy is shown in Table 6.5. A four-drug induction including VCR, PDN, L-ASP, and DNR is followed by an intensive consolidation phase including cyclophosphamide (CPM), cytosine arabinoside

(ARA-C), and 6-mercaptopurine (6-MP), and intensive intrathecal methotrexate (MTX) with or without cranial radiation.

Interim maintenance consists of high-dose methotrexate with rescue and 6-MP or intravenous (i.v.) VCR, i.v. MTX without rescue, and intramuscular L-ASP. Following interim maintenance, patients receive a delayed reinduction-reconsolidation phase (European – *protocol II*; American – *delayed intensification*) in which dexamethasone (DXM) replaces PDN, doxo-

rubicin (Dox) replaces DNR, and 6-thioguanine (6-TG) replaces 6-MP. Patients then receive maintenance therapy consisting of daily oral 6-MP and weekly oral MTX with or without VCR, PDN pulses and intrathecal MTX.

On the other hand, most adult protocols incorporate blocks of high-dose intermittent myelosuppressive chemotherapy including anthracyclines, CPM, etoposide (VP-16), and high doses of ARA-C and MTX [27, 28]. Few adult protocols incorporate a

Table 6.5 Children's Cancer Group (CCG)-modified Berlin-Frankfurt-Munster (BFM) therapy (CM-BFM). *PDN* Prednisone, *VCR* vincristine, *DNR* daunomycin, *l-ASP* l-asparaginase, *MTX* methotrexate, *IT ARA-C* intrathecal cytosine arabinoside, *IT MTX* intrathecal MTX, *CPM* cyclophosphamide, *6-MP* 6-mercaptopurine, *RT* radiation therapy, *DEX* dexamethasone, *DOX* doxorubicin, *6-TG* 6-thioguanine, *CNS* central nervous system, *p.o.* Per os, *bid* twice daily, *tid* three times daily, subg. subcutaneous *i.m.* intramuscular, *i.v.* intravenous, *qd* daily, gw weekly

Induction	PDN	60 mg/m² p.o. days 1–28 (bid or tid) then taper
	VCR	1.5 mg/m² i.v. days 1, 8, 15 and 22
	DNR	25 mg/m² i.v. days 1, 8, 15 and 22
	l-ASP	6000 U/m² i.m. 3 times per week × 3 weeks beginning day 3
	IT ARA-C	day 1 (age adjusted dosing)
	IT MTX	day 8 (age adjusted dosing)
Consolidation	PDN	Taper
	CPM	1000 mg/m² i.v. days 0, 14
	6-MP	60 mg/m² p.o. days 0–27
	ARA-C	75 mg/m² i.v. days 1–4, 8-11, 15–18, 22–25
	IT MTX	days 1, 8, 15, 22
	RT	1800 cGy cranial for no CNS disease at diagnosis / 2400 cGy cranial + 600 cGy spinal for CNS disease at diagnosis
Interim maintenance (8 weeks)	6-MP	60 mg/m² qd p.o. days 0–41
	MTX	15 mg/m² qw p.o. days 0, 7, 14, 21, 28, 35
Delayed intensification (7 weeks)		*Reinduction* (4 weeks)
	DEX	10 mg/m² p.o. qd days 0–20, then taper for 7 days
	VCR	1.5 mg/m² i.v. days 0, 7, 14
	DOX	25 mg/m² i.v. days 0, 7, 14
	l-ASP	600 U/m² i.m. days 3, 5, 7, 10, 12, 14
		Reconsolidation (3 weeks)
	CPM	1000 mg/m² i.v. day 28
	6-TG	60 mg/m² p.o. qd days 28–41
	ARA-C	75 mg/m² subq/i.v. days 29–32, 36-39
	IT MTX	days 29, 36
Maintenance (12-week cycles)	VCR	1.5 mg/m² i.v. days 0, 28, 56
	PDN	60 mg/m² p.o. qd days 0–4, 28-32, 56–60
	6-MP	75 mg/m² p.o. days 0–83
	MTX	20 mg/m² p.o. days 7, 14, 21, 28, 35, 42, 49, 56, 63, 70, 77
	IT MTX	day 0

delayed-intensification phase and duration of therapy is generally shorter compared to pediatric protocols. There is also increased usage of allogeneic bone marrow transplant in first remission for adults with ALL. There is a perception on the part of adult oncologists that older individuals have significantly greater toxicity associated with VCR and L-ASP.

A large number of pediatric trials have shown clearly that older adolescent and young adult ALL patients have a worse outcome compared to younger patients [29–36]. Older adolescent and young adult ALL patients have a higher incidence of induction deaths and deaths in remission compared to younger patients [37]. The fact that older adolescent and young adult patients have a low incidence of favorable cytogenetic abnormalities (t(12;21); hyperdiploidy) may account for some of the outcome difference.

Adolescents with leukemia may receive care from either pediatric or medical oncologists. Five studies have suggested that young adult patients with ALL entered on pediatric clinical trials have a significantly better event-free survival (EFS) and overall survival compared to adolescents treated on adult clinical trials [2–7].

In the first published experience, the CCG and Cancer and Acute Leukemia Group B (CALGB) compared outcome for young adult patients aged 16–21 years treated between 1988 and 1998 (CALGB) and between 1989 and 1995 (CCG) [2]. CALGB trials utilized a five-drug induction and a modified postremission BFM-type therapy. The majority of older adolescent and young adult patients treated on CCG protocols received either CCG-modified BFM or augmented BFM.

Compared to CCG-modified BFM, patients receiving augmented BFM received additional courses of VCR and L-ASP during initial consolidation and delayed intensification phases. "Capizzi" MTX was administered during interim maintenance phases. Patients received a second interim maintenance and delayed-intensification phase prior to beginning maintenance. The augmented BFM chemotherapy regimen is shown in Table 6.6. A comparison of dose intensity for various drugs in CCG-modified and augmented BFM is shown in Table 6.7.

For patients treated on CALGB trials, the induction rate was 93% and the 6-year EFS was 38%. For patients treated on CCG trials, the induction rate was 96% and the 6-year EFS was 64%. Thus, older adolescent and young adult patients with ALL had a significantly better outcome when treated on CCG versus CALGB trials.

Comparing the adult and pediatric therapies, patients treated on CCG protocols received significantly more VCR, steroid, and particularly more L-ASP, and significantly less CPM and ARA-C compared to patients treated on the CALGB protocols. Patients in both groups were well matched for major presenting features such as WBC, unfavorable cytogenetic features, and immunophenotype.

In a similar study design, French investigators compared outcomes for patients 15–20 years of age treated on either the FRALLE pediatric trial ($N = 77$) or the adult LALA trial ($N = 100$) between June 1993 and November 1999 [3]. FRALLE chemotherapy was similar to BFM therapy, but incorporated VP-16 into consolidation and delayed intensification, and included vindesine in reinduction. All patients received cranial radiotherapy. Adolescents treated on the LALA protocol received a four-drug induction consisting of PDN, VCR, idarubicin, and CPM without L-ASP. Patients were then randomized to an intensive consolidation (mitoxantrone, ARA-C) or a standard consolidation (CPM, ARA-C, 6-MP), followed by sequential courses of intermediate-dose MTX/ L-ASP, CPM/ARA-C, and VCR, DXM, and ADR. All patients received cranial radiation.

On both trials, patients with unfavorable prognostic features who achieved a remission were to receive an allograft if a matched sibling was available, or an autograft. For the FRALLE 93 trial, unfavorable features included WBC > 50 x 10^9/L, t(9:22), t(4:11), hypodiploidy (<45 chromosomes), tetraploidy, poor PDN response, and nonremission status at day 28. Unfavorable features for the LALA protocol included WBC > 30 x 10^9/L, t(9:22), t(1:19), t(4:11), CD10 and CD20 negativity, and myeloid marker positivity. There were no significant differences in presenting features for the two groups. Unfavorable cytogenetics (t(9:22), t(4:11), hypodiploidy) were found in 6% of the FRALLE patients and 5% of the LALA patients. Induction and 5-year EFS rates were 94% and 67%, respectively, for patients treated on FRALLE protocols compared to 83% and 41%, respectively, for patients treated on the LALA protocol.

Italian investigators studied the outcome of adolescent patients treated on either pediatric (AIEOP) or adult (GIMEMA) protocols [4]. Patients included were 14–18 years of age and enrolled between April 1996 and October 2003 (AIEOP – 150 patients; GIMEMA – 95 patients). AIEOP protocols were BFM based, while GIMEMA protocols include induction with high-dose anthracycline (550 mg/m^2) and high-dose ARA-C as consolidation. No high-dose MTX or a delayed intensification phase was given as in the BFM protocol. Maintenance consisted of courses of VCR, DNR, and CPM. Prognostic features such as immunophenotype and incidence of t(9:22) were similar between the two groups. Initial complete response rates were 94% for AIEOP vs. 89% for GIMEMA. The relapse rate was 17% in the AIEOP trial and 45% for the GIMEMA trial. Two-year overall survival was 80% for AIEOP and 71% for GIMEMA.

Dutch investigators compared the outcome for patients 15–20 years of age treated on either the pediatric ALL-9 trial or adult (HOVON) trial (1985–1999) [5]. Compared to the adult chemotherapy program, ALL-9 included a delayed intensification phase, therapy with either high-dose MTX and/or oral low-dose MTX, and maintenance therapy. Fifty-eight percent of patients on the Hovon trial received a bone marrow transplant in first remission compared to only 3% of patients treated on ALL protocols. Remission and 5-year EFS rates were 98% and 69% for patients treated on ALL-9 versus 91% and 34% for patients treated on the adult protocols.

CCG has presented preliminary outcome results for 262 older adolescent and young adult patients entered on the CCG 1961 trial between November 1996 and June 2002 [8]. Patients were assigned to either a rapid responder (MI Day 7 marrow) or slow responder subgroup (M2/3 Day 7 marrow). Rapid responders were randomized in a 2×2 design to augmented or standard-intensity BFM-type therapy and to one or two delayed intensification phases. Slow early responders received augmented BFM and were randomized to receive or not receive pulses of idarubicin and CPM in the two delayed intensification phases. Seventy three percent of patients had a WBC of <50 x 10^9/L and 21% of patients had T-cell immunophenotype. The 5-year EFS and overall survival for older adolescent and young adult patients were 70.3 ± 3% and 77 ± 3.2%, respectively.

6.7 Toxicity and Late Effects

It is well recognized that older patients with ALL have a higher rate of treatment-related morbidity and mortality compared to younger patients. There is a higher rate of death in induction and death in first remission for patients older than 10 years with ALL compared to younger patients [37]. The incidence of diabetes and pancreatitis during induction increases with age. Avascular necrosis of bone is a significant cause of morbidity for older patients with ALL.

On the CCG 1882 study, 14.2% of patients >10 years of age developed avascular necrosis (AVN) compared to a 1% incidence for patients <10 years of age [40]. In patients >10 years, the incidence was higher for females than for males, 17.4% vs. 11.7% ($p = 0.03$).

On CCG 1882, rapid early responders (Day 7 M1/M2 marrow) received CCG-modified BFM with or without cranial radiation. Slow responders (Day 7 M3 marrow) were randomized to receive CCG-modified BFM or augmented BFM. All slow responder patients received cranial radiation therapy. Patients receiving CCG-modified BFM received one delayed intensification phase, while patients receiving augmented BFM received two phases. Patients received 21 consecutive days of DXM during the delayed intensification phases. The incidence of AVN was 8.6% for rapid early responder patients, 16.2% for slow responder patients receiving one delayed intensification phase, and 23.2% for slow responder patients receiving two delayed intensification phases [38]. It is unclear why slow responder patients receiving one delayed intensification phase had a twofold increased risk of AVN compared to rapid responder patients receiving the same therapy.

Since continuous steroid exposure was thought to be associated with an increased risk for AVN, on the CCG 1961 protocol, rapid early responder patients randomized to two delayed intensification phases and all slow early responder patients (two delayed intensification phases) received DXM on days 0–6 and 14–20 of each delayed intensification phase. Rapid early

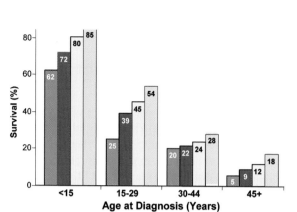

Figure 6.6

Five-year survival, ALL, by era during the period 1975–1998, United States SEER

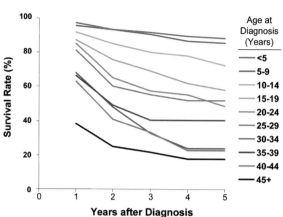

Figure 6.7

Survival, ALL, 1993–1998, by age, United States SEER

responder patients randomized to one delayed intensification phase received continuous DXM (days 0–20). For patients older than 10 years, rapid early responder patients receiving one delayed intensification (continuous DEX) had an AVN incidence of 13.4% compared to 7.5% for patients receiving two delayed intensification phases (discontinuous DXM; $p = 0.002$) [38, 39]. For patients receiving the augmented intensity regimens, the incidence of AVN was 15.2% for patients receiving continuous DXM vs. 5.3% for those receiving discontinuous DXM. In the older adolescent and young adult subgroup, the incidence of AVN was 12.4% for patients receiving discontinuous DXM vs. 28% for those receiving continuous DXM.

6.8 Outcome

Figure 6.6 illustrates the steady progress in survival that has been accomplished in ALL, with four equal 6-year eras from 1975 to 1998 represented. The 5-year age-dependent survival rates for ALL improved in each age category, with survival being correlated inversely with age.

For the population in general, and for both genders, 5-year survival rates for ALL declined with advancing

age. For the most recent interval evaluated, 1993–1998, the 5-year survival rates were highest among those younger than 10 years of age, both above 85% (Fig. 6.7). The 5-year rates decreased substantively for the next age group (10–14 years, 72%); and for the 15- to 19-year, 20- to 24-year, and 25- to 29-year age groups were 58%, 49% and 53%, respectively. For the older patients, the 5-year rate was 20–40% (Fig. 6.7).

Among females, the 5-year survival rates for the period 1993–1998 were 87%, 55%, 42%, and 14%, respectively, and for males, the corresponding values were 84%, 53%, 18%, and 20%, respectively (Figs. 6.8 and 6.9)

6.9 Summary and Conclusions

ALL represented 2.1% of all cancers that occurred in 15- to 29-year-olds in the United States over the time period 1975–1999. In the year 2000, approximately 530 persons 15–29 years of age were diagnosed as having ALL. In the years between adolescence and older adulthood, the incidence of ALL decreased gradually as the incidence of acute and chronic myeloid leukemias increased.

ALL was the most common type of leukemia in the 15- to 19-year group. In the 20- to 24-year age group,

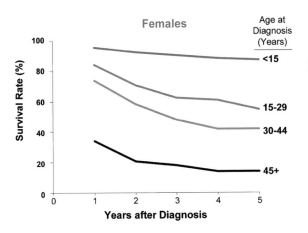

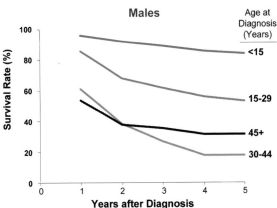

Figure 6.8

Survival, ALL, 1993–1998, females, by age, United States SEERdence of ALL by race/ethnicity, age 0–45 years, United States SEER registry, 1992–2000

Figure 6.9

Survival, ALL, 1993–1998, males, by age, United States SEER

ALL and acute myelogenous leukemia occurred at approximately equal rates; in the 25- to 29-year age group, acute myelogenous leukemia occurred at a rate 1.5 times that of ALL.

ALL occurred with greater frequency in males of all ages, with the male predominance greatest in 15- to 29-year-olds, essentially double that in females. At all ages Hispanics had the highest rate of ALL, and African Americans the lowest rate. Among 15- to 29-year-olds the incidence in Hispanics was 1.7-fold higher than in non-Hispanic whites, 2.8-fold greater than in African Americans/blacks, and 2.1 times increased over Asians/Pacific Islanders. Compared to younger patients, older adolescent and young adult patients with ALL have a higher incidence of T-cell immunophenotype, higher hemoglobin levels, a higher (although still low) rate of the t(9:22), a lower incidence of favorable cytogenetics such as high hyperdiploidy or the t(12:21), and a lower incidence of lymphomatous features.

During the period 1975–2000, the incidence of ALL increased significantly among those diagnosed before 30 years of age. Among 15- to 29-year-olds, most of the increase was in males, who had the greatest increase in this age group compared with all other ages.

Risk factors for ALL include male gender, young age (2–5 years), Caucasian race/ethnicity, pre- and postnatal radiation exposure; and constitutional syndromes including trisomy 21, neurofibromatosis type 1, Bloom syndrome, Shwachman syndrome, and ataxia-telangiectasia.

Survival rates for ALL declined dramatically with advancing age. For the period 1993–1998, the 5-year survival rates were 58, 49 and 53% for the 15- to 19-year, 20- to 24-year, and 25- to 29-year age groups, respectively.

An improvement in survival has occurred since 1975 in each category of leukemia, although the decrease in mortality among adolescent and young adult patients with ALL lags behind that of younger patients.

At present, EFS for older adolescent and young adult patients treated on pediatric trials is 60–70% and the overall survival is between 65 and 75%. Older adolescent and young adult patients have a higher incidence of induction death and death in remission compared to younger patients. The lower incidence of favorable cytogenetics in older adolescent and young adult patients with ALL may, in part, account for the worse outcome.

AVN is a serious treatment complication observed almost exclusively in patients >10 years of age, and the incidence is highest in the older adolescent and young adult subgroup. The use of discontinuous DXM in DI phases produces a significant decrease in the incidence of AVN.

In multiple comparisons of older adolescent and young adult patients with ALL treated on pediatric and adult protocols, there was a consistent and significant difference in both EFS and overall survival favoring patients treated on pediatric trials with the EFS advantage ranging from 20 to 30%.

In an editorial accompanying the presentation of the French FRALLE and LALA comparison [40], Dr. Charles Schiffer raised the issue whether the outcome difference favoring adolescents treated on pediatric protocols was a consequence of better regimens, better doctors, or both.

The most likely explanation for the EFS and overall survival difference favoring older adolescent and young adult patients with ALL treated on pediatric protocols is the significant differences in chemotherapy utilized by pediatric and adult oncologists, although other factors may also be operating. It appears that pediatric protocols which incorporate a DI, utilize more steroids, VCR and L-ASP; and use lower amounts of alkylating agents, high-dose ARA-C, and anthracyclines are more effective in treating older adolescent and young adult ALL than adult protocols. Among adult oncologists, there is a perception that older patients have significantly increased toxicity associated with the administration of VCR and L-ASP compared to younger patients. However, pediatric protocols have demonstrated that it is feasible to use intensive VCR and L-ASP in older adolescent and young adult patients with ALL.

The vast majority of older adolescent and young adult patients with ALL treated on pediatric trials are treated by university-based pediatric oncologists, while 25–40% of patients treated on adult trials are treated by community-based adult oncologists. However, a United Kingdom study suggested no difference in outcome for adults with ALL treated by university- or community-based adult oncologists [41], but this issue has not been examined in the United States adult ALL trials.

Physician compliance with drug administration as mandated by protocol may be an important issue. In his editorial [40], Dr. Schiffer commented on protocol compliance by pediatric oncologists as "military precision on the basis of a near religious conviction about the necessity of maintaining prescribed dose and schedule come hell, high water, birthdays, Bastille day, or Christmas." He concluded that, although there are few if any studies proving an advantage for such rigor, it is likely that neither adult university-based nor community-based oncologists meet the pediatric standard.

Currently, the three largest adult oncology groups in the United States are developing a clinical trial for young adult patients with ALL that will utilize one arm of the current CCG AALL0232 High Risk ALL protocol. On the AALL0232 trial, standard therapy for older adolescent and young adult patients with rapid morphological response, and <0.1% minimal residual disease on day 28 as measured by flow cytometry, will be "hemiaugmented" BFM therapy (augmented BFM with only one interim maintenance and one DI phase), which proved to be the best arm in the CCG 1961 trial for high-risk rapid responder patients [42]. On CCG 1961, this hemiaugmented BFM had an equivalent outcome to full augmented BFM (two interim maintenance and two delayed intensification phases). The AALL0232 trial is evaluating DXM at 10 mg/m2/day × 14 days versus PDN at 60 mg/m^2/day × 28 days during induction and high-dose MTX with Leucovorin rescue versus Capizzi MTX (no rescue) in the first interim maintenance phase. At present, the adult groups plan to utilize the DXM and Capizzi MTX arm for their trial.

To increase the cure rate for adolescents with ALL, we must decrease the incidence of induction deaths and deaths in remission by providing better supportive care or by identifying upfront those patients likely to experience severe toxicity with standard therapy. Identification of the key genetic polymorphisms that influence drug metabolism may play an important role. We must also develop more precise treatment response measures to predict which patients might achieve cure with standard or less aggressive treatment and which patients require either more intensive (BMT as a possibility) or novel therapies to improve cure. Determination of minimal residual disease by molecular or flow cytometric tools might be important

Table 6.6 Augmented BFM therapy (A-BFM)

Induction	PDN	60 mg/m^2 p.o. days 1–28 (bid or tid) then taper
	VCR	1.5 mg/m^2 i.v. days 1, 8, 15 and 22
	DNR	25 mg/m^2 i.v. days 1, 8, 15 and 22
	I-ASP	6000 U/m^2 i.m. 3 times per week × 3 weeks beginning on day 3
	IT ARA-C	day 1 (age adjusted dosing)
	IT MTX	day 8 (age adjusted dosing)
Consolidation (9 weeks)	CPM	1000 mg/m^2 i.v. days 0, 28
	ARA-C	75 mg/m^2 subq/i.v. days 1-4, 8-11, 29–32, 36–39
	6-MP	60 mg/m^2 p.o. days 0–13, 28–41
	VCR	1.5 mg/m^2 i.v. days 14, 21, 42, 49
	I-ASP	6000 U/m^2 i.m. days 14, 16, 18, 21, 23, 25, 42, 44, 46, 49, 51, 53
	IT MTX	days 1, 8, 15, 22
	RT	1800 cGy cranial, for no CNS disease at diagnosis 2400 cranial + 600 cGy + spinal for CNS disease
Interim maintenance I (8 weeks)	VCR	1.5 mg/m^2 i.v. days 0, 10, 20, 30, 40
	MTX	100 mg/m^2 i.v. days 0, 10, 20, 30, 40 (escalate by 50 mg/m^2/dose)
	I-ASP	15000 U/m^2 i.m. days 1, 11, 21, 31, 41
Delayed intensification I (8 weeks)		*Reinduction (4 weeks)*
	DEX	10 mg/m^2 p.o. qd days 0–20, then taper for 7 days
	VCR	1.5 mg/m^2 i.v. days 0, 14, 21
	DOX	25 mg/m^2 i.v. days 0, 7, 14
	I-ASP	6000 U/m^2 i.m. days 3, 5, 7, 10, 12, 14
		Reconsolidation (4 weeks)
	CPM	1000 mg/m^2 i.v. day 28
	6-TG	60 mg/m^2 p.o. days 28–41
	ARA-C	75 mg/m^2 subq/i.v. days 29–32, 36-39
	IT MTX	days 29, 36
	VCR	1.5 mg/m^2 i.v. days 42, 49
	I-ASP	6000 U/m^2 i.m. days 42, 44, 46, 51, 53
Interim maintenance II		See interim maintenance I except additional IT MTX on day 0, 20, 40
Delayed intensification II		See delayed intensification I
Maintenance (12-week cycles)	VCR	1.5 mg/m^2 i.v. days 0, 28, 56
	PRED	60 mg/m^2 p.o. qd days 0–4, 28–32, 56–60
	6-MP	75 mg/m^2 p.o. qd days 0–83
	MTX	20 mg/m^2 p.o. days 7, 14, 21, 28, 35, 42, 56, 63, 70, 77
	IT MTX	day 0

in this regard. We must also determine whether, utilizing similar if not identical treatment regimens, adult university-based or community-based oncologists can achieve similar EFS results obtained by pediatric oncologists for older adolescent and young adult patients with ALL. Answers to these important questions should be forthcoming in the next 5–10 years.

Table 6.7 CM-BFM vs A-BFM. Doses of chemotherapy in the 1st year

	CM-BFM	A-BFM
VCR	15	30
I-ASP	15	53
CPM	3	4
ARA-C	24	32
i.v. MTX	0	10
Dexamethasone courses	1	2

Table 6.8 Hyper CVAD Regimen

Cycles 1, 3, 5, 7a	
Cyclophosphamide	300 mg/m^2 i.v. every 12 h – 6 doses days 1–3
Vincristine	2 mg i.v. day 4, 11
Doxorubicin	50 mg/m2 i.v. day 4
Dexamethasone	40 mg daily p.o. days 1–4 and 11–14
IT Methotrexate	12 mg on day 2[b]
IT ARA-C	100 mg on day 8
Cycles 2, 4, 6, 8a	
Methotrexate	200 mg/m^2 i.v. over 2 h day 1
Methotrexate	800 mg/m^2 i.v. over 22 h day 1
Methylprednisolone	50 mg i.v. bid day 1 – 3
IT Methotrexate	12 mg on day 2 [b]
IT ARA-C	100 mg on day 2
Maintenance (to 2 years)	
Vincristine	2.0 mg i.v. day 1
6-MP	50 mg p.o. tid day 1–28
Methotrexate	20 mg/m^2 day 1, 8, 15, 22
Prednisone	200 mg p.o. days 1–5

[a]Courses given following recovery of CTS WBC > 3 × 109/l and platelet > 60 × 109/l
[b]High risk for CNS disease, cycles 1–8; low-risk patient, cycles 1, 2; unknown risk, cycles 1–4

References

1. Bleyer WA, O'Leary M, Barr R, Ries LAG (eds) (2006) Cancer Epidemiology in Older Adolescents and Young Adults 15 to 29 Years of Age, Including SEER Incidence and Survival, 1975–2000. National Cancer Institute, NIH Pub. No. 06-5767. Bethesda, MD, p 220
2. Stock W, Satner H, Dodge RK, et al. (2000) Outcome of adolescents and young adults with ALL: a comparison of Children's Cancer Group (CCG) and Cancer and Acute Leukemia Group B (CALGB) regimens. Blood 96:467a
3. Boissel N, Auclerc MF, Lheritier V, et al (2003) Should adolescents with acute lymphoblastic leukemia be treated as old children or young adults? Comparison of the French FRALLE-93 and LALA-94 trials. J Clin Oncol 21:774–780
4. Testi AM, Valsecchi MG, Conter V, et al (2004) Difference in outcome of adolescents with acute lymphoblastic leukemia (ALL) enrolled in pediatric (AIEOP) and adult (GIMEMA) protocols. Blood 104:539a
5. de Bont JM, van der Holt B, Dekker AW, et al (2003) Significant difference in outcome for adolescents with

acute lymphoblastic leukemia (ALL) treated on pediatric versus adult ALL protocols. Blood 102:222a

6. Ramanujachar R, Richards S, Hann IM, et al (2007) Adolescents with acute lymphoblastic leukaemia: outcome on UK national paediatric (ALL 97) and adult (UKALLXII/E2993) trials. Pediatr Blood Cancer, 48:254–261

7. Nachman J, Siebel N, Sather H, et al (2004) Outcome for adolescent and young adults 16–21 years of age (AYA) with acute lymphoblastic leukemia (ALL) treated on the Children's Cancer Group (CCG) 1961 study. Blood 104:196a

8. Bhatia S, Ross JA, Greaves MF, Robison LL (1999) Epidemiology and etiology. In: Pui CH (ed) Childhood Leukemias. Cambridge University Press Cambridge, UK, p 41

9. Narod SA, Stiller C, Lenoir GM (1991) An estimate of the heritable fraction of childhood cancer. Br J Cancer 63:993–999

10. Crispino JD (2005) GATA1 in normal and malignant hematopoiesis. Semin Cell Dev Biol 16:137–147

11. Hitzler JK, Zipursky A (2005) Origins of leukaemia in children with Down syndrome. Nat Rev Cancer 5:11–20

12. Ge Y, Stout ML, Tatman DA, et al (2005) GATA1, cytidine deaminase, and the high cure rate of Down syndrome children with acute megakaryocytic leukemia. J Natl Cancer Inst 97:226–231

13. Side L, Taylor B, Cayouette M, et al (1997) Homozygous inactivation of the NF1 gene in bone marrow cells from children with neurofibromatosis type 1 and malignant myeloid disorders. N Engl J Med 336:1713–1720

14. Duker NJ (2002) Chromosome breakage syndromes and cancer. Am J Med Genet 115:125–129

15. Eyfjord JE, Bodvarsdottir SK (2005) Genomic instability and cancer: networks involved in response to DNA damage. Mutat Res 592:18–28

16. Horwitz M, Li FQ, Albani D, et al (2003) Leukemia in severe congenital neutropenia: defective proteolysis suggests new pathways to malignancy and opportunities for therapy. Cancer Invest 21:579–587

17. Greaves MF (1988) Speculations on the cause of childhood acute lymphoblastic leukemia. Leukemia 2:120–125

18. Greaves MF, Alexander FE (1993) An infectious etiology for common acute lymphoblastic leukemia in childhood? Leukemia 7:349–360

19. Greaves MF (1997) Aetiology of acute leukaemia. Lancet 349:344–349

20. Gilham C, Peto J, Simpson J, et al (2005) Day care in infancy and risk of childhood acute lymphoblastic leukaemia: findings from UK case-control study. BMJ 330:1294

21. Jourdan-Da Silva N, Perel Y, Méchinaud F, et al (2004) Infectious diseases in the first year of life, perinatal characteristics and childhood acute leukaemia. Br J Cancer 90:139–145

22. Neglia JP, Linet MS, Shu XO, et al (2000) Patterns of infection and day care utilization and risk of childhood acute lymphoblastic leukemia. Br J Cancer 82:234–240

23. Chessells JM., Hall E, Prentice HG, et al (2004) The impact of age on outcome in lymphoblastic leukaemia; MRC UKALL X and XA compared: a report from the MRC Paediatric and Adult Working Parties. Leukemia 12:463–473

24. Plasschaert SLA, Kamps WA, Vellenga E, et al (2004) Prognosis in childhood and adult acute lymphoblastic leukaemia: a question of maturation? Cancer Treat Rev 30:3–51

25. Pieters R, Den Boer ML, Durian M, et al. (1998) Relation between age, immunophenotype and in vitro drug resistance in 395 children with acute lymphoblastic leukemia – implications for treatment of infants. Leukemia 12:1344–1348

26. Roman-Gomez J, Jimenez-Velasco A, Castillejo JA, et al. (2004) Promoter hypermethylation of cancer-related genes: a strong independent prognostic factor in acute lymphoblastic leukemia. Blood 104:2492–2498

27. Linker C, Damon L, Ries C , Navarro W (2002) Intensified and shortened cyclical chemotherapy for adult acute lymphoblastic leukemia. J Clin Oncol 20:2464–2471

28. Kantarijian H, Thomas D, O'Brien S, et al. (2004) Long-term follow-up results of hyperfractionated cyclophosphamide, vincristine, doxorubicin, and dexamethasone (Hyper-CVAD), a dose-intensive regimen, in adult acute lymphocytic leukemia. Cancer 101:2788–2801

29. Eden OB, Harrison G, Richards S, et al. (2000) on behalf of the Medical Research Council Childhood Leukaemia Working Party Long-term follow-up of the United Kingdom Medical Research Council protocols for childhood acute lymphoblastic leukaemia. Leukemia 14:1980–1997

30. Gaynon PS, Trigg ME, Heerema NA, et al. (2000) Children's Cancer Group trials in childhood acute lymphoblastic leukemia: 1983–1995. Leukemia 14:2223–2233

31. Harms DO, Janka-Schaub GE on behalf of the COALL Study Group (2000) Co operative study group for childhood acute lymphoblastic leukemia (COALL): long-term follow-up of trials 82, 85, 89 and 92. Leukemia 14:2234–2239

32. Kamps WA, Veerman AJP, Van Wering ER, et al (2000) Long-term follow-up of Dutch childhood leukemia study group (DCLSG) protocols for children with acute lymphoblastic leukemia, 1984–1991. Leukemia 14:2240–2246

33. Maloney KW, Shuster JJ, Murphy S, et al (2000) Long-term results of treatment studies for childhood acute lymphoblastic leukemia: Pediatric Oncology Group studies from 1986–1994. Leukemia 12:2276–2285

34. Pui CH, Boyett JM, Rivera GK, et al. (2000) Long-term results of total therapy studies 11, 12 and 13A for childhood acute lymphoblastic at St. Jude Children's Research Hospital. Leukemia 14:2286–2294

35. Schrappe M, Reiter A, Zimmermann M, et al. (2000) Long-term results of four consecutive trials in childhood ALL performed by the ALL-BFM study group from 1981 to 1995. Leukemia 14:2205–2222

36. Silverman LB, Declerck L, Gelber RD, et al. (2000) Results of Dana-Farber Cancer Institute Consortium protocols for children with newly diagnosed acute lymphoblastic leukemia (1981–1995). Leukemia 14:2247–2256

37. Rubnitz JE, Lensing S, Zhou Y, et al. (2004) Death during induction therapy and first remission of acute leukemia in childhood. Cancer 101:1677–1684

38. Mattano LA, Sather HN, La MK, et al (2003) Modified dexamethasone (DXM) reduces the incidence of treatment-related osteonecrosis (ON) in children and adolescents with higher risk acute lymphoblastic leukemia (HR ALL): a report of CCG-1961. Blood 102:221a (abstract 777)

39. Mattano LA, Sather HN, Trigg ME, Nachman JB (2000) Osteonecrosis as a complication of treating acute lymphoblastic leukemia in children: a report from the children's cancer group. J Clin Oncol 18:3262–3272

40. Schiffer CA (2003) Differences in outcome in adolescents with acute lymphoblastic leukemia: a consequence of better regimens? Better doctors? Both? J Clin Oncol 21:760–761

41. Benjamin S, Kroll ME, Cartwright RA, et al (2000) Haematologists' approaches to the management of adolescents and young adults with acute leukaemia. Br J Haematol 111:1045–1050

42. Seibel NL, Steinherz P, Sather H, et al (2003) Early treatment intensification improves outcome in children and adolescents with acute lymphoblastic leukemia presenting with unfavorable features who show a rapid early response to induction therapy: a report of CCG. Blood 102:A787

Acute Myelogenous Leukemia

Ursula Creutzig • William G. Woods

Contents

7.1 Abstract

After a peak during the first 2 years of life, the incidence of acute myelogenous leukemia (AML) is low (five per million 5- to 9-year-olds per year in the United States) until after 9 years of age, when it slowly increases during adolescence and adulthood (to nine per million 15- to 19-year-olds per year in the United States). Biological features of pediatric and young adult AML appear to be similar, albeit future studies in genomics and proteomics are likely to disclose differences. Treatment results in AML have improved during the last 20 years for all age groups; however, outcome decreases with advancing age even when risk factors are considered. In contrast to data about children and adults, data on biological features and outcome are scarce in the adolescent age group. This is partly due to the low number of patients of this age group participating in clinical trials. Differences in outcome for adolescents participating in pediatric or adult trials seem to be significant when different protocols are used, but minor with similar or identical protocols. As the needs of adolescents are different from those of young children and those of adults and elderly patients, it is recommended to treat these patients in special units whenever possible.

7.2 Introduction

AML represents approximately 15–20% of all leukemias in children, about one-third in adolescents and about 50% in adults (Fig. 6.2). In general, the biological features of pediatric and adult AML appear to be similar, but the differences have not been reviewed systematically. Treatment results in childhood AML have improved considerably over the last 20 years, with a 5-year survival in the range of 50–60% [1, 2]. In adults, outcome is less favorable, with overall cure rates of 30% or even less.

The number of adolescents and young adults included in clinical trials is relatively small, both in cooperative group studies of adults and in pediatric trials. Treatment protocols designed for children and adults often differ in various aspects from each other, and there are no data elucidating which kind of therapy could be particularly appropriate for young adults. It is our aim to describe the biological features, clinical symptoms and signs, treatment modalities, and outcome of this age cohort.

7.3 Epidemiology/Etiology

7.3.1 Incidence

Data herein were derived from United States SEER [3, 4] and the Automated Childhood Cancer Information System Europe (ACCIS 2003) [5] and the German Childhood Cancer Registry (GCCR 2003) [6]. The data are slightly different probably due to relatively low patient numbers or differences in race in different countries.

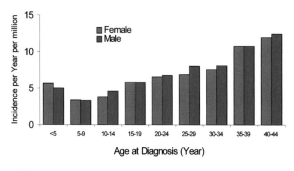

Figure 7.1

Incidence of acute myelogenous leu-kemia (AML) by gender (Surveillance, Epidemiology and End Results, United States SEER, 1975–1999)

Based on these data, the acute leukemias represent 31–34% of all cancer cases in children younger than 15 years of age; they account for 6% of cancer in 15- to 29-year-olds. Age-adjusted annual incidence rates (per million) of AML are given in Table 7.1. Fig. 7.1 shows the variation of incidence of AML in children and adolescents in different age groups. AML rates are highest in the first years of life, but subsequently decrease with a nadir at approximately 9 years of age followed by slowly increasing rates during adolescence and adulthood [4]. Therefore, with advancing age the percentage of AML increases within the total leukemias, resulting in an inversion of the frequency of acute lymphoblastic leukemia (ALL) and AML in late adolescence.

The incidence of AML is similar for males and females during adolescence (Fig. 7.1) [3, 4]. Slightly more affected female young adults were seen in the European studies (AML-CG; Table 7.2), but United States population data shows a male predominance from age 20 to 35 years (Fig. 7.1) [3, 4]. The incidence of AML, unlike that of ALL, was similar for white and black children for all age groups [4].

The SEER report [3, 4], the German Children Cancer Registry [7] and the Nordic countries [8] have not reported an increase in incidence in AML in children under 15 years. However, the rate of AML among adolescents and young adults does show some evidence of increase. In England the rate in 15- to 24-year-olds has increased from 6.6 per million per year in 1979–1983 to 8.1 per million per year in 1993–1997 [9]. It likewise appears to have increased among adolescent/young adults aged 15–24 years in The Netherlands [10] and in the United States among 20- to 24-year-olds in the period 1975–1998 [4].

7.3.2 Etiology

There are only a few proven etiologic factors for childhood AML, for example in utero exposure to alcohol, exposure to benzene, ionizing radiation, or different drugs that may contribute to AML in young children. The risk of AML is increased in children with congenital syndromes such as Fanconi anemia, Shwachman syndrome, and Down syndrome. Somatic mutations of the GATA 1 gene are seen in virtually all cases of AML associated with Down syndrome and may be implicated in

Table 7.1 Age-adjusted annual incidence rates per million for specific leukemia by age groups, all races, both sexes, United States SEER 1990–1999, Automated Childhood Cancer Information System Europe (ACCIS) [5] 1993–1997) and acute myelogenous leukemia (AML) – Germany (AML intergroup trials) [11]. *n.g.* Not given

Age (in years) at diagnosis	<5	5–9	10–14	15–19	<15[a]	Period
AML – US (estimated *n*=237) (% of total leukemias)	10.3 (14%)	5.0 (13%)	6.2 (24%)	9.3 (36%)	7.0 (16%)	1990–1995
AML – ACCIS[b]						1993–1997
AML – Germany (*n*=439)	9.1	5.2	5.8	n.g.	6.6	
AML – Germany (AML intergroup) [11]				6.2		
AML – UK, England and Wales (*n*=190)	8.2	4.4	6.5	n.g.	6.5	
AML – ACCIS[c] (*n*=29–71)				6.8–12.7		

[a]Rates are adjusted to the 1970 US standard population. Numbers in parentheses represent the percentage of the total cases for the specific age group.
[b]ACCIS = Automated Childhood Cancer Information System Europe
[c]ACCIS data from individual countries: Denmark, Ireland, The Netherlands, Slovakia and UK, and Scotland

Table 7.2 Initial clinical data according to age groups (Age: <2, 2–12, 13–21, 22–30 years). Data from the AML-Berlin-Frankfurt-Munster (BFM) Studies 93/98 and AML Cooperative Group (AMLCG)92 trial. *WBC* White blood cell count, *CNS* central nervous system

Age (years)	<2	2–12	13–21	22–30	p value
Gender male:female (%)	53:47	55:45	51:50	49:51	0.66
WBC median, range/µl	17900	17200	14000	19700	0.28
WBC >100,000/µl (%)	22	15	21	13	0.029
Hepatomegaly >5 cm (%)	24	25	27	35	0.36
Splenomegaly >5 cm (%)	28	27	34	26	0.61
CNS involvement (%)	17	8	10	n.g.	0.008
Extramedullary organ involvement (%)	36	19	26	n.g.	0.00001
Total (*n*)	231	448	210	72	

the 500-fold increased risk of megakaryoblastic AML seen in these patients [12, 13]. Such mutations may also confer enhanced leukemic sensitivity to cytarabine via dysregulation of cytidine deaminase gene expression [14]. AML as a secondary malignancy after intensive chemotherapy is quite often seen in older children and adults (cumulative incidence of 0.6% for children treated for ALL or solid tumors by 10 years follow-up, and 3.3–10% for adults treated for different types of solid tumors) [15, 16].

AML is most common and more likely to occur than ALL in the older age group (>65 years old), correlating to prolonged duration of exposure to environmental carcinogens proportional to age [17]. Only the incidence of acute promyelocytic leukemia (French-American-British, FAB, classification M3) appears approximately constant with respect to age after the first decade [18]. The FAB subtype M3 shows a high frequency (20–24%) in certain ethnic populations (e. g., Italian and Latin American) compared to other ethnic groups (5–8%), which may suggest a genetic predisposition for acute promyelocytic leukemia and/or specific environmental exposures [19].

7.3.3 Trends in survival

Survival rates in children under 20 years with AML have improved over the last three decades. Population-based estimates of 5-year survival increased from 23% in the period 1975–1984 to 41% in the period 1985–1994 [4]. Current 5-year survival in children, adolescents, and young adults enrolled in clinical trials (which tend to be higher estimates because trials may exclude patients with unfavorable features or patients from small hospitals) is in the range of 45–60% [1, 20–22]. Results from the AML-BFM studies (patients <18 years old) showed an improvement of 5-year survival from 49% (study AML-BFM 87, period 1987–1992) to 60% (period 1993–1998) [1]. The improvement in prognosis over the last decades in all age groups was made possible by intensified chemotherapy and supportive care. With intensive induction chemotherapy, 80–90% of young patients achieve complete remission (CR).

Little data specifically analyze survival for adolescents and young adults. Population-based data from regions of England and Wales showed that 5-year survival improved significantly from 36% in the period 1984–1988 to 46% in the period 1989–1994 for AML patients between 15 and 29 years old. For patients of this age group treated in the MRC-trials AML 9 and AML 10, 5-year survival increased from 35% to 55% (p=0.012) from the first to the second period [2].

According to SEER data on 15-to 29-year-olds, 5-year survival increased from 15% (1975–1980) to 40–42% between 1987 and 1998 [4].

7.3.4 Prognostic factors

Outcome for females with AML was somewhat better than that for males. Outcome was similar for white and for black children younger than 20 years of age [4], but recent data suggest that improvements in survival have preferentially favored whites, probably on a genetic basis [23].

Increasing age is a known poor prognostic factor in adults with AML [24]. In population studies, 5-year survival rates drop with age: 44% for patients aged 0–15 years, 42% for those aged 15–29 years, and 32% for those aged 30–44 years for the recent time period 1993–98 [4]. However, prognosis in different age groups of children and older adolescents treated similarly have rarely been reported.

The Children's Cancer Group (CCG) trials include children and adolescents less than 22 years old. Five-year survival in CCG trial 213 (1986–89) was 39% and therewith significantly higher than in the previous CCG 251 study (1979–83: 29%) [25]. In this study survival rates were not different in 2- to 10-year-old children and adolescents aged 10–21 years [26]. The same was seen in the recent CCG-2891 trial: in younger (0–16 years) and older (16–21 years) patients treated with intensive timing chemotherapy, survival at 5 years was 49% and 51%, respectively [27]. The British Medical Research Council (MRC) AML 10 trial (1988–1995) included AML patients up to age 35 years on the same treatment regimen. They achieved high CR rates for children under 15 years (91%) and young adults aged 15–34 years (85%). The induction death rate increased slightly, from 5% in children to 7% in young adults; a similar small increase in resistant disease was seen (5–7%). Survival at 5 years was 53% and 60% in children up to age 15 years (after daunorubicin-cytarabine-etoposide and daunorubicin-cytarabine-thioguanine induction, respectively) and 46–47% for the 15–24 year and 25–34 year age groups [20].

The same trend to decrease in survival with age was reported for the event-free survival (EFS) rates but not overall survival in more than 1,000 Japanese AML patients aged 1–29 years consecutively diagnosed in the period 1986–1999, who were treated in a variety of institutions and protocols. Seven-year probability of EFS (pEFS) for AML decreased from 34% in the age groups 10–15 years to 32% for 15- to 19-year-old adolescents, and to 26% in the 20- to 29-year-old young adults [28].

Treatment schedules and dosing of the AML-BFM 93/98 studies for children and adolescents (n=869) and the AMLCG92 study for adults (n=832) were similar during induction and consolidation [29]. In the adult study, 92 patients were 16–30 years old. A common analysis of patients of both studies showed that the CR rate was highest in the age group 2–12 years (89%) and lower in infants and patients of older age (<2 years, 80%; 13–<21 years, 83%; 21–30+ years, 75%). Long-term treatment results were also most favorable among 2- to 12-year-old children (5-year pEFS ±SE, 54±3%), slightly inferior in adolescents (46±4%, p=0.03), and unfavorable in young adults (28±5%, p=0.0001). Excluding patients with low-risk cytogenetics [t(8;21), inv16 and t(15;17)], results were inferior in adolescents (pEFS 32±5%) and young adults (pEFS 26±7%) compared with children aged 2–12 years (pEFS 47±4%) [30].

7.3.5 Treatment Differences

Adolescents and young adults, however, are not always treated on pediatric trials. Recently, adolescents of 16–21 years treated on CCG 2891 with intensive timing (1989–1995) were compared with patients of the same age group treated at the University of Texas MD Anderson Cancer Center on relatively less aggressive adult protocols (1980–2000). Patient characteristics were similar; however, 5-year survival for patients treated on the CCG-trials was 51% compared to 32% in the adult trial. Based on these results, the MD Anderson Cancer Center will now examine the role of intensive timing induction therapy in young adults with de novo AML [31].

7.4 Biology/Pathology

Biologic parameters across the entire age spectrum are reported rarely in the literature. Jeha et al. [29] reported on the influence of vascular endothelial growth factor (VEGF) in pediatric and adult patients. Unlike in adults, VEGF and VEGF-R2 levels in pediatric AML

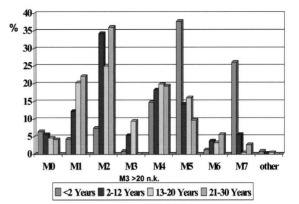

Figure 7.2

Distribution of FAB (French-American-British) classification subtypes of AML as a function of age group (data from the AML-BFM studies 93/98 and AMLCG92)

patients did not correlate with survival. Also contrary to the case in adults, expression of the multidrug resistance gene (*MRD1*) failed to define a poor prognostic group in childhood AML [32]. The frequency of cytogenetic subgroups of AML are age specific, certainly in adults, with an increase in the poor prognosis unbalanced aberrations with age [33].

We have analyzed the initial clinical, morphological, and cytogenetic data of children, adolescents, and young adults treated in the pediatric trials AML-BFM 93/98 (n=869) and of 92 young adults (<30 years) of the AMLCG92 study. Age classifications were infants (≤2 years), children between 2 and 12 years of age (because there were significant differences in biologic parameters in these age groups) [34], adolescents between 13 and 21 years of age, and young adults between 21 and 30 years. Results show (Fig. 7.2) that French-American-British (FAB) distribution was quite different in young children <2 years, 68% (147/213), who presented with FAB subtypes M5 or M7, compared to 18% (133/730) in the older age groups (χ^2 p<0.0001). However, apart from a trend toward increasing M1 and decreasing M7, there was no difference in FAB types for children (2–12 years) and patients 13–30 years old. The favorable karyotypes t(8;21), t(15;17), and inv16 were rarely seen in children

Table 7.3 Karyotypes in the different age groups. Data from the AML-BFM studies 93/98 and AMLCG92

Age (years)	<2	2–12	13–21	21–30	$p (\chi^2)$
t(8;21) (%)	1	18	10	5	0.0001
t(15;17) (%)	2	6	8	10	0.02
inv16 (%)	2	8	6	9	0.07
11q23 (%)	27	11	7	n.g.	0.0001
Total (n)	164	320	150	43	

<2 years (8/163=5%) compared to the 2- to ≤21-year-olds (141/580=24%; Fisher p=0.01; Table 7.3). With the limitation of the low patient number, it is of interest, that t(8;21) was seen less frequently in young adults compared to the 2- to 21-year-old group.

Our data do not show significant differences in biological parameters between the age groups of 2- to 12-year-old children, adolescents, and young adults, albeit there was a lower incidence of 11q23 and t(8;21) above age 12 years than below this age. Only patients younger than 2 years of age present with significant differences in comparison to older patients. Genomic and proteomic studies currently underway are likely to disclose other age differences, such has already been demonstrated for acute lymphoblastic leukemia.

One exception is the occurrence of the subtype M3, which has a high prevalence in Latinos [19]. In a single institute in Mexico, 20% of all AML patients and 30% of adolescents (11–21 years old) presented with FAB M3 [35]. A report from Japan ascertained a gradual increase of M3 in adolescence: 1–4 years, 5%; 5–9 years, 8%; 10–14 years, 12%; 15–19 years, 19%; 20–24 years, 22%; 25–29 years, 21% [28].

7.5 Diagnosis: Symptoms and Clinical Signs

The clinical presentation in children, adolescents, and young adults is mostly similar (Table 7.2). It reflects the degree to which the bone marrow has been infiltrated with leukemic blasts and the extent of extramedullary involvement, and can be both a reflection of tumor biology and health services factors (host- and provider-related delays in diagnosis). The most common symptoms and physical findings result from anemia, thrombocytopenia, and neutropenia, and include pallor and fatigue, anorexia, petechiae, purpura, bleeding, and infection. Occurrence of initial hyperleukocytosis (white blood cell count>100,000/µl) did not vary significantly in the different age groups. Initial involvement of the central nervous system (CNS) is seen less often in adolescents (~10%) and in children aged 2–13 years (~8%) than in infants (~17%) with AML (data not available for young adults, who rarely get diagnostic lumbar puncture). Infiltration of the skin, especially in monocytic leukemias, is also most frequent (~20%) in young children (<2 years) and rarely seen in older children and adolescents. Likewise, leukemic infiltrations of the periosteum and bone occur more often in young children than in adolescents.

7.6 Treatment/Management

Treatment regimens for AML are often but not always similar in children, adolescents, and adults, generally starting with intensive induction courses with cytarabine and anthracyclines of an adequate dosage to achieve remission. Induction therapy is followed by postremission phases to destroy residual blasts in the bone marrow or at other sites. The duration and the optimal type of postremission therapy remain to be established. In general, intensive chemotherapy cycles (referred to as consolidation and/or intensification courses) should include one or more courses of high-dose cytarabine. They are administered together with some kind of CNS prophylaxis and may be followed by a less intensive maintenance chemotherapy. Allogeneic

Table 7.4 Overall 5-year survival (%) in different age groups (only results of registries and trials with more than 100 patients reported). *MRC* Medical Research Council

Source	Treatment Period	Age 0–4 years	Age 5–9 years	Age 10–14 years	Age 15–19 years	Age 20–30 years
ACCIS Germany (n=439)	1993–1997	55	54	54		
ACCIS United Kingdom (n=190)	1993–1997	50	63	37		
MRC 10/12 trials (n=689)	1988–2000	64[a]	60	56		
AML BFM93/98 and AMLCG 92 (n=961)	1993–2001	62	66	59	51	40

[a] 2–4 years old

or autologous stem-cell transplantation may be included as another form of intensification, and indications and rates vary between countries, study groups, and between pediatric and adult providers.

For some specific subgroups, special treatment is available. The most successful special treatment was the introduction of the differentiating agent all-trans-retinoic acid (ATRA) for patients with AML-M3, inducing cell differentiation and maturation instead of cell destruction [36, 37]. A trial using this therapy for AML-M3 patients of all ages was the first biologically based clinical trial cooperation between adult and pediatric clinical trial groups in the United States.

Acute management and supportive care are required during all treatment phases, especially during the first few days and weeks of intensive induction therapy. With recent improvements in AML treatment results, the balance between treatment intensity and toxicity has become more important than in the past, requiring trials to perform risk-adapted therapy.

Generally speaking, the acute and chronic toxicity of chemotherapeutic agents has a similar impact on children, adolescents, and young adults. In adolescents, a higher degree of anticipatory vomiting is seen and, in our experience, a somewhat less rapid recovery from myeloablative treatment. Although the compliance during intensive treatment phases in the adolescent age group is not different from that in children and older patients, as most if not all chemotherapy is given in the

hospital, in our experience it may be lower during maintenance therapy, just as adherence to oral chemotherapy has been shown to be lower in adolescents with ALL.

Most difficult in the management of adolescents is the indispensable psychosocial care. The needs of adolescents are different from those of young children and are accompanied by the conventional problems that are associated with this age group (e.g., need of autonomy and independence, social development, sexual maturation, education, and employment) [39]. These problems are the same as for adolescents and young adults suffering from other types of cancer.

7.7 Participation in Clinical Trials

More than 90% of children less than 15 years of age with AML are treated within clinical trials in the Nordic countries [39], 67% in the United Kingdom [40], and more than 60% in the United States. However, for all cancer patients aged >15 years, the percent enrolled in clinical trials is much lower [41, 42]. This was true for AML patients aged 15–29 years in the United Kingdom from 1989 to 1994, where only 39% of patients aged >15 years were entered on clinical trials [2]. New data from the five German AML intergroup trials included in the Competence Network "Acute and Chronic Leukaemias" indicate that young adults are now generally included in clinical trials [11]. Benjamin et al. [40] reported on the percentages of patients with acute leukemia entered in the MRC trials from 1991 to 1995. Questionnaires were sent to 121 hospitals, and data from the 96 that responded showed that 82% of pediatric AML patients (61% aged between 15 and 19 years and 52% between 20 and 29 years) were entered "always" or "whenever possible" into MRC trials [40]. This low percentage is also a reason for the lack of data in clinical trials regarding the adolescent age group and a possible bias of results including comparisons in age groups.

Several authors state that the prognosis for adolescent leukemia sufferers may be improved by introducing pediatric trials that take into account the prognostic biological features [28]. Another point is the prognostic influence of referring these patients to centers with experience in the management of leukemia, or to centers that participate in clinical trials for children or adults. According to the data available, differences in outcome for patients treated in pediatric or adult trials were more pronounced for adolescent ALL than for AML patients [28, 43].

7.8 Expected Outcome, Including Late Effects

Late effects among survivors of AML during childhood and adolescence may have a significant impact on their quality of life. Long-term sequelae of treatments can include impaired intellectual and psychomotor functioning, neuroendocrine abnormalities, impaired reproductive capacity, and second malignancies [44]. However, most of these late effects, especially side effects after CNS irradiation (neurocognitive deficits, growth hormone deficiency, and secondary CNS tumor) given in the AML-BFM studies for all age groups, but not in other AML trials, affect the younger age group. Anthracycline cardiotoxicity is also seen at lower cumulative doses (<300 mg/m²) in patients younger than 18 years but rather at 550 mg/m² in those over 18 years [45].

The risk of endocrine dysfunction is relatively low in AML patients who are treated with standard chemotherapy only (without alkylating agents), however after stem-cell transplantation there is an increased risk of endocrine dysfunction [44]. Impairment of growth rates after busulfan/cyclophosphamide or cyclophosphamide/total body irradiation (TBI) conditioning regimens is a problem in children treated before or during their growth period. Gonadal toxicity is seen in all age groups, mainly as gonadal dysfunction; however, it is relatively low with modern conventional therapy [44]. Gonadal toxicity may cause disorder of pubertal development, infertility, sexual dysfunction, and the need for long-lasting hormone substitution. In adult women, high doses of alkylating agents and TBI increase the risk of ovarian failure and the probability of restoring the ovarian function decreases by a factor of 0.8 per year of age [46]. The addition of busulfan to cyclophosphamide causes permanent ovarian failure in nearly all female patients. In males the effects of both cytotoxic chemotherapy and TBI will damage the germinal epithelium of the testis, and for the majority of males in all age groups, permanent infertility is likely after TBI schedules [46].

Therefore, in the future, prior to stem-cell transplantation germ cells or gonadal tissue should be collected and stored with the aim of enabling patients to become parents later on [46].

Second malignant neoplasms have been described mainly in ALL patients, with a cumulative incidence of approximately 2–3% at 15 years of age [12, 44]. Data regarding second malignancies following treatment for AML are scarce, probably because the number of long-term survivors is much lower. Within the AML-BFM studies, only 12 second malignancies have been observed among 928 children, who were alive at least 3 years after treatment. Most of these patients had received chemotherapy only. After stem-cell transplantation, the risk of second malignancies is higher for any disease (standard incidence ratio from 6.7 to 11.6 in different studies compared to patients given chemotherapy only) [47]. AML and myelodysplastic syndrome are often reported as second malignancies after chemotherapy with alkylating agents or topoisomerase inhibitors, therefore it might be difficult to distinguish between relapse or second malignancy in primary AML patients.

In all age groups with leukemia and lymphoma, more depression and somatic distress were reported in comparison with sibling controls [44].

7.9 Summary

AML incidence increases with age, such that the frequency in adolescents lies in between that of children and adults. Biological factors vary by age, but the biology of AML in adolescents and young adults appear most similar to that of children. Outcome has improved for all age groups during the last 15–20 years, with the advent of better chemotherapy and supportive care. However, there continues to be a trend toward better survival in children than in young adults, which may be partly related to the intensity of treatment or to treatment in pediatric trials. Further research should be directed toward biologically based, not age-specific trials.

Acknowledgement

Thanks to Professor Thomas Büchner for generously providing data on young adults from the AMLCG Study

References

1. Creutzig U, Ritter J, Zimmermann M, et al (2001) Improved treatment results in high-risk pediatric acute myeloid leukemia patients after intensification with high-dose cytarabine and mitoxantrone: results of Study Acute Myeloid Leukemia-Berlin-Frankfurt-Munster 93. J Clin Oncol 19:2705–2713
2. Stiller CA, Benjamin S, Cartwright RA, et al (1999) Patterns of care and survival for adolescents and young adults with acute leukaemia – a population-based study. Br J Cancer 79:658–665
3. Bleyer WA, O'Leary M, Barr R, Ries LAG (eds) Cancer Epidemiology in Older Adolescents and Young Adults 15 to 29 Years of Age, including SEER Incidence and Survival, 1975–2000. National Cancer Institute, NIH Pub. No. 06-5767, Bethesda MD, June 2006; also available at www.seer.cancer.gov/publications
4. Ries LAG, Eisner MP, Kosary CL, et al (2003) National Cancer Institute SEER Cancer Statistics Review, 1975–2000. http://seercancergov/csr/1975_2000. National Cancer Institute, Bethesda, MD
5. ACCIS (2003) Automated Childhood Cancer Information System. http://www–depiarcfr/accis/datahtm
6. German Childhood Cancer Registry (GCCR) (2003) Annual Report 2002. http://infoimsduni–mainzde/K_Krebsregister/english/ . 14–10–2003
7. Kaatsch P, Spix C, Michaelis J (2002) Jahresbericht 2000 Deutsches Kinderkrebsregister (1st edn) Deutsches Kinderkrebsregister, Mainz
8. Hjalgrim LL, Rostgaard K, Schmiegelow K, et al (2003) Age- and sex-specific incidence of childhood leukemia by immunophenotype in the Nordic countries. J Natl Cancer Inst 95:1539–1544
9. Birch JM, Alston RD, Kelsey AM, et al (2002) Classification and incidence of cancers in adolescents and young adults in England 1979-1997. Br J Cancer 87:1267–1274
10. Reedijk AMJ, Janssen-Heijnen MLG, Louwman MWJ, et al (2005) Increasing incidence and improved survival of cancer in children and young adults in Southern Netherlands, 1973–1999. Eur J Cancer 41:760–769
11. Messerer D, Dugas M, Müller T, Hasford J (2003) How many patients with AML were treated in clinical trials in Germany? Rundbrief Kompetenznetz Leukämien 5:6–7
12. Crisphino JD (2005) GATA 1 in normal and malignant hematopoiesis. Semin Cell Dev Biol 16:137–147
13. Hitzler JK, Zipursky A (2005) Origins of leukaemia in children with Down syndrome. Nat Rev Cancer 5:11–20.
14. Ge Y, Stout ML, Tatman DA, et al. (2005) GATA 1, cytidine deaminase, and the high cure rate of Down syndrome children with acute megakaryocytic leukemia. J Natl Cancer inst 97:226–231
15. Löning L, Zimmermann M, Reiter A, et al (2000) Secondary neoplasms subsequent to Berlin-Frankfurt-Munster therapy of acute lymphoblastic leukemia in childhood: significantly lower risk without cranial radiotherapy. Blood 95:2770–2775
16. Pui CH, Hancock ML, Raimondi SC, et al (1990) Myeloid neoplasia in children treated for solid tumours. Lancet 336:417–421
17. Bleyer WA (2002) Cancer in older adolescents and young adults: epidemiology, diagnosis, treatment, survival, and importance of clinical trials. Med Pediatr Oncol 38:1–10
18. Vickers M, Jackson G, Taylor P (2000) The incidence of acute promyelocytic leukemia appears constant over most of a human lifespan, implying only one rate limiting mutation. Leukemia 14:722–726
19. Douer D, Preston-Martin S, Chang E, et al (1996) High frequency of acute promyelocytic leukemia among Latinos with acute myeloid leukemia. Blood 87:308–313
20. Hann IM, Stevens RF, Goldstone AH, et al (1997) Randomized comparison of DAT versus ADE as induction chemotherapy in children and younger adults with acute myeloid leukemia. Results of the Medical Research Council's 10th AML trial (MRC AML10). Adult and Childhood Leukaemia Working Parties of the Medical Research Council. Blood 89:2311–2318

21. Lie SO, Abrahamsson J, Clausen N, et al(2003) Treatment stratification based on initial in vivo response in acute myeloid leukaemia in children without Down's syndrome: results of NOPHO-AML trials. Br J Haematol 122:217–225

22. Stevens RF, Hann IM, Wheatley K, Gray RG, on behalf of the MRC Childhood Leukaemia Working Party (1998) Marked improvements in outcome with chemotherapy alone in paediatric acute myeloid leukaemia: results of the United Kingdom Medical Research Council's 10th AML trial. Br J Haematol 101:130–140

23. Davies SM, Robison LL, Buckley JD, et al (2001) Glutathione S-transferase polymorphisms and outcome of chemotherapy in childhood acute myeloid leukaemia. J Clin Oncol 19:1279–1287

24. Büchner T, Heinecke A (1996) The role of prognostic factors in acute myeloid leukemia. Leukemia 10:S28–S29

25. Wells RJ, Woods WG, Buckley JD, et al (1994) Treatment of newly diagnosed children and adolescents with acute myeloid leukemia: a Childrens Cancer Group Study. J Clin Oncol 12:2367–2377

26. Wells RJ, Arthur DC, Srivastava A, et al (2002) Prognostic variables in newly diagnosed children and adolescents with acute myeloid leukemia: Children's Cancer Group Study 213. Leukemia 16:601–607

27. Horibe K, Tsukimoto I, Ohno R (2001) Clinicopathologic characteristics of leukemia in Japanese children and young adults. Leukemia 15:1256–1261

28. Büchner T, Hiddemann W, Berdel WE, et al (2003) 6-Thioguanine, cytarabine, and daunorubicin (TAD) and high-dose cytarabine and mitoxantrone (HAM) for induction, TAD for consolidation, and either prolonged maintenance by reduced monthly TAD or TAD-HAM-TAD and one course of intensive consolidation by sequential HAM in adult patients at all ages with de novo acute myeloid leukemia (AML): a randomized trial of the German AML Cooperative Group. J Clin Oncol 21:4496–4504

29. Jeha S, Smith FO, Estey E, et al (2002) Comparison between pediatric acute myeloid leukemia (AML) and adult AML in VEGF and KDR (VEGF-R2) protein levels. Leuk Res 26:399–402

30. Creutzig U, Zimmermann M, Reinhardt D, Büchner T (2004) AML in adolescents compared to AML in children and young adults. Proceedings of the Fourth Biennial Hannover Symposium on Childhood Leukemia, May 3–5, 2004, Hannover, Germany

31 Woods WG, Alonzo TA, Lange BJ, et al (2001) Acute myeloid leukemia (AML) in adolescents and young adults (AYAs): a comparison of outcomes between patients treated on childhood or adult protocols (abstract). Blood 98:462a–463a

32. Steinbach D, Furchtbar S, Sell W, et al (2003) Contrary to adult patients, expression of the multidrug resistance gene (MDR1) fails to define a poor prognostic group in childhood AML. Leukemia 17:470–471

33. Bacher U, Kern W, Schnittger S, et al (2005). Population–based age-specific incidences of cytogenetic subgroups of acute myeloid leukemia. Haematologica 90:1502–1510

34. Vormoor J, Ritter J, Creutzig U, et al (1992) Acute myelogenous leukaemia in children under 2 years – experiences of the West German AML Studies BFM-78, -83 and -87. Br J Cancer 66:63–67

35. Ruiz-Arguelles GJ (1997) Promyelocytic leukemia in Mexican Mestizos. Blood 89:348–349

36. Douer D, Estey E, Santillana S, et al (2001) Treatment of newly diagnosed and relapsed acute promyelocytic leukemia with intravenous liposomal all-trans retinoic acid. Blood 97:73–80

37. Guidez F, Ivins S, Zhu J, et al (1998) Reduced retinoic acid-sensitivities of nuclear receptor corepressor binding to PML- and PLZF-RARalpha underlie molecular pathogenesis and treatment of acute promyelocytic leukemia. Blood 91:2634–2642

38. Penson RT, Rauch PK, McAfee SL, et al (2002) Between parent and child: negotiating cancer treatment in adolescents. Oncologist 7:154–162

39. Lie SO, Jonmundsson G, Mellander L, et al (1996) A population-based study of 272 children with acute myeloid leukaemia treated on two consecutive protocols with different intensity: best outcome in girls, infants, and children with Down's syndrome. Nordic Society of Paediatric Haematology and Oncology (NOPHO). Br J Haematol 94:82–88

40. Benjamin S, Kroll ME, Cartwright RA, et al (2000) Haematologists' approaches to the management of adolescents and young adults with acute leukaemia. Br J Haematol 111:1045–1050

41. Bleyer A (2002) Older adolescents with cancer in North America deficits in outcome and research. Pediatr Clin North Am 49:1027–1042

42. Bleyer WA, Tejeda H, Murphy SB, et al (1997) National cancer clinical trials: children have equal access; adolescents do not. J Adolesc Health 21:366–373

43. Schiffer CA (2003) Differences in outcome in adolescents with acute lymphoblastic leukemia: a consequence of better regimens? Better doctors? Both? J Clin Oncol 21:760–761

44. Robison LL, Bhatia S (2003) Late effects among survivors of leukaemia and lymphoma during childhood and adolescence. Br J Haematol 122:345–359

45. Buzdar AU, Marcus C, Smith TL, Blumenschein GR (1985) Early and delayed clinical cardiotoxicity of doxorubicin. Cancer 55:2761–2765

46. Brennan BM, Shalet SM (2002) Endocrine late effects after bone marrow transplant. Br J Haematol 118:58–66

47. Leiper AD (2002) Non-endocrine late complications of bone marrow transplantation in childhood: part II. Br J Haematol 118:23–43

Hodgkin Lymphoma

Tanya M. Trippett • Alexis Mottl •
Odile Oberlin • Archie Bleyer •
Louis S. Constine

Contents

8.1 Introduction

Hodgkin lymphoma is one of the most common cancers found in adolescents and young adults, accounting for 12% of all invasive cancer in the United States between 15 and 30 years of age [1]. It is a malignant lymphoma that is characterized by multinucleated giant cells, known as Reed-Sternberg cells. Treatment involves combination chemotherapy with or without radiation depending upon clinical stage and the treating institution. Hodgkin lymphoma is considered to be a highly curable neoplasm with 5-year survival rates of up to 90% with treatment. Adolescents and young adults are particularly susceptible to short- and long-term complications of treatment such as gonadal dysfunction, cardiomyopathy, pulmonary toxicity, and second malignancies.

8.2 Epidemiology

8.2.1 Incidence

8.2.1.1 Age-Specific Incidence

The most striking epidemiologic feature of Hodgkin lymphoma is its bimodal age distribution in developed countries, with incidence peaks at 20–24 years and at 75–79 years (Fig. 8.1) [2]. Among 15- to 29-year-olds in the United States, the incidence of Hodgkin lymphoma was approximately 44 per million per year between 1975 and 2000. In the time period 1975–2000, Hodgkin lymphoma accounted for 12% of cancers in 15- to 29-

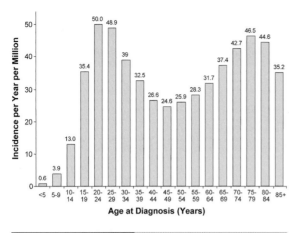

Figure 8.1

Incidence of Hodgkin lymphoma; United States Surveillance, Epidemiology and End Results (SEER) 1975–2000

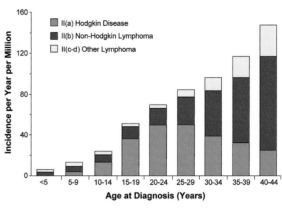

Figure 8.2

Incidence of Hodgkin lymphoma (International Classification of Childhood Cancer, ICCC II(a)) in comparison to non-Hodgkin lymphoma (ICCC II(b)) and other lymphoma (ICCC II(c), II(d) and II(e)); United States SEER 1975–2000

year-olds in the United States, and was the most common hematologic malignancy in the age group [3].

Table 8.1 depicts the incidence of Hodgkin lymphoma in the pediatric and adolescent/young adult age group. Average incidence in the United States increased with age until a peak occurred between 20 and 25 years of age. During the past quarter century, the incidence of Hodgkin lymphoma has declined in all age groups below age 20 years and increased in 20- to 29-year-olds. In Fig. 8.2, the incidence of Hodgkin lymphoma as a function of age is compared with non-Hodgkin and other lymphomas. The early age peak of Hodgkin lymphoma is contrasted with a steady increase in non-Hodgkin and other lymphomas.

8.2.1.2 Gender-Specific Incidence

The incidence of Hodgkin lymphoma in the period 1975–2000 was higher in females than males in the 15- to 19-year age group. In all older age groups the reverse

Table 8.1 Incidence of Hodgkin lymphoma in persons younger than 30 years of age in the United States, 1975–2000. *SEER* Surveillance, Epidemiology and End Results, *na* not available

Age at diagnosis (years)	<5	5–9	10–14	15–19	20–24	25–29
United States population, year 2000 census (in millions)	19.2	20.6	20.5	20.2	19.0	19.4
Hodgkin lymphoma						
Average incidence per million, 1975–2000, SEER	0.5	4.1	13.3	36.6	49.9	49.8
Average annual percent change in incidence, 1975–2000, SEER	na	−2.3%	−0.6%	−0.4%	0.2%	1.0%
Estimated incidence per million, year 2000, United States	na	2.5	12.2	34.7	51.3	55.3
Estimated number of persons diagnosed, year 2000, United States	10	84	273	702	973	1,072

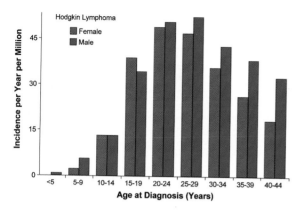

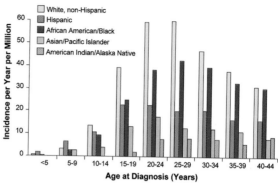

Figure 8.3

Incidence of Hodgkin lymphoma as a function of gender; United States SEER 1975–2000

Figure 8.4

Incidence of Hodgkin lymphoma as a function of race/ethnicity; United States SEER 1975–2000

was true, with the male:female ratio reaching nearly 2:1 by age 40 years (Fig. 8.3).

8.2.1.3 Racial/Ethnic Differences in Incidence

Figure 8.4 shows the racial/ethnic differences in the incidence of Hodgkin lymphoma among the young. Non-Hispanic whites had by far the greatest incidence among 15- to 29-year-olds, followed by African Americans/blacks, Hispanics, Asians/Pacific Islanders, and American Indians/Alaska Natives. The range in incidence of Hodgkin lymphoma according to race/ethnicity varied nearly tenfold in the 15- to 29-year age group. Above age 30 years, the incidence of Hodgkin lymphoma among whites and African Americans/blacks converged, but both races/ethnicities remained twofold or higher above the others. The higher incidence among white non-Hispanics in the adolescent and young adult group has been attributed to higher socioeconomic status [4] (cf. Section 8.3).

8.2.1.4 Trends in Incidence

The average annual percent change (AAPC) in incidence from 1975 to 1999 is shown in Fig. 8.5 for Hodgkin and non-Hodgkin lymphoma. Whereas non-Hodgkin lymphoma was reported to increase in the

United States in all age groups, Hodgkin lymphoma had an age-dependent pattern in incidence trend. In Hodgkin lymphoma, only those 30–44 years of age demonstrated a statistically significant increase in incidence; in patients over 45 years of age, a statistically significant decrease in incidence was seen (Fig. 8.5, yellow bars). The increase in Hodgkin lymphoma occurred predominantly in females (Fig. 8.6).

8.3 Etiology/Risk Factors

Evidence suggests that Hodgkin lymphoma represents several disease entities over the age spectrum, with different etiological factors for different age groups. Children acquire Hodgkin lymphoma at an earlier age in developing countries than in developed countries, and commonly show Epstein-Barr virus (EBV) genomic sequences in their Reed-Sternberg cells [5, 6]. The incidence of Hodgkin lymphoma in developed countries peaks in the adolescent and young adult years, and again in older adults [7]. This reflects the bimodal peak first noted by McMahon [2]. The increased risk of developing Hodgkin lymphoma at an early age has been linked to a higher socioeconomic status and standard of living during childhood, including factors such as low housing density, high

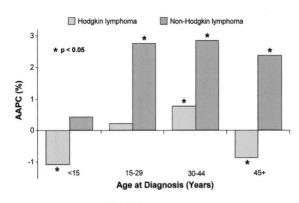

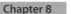

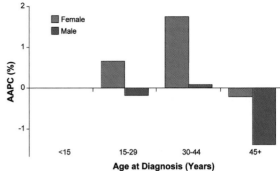

Figure 8.5

Average annual percent change (*AAPC*) in the incidence of non-Hodgkin lymphoma and Hodgkin lymphoma; United States SEER 1975–2000

Figure 8.6

Average annual percent change in the incidence of Hodgkin lymphoma by gender; United States SEER 1975–2000

maternal education, and few older siblings. These conditions may contribute to a delay in exposure to common childhood infections and a subsequent delay in maturation of cell immunity [8]. Yet in the younger (<10 years) and older (>45 years) age groups, the association with higher socioeconomic status is reversed [9]. Among the histologic subtypes of Hodgkin lymphoma, the nodular sclerosing subtype has a more favorable prognosis [10].

While the etiology of Hodgkin lymphoma remains unknown, it has long been thought that an infectious agent plays a role in the cause of the disease. There is growing evidence that the EBV contributes to the etiology of many cases of Hodgkin lymphoma [11]. This relationship, suggested by past medical history of infectious mononucleosis and serologic studies in patients with Hodgkin lymphoma, has been confirmed by immunohistochemistry and molecular biology. Approximately 40–50% of Hodgkin lymphoma cases are associated with the EBV in developed countries [12, 13]. The presence of the EBV genome in Reed-Sternberg cells is associated with the mixed-cellularity subtype [4]. As this subtype occurs infrequently in adolescents and young adults, childhood and older adult cases are more likely to be associated with EBV. Young adults are more commonly diagnosed with nodular sclerosis Hodgkin lymphoma, which is rarely associated with EBV, perhaps signifying a separate disease entity. This

variance in EBV incidence, histological subtypes, and the difference in gender ratios between young adults and children and older adults suggests that Hodgkin lymphoma has different etiologies in different age groups. The exact cause of non-EBV-associated Hodgkin lymphoma remains to be elucidated. Whereas the risk for Hodgkin lymphoma appears to be greater in young children from poorer socioeconomic conditions, the converse is seen for adolescents (Table 8.2). While the evidence points to EBV as a cofactor in the development of Hodgkin lymphoma, the exact relationship of the infection to the subsequent development of a tumor is not completely delineated.

The incidence of Hodgkin lymphoma is greatly increased in children with certain immunodeficiency disorders, specifically ataxia-telangiectasia, Wiskott-Aldrich syndrome, and Bloom syndrome. Given the broad spectrum of underlying genetic defects associated with these disorders and their association with the mixed-cellularity subtype, severely impaired immunity may be a likely etiology with consequent enhanced susceptibility to EBV.

Genetic susceptibility is also a factor for adolescents and young adults. The risk of developing Hodgkin lymphoma is significantly higher for those with relatives with the disease; the risk is higher for males than for females, and for siblings than for parents or offspring [14]. Familial clustering of Hodgkin lymphoma suggests a genetic predisposition. Identical twins of young adults with Hodgkin lymphoma are 100 times more likely to develop Hodgkin lymphoma than fraternal twins, supporting a genetic component to the development of Hodgkin lymphoma in young adulthood [15].

Adults with Hodgkin lymphoma are more likely to have children who develop the disease at a younger age, particulary during adolescence and young adulthood [16].

In patients with human immunodeficiency virus (HIV) infection, there is an increase in the incidence of both Hodgkin and non-Hodkgin lymphoma [17, 18]. Other risks associated with the development of Hodgkin lymphoma in this age group are a history of autoimmune disorder, a family history of cancer/hematopoietic disorder, and Jewish ethnicity [15, 16].

8.4 Pathology/Molecular Genetics

Hodgkin lymphoma is characterized histologically by the presence of Reed-Sternberg or Hodgkin cells, large, clonal, multinucleated cells that are B-cell in origin derived from a germinal center. The background environment consists of a pleomorphic inflammatory infiltrate comprised predominantly of lymphocytes. The World Health Organization modification of the Revised European-American Lymphoma classification is currently used for the histological classification of Hodgkin lymphoma, which is divided into classical and nodular lymphocyte-predominant Hodgkin lymphoma [19]. Classical Hodgkin lymphoma is divided into four subtypes, nodular sclerosis, mixed cellularity, lymphocyte rich, and lymphocyte depletion. Adoles-

Table 8.2 Epidemiology of Hodgkin lymphoma according to age at diagnosis. Adapted from Herbertson and Hancock (2005) [33]. *EBV* Epstein-Barr Virus

	Children <16 years	Adolescents 16–19 years	Adults >19 years
Histology	45% nodular sclerosis, 35% mixed cellularity In developed countries predominantly nodular sclerosis In undeveloped countries predominantly mixed cellularity/lymphocyte depleted	80% nodular sclerosis, 10–20% mixed cellularity	Nodular sclerosis peaks in young adults and declines with increasing age
EBV positivity	Increased incidence in developed and undeveloped countries Higher rate in mixed cellularity	Minority of nodular sclerosis in developed countries	Minority of young adults Majority of >50 years
Gender	Male:female 2:1 in Europe and America Male:female 3.5:1 in Asia	Male:female 1:1	Nodular sclerosis more common in females between 20 and 24 years in the West More common in males worldwide
Geographical area	Higher incidence rates in undeveloped countries Rare in developed countries	Peak incidence in developed countries	Second peak in older adults in developed countries
Socioeconomic status	Higher risks for lower status and large families	More common in high status urban areas	Twofold increased risk with higher status and education level

cents exhibit a higher incidence of the nodular sclerosis subtype as compared to younger children and adults (Table 8.3). This is correlated with the high incidence of mediastinal involvement in adolescents, similar to what is seen in young adults.

In the International Classification of Childhood Cancer (ICCC) [20], lymphoma is category II and Hodgkin lymphoma is category II(a). Hodgkin lymphoma in the ICCC corresponds to International Classification of Disease Morphology codes 9650–9667 and includes Hodgkin paragranuloma, Hodgkin granuloma, and Hodgkin sarcoma.

8.5 Symptoms and Clinical Signs

Hodgkin lymphoma is variable in its presentation in children and adolescents. Painless supraclavicular and/or cervical lymphadenopathy are the most common findings on presentation (80%). Axillary and inguinal lymph node enlargement is uncommon in children (15% and 10%, respectively in a French experience). Approximately 60% of pediatric patients present with mediastinal involvement at diagnosis, the incidence of which is significantly higher in adolescents compared to younger children, and is correlated with the higher incidence of nodular sclerosis histology observed in adolescents (Table 8.3). Mediastinal adenopathy may result in symptoms related to compression of the airway or vasculature structures, such as cough, dyspnea at rest or with exercise, or orthopnea. The presence of either hepatomegaly or splenomegaly at presentation is infrequent. Approximately one-third of patients initially have systemic symptoms (called "B" symptoms) including fever, night sweats, or weight loss due to chemokines released by the Hodgkin cells. Pruritus, another symptom of Hodgkin lymphoma, is relatively uncommon in children.

8.6 Diagnostic Testing

8.6.1 Hematology

Screening laboratory studies may include a complete blood count and measurement of the erythrocyte sedimentation rate (ESR). Anemia due to poor utilization of iron may be seen, particularly in patients with a high tumor burden. Additional causes may include mild chronic red cell destruction, or occasionally, a Coombs-positive hemolytic anemia. An elevated ESR is correlated with stage and the presence of systemic symptoms; its prognostic importance was recognized early and highlighted in multivariate analyses. Eosinophilia occurs in only 15% of patients, whereas neutrophilia is found frequently. Lymphopenia is often observed in advanced disease. Bone marrow involvement is not common (found in only 3% of subjects in

Table 8.3 Histological pattern, stage distribution and mediastinal involvement according to age (data from the French studies MDH82 and MDH90 [21])

	Total	<7 years	8–11 years	>12 years
Number	677	121	196	360
Histological subtype				
Nodular sclerosis	52%	27%	45%	64%
Mixed cellularity	28%	44%	31%	20%
Clinical stage				
I–II	63%	73%	60%	62%
III–IV	37%	27%	40%	38%
Mediastinal involvement	62%	36%	54%	76%

the French MDH82 study [21]). Bone marrow biopsy is the definitive method of detection of bone marrow involvement and should be performed in patients with advanced-stage disease, B symptoms, abnormal blood counts, or local bone involvement.

8.6.2 Imaging

Radiographic imaging by computed tomography scan is the preferred modality for determination of the sites of nodal and extranodal disease in the neck, chest, and abdomen. Gallium imaging was the standard method of detection for many years; however, this imaging has been replaced recently by positron emission tomography, which is a more sensitive imaging modality for Hodgkin lymphoma.

8.6.3 Surgery

The definitive diagnostic approach for detection of Hodgkin lymphoma is biopsy sampling of the largest accessible lymph node.

8.6.4 Clinical Staging

The Ann Arbor classification is currently used worldwide to stage Hodgkin lymphoma (Table 8.4). Stage is subclassified into two categories, A or B. Patients with asymptomatic disease are classified in category A. Patients in category B may present with any of the following symptoms: unexplained loss of more than 10% of their body weight in the 6 months prior to diagnosis, unexplained fever (>38°C for more than 3 days), or drenching night sweats. Subclassification E represents involvement of an extranodal site contiguous to the known nodal site. Stage I disease denotes involvement of a single nodal region, which in the majority of cases is the cervical region (85%). Inguinal node involvement is noted in 10% of the cases. Isolated axillary and mediastinal involvement is rare (2%). Stage II represents involvement of two or more lymph node regions on the same side of the diaphragm, which in two-thirds may comprise cervical and mediastinal involvement, in 20% bilateral cervical involvement, and in 4% cervical and axillary involvement. Only 5% of patients with stage II disease present in subdiaphragmatic sites. Stage III includes involvement above and below the diaphragm. Stage IV disease denotes metastatic disease at extranodal sites including lung involvement (occurring most frequently in 73% of cases), bone marrow (20%), liver (18%), bone (15%), and kidney (4%). Adolescents and children above 8 years of age tend to have more advanced stages than younger children.

Table 8.4 Ann Arbor staging classification of Hodgkin Lymphoma

Stage I	Involvement of a single lymph node region (I) or of a single extralymphatic organ or site (IE)
Stage II	Involvement of two or more lymph node regions on the same side of the diaphragm (II) or localized involvement of an extralymphatic organ or site and of one or more lymph node regions on the same side of the diaphragm (IIE)
Stage III	Involvement of lymph node regions on both sides of the diaphragm (III), which may also he accompanied by localized involvement of an extralymphatic organ or site (IIIE) or by involvement of the spleen (HIS) or both (HISE)
Stage IV	Diffuse or disseminated involvement of one or more extralymphatic organs or tissues with or without associated lymph node enlargement
Each stage is subdivided into A and B categories	
A	No systemic symptoms
B	Unexplained weight loss greater than 10% of the body weight in the previous 6 months and/or unexplained fever with temperatures above 38°C and/or night sweats

8.7 Treatment/Management

8.7.1. General Treatment Consideration

Hodgkin lymphoma is highly curable in the adolescent and young adult patient population. The challenge faced by oncologists today is to find the balance between maximizing cure and minimizing the late effects in this population. Adolescents with Hodgkin lymphoma are not treated as a distinct patient population and are routinely placed on either pediatric or adult treatment regimens, without a strong foundation for the decision. Several studies, however, have reported a poorer outcome in adolescent patients treated on adult clinical trials.

Salient differences exist currently between adult and pediatric treatment strategies for Hodgkin lymphoma. The adult treatment approach stratifies stage into early (stages I and II) and advanced (stages III and IV) disease. Adolescents treated on adult regimens for advanced-stage Hodgkin lymphoma will most commonly receive six cycles of doxorubicin + bleomycin + vinblastine + dacarbazine (ABVD) chemotherapy alone rather than the combined-modality therapy used in the pediatric approach, which alternates an alkylating agent regimen with ABVD in order to decrease the ABVD-related risk of cardiopulmonary toxicity. Until recently, treatment for favorable disease presentation (stages I and II and the absence of B symptoms and nodal bulk) in both children and adults has relied on radiation alone, a practice that originated in the 1950s. The most common method was to employ mantle field irradiation (including the neck, chest, and axilla nodes) with doses of 40–44 Gy followed by inverted Y irradiation to the spleen, para-aortic and pelvic nodes. The use of radiation therapy as a single-therapeutic modality has gradually declined given that the initial effectiveness of extended-field, high-dose radiotherapy is counterbalanced by unsatisfactory risk of relapse, late side effects, and poor quality of life, especially in children and adolescents. The introduction of combined-modality therapy allows for dose and volume reduction of the radiation field and is now the preferred treatment for favorable Hodgkin lymphoms in both adults and children.

Chemotherapy alone for localized disease has been used in developing countries with some success [22].

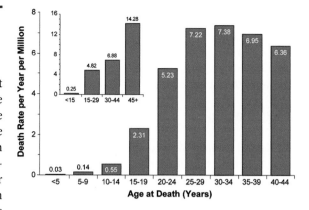

Figure 8.7

National mortality for Hodgkin lymphoma; United States SEER, 1975–2000

Risk-adapted therapeutic strategies have been used in the pediatric trials that employ variations of combined-modality therapy dependent upon stage, symptoms, and gender. Prognostic factors specifically for children and young adults treated with combined-modality therapy have been developed [23]. A series of 328 patients, aged 2–20 years, were analyzed and five pretreatment factors were found to correlate by multivariate analysis with inferior disease-free survival; male sex, stage IIB, IIIB, or IV disease, bulk mediastinal disease, hemoglobin <11 g/dl, and white blood cell count of >13,500/ul. Response to therapy was also shown to be a predictor of outcome. Age was not a significant factor in the comparison of patients greater or less than 14 years of age. In other studies, nodular sclerosis histology and the presence of B symptoms correlated with an inferior outcome [24]. Based upon these findings, tailored risk-adapted strategies have been explored. These strategies have incorporated stratification by stage into three risk groups: (1) early/favorable, including localized disease involving less than three or four nodal regions in the absence of B symptoms, bulky disease, or extranodal extension, (2) intermediate/localized unfavorable, defined as localized disease involving less than or equal to three or four nodal regions in the presence of bulky lymphadenopathy, and (3) advanced/unfavorable, which includes

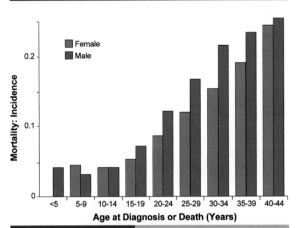

Figure 8.8

Ratio of national mortality to SEER incidence for Hodgkin lymphoma, by gender; United States SEER, 1975–2000

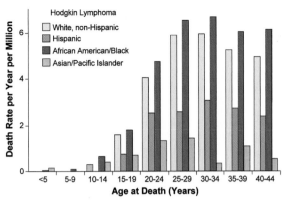

Figure 8.9

National mortality for Hodgkin lymphoma by race/ethnicity; United States SEER, 1975–2000

patients with stage II disease who experience constitutional symptoms of fever or weight loss, and patients with stage III or IV disease. It is believed that each pediatric patient presents with a unique combination of factors that should be evaluated in determining optimal treatment. Issues such as gender- and age-related susceptibilities to treatment toxicities have also been considered in the development of therapeutic strategies to minimize late effects.

Accumulating experience with risk-adapted approaches suggest that survival is excellent for all risk groups, and that low-risk patients may not require adjuvant radiation therapy [25]. This finding is suggested by a large recent adult study that indicates that consolidation radiation therapy increased the overall survival, especially in the subgroup of patients with B symptoms, stage III–IV disease, and patients younger than 15 years [26]. The trials that show no benefit of a consolidation radiation therapy for advanced disease were those using eight cycles of chemotherapy [alternating mechlorethamine + vincristine + procarbazine + prednisolone (MOPP), and ABVD or "hybrid" MOPP/doxorubicin + bleomycin + vinblastine (ABV) or bleomycin + etoposide + doxorubicin + cyclophosphamide + vincristine + procarbazine + prednisolone (BEACOPP), or doxorubicin + bleomycin + vinblastine + procarbazine + prednisolone (ABVPP). It is likely that the patients in com-

plete remission after 3–6 cycles of chemotherapy received some sort of consolidation therapy in the form of additional chemotherapy, obviating the benefit of radiation. However, such strategies lead to high cumulative doses of chemotherapy and the risk of male infertility due to the use of alkylating agents, cardiomyopathy from anthracyclines, pulmonary fibrosis from bleomycin, and of secondary leukemia and lung cancer after alkylating agents and etoposide.

8.7.2 Specific Treatment Trials

There have been no prospective randomized trials for adolescents and young adults with Hodgkin lymphoma per se. It has been shown that adolescents experience disease outcomes superior to older adults; however, it remains inconclusive whether adolescents experience a similar prognosis as do younger children where 5-year event-free survival is greater than 90%. A recent review of 79 treatment trials published in the past 15 years revealed only four major studies evaluating the outcome of the adolescent subgroup. Two of these trials reveal a significant difference in treatment outcome compared to the entire study population. These studies are summarized in Table 8.5.

The Stanford, Dana Farber, and St. Jude teams treated a selected group of patients (clinical stage I and

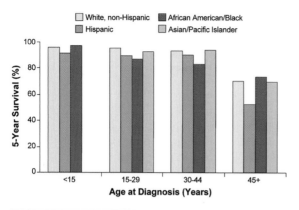

Figure 8.10

Five-year survival rate for Hodgkin lymphoma by race/ethnicity; United States SEER, 1975–2000

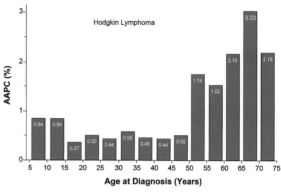

Figure 8.12

Average annual percent change in the 5-year survival rate for Hodgkin lymphoma by gender; United States SEER, 1975–2000

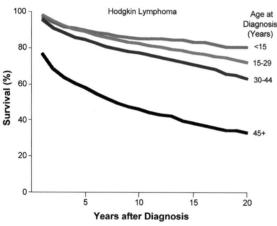

Figure 8.11

Survival rates for Hodgkin lymphoma as a function of years after diagnosis for different age groups: <15 years, 15–29 years, 30–44 years, and 45+ years; United States SEER, 1975–2000

II, without bulky disease or B symptoms, representing one-third of the whole cohort of children with Hodgkin disease) with four cycles of vinblastine + adriamycin + methotrexate + prednisone (VAMP) before involved-field radiation. Five-year survival and event-

free survival were respectively 100% and 97%. Little difference was seen in outcome on the basis of age (cut point being 13 years; not statistically significant) [27]. The German Austrian Pediatric Oncology Group tailored the length of the chemotherapy to the extent of the disease by using two cycles of vincristine + procarbazine + prednisone + doxorubicin (OPPA) for stages IA-IB-IIA, two cycles of OPPA + two cycles cyclophosphamide + vincristine + procarbazine + prednisone (COPP) for stages IIB-IIIA, and two cycles of OPPA + four cycles of COPP for stages IIIB and IV. In 1990, treatment was modified to reduce the amount of procarbazine administered to males with two cycles of OPPA replaced by two cycles of vincristine + etoposide + prednisone + doxorubicin (OEPA). The results of this study demonstrated that there was no difference in outcome according to gender or age (grouped by ages: less than 10 years, from 10 to 15 years and older than 15 years) [28]. The French Pediatric Group introduced a novel combination devoid of both alkylating agents and anthracyclines consisting of vinblastine + bleomycin + etoposide + prednisone (VBEP) followed by 20 Gy of radiotherapy for good responders. Poor responders to the VBEP regimen were given OPPA as second-line chemotherapy. Event-free survival was 96% among patients under 9 years of age at diagnosis compared with 87% in older children, but this differ-

Table 8.5 Publications reporting outcome for adolescent subgroup. *ChlVPP* Chlorambucil + vinblastine + procarbazine + prednisolone, *RT* radiation therapy, *MOPP* mechlorethamine + vincristine + procarbazine + prednisolone, *ABVD* doxorubicin + bleomycin + vinblastine + dacarbazine, *OEPA* vincristine + etoposide + prednisone + doxorubicin, *COPP* cyclophosphamide + vincristine + procarbazine + prednisone, *IFRT* involved-field radiation therapy, *OPPA* vincristine + procarbazine + prednisone + doxorubicin, *VAMP* vinblastine + doxorubicin + methotrexate + prednisone, *ABV* doxorubicin + bleomycin + vinblastine, *CVPP* cyclophosphamide + vinblastine + procarbazine + prednisone, *G-SCF* granulocyte stem-cell factor, *DFS* disease-free survival, *OS* overall survival, *EFS* event-free survival, *CMT* combined-modality therapy, *CT* chemotherapy alone

Reference number	Primary population	N	No. of adolescents	Treatment	Stage	Overall outcome	Adolescent outcome	Analysis
18	Adult	229	74 between age 16 and 26 years	ChlVPP ± RT	I–IV	5-year DFS/OS: 74.4%/73.1%	5-year DFS/OS: 82.4%/86.0%	Age 16–26 years associated with significantly superior OS (p=0.030)
21	Pediatric	179	103 between age 14 and 20 years	8 cycles MOPP-ABVD; ± total nodal RT	IIB–IV	EFS/OS: CMT: 80%/87% CT: 79%/96%	EFS: 72%	Age greater than 13 years associated with significantly worse EFS (p=0.006)
17	Pediatric	578	138 between age 15 and 18 years	Males: 2 cycles OEPA + 2 or 4 cycles COPP, followed by 20–25 Gy IFRT Females: 2 cycles OPPA + 2 or 4 cycles COPP, followed by 20–25 Gy IFRT.	I–IV	5-year EFS/OS: 91%/98%	5-year EFS/OS: 92%/97%	Age not significant factor in treatment outcome
3	Pediatric	110	56 between age 13 and 20 years	4 cycles VAMP + 15–25.5 Gy IFRT	I–II favorable	5-year EFS/OS: 93%/99%	5-year EFS/OS: 92%/100%	Age not significant factor in treatment outcome
2	Pediatric	72	40 between age 15 and 19 years	3–6 cycles MOPP or 3 cycles CVPP followed by 35–40 Gy RT or 40 Gy IFRT	IA–IIB	5-year EFS/OS 87.6%/91.6%	12-year EFS/OS: 88%/92.4%	Age not significant factor in treatment outcome
14	Pediatric	829	328 between age 15 and 19 years	4–6 cycles COPP/ABV or 2 cycles intensive multidrug chemo-therapy with G-SCF followed by +/- LD-IFRT	I–IV	3-year EFS/OS 87%/95%		

ence did not reach significance and age was not a prognostic variable in multivariate analysis [21].

A retrospective outcome analysis performed by Yung et al. reviewed this controversy surrounding treatment for adolescents with Hodgkin lymphoma [29]. A review of the British National Lymphoma Investigation database of 209 adolescents, aged 15–17 years, treated on previous adult regimens for Hodgkin lymphoma between 1970 and 1997, showed a 5-year event-free survival of 50% for all stages combined. This was compared to other pediatric trials with the patient populations experiencing between 79% and 86% event-free survival. They concluded that the poor outcome in adolescents was attributed to treatment on adult protocols rather than the risk-adapted combined-modality regimens used in the pediatric setting.

8.8 Outcome

8.8.1 Mortality

Mortality in 15- to 29-year-olds with Hodgkin lymphoma during the time period 1975–1999 was 4.82 deaths per year per million (Fig. 8.7; inset). The death rate doubled for 20- to 24-year-olds when compared to 15- to 19-year-olds; rates for 25- to 29-year-olds reached nearly the maximum, as seen in Fig. 8.7.

For Hodgkin lymphoma, a male excess in mortality occurred over age 15 years (Fig. 8.8), and the comparison with incidence showed that there were more males than females dying of the disease between 15 and 40 years of age than expected from the incidence pattern (Fig. 8.3). This analysis suggests that male gender was an adverse prognostic factor in patients between 15 and 40 years of age. Females are known to present with more favorable histology and lesser stage disease [4].

Analysis of Hodgkin lymphoma mortality by race/ethnicity as a function of age indicates that African Americans/blacks had the highest death rate for those over 20 years of age (Fig. 8.9). When compared with incidence patterns (Fig. 8.4), the excess death rate among African Americans/blacks was not explained by differences in incidence.

8.8.2 Survival

Since 1990, there have been no significant differences in 5-year survival rates among whites of either Hispanic or non-Hispanic ethnicity, African Americans/blacks, or Asians/Pacific Islanders with Hodgkin lymphoma (Fig. 8.10). The suggestion from comparisons of death rates to incidence that show a deficit among African Americans/blacks applies to the period 1975–1998. It appears that this racial inequity may have been overcome by 1990.

Survival curves for Hodgkin lymphoma indicate that 15- to-29-year-old patients did not fare as well as younger patients, with a continued fall-off in mortality and no evidence for a plateau (Fig. 8.11).

The AAPC in 5-year survival rates from 1975 to 1997 for Hodgkin lymphoma are shown in Fig. 8.12. As suggested by the mortality versus incidence comparisons described above, the least amount of progress occurred in 15- to 50-year-olds with Hodgkin lymphoma (Fig. 8.12).

8.9 Follow-up/Late Effects

Adolescents treated for Hodgkin lymphoma experience a higher incidence of secondary complications from treatment, including secondary malignancies, compared to adult patients [30]. Many patients survive for decades after treatment, allowing a greater window of observation of the late damaging effects of chemotherapy and radiation. Young adults do not suffer the radiation-induced growth retardation observed in children who were not fully grown up at the time of therapy. However, children and adolescents share the adult experience of an increased mortality rate related to radiation and anthracycline-induced cardiotoxicity [31] and secondary radiation-induced solid tumors [32]. Studies have shown that girls who are between the ages of 10 and 16 years at the time of radiation treatment are at greater risk of breast cancer than younger patients. In these cases, it is hypothesized that the radiation therapy was delivered during a period of breast tissue proliferation. This finding is confounded by the fact that the female survivors of Hodgkin lymphoma who were older at their childhood cancer diagnosis, were at higher risk because the overall breast cancer risk increases with age. Regardless, this terribly high cumulative incidence of secondary breast cancer (13.9% at age 40 years and 20.1% at age 45 years) is a matter of concern and calls for limitation of the radiation fields and doses. MOPP was the first effective systemic therapy for patients with Hodgkin lymphoma, and treatment with this regimen resulted in late effects including gonadal damage in males and increased risk of secondary myelodysplastic syndrome/acute myelogenous leukemia due to the use of alkylating agents. In an effort to reduce these effects, a variety of MOPP derivatives has been developed. The introduction of ABVD provided improved disease-free survival without leukemogenic and gonadotoxic effects. ABVD-associated late effects include cardiomyopathy, which is attributable to anthracyclines, and lung fibrosis, which is caused by bleomycin. Thoracic radiation amplifies these toxicities.

The key to limiting toxicity in current approaches of this disease is to adapt the intensity of the therapy to the risk factors of the patient. Toward this goal, combined-modality, risk-adapted therapies have explored the reduction in dose, intensity, and field of irradiation, as well as a reduction in the cumulative dose of cytotoxic chemotherapy.

8.10 Conclusions

Adolescents and young adults with Hodgkin lymphoma represent a unique patient population with this disease. They experience the highest incidence rates of any age group, distinctive pathological characteristics including an elevated incidence of nodular sclerosis subtype, and suspected etiologies that differ from that of adults and younger children.

Hodgkin lymphoma accounts for 12% of all cancers in 15- to 29-year-olds in the United States during the past quarter century. The incidence of Hodgkin lymphoma as a function of age is bimodal, with a peak at between 20 and 25 years of age and a second peak between 75 and 80 years of age.

In the period 1975–2000, females had a higher incidence of Hodgkin lymphoma in the 15- to 19-year age group. Males had a higher incidence of all lymphomas in all other age groups. The incidence of Hodgkin lymphoma in the adolescent and young adult age group was highest among white non-Hispanics.

Factors associated with a high standard of living may contribute to delayed exposure to childhood infections and subsequent delay in maturation of cell immunity. EBV infection acquired in adolescence, with subsequent development of infectious mononucleosis, may increase the risk of Hodgkin lymphoma in adolescents and young adults. A history of autoimmune disorder, family history of malignancy/hematopoietic disorder, and Jewish ethnicity are all risk factors for Hodgkin lymphoma. HIV infection also predisposes to Hodgkin lymphoma.

Males had higher mortality from Hodkgin lymphoma than females at all ages above 10 years. Mortality for all Hodgkin lymphoma was comparable for 15- to 19-year-old whites and African Americans/blacks, but was higher for African Americans/blacks at all ages above 20 years. Of all age groups, 15- to 49-year-olds with Hodgkin lymphoma have had the least improvement in survival during the past quarter century. Five-year survival for Hodgkin lymphoma in the 15- to 29-year age group was similar for all racial/ethnic groups.

Adolescents and young adults experience higher rates of toxicities and malignancies secondary to treatment than do older adult patients. Currently, adolescents are treated on either pediatric or adult treatment regimens, which differ in risk stratification and their use of radiation and chemotherapy. The goal of modern therapy for adolescents and young adults with Hodgkin lymphoma is to improve disease outcome while minimizing dangerous late effects.

As past treatment protocols were not designed specifically for adolescents, this population is consequently treated either on adult or pediatric treatment regimens, with similar outcomes for disease control. Whether the late effects of therapy differ according to adult vs. pediatric approaches has not been adequately studied. Current trials are focused on tailored regimens based upon prognostic risk factors in an effort to maintain high cure rates while reducing the damaging late effects of treatment. Clinical treatment trials focusing on optimal treatment for adolescents and young adults with Hodgkin lymphoma are needed.

References

1. Bleyer WA, O'Leary M, Barr R, Ries LAG (eds) (2006) Cancer Epidemiology in Older Adolescents and Young Adults 15 to 29 Years of Age, Including SEER Incidence and Survival, 1975–2000. National Cancer Institute, NIH Pub. No. 06-5767. Bethesda, MD

2. McMahon B (1957) Epidemiological evidence on the nature of Hodgkin Disease. Cancer 10:1045–1054

3. O'Leary M, Sheaffer JW, Keller FG, et al (2006) Lymphomas and reticuloendothelial neoplasms. In: Bleyer WA, O'Leary M, Barr R, Ries LAG (eds) Cancer Epidemiology in Older Adolescents and Young Adults 15 to 29 Years of Age, including SEER Incidence and Survival, 1975–2000. National Cancer Institute, NIH Pub. No. 06-5767. Bethesda, MD

4. Mueller NE, Grufferman S (1999) The epidemiology of Hodgkin Disease. In: Mauch PM, Armitage JO, Diehl V, Hoppe RT, Weiss LM (eds) Hodgkin Disease. Lippincott Williams & Wilkins, Philadelphia, pp 61–78

5. Sleckman BG, Mauch PM, Ambinder RF, et al (1998) Epstein-Barr virus in Hodgkin disease: correlation of risk factors and disease characteristics with molecular evidence of viral infection. Cancer Epidemiol Biomarkers Prev 7:1117–1121

6. Glaser SL, Lin RJ, Stewart SL, et al (1997) Epstein-Barr virus-associated Hodgkin disease: epidemiologic characteristics in international data. Int J Cancer 70:375–382

7. Chang ET, Montgomery SM, Richiardi L, et al (2004) Number of siblings and risk of Hodgkin lymphoma. Cancer Epidemiol Biomarkers Prev 13:1236–1243

8. Chang ET, Zheng T, Weir EG, et al (2004) Childhood social environment and Hodgkin lymphoma: new findings from a population-based case-control study. Cancer Epidemiol Biomarkers Prev 13:1361–1370

9. Ambinder RF, Weiss LM (1999) Association of Epstein-Barr virus with Hodgkin disease. In: Mauch PM, Armitage JO, Diehl V, Hoppe RT, Weiss LM (eds) Hodgkin Disease. Lippincott Williams & Wilkins, Philadelphia, pp 79–100

10. Henderson BE, Dworsky R, Pike MC, et al (1979) Risk factors for nodular sclerosis and other types of Hodgkin Disease. Cancer Res 39:4507–4511

11. Jarrett RF (2003) Risk factors for Hodgkin lymphoma by EBV status and significance of detection of EBV genomes in serum of patients with EBV-associated Hodgkin lymphoma. Leuk Lymphoma 44:S27–32

12. Hjalgrim H, Askling J, Rostgaard K, et al (2003) Characteristics of Hodgkin lymphoma after infectious mononucleosis. N Engl J Med 349:1324–1332

13. Thorley-Lawson DA, Gross A (2004) Persistence of the Epstein-Barr virus and the origins of associated lymphomas. N Engl J Med 350:1328–1337

14. Goldin LR, Pfeiffer RM, Gridley G, et al (2004) Familial aggregation of Hodgkin lymphoma and related tumors. Cancer 100:1902–1908

15. Mack TM, Cozen W, Shibata DK, et al (1995) Concordance for Hodgkin disease in identical twins suggesting genetic susceptibility to the young-adult form of the disease. N Engl J Med 332:413–418

16. Staratschek-Jox A, Shugart YY, Strom SS, et al (2002) Genetic susceptibility to Hodgkin lymphoma and to secondary cancer: workshop report. Ann Oncol 13:30–33

17. Calza L, Manfredi R, Colangeli V, et al (2003) Hodgkin disease in the setting of human immunodeficiency virus infection. Scand J Infect Dis 35:136–141

18. Westergaard T, Melbye M, Pedersen JB, et al (1997) Birth order, sibship size and risk of Hodgkin disease in children and young adults: a population-based study of 31 million person-years. Int J Cancer 72:977–981

19. Harris NL (1999) Hodgkin lymphomas: classification, diagnosis, and grading. Semin Hematol 36:220–232

20. Steliarova-Foucher E, Stiller C, Lacour B, Kaatsch P (2005) International Classification of Childhood Cancer, third edition. Cancer 103:1457–1467

21. Landman-Parker J, Pacquement H, Leblanc T, et al (2000) Localized childhood Hodgkin disease: response-adapted chemotherapy with etoposide, bleomycin, vinblastine, and prednisone before low-dose radiation therapy – results of the French Society of Pediatric Oncology Study MDH90. J Clin Oncol 18:1500–1507

22. Lobo-Sanahuja F, Garcia I, Barrantes JC, et al (1994) Pediatric Hodgkin disease in Costa Rica: twelve years experience of primary treatment by chemotherapy alone, without staging laparotomy. Med Pediatr Oncol 22:398–403

23. Smith M, Gurney J, Ries L (1999) Cancer among adolescents 15–19 years old. In: Ries LAG (ed) Cancer Incidence and Survival among Children and Adolescents: United States SEER Program 1975–1995. National Cancer Institute, Bethesda, MD, pp 157–164

24. Selby P, Pate P, Milan S, et al (1990) ChlVPP combination chemotherapy for Hodgkin disease: long-term results. Br J Cancer 62:279–285

25. Nachman JB, Sposto R, Herzog P, et al (2002) Randomized comparison of low-dose involved-field radiotherapy and no radiotherapy for children with Hodgkin disease who achieve a complete response to chemotherapy. J Clin Oncol 20:3765–3771

26. Laskar S, Gupta T, Vimal S, et al (2004) Consolidation radiation after complete remission in Hodgkin disease following six cycles of doxorubicin, bleomycin, vinblastine, and dacarbazine chemotherapy: is there a need? J Clin Oncol 22:62–68

27. Donaldson SS, Hudson MM, Lamborn KR, et al (2002) VAMP and low-dose, involved-field radiation for children and adolescents with favorable, early-stage Hodgkin disease: results of a prospective clinical trial. J Clin Oncol 20:3081–3087

28. Schellong G, Potter R, Bramswig J, et al (1999) High cure rates and reduced long-term toxicity in pediatric Hodgkin disease: the German-Austrian multicenter trial DAL-HD-90. The German-Austrian Pediatric Hodgkin Disease Study Group. J Clin Oncol 17:3736–3744

29. Yung L, Smith P, Hancock BW, et al (2004) Long-term outcome in adolescents with Hodgkin lymphoma: poor results using regimens designed for adults. Leuk Lymphoma 45:1579–1585

30. Ng AK, Bernardo MVP, Weller E, et al (2002) Second malignancy after Hodgkin Disease treated with radiation therapy with or without chemotherapy: long-term risks and risk factors. Blood 100:1989–1996

31. Hancock SL, Donaldson SS, Hoppe RT (1993) Cardiac disease following treatment of Hodgkin disease in children and adolescents. J Clin Oncol 11:1208–1215

32. Bhatia S, Yasui Y, Robison LL, et al (2003) High risk of subsequent neoplasms continues with extended follow-up of childhood Hodgkin disease: report from the Late Effects Study Group. J Clin Oncol 21:4386–4394

33. Herbertson R, Hancock BW (2005) Hodgkin lymphoma in adolescents. Cancer Treatment Rev 31:339–360

Non-Hodgkin Lymphoma

Catherine Patte · Archie Bleyer ·
Mitchell S. Cairo

Contents

9.1 Introduction

Non-Hodgkin lymphoma is a heterogeneous group of lymphoid malignancies. The overall incidence and frequency of the different histological subgroups varies according to age at diagnosis. Adolescence is at the junction of childhood and adulthood in the sense that, in adolescents, the lymphomas frequent in children and rare in adults may still be seen (the Burkitt and the lymphoblastic types), but the incidence of the large cell subtypes, especially the diffuse large B-cell lymphomas, frequent in adults, increases greatly in young adults (to 30 years of age).

In many countries, the minority of adolescents are referred to pediatric departments where they are generally included in trials, but the majority are referred to adult departments where a minority are registered in trials. So far, there are few data on adolescents and young adults with non-Hodgkin lymphoma. The questions are: is there a difference in results when patients are treated with childhood versus adult non-Hodgkin lymphoma protocols and in their respective departments? If yes, is it related to the type of treatment? Is there a prognostic value of age of onset and treatment with similar therapeutic strategies? Is this related to different biology? In this chapter we will present what is presently known, but many questions are still without answers, which indicates the need for further studies directed specifically toward adolescents and young adults with non-Hodgkin lymphoma.

9.2 Epidemiology

9.2.1 Age-Specific Incidence

The overall incidence of non-Hodgkin lymphoma increases steadily with age (Table 9.1 and Fig. 9.1), in contrast to Hodgkin lymphoma, which peaks in early adulthood, declines in incidence with age, and increases again in late adulthood (Fig. 9.1) [1]. During the past quarter century in the United States, the incidence of non-Hodgkin lymphoma has increased in each age group through to age 30 years (Table 9.1). In 20- to 29-year-olds, the increase was dramatic, averaging 4–19% per year over 25 years. Most of the increase was in the non-Burkitt, non-Hodgkin Lymphoma category II(b), according to the International Classification of Childhood Cancer (ICCC), which was in part due to the human immunodeficiency virus (HIV) epidemic that occurred during the 1980s and early 1990s (Table 9.1). In the 1979–1997 English registry, non-Hodgkin lymphoma represented 7% of all cancers in adolescents, very similar to the corresponding proportion in the United States.

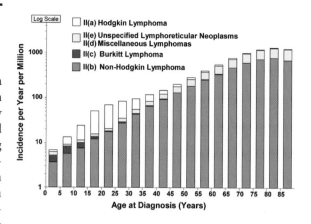

Figure 9.1

Incidence of malignant lymphoma in the United States by age in persons younger than 45 years, according to the International Childhood Cancer Classification (ICCC), United States SEER, 1975–2000

Table 9.1 Incidence of non-Hodgkin lymphoma in persons younger than 30 years of age, United States, 1975–2000. *ICCC* International Classification of Childhood Cancer, *SEER* Surveillance, Epidemiology and End Results, *na* not available

Age at diagnosis (years)	<5	5–9	10–14	15–19	20–24	25–29
United States population, year 2000 census (in millions)	19.176	20.550	20.528	20.220	18.964	19.381
Non-Hodgkin lymphoma, ICCC II(b)						
Average incidence per million, 1975–2000, SEER	3.4	5.4	7.1	11.7	16.5	27.3
Average annual % change in incidence, 1975–2000, SEER	na	0.2%	2.2%	2.3%	3.6%	6.2%
Estimated incidence per million, year 2000, United States	2.8	5.5	8.8	14.3	21.8	39.3
Estimated number of persons diagnosed, year 2000, U.S.	66	110	147	290	413	762
Burkitt and other non-Hodgkin lymphoma, ICCC II(c), II(d), and II(e)						
Average incidence per million, 1975–2000, SEER	2.8	3.7	3.9	3.1	3.6	7.5
Average annual % change in incidence, 1975–2000, SEER	na	–1.0%	–0.7%	1.6%	9.8%	18.5%
Estimated incidence per million, year 2000, United States	1.9	3.2	3.6	3.5	5.6	12.5
Estimated number of persons diagnosed, year 2000, U. S.	54	76	81	72	108	243

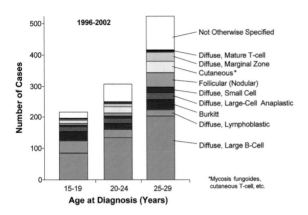

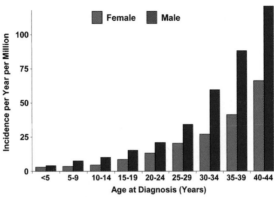

Figure 9.2

Incidence of non-Hodgkin lymphoma in the United States by histologic type; United States SEER, 1992–2000

Figure 9.3

Incidence of non-Hodgkin lymphoma in the United States by gender; United States SEER, 1975–2000

9.2.2 Incidence of Histologic Types

When analyzed according to histologic type of non-Hodgkin lymphoma, the greatest change in the distribution of the subtypes over the 15- to 29-year age span is the appearance of follicular (nodular) lymphoma which, during the period 1992–2002, was virtually nonexistent before age 15 years and increased in relative proportion to 11% among 25- to 29-year-olds (Fig. 9.2). Diffuse small-cell lymphoma also increased, and mantle cell lymphoma made its appearance in 15- to 29-year olds. The incidence of lymphoblastic lymphoma (LL) and Burkitt lymphoma decreased as a function of age from the 15- to 19-year age interval to the 25- to 29-year interval.

The French-American-British (FAB) LMB96 study, a 5-year prospective international study for the treatment of B-cell lymphoma in children and adolescents, was not a population-based registry, but interestingly some differences were observed between the three countries in terms of repartition of the two subgroups of B-cell non-Hodgkin lymphoma. After adjusting for age, diffuse large B-cell lymphoma (DLBCL) was more frequent in the United States than in the European countries, especially in France [2, 3].

9.2.3 Gender-Specific Incidence

Non-Hodgkin lymphoma was more common among males than females for all ages up to 45 years. In non-Burkitt, non-Hodgkin lymphoma (ICCC category IIb), the male:female ratio increased over this age interval to nearly twofold greater in males (Fig. 9.3).

In Burkitt lymphoma, the male predominance is striking, with male:female ratios approaching 6 for the 5- to 14-year and 25- to 44-year age groups (Fig. 9.4). Females in the 15- to 24-year age group had a higher incidence of Burkitt lymphoma relative to males than in younger or older age groups, with a male:female ratio at a nadir of 2.6–3.2 (Fig. 9.4).

9.2.4 Racial/Ethnic Differences in Incidence

Figure 9.5 displays the incidence of all non-Hodgkin lymphoma as a function of race/ethnicity. Incidence increased for all groups as a function of age. A switchover from the highest rate among non-Hispanic whites and Asians/Pacific Islanders to the highest rate among African Americans/blacks occurred at about 20 years of age. At all ages, American Indians/Alaska Natives had the lowest incidence of non-Hodgkin lymphoma.

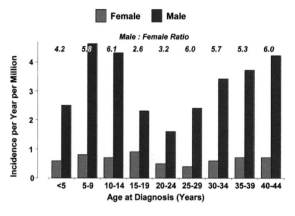

Figure 9.4

Incidence of Burkitt lymphoma (ICCC IIc) in the United States by gender; United States SEER, 1975–2000

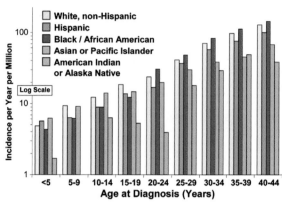

Figure 9.5

Incidence of non-Hodgkin lymphoma (ICCC IIb, IIc, IId, and IIe) by race/ethnicity; United States SEER, 1992–2000

9.3 Etiology/Risk Factors

Whatever the age, it is known that a few patients are at increased risk of developing non-Hodgkin lymphoma: those with congenital or acquired immunodeficiency and those receiving immunosuppressive therapy (such as after organ transplantation). The incidence is significantly higher in males than in females, and is higher in whites than African Americans/blacks, as reviewed earlier. Specific geographical areas are also recognized for particular types of lymphoma, such as the "endemic" (African) Burkitt lymphoma. Other risk factors include Epstein-Barr virus (EBV) or *Helicobacter pylori* infection, tobacco, and chemical or other environmental exposure. In underdeveloped countries, there is a documented link between EBV and Burkitt lymphoma, while in the developed world EBV is also associated with other subtypes of non-Hodgkin lymphoma. Secondary neoplasms are well-documented sequelae of HIV infection, and account for an increase in non-Hodgkin lymphoma incidence, particularly in males. The increase in non-Hodgkin lymphoma has persisted in the face of a stabilization of the incidence of new cases of HIV and with improved treatments for the infection. A few familial cases of lymphoid malignancies have been observed, without apparent recognized genetic abnormalities.

9.4 Histology/Cytogenetics

Classification of non-Hodgkin lymphoma has changed many times over the years and became more distinct with the increased understanding of lymphomagenesis and the development of new diagnostic tools (immunophenotyping, cytogenetics, molecular biology, and now gene profiling). The current World Health Organization (WHO) classification [4], preceded by the Revised American European Lymphoma (REAL) classification [5], is now widely used. Microarray technologies, by studying the expression of many genes at once, are very promising [6], but their implication for diagnosis and prognosis, and their further utility in clinical practice, especially in adolescence and young adults, require further investigation. The characteristics of the four categories of lymphoma most frequently encountered in adolescents and young adults (Burkitt, LL, DLBCL and anaplastic large cell, ALCL) are demonstrated in Table 9.2.

Table 9.2 Different subtypes of non-Hodgkin lymphoma in adolescents and young adults and their clinical and biologic characteristics. *FAB* French-American-British, *NPM* nucleophosmin, *ALK* anaplastic lymphoma kinase, *EMA* epithelial membrane antigen, *NA* not applicable

	Burkitt	Lymphoblastic	Large B-cell	Anaplastic large cell
Preferential tumor site	abdomen head and neck	mediastinum (T cell) bone, (sub)cutaneous (B cell)	abdomen, thymus, bone	node, skin
Histology				
cell size	medium,	medium	large	voluminous
cytoplasm	narrow basophilic, with vacuoles	narrow, pale		abundant and clear erythrophagocytosis
nucleus	round,	convoluted or not,	cleaved or not, vesicular distinct, often adherent to nucleus membrane	irregular, clear
nucleoli	several nucleoli	poorly discernable nucleoli		voluminous
chromatin	coarse and irregular	finely stippled		
FAB equivalent	L3	L1, L2	NA	NA
Immunophenotyping	CD20+ CD79a+ SIg+ Ki 67+>95%	TdT+ B lineage T lineage CD19+, CD7+ CD 79a+, CD2+ S Ig−, CD3c+ cMu −/+	CD20+ CD79a+ SIg +/− bcl6 +/− Ki 67 : 60 – 90%	CD30+ EMA+ ALK+ (T or "null" markers)
Cytogenetics	t (8;14)(q24;q32) or variant t(2;8) (p11;q24) t(8;22) (q24;q11)	no specific abnormalities, sometimes involvement of T-cell antigene receptor genes (TCR) on chromosome 7(q34) or 14(q11)	Sometimes t(8;14)(q24;q32) der (3)(q27) (bcl6)	t(2 ;5) (p23 ;q35) or variant
Result	transcriptional deregulation of c-MYC		transcriptional deregulation of bcl6	NPM/ALK fusion protein; ALK is a tyrosine kinase receptor located on 2p23

9.5 Clinical Features

The clinical presentation of non-Hodgkin lymphoma in adolescents and young adults, as in other age classes, varies and depends on the primary site of the disease, the histological subtype, and the extent of the disease. Burkitt lymphoma generally arises in the abdomen (digestive track) and in the Waldeyer ring, while LL generally arises from the thymus. Burkitt abdominal lymphoma generally presents as a large and rapidly growing abdominal mass that is often associated with ascites and other intra- or extraabdominal involvement. Intussusception leading to the discovery of a small excisable abdominal tumor is a rare presentation that is related to Burkitt or DLBCL. Extensive abdominal surgery should be avoided. The diagnosis can be made on surgical biopsy, but also on cytological examination of a serous effusion or on percutaneous needle biopsy of the tumor.

Lymphoblastic mediastinal lymphoma leads to mediastinal compression, which may be life threatening (general anesthesia should be avoided if possible) and is often associated with a concomitant pleural effusion. Therefore, the diagnosis should be made using cytological examination of effusions or bone marrow smears. If a tumor biopsy is needed, then this should be done by percutaneous needle biopsy or by mediastinoscopy. Another lymphoma arising in the thymus is the primary mediastinal B-cell lymphoma of thymus origin, which may present with pericarditis, pulmonary nodules and/or subdiaphragmatic involvement such as the kidney and pancreas.

Head and neck primary sites including Waldeyer's ring and the facial bones are more often seen in Burkitt lymphoma. In the less frequent sites such as superficial lymph nodes, bone, skin, thyroid, orbit, eyelid, kidney, and epidural space, any subtype of lymphoma can be seen, emphasizing the necessity of a good-quality sample for histology and immunophenotyping.

ALCLs present with more unique features: usually nodal involvement, sometimes painful, which is characteristic of this disease; frequent skin involvement with inflammatory symptoms of the involved nodes, distant macular lesions, or general skin modification resembling ichthyosis; frequent general symptoms with widely fluctuating fever; and "wax and wane"

evolution in a few cases with previous episode(s) of spontaneous regression.

9.6 Initial Work-Up and Staging

Diagnosis can be obtained utilizing biopsy material including tumor-touch preparations, but also cytological examination of effusion fluids or bone marrow smears, so surgical procedures can be avoided in diffuse Burkitt and lymphoblastic diseases. Also strongly recommended are the immunological and cytogenetic or molecular biology studies.

Once the diagnosis of non-Hodgkin lymphoma has been made, a speedy assessment of diagnosis, staging, and general evaluation must be done in order to commence appropriate treatment as soon as possible. This is particularly important in Burkitt lymphoma and LL, which have a great propensity to spread rapidly both regionally and systemically, especially in the bone marrow and in central nervous system (CNS).

Staging classifications are different in children, where the St Jude (also called Murphy) classification [7] is used because of the predominance of extranodal primaries, and in adults where the Ann Arbor classification, more adapted to nodal disease, is used (Table 9.3). These two different staging systems between children and adults make comparisons between pediatric and adult studies difficult, particularly in the adolescent and young adult age range. Also utilized for therapeutic classification in adults is the International Prognostic Index (IPI) based on stage, serum lactate dehydrogenase (LDH) levels, and Performance Status (PS). PS does not seem appropriate for very fast-growing tumors such as Burkitt and lymphoblastic, and is often not documented in pediatric lymphoma trials. This might make comparisons difficult between childhood and adult studies, especially in large-cell lymphoma. PS should be included in future studies that include adolescents. In spite of being an unspecific marker and of different methods of dosage with different "norms", serum LDH level is a very good indicator of tumor burden and generally has prognostic significance.

The traditional boundary between leukemia and lymphoma has been defined arbitrarily by more or less

Table 9.3 Non-Hodgkin Straging Systems and Prognostic Index. *CNS* Central nervous system. *LDH* Lactate dehydrogenase

St Jude (Murphy) staging used in childhood non-Hodgkin lymphoma.

Stage I	A single tumor (extranodal) or single anatomical area (nodal) with the exclusion of the mediastinum or abdomen.
Stage II	A single tumor (extranodal) with regional node involvement. Two or more nodal areas on the same side of the diaphragm. Two single (extranodal) tumors with or without regional node involvement on the same side of the diaphragm. A primary gastrointestinal tract tumor, usually in the ileocecal area, with or without involvement of associated mesenteric nodes only, grossly completely resected.
Stage III	Two single tumors (extranodal) on opposite sides of the diaphragm. Two or more nodal areas above and below the diaphragm. All the primary intrathoracic tumors (mediastinal, pleural, thymic). All extensive primary intra-abdominal disease, unresectable. All paraspinal or epidural tumors, regardless of other tumor site(s).
Stage IV	Any of the above with initial CNS and/or bone marrow involvement.

Ann Arbor classification used in adult non-Hodgkin lymphoma

Stage I	Involvement of a single lymph node region (I) or a single extralymphatic organ or site (I$_E$).
Stage II	Involvement of two or more lymph node regions on the same side of the diaphragm (II), which may be accompanied by a contiguous involvement of an extralymphatic organ or site (II$_E$).
Stage III	Involvement of lymph node regions on opposite sides of the diaphragm, which may be accompanied by involvement of the spleen (III$_S$) or by a localized involvement of an extralymphatic organ or site (III$_E$) or both (III$_{SE}$).
Stage IV	Disseminated involvement of one or more extralymphatic organ or tissues, with or without associated lymph node involvement.

International prognostic index used in adult non-Hodgkin lymphoma (patients <60 years)

Factors	**Risk classification**	
Performance status > 2		
LDH > normal	Low:	0 factor
Stage III – IV	Low– intermediate:	1 factor
	High–intermediate:	2 factors
	High:	3 factors

than 25% blast cells in the bone marrow, but this does not correspond to either clinical or biological differences. CNS involvement is defined by the presence of unequivocal malignant cells in a cytocentrifuged specimen of spinal fluid and/or the presence of obvious neurological deficits, such as cranial nerve palsies.

Experience with positron emission tomography in childhood and adolescent non-Hodgkin lymphoma is in the early stages of investigation. It is hoped that this diagnostic tool will help to predict the presence of active tumors in a residual mass.

Patients often have other problems at diagnosis, such as malnutrition, infection, postsurgical complications, and respiratory and metabolic abnormalities; these may be life threatening or compromise the onset of therapy. Tumor lysis syndrome may be present at diagnosis or may develop during treatment. In advanced diseases, especially in Burkitt lymphoma and LL, preventive measures must always be instituted: hyperdiuresis and "uricolytic" drugs (allopurinol or urate oxidase). Urate oxidase should be utilized in cases of high tumor burden [8–11]. Urate oxidase converts uric acid into allantoin, which is highly soluble in urine. It is an efficient way of promptly reducing serum uric acid levels, thus preventing uric acid nephropathy and preserving renal function, allowing a better excretion of the other cell metabolites such as potassium and phosphorus. Strict clinical and metabolic monitoring of patients during the lysis phase is essential.

9.7 B-Cell non-Hodgkin Lymphoma

The two main entities of B-cell non-Hodgkin lymphoma are Burkitt and DLBCL. The other B-cell non-Hodgkin lymphomas, such as the follicular, mantle cell, or the mucosa-associated lymphoid tissue lymphomas, are not often encountered in adolescents and young adults and will not be discussed in this chapter.

9.7.1 Burkitt Lymphoma

Burkitt lymphoma is characterized by a high proliferation rate and a short doubling time, so it generally presents with a high tumor burden in advanced stages. General guidelines for treatment are as follows. Chemotherapy must be intensive, although adapted to tumor burden, combining several drugs, and given as pulse courses. The most frequently used drugs are cyclophosphamide (CPM), high-dose (HD) methotrexate (MTX), and cytarabine (ARA-C). Other effective drugs are doxorubicin, vincristine (VCR), VP16 (etoposide), ifosfamide, and corticosteroids. CNS prophylaxis is essential and is achieved by intrathecal injections of MTX and/or ARA-C, and by HD MTX ± HD ARA-C. CNS treatment is done with the same drugs at a higher dose. Cranial irradiation is thought to be ineffective in Burkitt and is therefore unnecessary. Treatment is of short duration, usually a few months. Relapses in Burkitt usually occur within the 1st year of treatment; therefore, a patient who is alive in first complete remission after 1 year can be considered as cured.

With the LMB protocols developed by the Societe Francaise d'Oncologie Pediatrique (SFOP) [12–14] and the Berlin-Frankfurt-Munster (BFM) protocols developed in Germany [15, 16], survival reaches an average of 90%. The lessons from these studies, but also from others [17–20], are:

1. Resected localized tumors (the minority) can be treated with very short treatment, some of them without any CNS prophylaxis [14, 16, 21–24].
2. The absence of tumor response at D7 after the prephase combining a low dose of VCR and CPM, and corticosteroids, indicates a bad prognosis and the need for intensifying treatment (LMB84 and LMB89 studies) [13, 14].
3. The introduction of HD ARA-C + VP16 increased the event-free survival (EFS) of patients with L_3ALL and who were CNS positive in the LMB86 and LMB89 group C studies (CYVE courses) [14] and that of patients with advanced stages in the BFM90 and BFM95 studies (course CC) [16, 25].
4. Treatment with HD MTX is very important in Burkitt. The more advanced the stage, the more treatment with HD MTX is important. The prognosis of stage III with high LDH and of any stage IV was greatly improved when MTX was increased from 0.5 to 5 g/m^2 in BFM86 and BFM90 [15, 16]. Results were also better in higher-risk patients when the infusion duration of HD MTX was longer (BFM95 study) [25].
5. Dose intensity during the 1st month is of great importance, as demonstrated in the FAB LMB96 study in which the outcome of the intermediate-risk patients was inferior when the second induction course was commenced more than 21 days after the first course [16, 26].

A few adolescents were included in these pediatric studies. There was a tendency in some studies toward an inferior EFS of patients older than 15 years [14, 27], but the numbers were too small to draw any definitive conclusions.

The LMB and the BFM regimens have been used in France and Germany, respectively, for young adult and older adult patients, but often with dose reduction of HD MTX because of poor tolerance of this drug in older patients. Does this explain the inferior results, or are they attributable to a different biology? It is interesting to note that the prognostic factors are the same in the LMB pediatric and adult studies: the absence of tumor response at Day 7 of therapy, LDH level, CNS involvement, and higher age. A study combining both children and adult databases will need to be performed to determine the prognosis of adolescents and young adults with Burkitt lymphoma and to determine the best course of management with either a pediatric or adult non-Hodgkin-lymphoma-based therapy.

Only two institutional studies (National Cancer Institute and Bologna) have addressed the question of outcome of adults and children treated in the same department with the same protocol. In a very small number of patients (41 and 21, respectively), they showed similar outcomes [17, 28].

Until further studies provide evidence to the contrary, adolescents and young adults probably should be treated with the pediatric regimens, without dose reductions.

One question concerns the use of rituximab in Burkitt. Some adult hematologists tend to use it systematically. There have been only a few case reports on the response in relapsed Burkitt [29, 30]. Currently, there is no published study demonstrating the benefit of rituximab in Burkitt. A study has just opened in France for adults comparing the LMB regimen with or without rituximab. A Children's Oncology Group (COG) study investigating the safety and efficacy of rituximab in combination with FAB therapy has just opened.

9.7.2 Diffuse Large B-Cell Lymphoma

Depending on the country, DLBCL is included either in studies designed for Burkitt (LMB and BFM studies) [14, 16] or in studies designed for large cells in general (Pediatric Oncology Group, POG, studies) [31, 32]. In the LMB89 study, DLBCL represented 10% of all registered patients. As with Burkitt, they are treated according to initial resection and stage. The EFS is similar to that of Burkitt (Fig. 9.6), but it should be noted that the proportion of patients with advanced stages is lower than in Burkitt. However, by stage, EFS is not significantly different [33]. In the BFM90 study, the EFS of DLBCL is also similar to that of Burkitt. The criticism of such an approach is that too much CNS-directed therapy is given in DLBCL, in which the risk of CNS disease is lower than in Burkitt.

In a POG study, all advanced-stage large-cell lymphomas, by histology and/or immunophenotype, were treated with an APO (adriamycin + prednisone + onc-

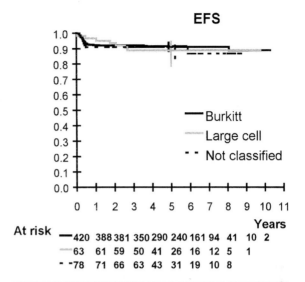

Figure 9.6

Event-free survival of patients treated in the Societe Francaise d'Oncologie Pediatrique LMB89 protocol according to histology (Burkitt vs. diffuse large B-cell lymphoma). From Patte et al. [14]

ovin)-based regimen. The addition of CPM did not change the outcome [32]. In another study, the addition of HD MTX and ARA-C was randomized. Results indicate a benefit to DLBCL, but not to ALCL [34].

In adults, recognized prognostic factors are age, IPI, LDH, stage, and to a lesser extent, number of extranodal sites and tumor size. Treatment is stratified according to these factors, including HD chemotherapy followed by autologous hematopoietic stem-cell rescue in poor-risk patients. Biologic characteristics may also have prognostic value, such as the presence of t(14;18)(q32;q21) involving bcl-2. Microarray studies have recognized two subtypes of DLBCL, the activated B-like and the germinal center-like ones, with different outcomes [35]. Overall therapeutic results in adults are not as satisfactory as in children. This raises the question of a different biology of DLBCL in children, where t(14;18)(q32;q21) is not seen, versus adults. What is the biology of adolescent and young adult DLBCL? Is it intermediate between that of adults and children, or closer to one or other of them?

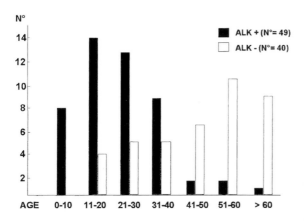

Figure 9.7

The different age distributions of anaplastic lymphoma kinase gene (*ALK*)⁺ anaplastic large-cell lymphoma (ALCL) and ALK⁻ ALCL. From Stein et al. [52]

The current main question is the addition of rituximab to chemotherapy. It was first shown in elderly patients with DLBCL that the addition of rituximab to CHOP (CPM + doxorubicin + VCR + prednisone) increased by 10–15% the complete response rate and the 3-year EFS and overall survival (OS) [36]. Recently, a European study in younger adults (18–59 years) also showed the benefit of adding rituximab to CHOP [37]. Consequently, it is now recommended that rituximab should be given with first-line chemotherapy in the treatment of adult DLBCL. Pediatricians who want to treat adolescents will have to take a position for their patients with DLBCL, knowing that their global results are better than in adults, that they use chemotherapy regimens different from CHOP, and that randomized studies addressing the question of rituximab are not possible due to the small number of patients.

One particular subtype of DLBCL is the primary mediastinal large B-cell lymphoma (PMLBCL), which has a different biology [38]. In the adult literature, there are controversies on their similarity or difference with other DLBCLs. The best therapeutic approach is not clearly defined, especially the potential role of radiotherapy. In the pediatric BFM and FAB LMB96

series, PMLCBL had a worse prognosis than other DLBCL, with an EFS of approximately 65–75% [39, 40]. Conversely, the Children's Cancer Group (CCG) claimed that the outcome of these lymphomas was better than for other DLBCLs [41]. In fact, the number of patients is small and there is a need to combine these data to find prognostic factors and to adapt therapy.

9.7.3 Anaplastic Large Cell Lymphoma

ALCL was first described as a distant clinicopathological entity in 1985 by Stein et al. [42] CD30 (Ki-1) expression was the hallmark feature that distinguished this lymphoma from the other forms of non-Hodgkin lymphoma. The characteristic t(2;5)(p23;q35) cytogenetic translocation was identified in 1989 to be associated with ALCL [43]. In 1994, Morris et al. cloned the translocation breakpoints of the nucleophosmin (*NPM*) gene on chromosome 5 and the anaplastic lymphoma kinase gene (*ALK*) on chromosome 2 [44]. The median age of presentation ranges between 17 and 50 years, with a bimodal age of distribution with a larger peak in the 20- to 30-year-old range and a smaller peak in the sixth and seventh decades of life [45–48]. *ALK*-positive ALCL tends to occur in the adolescent and young adult age range, whereas *ALK*-negative cases tend to occur in an older age group (43–61 years; Fig. 9.7) [49–51]. Cutaneous ALCL (C-ALCL) rarely occurs in the adolescent and young adult age group and is usually manifested in the sixth and seventh decades of life. There is a male predominance (6–7:1) in ALCL in the adolescent and young adult age group and patients tend to present with advanced-stage disease (stage III/IV) and extranodal involvement [51, 52]. Bone marrow involvement ranges between 11% (hematoxylin and eosin stains) and upwards to 34% when analyzed by immunohistochemistry [52, 53]. CNS involvement occurs in less than 3–5% of adolescent and young adult cases of ALCL [52].

9.7.3.1 Biology/Pathology

ALCL is the least common form of adolescent non-Hodgkin lymphoma (<10%), is characterized by the expression of CD30 (Ki-1), and consists of two major histological subtypes, systemic (S-ALCL) and primary

C-ALCL [4]. ALCL is defined by large, pleomorphic, multinucleated cells or cells with eccentric horseshoe-shaped nuclei and abundant clear to basophilic cytoplasm with an area of eosinophilia near the nucleus (termed "hallmark cells") [54]. These hallmark cells commonly resemble Reed-Sternberg cells (characteristic of Hodgkin lymphoma), although they tend to have less conspicuous nucleoli.

There are several morphologic variants of ALCL that have been identified in the REAL and WHO classifications [4, 5]. These variants include the common variety (75%), which is composed primarily of hallmark cells, the lymphohistiocytic variety (10%), which has a large number of benign histiocytes admixed with neoplastic cells, and the small-cell variety (10%), which is composed of small neoplastic cells and only scattered hallmark cells. Other (<5%) less well described variants include sarcomatoid, signet-ring, neutrophil-rich, and giant-cell variants [52, 55]. Neoplastic cells tend to infiltrate in a sinusoidal pattern in regional lymph nodes, mimicking metastatic disease, although diffuse effacement of nodes may also be demonstrated. There is a high propensity of S-ALCL to spread to extranodal tissues (skin, bone, soft tissues) either as the only sites of disease or, more commonly, in association with nodal disease [55].

C-ALCL is part of a spectrum of CD30-positive, T-cell lymphoproliferative disorders [52, 56, 57]. CD30-positive cutaneous lymphoproliferative disorders share overlapping pathologic and clinical features, and so diagnosis requires careful assessment of clinical, histologic, immunophenotypic, and genetic features. C-ALCL is a peripheral T-cell lymphoma of large, anaplastic, CD30-positive cells that is limited to the skin. C-ALCL usually presents as a solitary tumor, nodule, or papule that is composed of larger, pleomorphic cells that infiltrate the upper and deep dermis and extend into the subcutaneous tissues. Epidermal invasion is uncommon and surrounding inflammation is usually present [57].

Both S-ALCL and C-ALCL express CD30, as evidenced by immunohistochemistry [51]. The majority of ALCLs have been shown to be of the T-cell phenotype (CD2, CD3, CD5, CD7, CD45RO, CD43) or fail to stain with either T- or B-cell markers (null cell). Expression of cytotoxic antigens, such as TIA-1 or

granzyme, and epithelial membrane antigen (EMA) is commonly observed in ALCL. ALK expression (P80) detects the fusion protein generated by translocations associated with S-ALCL. ALK staining is absent in C-ALCL, and, if observed, indicates the likelihood that systemic disease is present [58].

Most cases of S-ALCL and C-ALCL demonstrate T-cell receptor gene rearrangements, even when immunophenotypic analysis fails to demonstrate expression of T-cell antigens [52]. Cytogenetic and molecular analyses often demonstrate a characteristic genetic alteration involving the ALK locus on chromosome 2. Classically this is manifested as the t(2;5)(p23;q35) translocation, which includes a rearrangement of a nucleolar phosphoprotein gene (*NPM1*) adjacent to the *ALK* tyrosine kinase gene [44]. Less common translocations include translocation of *ALK* to partner genes on chromosomes 1, 2, 3, and 17, which also results in upregulation of ALK expression [59, 60]. The pattern of ALK staining is usually nuclear with or without cytoplasmic staining for t(2;5), and is only in the cytoplasm for many of the alternative translocations [52]. Greater than 90% of advanced adolescent and young adult cases of S-ALCL are associated with *ALK* translocations, which are commonly absent in C-ALCL and seen with lower frequency in adults with S-ALCL [52, 59, 60]. The presence of an *ALK* translocation or ALK protein expression, however, appears to be associated with a better prognosis in adults [52, 61].

9.7.3.2 Treatment/Management of S-ALCL

Optimal therapeutic approaches for limited S-ALCL have not been well defined [62]. In a recent report, children and adolescents with localized (stage I/stage II resected) ALCL with a median age of 10.5 years (0.8–17.3) achieved 100% EFS with 2 months of chemotherapy including dexamethasone, ifosfamide, MTX, ARA-C, etoposide, and prophylactic intrathecal therapy [63]. A 75% EFS has been reported in a small number of children and adolescents with localized CD30-positive large-cell lymphoma, presumably S-ALCL, who had a median age of 13 years (0.2–19.9 years) and were treated at St. Jude Children's Research Hospital with three courses of CHOP, either with or without maintenance with 6-mercaptopurine

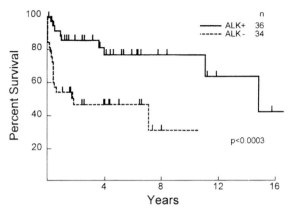

Figure 9.8

A comparison of probability of overall survival of patients with systemic ALCL (S-ALCL) expressing *ALK⁺* or no *ALK* expression (*ALK⁻*). From Gascoyne et al. [50]

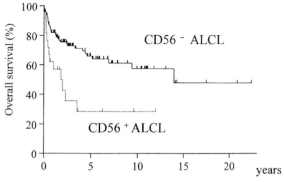

Figure 9.10

A comparison of probability of overall survival in patients with S-ALCL with CD56⁺ vs. CD56⁻ expression. From Suzuki et al. [68]

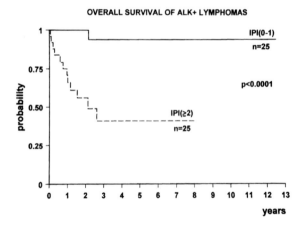

Figure 9.9

A comparison of probability of overall survival of *ALK⁺* ALCL according to age-adjusted Intermediate Prognostic Index (*IPI*). Score 0–1 (low/low intermediate) vs. score >2 (high/high intermediate). From Falini et al. [51]

and MTX [64]. Similarly, in small numbers of children with limited-stage S-ALCL treated on United Kingdom Children's Cancer Study Group studies 9001, 9002, and 9602, the 5-year EFS was 62% (39–82%) [65].

Poor-risk prognostic factors in childhood and adolescent advanced-disease S-ALCL that have been identified include organ involvement (liver, lung, spleen), mediastinal involvement, an elevated LDH, and/or disseminated skin disease [66, 67]. Adolescent and young adult patients with advanced-disease S-ALCL are commonly treated with anthracycline (doxorubicin)-containing chemotherapy regimens. The prognosis is significantly improved in patients with ALK expression and lower IPI scores [50, 51]. Gascoyne et al. demonstrated that the 5-year EFS and OS was 88% and 93%, respectively for *ALK*-positive S-ALCL patients compared to 37% and 37%, respectively for *ALK*-negative S-ALCL patients ($p<0.0001$; Fig. 9.8) [50]. Falini et al. further demonstrated that the 10-year disease-free survival (DFS) and OS of *ALK*-positive versus *ALK*-negative patients were significantly different (82±6% vs. 28±14%, $p<0.0001$) [51]. Similarly, patients with S-ALCL and an elevated IPI score (≥2) at diagnosis also had a significantly inferior outcome compared to patients with S-ALCL and IPI 0–1 (OS 41±5% vs. 94±5%, $p<0.0001$; Fig. 9.9) [51]. Furthermore, patients with CD56-positive, *ALK*-positive, and *ALK*-negative S-ALCL have an inferior prognosis compared to CD56-negative (*ALK*-negative) S-ALCL patients (5-year OS 70% vs. 35%, $p<0.002$) (Fig. 9.10) [68].

The use of CHOP-based therapies over a 6-month period in childhood S-ALCL has resulted in greater than 75% 3-year OS [64, 69]. Cooperative European studies using either BFM-NHL or SFOP HM89-91, and the POG study using an APO regimen (doxorubicin + prednisone + VCR) in children with advanced-disease S-ALCL have demonstrated a 65–75% 3- to 5-year EFS (Table 9.4) [63, 67, 70–73]. Children with advanced-disease S-ALCL treated on NHL-BFM 90 have achieved EFS rates of 76% after receiving short courses of intensive B-cell non-Hodgkin lymphoma therapy, stratified according to disease stage. The COG recently reported the results of a pilot study (CCG-5941) in children with stage III/IV S-ALCL [73]. CCG-5941 was a T-cell lymphoblastic protocol that was utilized as a pilot for advanced ALCL. Induction therapy consisted of VCR, prednisone, daunomycin, CPM, and L-asparaginase. Intensification phase followed with VCR, ARA-C, VP16, HD MTX, 6-thioguanine (6TG), and L-asparaginase. Maintenance therapy consisted of alternating pulses of: (1) CPM and 6TG; (2) VCR, prednisone, and doxorubicin; (3) VCR and HD MTX; and (4) ARA-C and VP16. The 3-year EFS and OS were 73±6% and 83±5%, respectively [73].

The treatment for adolescents and young adults with advanced-disease S-ALCL usually involves an anthracycline-containing adult, non-Hodgkin lymphoma chemotherapy regimen (Table 9.4). Gascoyne et al. reported on the results of 70 adults with S-ALCL (36 ALK-positive with a median age of 30 years) with anthracycline-containing regimens [50]. The 5-year OS and EFS for all 70 patients was 65% and 63%, respectively [50]. In the adolescent and young adult age group (median age 30 years) with ALK-positive S-ALCL, the 5-year OS was 79%, compared to 46% for ALK-negative patients (p<0.0003) [50]. Falini et al. similarly reported the results in 78 adults with S-ALCL (53 ALK-positive and 25 ALK-negative) treated on anthracycline-containing regimens [51]. OS was significantly improved in ALK-positive vs. ALK-negative patients (71±6 vs. 15±11%, p<0.0007; Table 9.4) [51]. A subpopulation of adult patients with advanced-disease S-ALCL has been treated with aggressive chemotherapy (F-MACHOP: 5-fluorouracil, MTX with leucovorin rescue, ARA-C, CPM, doxorubicin, VCR, and prednisone), involved-field radiotherapy, and mye-

Table 9.4 Treatment and prognosis of advanced anaplastic large-cell lymphoma in children, adolescents and young adults. *EFS* Event-free survival, *Est* estimate, *BFM* Berlin Frankfurt Munster, *POG* Pediatric Oncology Group, *SFOP* Societe Francaise d'Oncologie Pediatrique, *CCG* Children's Cancer Group, *NHL* non-Hodgkin lymphoma

	BFM Seidemann et al. [63]	POG Laver et al. [34]	SFOP Brugieres et al. [67]	CCG Abromovich et al. [73]	Vancouver Gascoyne et al. [50]	Italian Falini et al. [105]
Patients (N)	89	67	82	80	36 (ALK+)	53 (ALK+)
Age: median years (range)	11 (1–17)	15 (1–22)	10 (1.5–17)	11 (3–21)	30 (ALK+)	23 (3–52)
Protocol	NHL-BFM 90	POG 9315	HM89-91	CCG-5941	Anthracycline based	Anthracycline based
Duration (months)	2–5	12	7–8	12	3–6	3–6
EFS (Est) 2–10 years	76%	73%	66%	73%	88%	82%

loablative chemotherapy and autologous stem-cell transplantation [74]. Although the numbers are small (N=16; median age 35 years), the results are encouraging, with 100% DFS and OS [74]. It remains to be determined which subsets of newly diagnosed patients in the adolescent and young adult age group with *ALK*-positive disease require such aggressive and intensive therapy.

9.8 Lymphoblastic Lymphoma

LL was initially described as a distinct pathological entity by Sternberg in 1916 [75]. In 1975, Barcos and Lukes defined this pathological entity as "lymphoblastic lymphoma" because of its close morphologic similarity to blasts of acute lymphoblastic leukemia (ALL) [76]. LL is considered an aggressive form of non-Hodgkin lymphoma by the REAL and WHO classifications. The majority of LL cases (≥75%) express a T-cell lineage and the remainder express a pre-B or B-cell immunophenotype. The most typical cytogenetic abnormalities, especially of the T-cell immunophenotype, commonly include *TCR* gene rearrangement, including *TCRα/β* (14q11-13), *TCRβ* (7q32-36) and *TCRγ* (7p15). Other commonly abnormal rearranged genes that have been described in LL include *TAL-1, TAL-2, TCL-1, TCL-2, TCL-3, HOX-11, RHOM-1, RHOM-2, LYL-1, TAN-1, LCK, PBX-1,* and *E2A* among others. There is a high incidence of LL in children with a median age of onset at around 9 years [77–80], and more importantly, LL also has a peak incidence in the adolescent and young adult group (15–30 years) with a median onset of approximately 25 years of age [81, 83]. There is a predominant male to female ratio ranging in different studies from 2:1 to 3:1. LL tends to present most commonly as a mediastinal mass in the adolescent and young adult age group (≥90%), may involve the bone marrow at diagnosis (25%), tends to present with advanced-stage disease (≥III; 75%), and less often involves the CNS (5%) [84, 85].

9.8.1 Biology/Pathology

LL has been well described in both the REAL and WHO classifications, including precursor T (and B) lymphoblastic lymphoma. Precursor B-cell disease

predominates in ALL compared to most of the LLs that are of precursor T-cell origin (80–90% T cell vs. 10–20% B cell). Precursor T-cell LL tends to present as mediastinal or upper torso nodal masses, whereas precursor B-cell LL is more likely to present in skin, soft tissue, bone, tonsil, and peripheral lymph nodes [86].

The morphologic features of LL include diffuse or partial effacement of lymph nodes that usually infiltrate interfollicular zones with sparing of benign, reactive follicles. A starry-sky pattern derived from the presence of macrophages ingesting apoptotic debris occurs commonly. Cytologically, the neoplastic cells are indistinguishable from those seen in precursor B-cell or T-cell ALL. The cells have an immature, blast-like appearance with fine chromatin, inconspicuous or absent nucleoli, and scanty cytoplasm that ranges from pale to slightly basophilic in color, and most LL have a high proliferative rate [86].

Immature B- or T-lymphoid blasts express terminal deoxynucleotidyl transferase (TdT). T-LL commonly expresses CD1, CD2, CD5, and CD7 along with coexpression of CD4 and/or CD8. Occasionally, both CD4 and CD8 may be absent. CD10 is expressed in 15–40% of cases, and occasionally natural killer antigens such as CD57 or CD16 may be seen [86]. Precursor B-cell LL most often displays the immunophenotype of early pre-B or pre-B phenotypes (CD19, CD10, and TdT with variable CD20, CD22, HLA-Dr, and cytoplasmic immunoglobulin) [86].

T-LL will commonly display early T-cell gene rearrangements (*TCRδ, TCRγ, TCRα,* and/or *TCRβ*) [81, 87]. Precursor B-LL commonly demonstrates clonal immunoglobulin gene rearrangements and lacks evidence of somatic hypermutation [88]. Cytogenetic abnormalities are common (50–80%) in both B- and T-LL [81]. T-LL chromosomal breakpoints have included T-cell receptor (TCR) genes or specific oncogenes *TCRα/δ* (14q11), *TCRβ* (7q32-36), and *TCRγ* (7p15). Often the TCR enhancer or promoter elements are translocated and juxtaposed to putative transcription factors [81, 87]. Specific oncogenes associated with T-LL include *TCL-1* (14q32), which is involved in t(7;14)(q35;q32) or t(14;14)(q11;q32), *TCL-2* (11p13), which is involved in t(11;13)(p13;q11), *TCL-3* (10q24), which is seen in t(8;14)(q24;q11), and *TAL-1* (1p32), which is involved in t(1;14)(q32;q11).

9.8.2 Treatment and Management

Children with limited-disease LL, Murphy stages I and II, have a favorable prognosis with a long-term OS of 85–90%, but DFS rates of only 63–73%. The excellent OS rates have been attributed to effective salvage strategies for children who have relapsed after initial less-intensive therapies. Over the past 20 years, the need for local radiotherapy in children with LL, especially to the mediastinum, has been virtually eliminated [89]. Successful therapeutic approaches in children with LL have varied and have included CHOP with mercaptopurine and MTX maintenance (POG) [22, 89], LSA$_2$L$_2$ (Memorial Sloan-Kettering Cancer Center) [79], COMP (CPM + oncovin + MTX + prednisone; CCG) [23, 90], and modified LSA$_2$L$_2$ with the addition of HD MTX [91].

The treatment for limited-stage disease (I/II) LL in the adolescent and young adult group has been quite varied [91]. Most adolescent and young adult patients, with both limited stage and advanced stage (III/IV), have received similar treatment regardless of initial staging [91]. The probability of OS of limited-stage LL in the adolescent and young adult group varies from 40 to 60% [81]. Hoelzer et al. reported a 5-year OS rate for stage I/II LL in adolescents and young adults of 56±24% (Fig. 9.11) in the German ALL studies (GMALL) [83]. Few studies of LL in the adolescent and young adult age group have utilized involved-field radiotherapy, and most studies have utilized either CHOP, BFM, LSA$_2$L$_2$, BACOP (bleomycin + epidoxorubicin + CPM + VCR + prednisone), and/or M-BACOD (MTX + bleomycin + doxorubicin + CPM + VCR + dexamethasone)-type multiagent chemotherapy regimens.

The prognosis for children with advanced LL has improved significantly since the introduction of the 10-drug LSA$_2$L$_2$ regimen by Wollner et al. at MSKCC [91]. The CCG subsequently compared LSA$_2$L$_2$ with COMP in advanced LL in children [92]. The 5-year EFS for children with advanced-disease LL treated with LSA$_2$L$_2$ in comparison with COMP was significantly better (64% vs. 34%, p<0.001) [92]. Recent excellent results have also been demonstrated without the requirement of involved-field radiotherapy [80]. Treatment approaches for childhood advanced LL have varied, with many pediatric cooperative groups investigating

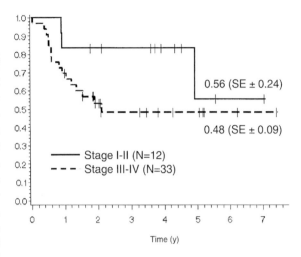

Figure 9.11

A comparison of probability of overall survival in lymphoblastic lymphoma patients with stage I/II versus stage III/IV disease. From Hoelzer D et al. [83]

ALL-based therapeutic regimens. An OS of 60–90% has been demonstrated using a variety of multiagent chemotherapy regimens raging from 12 to 32 months of therapy (Table 9.5) [15, 77–81, 91–98]. More recently, excellent results (including a 90% EFS) have been demonstrated with the BFM NHL90 protocol, which utilizes HD MTX, dexamethasone, moderate doses of anthracyclines, and CPM, as well as prophylactic cranial radiation, with a treatment stratification based upon tumor response to induction therapy [80].

The treatment for advanced-stage (III/IV) LL in the adolescent and young adult group has also been varied. The probability of DFS in advanced-stage (III/IV) LL in the adolescent and young adult group has ranged from 30 to 60% [81]. Initial results with an LSA$_2$L$_2$-like regimen by Coleman et al. [99] and the Stanford group in 44 patients with LL yielded a 56% 3-year DFS. Morel et al. in a French cooperative series of studies utilizing CHOP, LNH-84, FRALLE, and LALA, demonstrated a 33–53% DFS in adolescent and young adult patients with advanced LL [100]. Zinzani et al. reported for the Italian cooperative studies an overall 56% 10-year DFS in patients with advanced LL treated on successive Italian studies (L17, L0288, L20) [101]. More recently,

Table 9.5 Outcome results in adolescents/young adults with advanced lymphoblastic lymphoma. *DFS* Disease-free survival, *ECOG* Eastern Cooperative Oncology Group, *CHOP* cyclophosphamide + doxorubicin + vincristine + prednisone, *LASP* l-asparaginase

	German Hoelzer et al. [83]	ECOG Colgan et al. [82]	Stanford Coleman et al. [99]	French Morel et al. [100]	Italian Zinzani et al. [101]
Patients (N)	45	39	44	80	106
Protocol	GMALL 89 GMALL 93	CHOP/LASP	LSA_2L_2	CHOP, LNH-84, FRALLE, LALA	L17, L0288, L20
Duration (months)	12	15	12	12–15	12–15
DFS (Est) (3–10 years)	57%	49%	56%	33–53%	56%

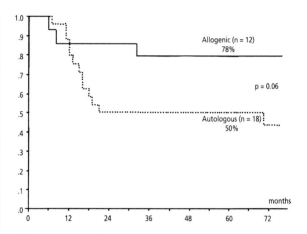

Figure 9.12

A comparison of probability of overall survival for patients with lymphoblastic lymphoma treated with either allogeneic stem-cell transplantation (*solid line*) or autologous stem-cell transplantation (*dashed line*). From Bouabdallah et al. [102]

Hoelzer et al., utilizing two German ALL protocols (GMALL89 and GMALL93), reported a 57% 3-year DFS in adolescent and young adult patients with advanced LL (Table 9.5) [83]. Finally, Thomas et al. at the MD Anderson Cancer Center have piloted the use of hyperfractionated-CVAD (CPM + doxorubicin + VCR + dexamethasone) in adolescents and young adults with advanced LL and demonstrated in early results a 3-year DFS of 72% [81]. In comparison with the results with treatment for advanced LL in children vs. adolescents and young adults, the outcome appears to be superior in children with the use of pediatric-designed treatment protocols (Table 9.5).

Additional approaches for advanced LL in the adolescent and young adult group have been the use of high-dose therapy and autologous or allogeneic stem-cell transplantation [81]. Bouabdallah et al. reported the results of allogeneic stem-cell transplantation (*n*=12; 11 underwent the procedure during their first complete remission, CR1) and autologous stem-cell transplantation (*n*=18; 16=CR1) in adolescent and young adult patients with advanced LL [102]. The overall 5-year EFS for all transplant patients was 66%,

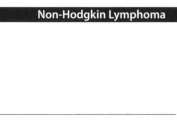

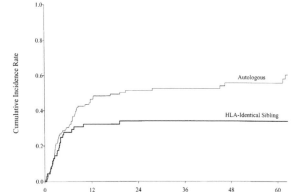

Patients at risk

ASCT	31	19	14	13	13	12	10	9	7
Conv.	34	19	15	13	9	9	5	3	2

Figure 9.13

A comparison of probability of actuarial relapse-free survival for patients with lymphoblastic lymphoma randomized to autologous stem-cell transplantation (*ASCT; solid line*) or conventional-dose (*Conv.*) consolidation/maintenance therapy (*dashed line*). From Sweetenham et al. [103]

Figure 9.14

A comparison of probability of relapse in patients with lymphoblastic lymphoma treated with human leukocyte antigen (HLA)-identical sibling allogeneic transplantation group vs. autologous transplantation. From Levine et al. [104]

compared to 33% in a similar group of patients not transplanted (*p*<0.01; Fig. 9.12) [102]. The allogeneic subgroup had an OS of 78%, compared to 50% in the autologous transplant group (*p*<0.06) [102]. Sweetenham et al. randomized adolescent and young adult patients (median age=26 years) with advanced LL in CR1 to high-dose therapy and autologous peripheral blood stem-cell transplantation (PBSCT) vs. continued chemotherapy [103]. The relapse-free survival was 55%, in the autologous PBSCT group compared with 24% in the chemotherapy group (Fig. 9.13). In a retrospective analysis of autologous PBSCT vs. allogeneic stem-cell transplantation in patients with LL reported to the International Bone Marrow Transplant Registry and Autologous Blood and Marrow Transplant Registry, Levine et al. demonstrated that the relapse rate was significantly higher in the autologous vs. allogeneic subgroups (34% vs. 56%, *p*<0.004; Fig. 9.14) [104]. These results suggest that there may be an allogeneic graft vs. lymphoma effect in adolescent and young adult patients with advanced LL.

In summary, adolescent and young adult patients with advanced LL have benefited from the use of pedi-

atric ALL-type chemotherapy regimens, long-term maintenance chemotherapy (12–24 months), aggressive intrathecal CNS prophylaxis, and high-dose therapy and stem-cell transplantation in selected patients in CR1 and responders in their first partial remission or in their second complete remission. Additional research is required to determine the molecular basis of adolescent and young adult LL, its relationship to pediatric LL, comparison to adolescent and young adult T-ALL, mechanisms of drug resistance, and the development of novel targeted therapeutic approaches.

9.9 Overall Survival

Overall 5-year survival rates of patients with all types of non-Hodgkin lymphoma by era during the past quarter century are shown in Fig. 9.15 as a function of age at diagnosis. Progress was most significant in children and young adolescents, with an increase from about 50% to over 89%. Among 15- to 29-year-olds, little progress was achieved until the 1990s, when the 5-year survival rate increased from about 55% to 65%.

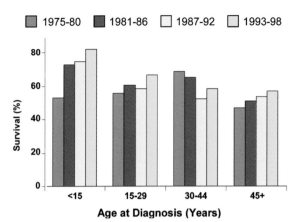

Figure 9.15

Five-year survival of non-Hodgkin lymphoma patients (ICCC IIb, IIc, IId and IIe) by era between 1975 and 1998; data from SEER [1]

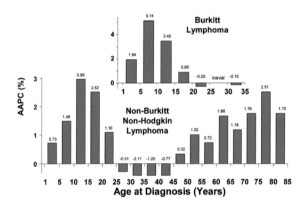

Figure 9.16

Average annual percent change (*AAPC*) in 5-year survival of patients with newly diagnosed non-Burkitt, non-Hodgkin lymphoma (ICCC IIb) and Burkitt lymphoma (ICCC IIc) during the period 1975–1997, as a function of age at diagnosis. Data from SEER

Transient reductions in the 5-year survival rate noted among 15- to 44-year-olds in the late 1980s and early 1990s were related, at least in part, to the HIV/acquired immune deficiency syndrome (AIDS) epidemic in the United States.

For 25- to 45-year-olds in the United States with non-Burkitt, non-Hodgkin lymphoma, there was no improvement in 5-year survival rate when it was averaged over the past quarter century (Fig. 9.16). Both younger and older patients have had a much greater survival improvement. For Burkitt lymphoma, a similar lack of progress is evident (Fig. 9.16, inset), at least in comparison to children (the incidence of Burkitt lymphoma is too uncommon in older persons to allow for a comparison). Burkitt lymphoma has not been associated with HIV infection, and yet shows a similar adult survival improvement deficit. It thus is not likely that the HIV/AIDS era explains the relative lack of progress in lymphoma survival in young adults.

9.10 Conclusions

The incidence of non-Hodgkin lymphoma has increased in all age groups through to age 30 years, and in 20- to 29-year-olds, the increase has been dramatic, averaging 4–19% per year over 25 years. Follicular (nodular) and mantle cell lymphoma, virtually nonexistent before age 15 years, increases to represent 11% of all non-Hodgkin lymphomas among 25- to 29-year-olds. Males are far more likely than females to develop non-Hodgkin lymphoma, especially Burkitt lymphoma. For 15- to 29-year-olds with either Burkitt or non-Burkitt non-Hodgkin lymphoma, survival improvement has significantly lagged behind that achieved in children and older adults with the same diseases, a deficit that can not be attributed solely to the HIV era.

The biology, prognosis and best treatment regimen for adolescents and young adults with non-Hodgkin lymphoma is still currently largely unknown. Few comparative studies have been performed to determine if the genetics and/or biology of adolescent and young adult non-Hodgkin lymphoma are similar to those of childhood or adult non-Hodgkin lymphoma, or whether it is a distinct biological entity. The pediatric approach may be more beneficial for certain subtypes of adolescent and young adult non-Hodgkin lymphoma and with other subtypes there is little data to support either pediatric or adult approaches as being superior. Further research and collaboration with pediatric and adult oncology cooperative groups is required to improve our understanding of the biology and best treatment approach for this subset of adolescents and young adults with non-Hodgkin lymphoma.

Acknowledgements

The authors would like to thank Linda Rahl for her expert editorial assistance in the development of this chapter. Supported in part by the Pediatric Cancer Research Foundation (MSC) and the National Cancer Institute (P30 CA13693) (MSC).

References

1. Bleyer WA, O'Leary M, Barr R, Ries LAG (eds) (2006) Cancer Epidemiology in Older Adolescents and Young Adults 15 to 29 Years of Age, including SEER Incidence and Survival, 1975–2000. National Cancer Institute, NIH Pub. No. 06-5767, Bethesda MD; also available at www.seer.cancer.gov/publications
2. Birch JM, Alston RD, Quinn M, Kelsey AM (2003) Incidence of malignant disease by morphological type, in young persons aged 12–24 years in England, 1979–1997. Eur J Cancer 39:2622–2631
3. Perkins SL, Raphael M, McCarthy K, et al (2003) Pediatric mature B-cell lymphoma: distribution of lymphoma subtype varies between national groups. Results from the FAB/LMB96 International Cooperative Group Study. Blood 102:1428 (abstract)
4. Jaffe E, Harris N, Stein H, Vardiman J (eds) (2000) World Health Organization Classifiction of Tumors. Tumours of Haematopoietic and Lymphoid Tissues. IARC Press, Washington DC
5. Harris N, Jaffe E, Stein H, et al (1994) A revised European-American classification of lymphoid neoplasms: a proposal from the International Lymphoma Study Group. Blood 84:1361–1392
6. Shipp MA, Ross KN, Tamayo P, et al (2002) Diffuse large B-cell lymphoma outcome prediction by gene-expression profiling and supervised machine learning. Nat Med 8:68–74
7. Murphy SB (1980) Classification, staging and end results of treatment of childhood non-Hodgkin lymphoma: dissimilarities from lymphomas in adults. Semin Oncol 7:332–339
8. Patte C, Sakiroglu C, Ansoborlo S, et al (2002) Urate-oxidase in the prevention and treatment of metabolic complications in patients with B-cell lymphoma and leukemia, treated in the Société Francaise d'Oncologie Pédiatrique LMB89 protocol. Ann Oncol 13:789–795
9. Pui CH, Mahmoud HH, Wiley JM, et al (2001) Recombinant urate oxidase for the prophylaxis or treatment of hyperuricemia in patients with leukemia or lymphoma. J Clin Oncol 19:697–704
10. Goldman SC, Holcenberg JS, Finklestein JZ, et al (2001) A randomized comparison between rasburicase and allopurinol in children with lymphoma or leukemia at high risk for tumor lysis. Blood 97:2998–3003
11. Coiffier B, Mounier N, Bologna S, et al (2003) Efficacy and safety of rasburicase (recombinant urate oxidase) for the prevention and treatment of hyperuricemia during induction chemotherapy of aggressive non-Hodgkin lymphoma: results of the GRAAL1 (Groupe d'Etude des Lymphomes de l'Adulte Trial on Rasburicase Activity in Adult Lymphoma) study. J Clin Oncol 21:4402–4406
12. Patte C, Philip T, Rodary C, et al (1986) Improved survival rate in children with stage III and IV B cell non-Hodgkin lymphoma and leukemia using multi-agent chemotherapy: results of a study of 114 children from the French Pediatric Oncology Society. J Clin Oncol 4:1219–1226
13. Patte C, Philip T, Rodary C, et al (1991) High survival rate in advanced-stage B-cell lymphomas and leukemias without CNS involvement with a short intensive polychemotherapy: results from the French Pediatric Oncology Society of a randomized trial of 216 children. J Clin Oncol 9:123–132
14. Patte C, Auperin A, Michon J, et al (2001) The Societe Francaise d'Oncologie Pediatrique LMB89 protocol: highly effective multiagent chemotherapy tailored to the tumor burden and initial response in 561 unselected children with B-cell lymphomas and L3 leukemia. Blood 97:3370–3379
15. Reiter A, Schrappe M, Parwaresch R, et al (1995) Non-Hodgkin lymphomas of childhood and adolescence: results of a treatment stratified for biologic subtypes and stage – a report of the Berlin-Frankfurt-Munster group. J Clin Oncol 13:359–372
16. Reiter A, Schrappe M, Tiemann M, et al (1999) Improved treatment results in childhood B-cell neoplasms with tailored intensification of therapy: a report of the Berlin-Frankfurt-Munster Group Trial NHL-BFM 90. Blood 94:3294–3306
17. Magrath I, Adde M, Shad A, et al (1996) Adults and children with small non-cleaved-cell lymphoma have a similar excellent outcome when treated with the same chemotherapy regimen. J Clin Oncol 14:925–934
18. Atra A, Gerrard M, Hobson R, et al (1998) Improved cure rate in children with B-cell acute lymphoblastic leukaemia (B-ALL) and stage IV B-cell non-Hodgkin lymphoma (B-NHL) – results of the UKCCSG 9003 protocol. Br J Cancer 77:2281–2285
19. Atra A, Imeson JD, Hobson R, et al (2000) Improved outcome in children with advanced stage B-cell non-Hodgkin lymphoma (B-NHL): results of the United

Kingdom Children Cancer Study Group (UKCCSG) 9002 protocol. Br J Cancer 82:1396–1402

20. Spreafico F, Massimino M, Luksch R, et al (2002) Intensive, very short-term chemotherapy for advanced Burkitt lymphoma in children. J Clin Oncol 20:2783–2788

21. Murphy SB, Hustu HO, Rivera G, Berard CW (1983) End results of treating children with localized non-Hodgkin lymphomas with a combined modality approach of lessened intensity. J Clin Oncol 1:326–330

22. Link MP, Shuster JJ, Donaldson SS, et al (1997) Treatment of children and young adults with early-stage non-Hodgkin lymphoma. N Engl J Med 337:1259–1266

23. Meadows AT, Sposto R, Jenkin RD, et al (1989) Similar efficacy of 6 and 18 months of therapy with four drugs (COMP) for localized non-Hodgkin lymphoma of children: a report from the Childrens Cancer Study Group. J Clin Oncol 7:92–99

24. Gerrard M, Cairo MS, Patte C, et al (2003) Results of the FAB international study in children and adolescents (C+A) with localised B-NHL (large cell [LCL], Burkitt [BL] and Burkitt-like [BLL]). Proc ASCO 22:795 (abstract)

25. Reiter A, Schrappe M, Zimmermann M, et al (2003) Randomized trial of high dose methotrexate I.V. infusion over 24 hours versus 4 hours as part of combination chemotherapy for childhood and adolescent B-cell neoplasms. A report of the BFM Group. J Pediatr Hematol Oncol 25:S2 (abstract)

26. Patte C, Gerrard M, Auperin A, et al (2003) Early treatment intensity has a major prognostic impact in the "intermediate risk" childhood and adolescent B-cell lymphoma: results of the international FAB LMB 96 trial. Blood 102:491 (abstract)

27. Pusill-Wachtsmuth B, Zimmermann M, Seidemann K, et al (2003) Non-Hodgkin-lymphoma of adolescence: treatment results in the pediatric multicenter studies NHL-BFM. J Pediatr Hematol Oncol 25:S2 (abstract)

28. Todeschini G, Tecchio C, Degani D, et al (1997) Eighty-one percent event-free survival in advanced Burkitt lymphoma/leukemia: no differences in outcome between pediatric and adult patients treated with the same intensive pediatric protocol. Ann Oncol 8:77–81

29. Corbacioglu S, Eber S, Gungor T, et al (2003) Induction of long-term remission of a relapsed childhood B-acute lymphoblastic leukemia with rituximab chimeric anti-CD20 monoclonal antibody and autologous stem cell transplantation. J Pediatr Hematol Oncol 25:327–329

30. de Vries MJ, Veerman AJ, Zwaan CM (2004) Rituximab in three children with relapsed/refractory B-cell acute lymphoblastic leukaemia/Burkitt non-Hodgkin lymphoma. Br J Haematol 125:414–415

31. Cairo MS, Sposto R, Hoover-Regan M, et al (2003) Childhood and adolescent large-cell lymphoma (LCL): a review of the Children's Cancer Group experience. Am J Hematol 72:53–63

32. Laver JH, Mahmoud H, Pick TE, et al (2002) Results of a randomized phase III trial in children and adolescents with advanced stage diffuse large cell non-Hodgkin lymphoma: a Pediatric Oncology Group study. Leuk Lymphoma 43:105–109

33. Patte C, Auperin A, Bergeron C, et al (2002) Large B-cell lymphoma (LBCL) in children: similarities and differences with Burkitt (BL) in children and LBCL in adults. Experience of the SFOP LMB89 study. Ann Oncol 13:110 (abstract #379)

34. Laver JH, Weinstein HJ, Hutchison RE, et al (2001) Lineage-specific differences in outcome for advanced stage large cell lymphoma in children and adolescents: results of a randomized phase III Pediatric Oncology Group Trial. Blood 98:345a (abstract)

35. Alizadeh AA, Eisen MB, Davis RE, et al (2000) Distinct types of diffuse large B-cell lymphoma identified by gene expression profiling. Nature 403:503–511

36. Coiffier B, Lepage E, Briere J, et al (2002) CHOP chemotherapy plus rituximab compared with CHOP alone in elderly patients with diffuse large-B-cell lymphoma. N Engl J Med 346:235–242

37. Pfreundschuh MG, Trumper L, Ma D, et al (2004) Randomized intergroup trial of first line treatment for patients <= 60 years with diffuse large B-cell non-Hodgkin lymphoma (DLBCL) with a CHOP-like regimen with or without the anti-CD20 antibody rituximab – early stopping after the first interim analysis. Proc ASCO 23:6500 (abstract)

38. Savage KJ, Monti S, Kutok JL, et al (2003) The molecular signature of mediastinal large B-cell lymphoma differs from that of other diffuse large B-cell lymphomas and shares features with classical Hodgkin lymphoma. Blood 102:3871–3879

39. Patte C, Gerrard M, Auperin A, et al (2003) Results of the randomised international trial FAB LMB 96 for the "intermediate risk" childhood and adolescent B-cell lymphoma: reduced therapy is efficacious. Proc ASCO 22:796 (abstract)

40. Seidemann K, Tiemann M, Lauterbach I, et al (2003) Primary mediastinal large B-cell lymphoma with sclerosis in pediatric and adolescent patients: treatment and results from three therapeutic studies of the Berlin-Frankfurt-Munster Group. J Clin Oncol 21:1782–1789

41. Lones MA, Perkins SL, Sposto R, et al (2000) Large-cell lymphoma arising in the mediastinum in children and adolescents is associated with an excellent outcome: a Children's Cancer Group report. J Clin Oncol 18:3845–3853

42. Stein H, Mason DY, Gerdes J, et al (1985) The expression of the Hodgkin disease associated antigen Ki-1 in reactive and neoplastic lymphoid tissue: evidence that Reed-Sternberg cells and histiocytic malignancies are derived from activated lymphoid cells. Blood 66:848–858

43. Rimokh R, Magaud JP, Berger F, et al (1989) A translocation involving a specific breakpoint (q35) on chromosome 5 is characteristic of anaplastic large cell lymphoma ('Ki-1 lymphoma'). Br J Haematol 71:31–36

44. Morris SW, Kirstein MN, Valentine MB, et al (1994) Fusion of a kinase gene, ALK, to a nucleolar protein gene, NPM, in non-Hodgkin lymphoma. Science 263:1281–1284

45. Chott A, Kaserer K, Augustin I, et al (1990) Ki-1-positive large cell lymphoma. A clinicopathologic study of 41 cases. Am J Surg Pathol 14:439–448

46. Delsol G, Al Saati T, Gatter KC, et al (1988) Coexpression of epithelial membrane antigen (EMA), Ki-1, and interleukin-2 receptor by anaplastic large cell lymphomas. Diagnostic value in so-called malignant histiocytosis. Am J Pathol 130:59–70

47. Nakamura S, Takagi N, Kojima M, et al (1991) Clinicopathologic study of large cell anaplastic lymphoma (Ki-1-positive large cell lymphoma) among the Japanese. Cancer 68:118–129

48. Greer JP, Kinney MC, Collins RD, et al (1991) Clinical features of 31 patients with Ki-1 anaplastic large-cell lymphoma. J Clin Oncol 9:539–547

49. Shiota M, Nakamura S, Ichinohasama R, et al (1995) Anaplastic large cell lymphomas expressing the novel chimeric protein p80NPM/ALK: a distinct clinicopathologic entity. Blood 86:1954–1960

50. Gascoyne RD, Aoun P, Wu D, et al (1999) Prognostic significance of anaplastic lymphoma kinase (ALK) protein expression in adults with anaplastic large cell lymphoma. Blood 93:3913–3921

51. Falini B, Pileri S, Pizzolo G, et al (1995) CD30 (Ki-1) molecule: a new cytokine receptor of the tumor necrosis factor receptor superfamily as a tool for diagnosis and immunotherapy. Blood 85:1–14

52. Stein H, Foss HD, Durkop H, et al (2000) CD30(+) anaplastic large cell lymphoma: a review of its histopathologic, genetic, and clinical features. Blood 96:3681–3695

53. Fraga M, Brousset P, Schlaifer D, et al (1995) Bone marrow involvement in anaplastic large cell lymphoma. Immunohistochemical detection of minimal disease and its prognostic significance. Am J Clin Pathol 103:82–89

54. Benharroch D, Meguerian-Bedoyan Z, Lamant L, et al (1998) ALK-positive lymphoma: a single disease with a broad spectrum of morphology. Blood 91:2076–2084

55. Jaffe ES (2001) Anaplastic large cell lymphoma: the shifting sands of diagnostic hematopathology. Mod Pathol 2001;14:219–228

56. Willemze R, Beljaards RC (1993) Spectrum of primary cutaneous CD30 (Ki-1)-positive lymphoproliferative disorders. A proposal for classification and guidelines for management and treatment. J Am Acad Dermatol 28:973–980

57. Vergier B, Beylot-Barry M, Pulford K, et al (1998) Statistical evaluation of diagnostic and prognostic features of CD30+ cutaneous lymphoproliferative disorders: a clinicopathologic study of 65 cases. Am J Surg Pathol 22:1192–1202

58. DeCoteau JF, Butmarc JR, Kinney MC, Kadin ME (1996) The t(2;5) chromosomal translocation is not a common feature of primary cutaneous CD30+ lymphoproliferative disorders: comparison with anaplastic large-cell lymphoma of nodal origin. Blood 87:3437–3441

59. Drexler HG, Gignac SM, von Wasielewski R, et al (2000) Pathobiology of NPM-ALK and variant fusion genes in anaplastic large cell lymphoma and other lymphomas. Leukemia 14:1533–1559

60. Duyster J, Bai RY, Morris SW (2001) Translocations involving anaplastic lymphoma kinase (ALK). Oncogene 20:5623–5637

61. Gascoyne RD, Adomat SA, Krajewski S, et al (1997) Prognostic significance of Bcl-2 protein expression and Bcl-2 gene rearrangement in diffuse aggressive non-Hodgkin lymphoma. Blood 90:244–251

62. Murphy SB (1994) Pediatric lymphomas: recent advances and commentary on Ki-1-positive anaplastic large-cell lymphomas of childhood. Ann Oncol 5:31–33

63. Seidemann K, Tiemann M, Schrappe M, et al (2001) Short-pulse B-non-Hodgkin lymphoma-type chemotherapy is efficacious treatment for pediatric anaplastic large cell lymphoma: a report of the Berlin-Frankfurt-Munster Group Trial NHL-BFM 90. Blood 97:3699–3706

64. Sandlund JT, Pui CH, Santana VM, et al (1994) Clinical features and treatment outcome for children with CD30+ large-cell non-Hodgkin lymphoma. J Clin Oncol 12:895–898

65. Williams DM, Hobson R, Imeson J, et al (2002) Anaplastic large cell lymphoma in childhood: analysis of 72 patients treated on The United Kingdom Children's Cancer Study Group chemotherapy regimens. Br J Haematol 117:812–820

66. Massimino M, Spreafico F, Luksch R, Giardini R (2001) Prognostic significance of p80 and visceral involvement in childhood CD30 anaplastic large cell lymphoma (ALCL). Med Pediatr Oncol 37:97–102

67. Brugieres L, Deley MC, Pacquement H, et al (1998) CD30(+) anaplastic large-cell lymphoma in children: analysis of 82 patients enrolled in two consecutive studies of the French Society of Pediatric Oncology. Blood 92:3591–3598

68. Suzuki R, Kagami Y, Takeuchi K, et al (2000) Prognostic significance of CD56 expression for ALK-positive and ALK-negative anaplastic large-cell lymphoma of T/null cell phenotype. Blood 96:2993–3000

69. Sandlund JT, Pui CH, Roberts WM, et al (1994) Clinicopathologic features and treatment outcome of children with large-cell lymphoma and the t(2;5)(p23;q35). Blood 84:2467–2471

70. Cairo MS, Krailo MD, Morse M, et al (2002) Long-term follow-up of short intensive multiagent chemotherapy without high-dose methotrexate ("Orange") in children with advanced non-lymphoblastic non-Hodgkin lymphoma. A Children's Cancer Group report. Leukemia 16:594–600

71. Reiter A, Schrappe M, Tiemann M, et al (1994) Successful treatment strategy for Ki-1 anaplastic large-cell lymphoma of childhood: a prospective analysis of 62 patients enrolled in three consecutive Berlin-Frankfurt-Munster group studies. J Clin Oncol 12:899–908

72. Mora J, Filippa DA, Thaler HT, et al (2000) Large cell non-Hodgkin lymphoma of childhood: Analysis of 78 consecutive patients enrolled in 2 consecutive protocols at the Memorial Sloan-Kettering Cancer Center. Cancer 88:186–197

73. Abromowitch M, Sposto R, Perkins SL, et al (2002) Preliminary results of CCG-5941: a pilot study in children and adolescents with anaplastic large cell lymphoma. Ann Oncol 13:erratum

74. Fanin R, Silvestri F, Geromin A, et al (1996) Primary systemic CD30 (Ki-1)-positive anaplastic large cell lymphoma of the adult: sequential intensive treatment with the F-MACHOP regimen (+/– radiotherapy) and autologous bone marrow transplantation. Blood 87:1243–1248

75. Sternberg C (1916) Leukosarkomatose and myeloblastenleukaamie. Beitr Pathol 61:75

76. Barcos MGP, Lukes RJ (1975) Malignant lymphoma of the convoluted lymphocytes: a new entity of possible T-cell type. In: Sinks L, Godden J (eds) Conflicts in Childhood Cancer: An Evaluation of Current Management. Liss, New York, p 147

77. Amylon MD, Shuster J, Pullen J, et al (1999) Intensive high-dose asparaginase consolidation improves survival for pediatric patients with T cell acute lymphoblastic leukemia and advanced stage lymphoblastic lymphoma: a Pediatric Oncology Group study. Leukemia 13:335–342

78. Tubergen DG, Krailo MD, Meadows AT, et al (1995) Comparison of treatment regimens for pediatric lymphoblastic non-Hodgkin lymphoma: a Childrens Cancer Group study. J Clin Oncol 13:1368–1376

79. Mora J, Filippa DA, Qin J, Wollner N (2003) Lymphoblastic lymphoma of childhood and the LSA2-L2 protocol: the 30-year experience at Memorial-Sloan-Kettering Cancer Center. Cancer 98:1283–1291

80. Reiter A, Schrappe M, Ludwig WD, et al (2000) Intensive ALL-type therapy without local radiotherapy provides a 90% event-free survival for children with T-cell lymphoblastic lymphoma: a BFM group report. Blood 95:416–421

81. Thomas DA, Kantarjian HM (2001) Lymphoblastic lymphoma. Hematol Oncol Clin North Am 15:51–95

82. Colgan JP, Andersen J, Habermann TM, et al (1994) Long-term follow-up of a CHOP-based regimen with maintenance therapy and central nervous system prophylaxis in lymphoblastic non-Hodgkin lymphoma. Leuk Lymphoma 15:291–296

83. Hoelzer D, Gokbuget N, Digel W, et al (2002) Outcome of adult patients with T-lymphoblastic lymphoma treated according to protocols for acute lymphoblastic leukemia. Blood 99:4379–4385

84. Cairo MS, Raetz E, Perkins SL (2003) Non-Hodgkin lymphoma in children. In: Kufe DW, Pollock RE, Weichselbaum RR, et al (eds) Cancer Medicine (6th edition). Decker, London, pp 2337–2348

85. Sandlund JT, Downing JR, Crist WM (1996) Non-Hodgkin lymphoma in childhood. N Engl J Med 334:1238–1248

86. Perkins SL (2000) Work-up and diagnosis of pediatric non-Hodgkin lymphomas. Pediatr Dev Pathol 3:374–390

87. Pilozzi E, Muller-Hermelink HK, Falini B, et al (1999) Gene rearrangements in T-cell lymphoblastic lymphoma. J Pathol 188:267–270

88. Hojo H, Sasaki Y, Nakamura N, Abe M (2001) Absence of somatic hypermutation of immunoglobulin heavy chain variable region genes in precursor B-lymphoblastic lymphoma: a study of four cases in childhood and adolescence. Am J Clin Pathol 116:673–682

89. Link MP, Donaldson SS, Berard CW, et al (1990) Results of treatment of childhood localized non-Hodgkin lymphoma with combination chemotherapy with or without radiotherapy. N Engl J Med 322:1169–1174

90. Anderson J, Jenkin R, Wilson J, et al (1993) Long-term follow-up of patients treated with COMP or LSA$_2$L$_2$ therapy for childhood non-Hodgkin lymphoma: a report of CCG-551 from the Childrens Cancer Group. J Clin Oncol 11:1024–1032

91. Wollner N, Burchenal JH, Lieberman PH, et al (1976) Non-Hodgkin lymphoma in children. A comparative study of two modalities of therapy. Cancer 37:123–134

92. Anderson J, Wilson J, Jenkin D, et al (1983) Childhood non-Hodgkin lymphoma. The results of a randomized therapeutic trial comparing a 4-drug regimen (COMP) with a 10-drug regimen (LSA$_2$-L$_2$). N Engl J Med 308:559–565

93. Asselin B, Shuster JJ, Amylon M, et al (2001) Improved event-free survival (EFS) with high dose methotrexate (HDM) in T-cell lymphoblastic leukemia (T-ALL) and advanced lymphoblastic lymphoma (T-NHL): a Pediatric Oncology Group (POG) study. Proc Am Soc Clin Oncol 20:1464 (abstract)

94. Millot F, Suciu S, Philippe N, et al (2001) Value of high-dose cytarabine during interval therapy of a Berlin-Frankfurt-Munster-based protocol in increased-risk children with acute lymphoblastic leukemia and lymphoblastic lymphoma: results of the European Organization for Research and Treatment of Cancer 58881 randomized phase III trial. J Clin Oncol 19:1935–1942

95. Weinstein HJ, Cassady JR, Levey R (1983) Long-term results of the APO protocol (vincristine, doxorubicin [adriamycin], and prednisone) for treatment of mediastinal lymphoblastic lymphoma. J Clin Oncol 1:537–541

96. Hvizdala EV, Berard C, Callihan T, et al (1988) Lymphoblastic lymphoma in children – a randomized trial comparing LSA2-L2 with the A-COP+ therapeutic regimen: a Pediatric Oncology Group Study. J Clin Oncol 6:26–33

97. Eden OB, Hann I, Imeson J, et al (1992) Treatment of advanced stage T cell lymphoblastic lymphoma: results of the United Kingdom Children's Cancer Study Group (UKCCSG) protocol 8503. Br J Haematol 82:310–316

98. Abromowitch M, Sposto R, Prkins S, et al (2000) Outcome of Children's Cancer Group (CCG) 5941: A pilot study for the treatment of newly diagnosed pediatric patients with disseminated lymphoblastic lymphoma. Proc Am Soc Clin Oncol 19:2295 (abstract)

99. Coleman CN, Picozzi VJ Jr, Cox RS, et al (1986) Treatment of lymphoblastic lymphoma in adults. J Clin Oncol 4:1628–1637

100. Morel P, Lepage E, Brice P, et al (1992) Prognosis and treatment of lymphoblastic lymphoma in adults: a report on 80 patients. J Clin Oncol 10:1078–1085

101. Zinzani PL, Bendandi M, Visani G, et al (1996) Adult lymphoblastic lymphoma: clinical features and prognostic factors in 53 patients. Leuk Lymphoma 23:577–582

102. Bouabdallah R, Xerri L, Bardou VJ, et al (1998) Role of induction chemotherapy and bone marrow transplantation in adult lymphoblastic lymphoma: a report on 62 patients from a single center. Ann Oncol 9:619–625

103. Sweetenham JW, Santini G, Qian W, et al (2001) High-dose therapy and autologous stem-cell transplantation versus conventional-dose consolidation/maintenance therapy as postremission therapy for adult patients with lymphoblastic lymphoma: results of a randomized trial of the European Group for Blood and Marrow Transplantation and the United Kingdom Lymphoma Group. J Clin Oncol 19:2927–2936

104. Levine JE, Harris RE, Loberiza FR, Jr., et al (2003) A comparison of allogeneic and autologous bone marrow transplantation for lymphoblastic lymphoma. Blood 101:2476–2482

105. Falini B, Pileri S, Zinzani PL, et al (1999) ALK+ lymphoma: clinico-pathological findings and outcome. Blood 93:2697–2706

Central Nervous System Tumors

David A. Walker • Anne Bendel •

Charles Stiller • Paul Byrne • Michael Soka

Contents

10.1 Introduction

We suggest that central nervous system (CNS) tumors present unique clinical and scientific challenges in the adolescent and young adult age group due to the intricacies of development, presentation, management, and rehabilitation for patients with these tumors. These challenges compound the complexity of a cancer diagnosis and the risk of neurological insult during the journey from childhood to adulthood. The cancer diagnosis and tumor-related brain injury not only shocks the patient, family, and friends, but also affects the physiological processes driving development itself. Neurological damage and physical disability may occur, and cognitive deficits may develop that slow down training and education, change work ambitions and life plans and, at worst, set the individual on a course for life-long dependent living.

Neurooncology is an emerging subspecialty. In the childhood age range (0–15 years), dramatic improvements in management and outcome have been achieved by multidisciplinary teams working in specialist centers, recruitment of patients to multicenter trials of novel therapies, and the establishment of links to community-based rehabilitation services. Adult neurooncology, on the other hand, is well established as a subspecialty, and great advances have been made in diagnostic imaging, neuropathology, neurosurgery, and radio- and chemotherapeutic approaches to tumor-related management.

The incidence of CNS tumors in the 15- to 29-year age group is ranked sixth compared to other tumor types and accounts for 6% of all neoplasms [1]. Adolescent and young adults with CNS tumors have a better overall life expectancy than older adults, but age and disease-specific comparisons are rare and the poor track record for recruiting adolescent and young adults to cancer trials [2] suggests that this favorable comparison does not justify a complacent approach.

In the first section of this chapter we will outline the classification of histological subtypes, consider the

Table 10.1 Annual incidence per 100,000 for malignant tumors of the brain and nervous system (ICD-10 C70-72) diagnosed in the 1990s. Populations ranked according to incidence in males aged 15–29 years. *SEER* Surveillance, Epidemiology and End Results, *IARC* International Agency for Research and Cancer

	Male age (years)			Female age (years)		
	15–19	20–24	25–29	15–19	20–24	25–29
Algeria, four registries [3]	0.5	0.7	1.0	0.4	0.6	0.9
Japan, Osaka [4]	0.7	0.7	1.2	0.5	0.7	1.1
India, Mumbai (Bombay) [4]	0.8	1.5	1.3	1.1	0.9	1.1
Zimbabwe, Harare: African [3]	1.2	1.0	0.9	0.3	0.1	0.8
Singapore: Chinese [4]	1.2	1.8	1.3	0.3	0.7	0.9
UK, Scotland [4]	1.6	1.9	3.0	2.0	0.9	2.4
Colombia, Cali [4]	1.9	2.0	3.5	0.5	1.3	1.7
USA, SEER: Black [4]	1.9	2.2	1.8	1.2	1.4	1.3
Australia [4]	1.9	2.3	4.2	1.8	2.1	2.5
USA, SEER: White [4]	2.0	3.3	3.5	1.9	1.3	2.7
Czech Republic [4]	2.0	2.2	2.8	1.0	1.4	2.2
Lithuania [4]	2.1	2.6	3.2	2.0	1.8	1.7
Netherlands [4]	2.1	2.6	3.1	2.0	2.0	2.1
Sweden [4]	2.2	3.3	4.3	2.0	2.6	2.5

incidence and complex age-incidence patterns of histology in this age group, and describe the recognized clinical predisposition syndromes and factors. In the second section of this chapter we will describe the clinical presentation and assessments needed for planning approaches to CNS tumor management in general. We have chosen to concentrate discussion of evidence-based clinical management on germ cell tumors (GCT) as the model adolescent and young adult CNS tumor. From this, several general principles will be identified that will be proposed as a focus of study for adolescent and young adult clinical neurooncology.

10.2 Incidence, Pathology, and Etiology of CNS Tumors

10.2.1 Incidence of CNS Tumors in the Adolescent and Young Adult

Table 10.1 shows the annual incidence of malignant brain and nervous system tumors among people diagnosed at 15–29 years of age in 13 countries. Males had consistently higher incidence than females. The ratio of cumulative incidence for males to that for females ranged from 1.1 in Japan to 2.6 in Zimbabwe, although for most populations it was in the range 1.2–1.5. Incidence usually increased with age in both genders. This increase was more marked for males. The highest incidence for both males and females was in Sweden; the lowest was in Algeria. In the USA, African Americans/blacks had a lower incidence than whites, and their incidence did not increase with age. These data undoubtedly underestimate the total risk of CNS tumors. This is due in part to underdiagnosis, especially in some less-developed countries where there is severely restricted access to neurological and neurosurgical facilities. Certain categories of tumors, however, are systematically excluded from these data. Numerically, the most important are nonmalignant tumors. In the United States it has been estimated that inclusion of nonmalignant tumors would increase the incidence among adolescents aged 15–19 years by 57% [5]. United States Surveillance, Epidemiology, and End Results (SEER) data for CNS tumors does not include brain lymphomas, which are grouped with lymphomas of all other sites, and CNS GCTs, which are grouped with gonadal malignancies.

10.2.2 United States Population Databases: SEER and CBTRUS

Population-based incidence data by histological subgroup is available from two large United States databases, namely the SEER Program, the data for which were collected from 1975 to 1998 [1], and the Central Brain Tumor Registry of the United States (CBTRUS), for which data were gathered from 1997 to 2001 (CBTRUS 2004–2005) [6]. There are important differences, however, between the two sources in scope and reporting. The SEER data are reported by 5-year age groups, allowing results to be presented for adolescents and young adults defined as people who are 15–29 years of age; the CBTRUS data are divided into adolescents 15–19 years of age and young adults 20–34 years of age (CBTRUS 2004–2005). The SEER data include mainly malignant tumors, but also includes some benign CNS tumors, and "lumps" CNS tumors into five somewhat broad categories: astrocytoma, other gliomas, medulloblastoma/primitive neuroectodermal tumors (PNETs), ependymoma, and miscellaneous. Therefore, SEER data are not available specifically for meningioma, adenomas, or craniopharyngioma (which are included under miscellaneous), limiting the discussion about these tumors. SEER data are available for malignant CNS GCTs, but they are not included in the overall group of CNS tumors, instead being categorized with "Germ Cell, Trophoblastic, and Other Gonadal Malignancies". The CBTRUS uses a more detailed histological classification and includes nonmalignant tumors. SEER incidence data for 5-year age groups up through 44 years of age is shown in Fig. 10.1, and CBTRUS incidence data for the age group 15–19 years is displayed in Fig. 10.2. The World Health Organization (WHO) classification will be used to describe tumors throughout this chapter.

10.2.3 Data from the United Kingdom

Incidence data for people aged 15–24 years in England (United Kingdom) have been published recently in more detail [7]. The results are shown in Table 10.2.

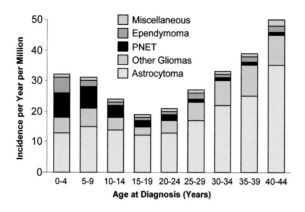

Figure 10.1

Incidence of central nervous system (CNS) tumors in American children, adolescents, and young adults by tumor type according to age at diagnosis. Data from the United States SEER Program [1]

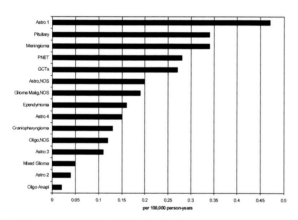

Figure 10.2

Ranked incidence by histological subtype in patients diagnosed with a brain tumor between 15 and 19 years of age, inclusive. Data from the Central Brain Tumor Registry of the United States (CBTRUS), 2004–2005 [6]. *AYA* adolescents/young adults, *Astro 1* grade I astrocytoma, *Astro 2* grade II astrocytoma, *Astro 3* grade III astrocytoma, *Astro 4* grade IV astrocytoma, *PNET* primitive neuroectodermal tumor, *GCT* germ-cell tumor, *Malig* malignant, *Oligo* oligodendroglioma, *Anapl* anaplastic, *NOS* not otherwise specified

Table 10.2 Incidence per 100,000 of malignant central nervous system (CNS) tumors at age 15–24 years in England, 1979–1997 [7]. *PNET* Primitive neuroectodermal tumor

	Age 15–19 years	Age 20–24 years
Astrocytoma	0.83	0.86
Low grade	0.18	0.10
High grade	0.12	0.14
Unspecified	0.53	0.61
Other glioma	0.29	0.44
Ependymoma	0.10	0.12
PNET	0.15	0.15
Germ cell	0.08	0.05
Other specified	0.04	0.04
Unspecified	0.16	0.16
Total	1.64	1.82

Total incidence was somewhat lower than in the SEER data, but the relative frequencies of the histological subtypes were similar. Among astrocytomas of specified grade, low-grade tumors accounted for a higher proportion at age 15–19 years, whereas high-grade tumors were more frequent at age 20–24 years. In both age groups, more than 60% of astrocytomas were of unspecified subtype. Variations in incidence of specific histological types in other regions of the world are generally poorly documented.

10.2.4 Histology Age-Incidence Patterns

The pattern of age-incidence of primary CNS tumors arising in the adolescent and young adult period suggests that their development is driven, in part, by factors linked to the completion of the brain's growth and development, its central role in sexual maturation, and the influence of adult aging. How such factors influence the proliferative processes, harnessed by tumor-driven tissue growth, is poorly understood. However, the ranked tumor incidences from the 15- to 19-year category (Fig. 10.2), together with patterns of age inci-

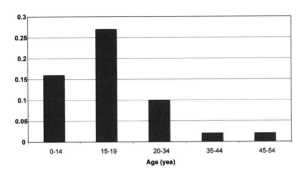

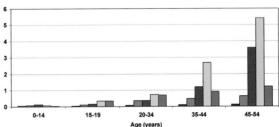

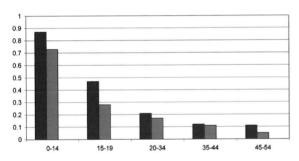

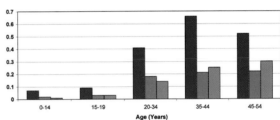

Figure 10.3

Incidence of CNS germ-cell tumors by age in American patients younger than age 55 years who were diagnosed between 1997 and 2001, inclusive. Data from the CBTRUS, 2004–2005 [6].

Figure 10.5

Incidence of grade II astrocytoma (*blue bars*), grade III astrocytoma (*green bars*), grade IV astrocytoma (*purple bars*), meningioma (*yellow bars*), and pituitary tumors (*red bars*) by age in American patients younger than age 55 years who were diagnosed between 1997 and 2001, inclusive. Data from the CBTRUS, 2004–2005 [6].

Figure 10.4

Incidence of grade I astrocytoma (*blue bars*) and CNS PNETs (*red bars*) by age in American patients younger than age 55 years who were diagnosed between 1997 and 2001, inclusive. Data from the CBTRUS, 2004–2005 [6].

Figure 10.6

Incidence of nonspecified oligodendroglioma (*blue bars*), anaplastic oligodendroglioma (*red bars*), and oligoastrocytoma (*green bars*) by age in American patients younger than age 55 years who were diagnosed between 1997 and 2001 inclusive. Data from the CBTRUS, 2004–2005 [6].

dence for these tumor types (Figs. 10.3–10.7) provide clues to developmental and aging factors, which may influence tumor initiation and progression. Four patterns of tumor incidence can be recognized from the SEER and CBTRUS databases: peak incidence in the 15–19 year age group, decreasing incidence with age, rising incidence with age, and varying incidence with age.

The peak incidence of GCTs, with a male preponderance that is also seen in extracranial GCTs, is considered to be a consequence of pubertal development and the tumor growth promoting consequences of the associated surge in sex hormones. For this reason, intracranial GCTs in our view are the "model" CNS tumor for an adolescent and young adult neurooncology service. The falling incidence of grade 1 astrocyto-

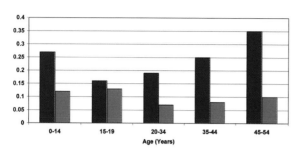

Figure 10.7

Incidence of ependymoma (*blue bars*) and craniopharyngioma (*red bars*) by age in American patients younger than age 55 years who were diagnosed between 1997 and 2001, inclusive. Data from the CBTRUS, 2004–2005 [6.]

mas and PNETs suggests that tumor development and progression in these tumors are linked to factors related to early brain growth and development, which recede as adolescent brain growth slows and developmental processes finalize. The large category of predominantly astrocytic tumors that demonstrate a rising incidence with increasing age would be compatible with adult type, age-related genetic dysregulation or environmental insult as etiological factors reflected in the complex genetic mutations typically seen in these tumor types. The relationship between low-grade and higher-grade astrocytomas supports the hypothesis that the benign variant can transform into the malignant phenotype in a proportion of cases. The accelerated development of meningiomas and grade 4 astrocytomas in young people after prior CNS radiation therapy (RT) for childhood cancers suggests that RT can accelerate or mimic this aging/environmental effect. Finally, ependymomas and craniopharyngiomas show stable incidence across age groups, suggesting that their etiology is independent of aging. Ependymomas arise from the ependymal lining of ventricles; they remain deficient in reliable biological markers of tumor behavior. Craniopharyngiomas are tumors that arise as a result of the developmental malformations associated with Rathke's pouch and are therefore not tumors in the strictest sense, although they are space occupying, have the capacity to grow, and respond to radiotherapy.

10.2.5 Etiology of CNS Tumors Adolescent and Young Adult

10.2.5.1 Environmental and Exogenous Risk Factors

Environmental and genetic factors are the most commonly considered potential causes of brain tumors and have been the focus of much research. The most comprehensive review of environmental and exogenous risk factors was published in 1996 [8, 9]. The authors candidly stated: "We simply have no idea what causes most nervous system tumors." Despite the subsequent publication of numerous etiological studies and reviews, this is still true. The evidence is summarized below.

Ionizing Radiation

The only established environmental risk factor for CNS tumors is ionizing radiation. RT for cancer, including prophylactic CNS irradiation as part of the treatment for childhood leukemia, increases the risk of CNS tumors in young people [9]. The predominant tumor types are meningiomas and grades 3 and 4 astrocytomas. Radiotherapy for nonmalignant conditions such as tinea capitis also carries an increased risk of CNS tumors [10], although this practice ceased so long ago that all the CNS tumors attributable to it in those under age 30 years should have already occurred.

Electromagnetic Fields and Radiofrequencies

There is little evidence that residential exposure to electric and magnetic fields (EMF) is a risk factor for brain tumors at any age [11–14]. There is no consistent association between parental exposure to EMF and brain tumors in their offspring [13, 15]. Electrical workers themselves may be at slightly increased risk for brain tumors, but exposure misclassification and the absence of a dose–response relationship in most studies make the results hard to interpret [13]. Epidemiological studies of exposure to radiofrequency emissions from use of mobile telephones suggest that a large risk over a short time of use is unlikely, but there is insufficient evidence regarding the possibility of increased risks that are relatively small or related to longer follow-up periods [16].

N-Nitroso Compounds, Diet, and Smoking

Since N-nitroso compounds (NOCs) were found to be potent experimental carcinogens more than 20 years ago, a succession of epidemiological studies has investigated the hypothesis that exposure to preformed NOCs or their precursors can cause brain tumors in humans [8]. The results of a meta-analysis of seven case-control studies suggest that maternal consumption of cured meat during pregnancy may be a risk factor for childhood brain tumors, especially astrocytomas [17]. An earlier review of the same studies, however, noted that some were based on rather small numbers of cases, the dietary information was apparently not validated, and selection bias could not be ruled out [18]. A pooled analysis of nine studies of adults did not show clear evidence for an elevated risk of brain tumors with ingestion of NOCs from cured meat in adulthood [19]. There is limited evidence for a reduction in risk of CNS tumors with increased fruit and vegetable consumption and with use of vitamin supplements, although studies have not been consistent [8]. These results may support the N-nitroso hypothesis insofar as these nutrients inhibit the endogenous formation of nitrosamines, but any protective effect could be due to other mechanisms [8].

Tobacco smoke is a potent source of NOCs and polycyclic aromatic hydrocarbons (PAHs), among other carcinogens. Meta-analyses have provided little evidence of an association between maternal smoking during pregnancy and childhood brain tumors [20, 21]. Preconception and childhood exposure to paternal tobacco smoke revealed a raised risk, but confounding with other risk factors could not be ruled out [20]. The results of studies of smoking as a risk factor for CNS tumors in adults have been inconsistent [8]. Likewise, there is no consistent evidence for an elevated risk associated with alcohol consumption [8].

Pesticides and Agriculture

Exposure to pesticides has been analyzed in many studies of childhood CNS tumors and several studies have investigated exposure to animals and residence on farms as a risk factor. Elevated risks have been found for at least one measure of pesticide exposure in half the studies, more markedly for domestic exposure during pregnancy, although there have also been numerous nonsignificant results and few studies have provided risks for specific histological types [22]. Childhood farm residence and maternal or child exposure to farm animals tended to be associated with higher risk [23]. If the latter associations are real, they might be related to oncogenic animal viruses, but there is also likely to have been a high degree of confounding with pesticide exposure. In the International Adult Brain Tumor Study there was little evidence that gliomas or meningiomas were associated with contact with animals or with occupations involving high levels of contact with animals or humans [24].

Other Occupational Factors

There has been little consistency in studies of other parental occupations in relation to childhood brain tumors [15, 25, 26]. A large international study found a raised risk for astroglial tumors associated with paternal occupations before conception that were likely to involve relatively high exposure to PAHs [27]. This result, together with earlier findings of a raised risk among children of fathers who smoked, tends to support the hypothesis that paternal preconception exposure to PAHs is a risk factor for brain tumors, but confirmation based on more direct assessment of PAH exposure is required. The incidence of brain tumors increases with increasing socioeconomic status, but there has only been limited consistency in studies of occupation and brain tumors in adults [8]. Several studies, however, have found raised risks for workers in the petrochemical and rubber industries [8, 28–31], although odds ratios were often not statistically significant. Raised risks have also been found among health-care professionals [8, 28–30], but this may reflect a social class effect rather than a risk associated with any specific exposure.

Protective Factors

Decreased risks of glioma that have been found in association with past history of allergies [32–34], autoimmune diseases [32] or certain common viral infections [33, 35] may all indicate a role for immunological factors in the etiology of glioma. These results should be treated with caution, however, as they were based on questionnaires in case-control studies without validation from medical records. Moreover, proxy respondents supplied information on a substantial proportion of cases, usually because the subject was too ill to respond or had died. For allergies, the odds ratios in different studies were inversely correlated with the percentage of proxy respondents, indicating possible bias [36]. Two studies, however, that were not susceptible to recall bias also provide support for an immune-related etiology of glioma. A large cohort study in Sweden, involving record linkage between the population-based Twin Registry, Hospital Discharge Registry, and Cancer Registry, found an inverse association between immune-related discharge diagnoses and glioma [36]; the hazard ratio of 0.46 was not statistically significant, but was similar to the odds ratio in earlier case-control studies. In the San Francisco Bay Area Adult Glioma Study, glioblastoma cases diagnosed during two separate calendar periods were significantly less likely than their respective controls to have immunoglobulin G antibodies to varicella-zoster virus [37, 38].

Acquired Immune Deficiency Syndrome

Primary non-Hodgkin lymphoma (NHL) of the brain has occurred consistently as an acquired immune deficiency syndrome (AIDS)-defining illness in around 0.5% of AIDS patients [39]. A population-based study in Italy during the period 1985–1994 found that 22 out of 40 (55%) cases of brain NHL at age 15–49 years occurred in people with AIDS, giving a standardized incidence ratio of over 2,000 [40]. In an analysis of cancer incidence among nearly 48,000 human immunodeficiency virus (HIV)-seropositive people from North America, Europe, and Australia, the adjusted annual incidence of cerebral NHL fell significantly from 1.7 per 1,000 during the period 1992–1996, to 0.7 per 1,000 during the years 1997–1999, indicating a

substantial reduction in risk with the introduction of highly active antiretroviral therapy (International Collaboration on HIV and Cancer 2000) [41].

Noncontributory Effects of Simian Virus 40 (SV40) Immunization Contamination

Large quantities of polio vaccine administered during the period 1955–1963 were contaminated with SV40. SV40 DNA sequences have been detected in large proportions of ependymomas and choroid plexus tumors in some laboratory studies [42], suggesting a role for SV40 in their etiology. No such association has been found in other series, however, including one of 33 ependymomas and 14 choroid plexus tumors from northern India, where the population has frequent contact with SV40-infected rhesus macaques [43]. Cohort studies of populations exposed to contaminated vaccines have failed to detect an increased risk. In some of these studies, not all vaccine was contaminated or the extent of use was poorly documented, but these criticisms do not apply to the most recent, large national study from Denmark [44].

Nonsteroidal Anti-Inflammatory Drugs

A recent case-control study found a protective effect of self-reported use of nonsteroidal anti-inflammatory drugs (NSAIDs) against glioblastoma [45]. A previous cohort study of low-dose aspirin users had found a significantly increased risk of brain cancer [46]. This does not contradict the hypothesis that NSAIDs could protect against glioma, however, as the excess was entirely in the 1st year of follow-up and could well have been an artifact resulting from use of aspirin to relieve symptoms of an as yet undiagnosed tumor, and for follow-up in excess of 5 years there was in fact a nonsignificantly reduced risk similar to that observed in the case-control study.

Epilepsy and Head Injury

Raised risks of glioma in association with a history of epilepsy have been found in several studies of children [47] and adults [33, 35]. It seems likely, however, that this reflects, at least in part, the fact that epilepsy can be an early symptom of a brain tumor, especially low-grade astrocytomas of childhood [47]. There is little consistent evidence that head injury is a risk factor for CNS tumors. In a national population-based cohort study in Denmark, a raised risk was found only in the 1st year after head injury [48]. The excess was most marked for people who also had epilepsy and could well reflect an increased risk of head injury in the presence of an asymptomatic brain tumor. A borderline significant increased odds ratio for head injury was found in the San Francisco Bay Area Adult Glioma Study, but this was most likely an artifact of incomplete recall by the subset of controls who only completed a brief telephone interview [49]. In the International Adult Brain Tumor Study there was little evidence that head injury was a risk factor for glioma [50]. There was a suggestion that meningioma might be associated with head trauma, but this was based on small numbers, and patients aged under 25 years were excluded [50].

10.2.5.2 Predisposing Conditions

An appreciable proportion of adolescent and young adults with CNS tumors may be associated with predisposition syndromes that in some instances may not be diagnosed until the CNS tumor presents. Their recognition is critical as the predisposing condition may: (1) determine the diagnostic process, (2) affect the prognosis for the tumor, (3) play a part in treatment selection, (4) provide novel genetically determined approaches for therapy, and (5) be the presenting symptom of a previously unrecognized genetic disease and provide an opportunity for participation in important tumor-related research, which, with current rates of progress, may influence treatment options in the foreseeable future. The range of currently recognized predisposing genetic conditions is listed in Table 10.3.

CNS Tumor Risk

Neurofibromatosis

Neurofibromatosis (NF) type 1 is associated with optic glioma and other tumors of the CNS [51–55]. NF type 2 (NF2) is associated with a high risk of intracranial

meningioma, affecting 18–58% of patients in four large studies [56]. Astrocytomas and ependymomas are rarer, but each is seen in about 3% of patients [56].

Meningiomas

Multiple meningiomas are the second hallmark of NF2, occur earlier in life than sporadic meningiomas, and are usually WHO grade 1 tumors. There is no increased frequency of atypical or malignant meningiomas, although they are more frequently fibroblastic.

Schwannomas

NF2-associated schwannomas are WHO grade 1 tumors that differ from sporadic schwannomas by presenting at an earlier age and at multiple sites (e.g., bilateral vestibular schwannomas occurring in the third decade of life). They affect multiple cranial and spinal nerves, predominantly sensory (5th and 8th), although motor roots such as the 12th are reported. They may present as either multilobular tumors or as multiple schwannomatous tumorlets with potential to progress to schwannomas. Vestibular schwannomas may entrap several cranial nerves, exhibiting high proliferative activity.

Gliomas

The overwhelming majority (80%) of gliomas associated with NF2 are intramedullary, either within the spinal cord or the spinal cauda equina. A further 10% affect the medulla. Up to 75% are ependymomas, frequently multiple., the remainder being diffuse or pilocytic astrocytomas.

Neurofibromas

Although these occur, they are frequently found to be schwannomas upon review. Plexiform neurofibromas are not seen in NF2.

10.2.5.3 Von Hippel-Lindau Syndrome

Von Hippel-Lindau (VHL) syndrome is an autosomal dominant disorder with an incidence of between

Table 10.3 Genetic predisposing conditions. *CHRPE* Congenital hypertrophy of the retinal pigment epithelium, *MPNST* malignant peripheral nerve sheath tumor

Syndrome	Gene	Chromosome	Nervous system	Skin	Other tissues
Neurofibromatosis type 1 (OMIM 162200)	*NF1*	17q11	Neurofibromas, optic nerve gliomas, astrocytomas, MPNST	Café au lait spots, axillary freckling	Iris hamartomas, osseous lesions, phaeochromocytoma, leukemia, soft-tissue sarcoma
Neurofibromatosis type 2 (OMIM 101000)	*NF2*	22q12	Vestibular and peripheral schwannomas, meningioma(s), meningiomatosis, spinal ependymomas, astrocytomas, glial hamartomas, cerebral calcification		Posterior capsular cataract or opacity
Von Hippel-Lindau (OMIM 193300)	*VHL*	3p25	Hemangioblastoma		Retinal hemangioblastoma, renal cell carcinoma, phaeochromocytoma, visceral cysts
Tuberous sclerosis (OMIM 191100)	*TSC1* *TSC2*	9q34 16p13	Subependymal giant cell astrocytoma, cortical tubers	Cutaneous angiofibroma, peau chagrin, subungual fibromas	Cardiac rhabdomyomas, adenomatous polyps of the small intestine, cysts of the lung and kidney, lymphangioleiomyomatosis, renal angiomyolipoma
Li-Fraumeni syndrome (OMIM 151623)	*TP53*	17p13	Astrocytomas, PNET		Breast carcinoma, bone and soft-tissue sarcoma, adrenocortical carcinoma, leukemia
Cowden disease (OMIM 158350)	*PTEN* (*MMAC1*)	10q23	Dysplastic gangliocytoma of the cerebellum (Lhermitte Duclos), megencephaly	Multiple trichilemmomas fibromas	Hamartomatous colon, polyps, thyroid, neoplasms, breast carcinoma
Gardner's syndrome Familial adenomatous polyposis (OMIM 175100)	*APC*	5q21	Medulloblastoma	Epidermal cysts	Osteomas, supernumerary teeth, desmoid tumors, colorectal and gastroduodenal polyps and carcinomas, CHRPE, thyroid carcinoma
Turcot syndrome Hereditary nonpolyposis colorectal cancer (OMIM 114500)	*MSH2* *MLH1* *PMS2*	2p22–21 3p21 7p22	Glioblastoma	Café au lait spots	Colorectal carcinoma
Multiple endocrine neoplasia type 1 (OMIM 131100)	*MEN1*	11q13	Pituitary tumors, ependymoma		Parathyroid adenoma, gastroenteropancreatic neuroendocrine tumors
Down's syndrome (OMIM 190685)		Trisomy 21	Reduced risk overall, enhanced risk for germ-cell tumors		Leukemia

1:36,000–45,500. Diagnostic criteria are based upon: (1) capillary hemangioblastoma in the CNS or retina, and (2) the presence of one of the typical VHL-associated tumors, or (3) a previous family history.

Among 83 subjects in a genetic register for VHL disease in northwest England, cerebellar hemangioblastoma affected 60% and was the presenting manifestation in 35% [57]. Hemangioblastoma was diagnosed at a mean age of 30 years (range 15-56 years), so a sizeable proportion of diagnoses must have been at age 15–29 years. Spinal hemangioblastoma occurred in 14% of subjects, at slightly more advanced ages. Of 86 people with a CNS hemangioblastoma in the regional cancer registry, 13% were on the VHL register.

Capillary Hemangioblastoma

A WHO grade 1 tumor of stromal cells and abundant capillaries, uncertain histogenesis, and a preferential cerebellar location, capillary hemangioblastoma, has been reported in the brainstem, spine, and, rarely, supratentorially. When associated with VHL, these tumors are frequently multiple in number. They occur with increasing frequency during development, the peak incidence occurring in middle age (30–39 years). Success of surgical resection means that life-limiting tumor problems of VHL relate to malignancy at other sites (e.g., renal cell carcinoma), justifying surveillance at regular intervals.

Other CNS Manifestations

Ependymomas and choroid plexus papillomas have been reported in association with VHL.

10.2.5.4 Tuberous Sclerosis

Tuberous sclerosis (TS) is an autosomal dominant disorder with an estimated incidence of 1:5,000–10,000. Diagnostic criteria are divided into: definitive features, typical TS lesions involving the CNS, retina, skin, heart and kidneys; and provisional or suspect features, multiple cutaneous angiofibromas or their detection early in life, involvement of other organs with TS lesions including the lungs, spleen, pancreas, bones, teeth, gingival, and gastrointestinal tract [58].

Subependymal Giant Cell Astrocytoma

Patients with either type of TS have a high risk of brain tumors. Among a population-based series of 131 patients, 7 (5%) had developed giant cell astrocytoma by age 30 years [59]. The earliest age at diagnosis was 13 years and incidence at age 15–29 years is likely to exceed 5%, as some subjects were still children at last follow-up. Subependymal giant cell astrocytoma (SEGA) is typically a WHO grade 1 tumor that arises in the wall of the lateral ventricles and is composed of large ganglioid astrocytes. Malignant transformation even at relapse is not reported. Worsening epilepsy and raised intracranial pressure due to obstruction of the lateral/third ventricles are common presenting symptoms; occasionally, massive spontaneous hemorrhage can occur. The currently preferred treatment is surgical resection when possible. The use of chemotherapy or other medical treatments is not currently reported. The possibility of harnessing knowledge of biological consequences of TS mutations may provide novel methods for treatment that would require careful evaluation. The tuberous sclerosis complex gene product TSC2 mediates the cellular energy response to control cell growth and survival [60, 61]. Such new approaches are worthy of trial in patients with well-defined disease not amenable to a surgical approach. In considering this, balancing the risks of treatment-related neurotoxicity is critical, given the inherent cognitive consequences of TS due to cortical lesions and associated epilepsy.

10.2.5.5 Li-Fraumeni Syndrome

Li-Fraumeni syndrome (LFS) is an autosomal dominant disorder; its population incidence is unknown, although 108 families with TP53 germ-line mutations were reported from 1990 to 1996 [62]. Diagnostic criteria are: (1) occurrence of sarcoma before age 45 years, (2) at least one first-degree relative with any tumor before age 45 years, or (3) a second- (or first-) degree relative with cancer before 45 years or a sarcoma at any age [63–65].

Brain tumors are a recognized component of LFS [66]. In a cohort study of 28 LFS families with germline TP53 mutations, the risk of CNS tumors at age

15–29 years was 32 times that in the general population [67]. The spectrum of CNS tumors associated with LFS reflects the age incidence of other tumors in the adolescent and young adult population, with astrocytomas predominating [62]. The mean age at presentation of a CNS tumor in patients with LFS is 25.9 years – the third youngest age category. Sarcomas (mean age 16.7 years) and adrenal tumors (mean age 4.7 years) present earlier in life. Multiple tumors in those with LFS are well recognized; prior CNS irradiation may confer additional risk.

Of those CNS tumors reported to be associated with LFS, the age-incidence pattern is preserved, with childhood embryonal (PNET), ependymal and choroid plexus tumors arising in childhood, and the astrocytic tumors (low-grade, anaplastic, glioblastoma, oligoastrocytoma, and gliosarcoma) arising in the adolescent and young adult and adult years.

10.2.5.6 Multiple Endocrine Neoplasia

Pituitary tumors are a frequent component of multiple endocrine neoplasia (MEN) type 1. In a multicenter series of 220 affected members of 98 MEN type 1 families, 30% had a pituitary tumor [68]; these tumors were nearly always diagnosed before age 40 years.

10.2.5.7 Cowden Disease

This is an autosomal dominant condition in which the population incidence is unknown; it is thought to have a relatively high rate of novel mutations and a variable severity of phenotype, making its hereditary pattern obscure. Diagnostic criteria include multiple trichilemmomas (benign skin appendage tumors; 85%), thyroid tumors (70%), malignant breast tumors (30%), oral papillomatosis, cutaneous keratoses, hamartomatous soft-tissue tumors, and benign breast tumors.

The CNS manifestation of this condition is dysplastic gangliocytoma of the cerebellum (Lhermitte-Duclos disease), which is a diffuse enlargement of the cerebellum [69]. The histology is a WHO grade 1 lesion consisting of large neuronal cells expanding the granular and molecular layers. It is unclear whether this is a hamartomatous or neoplastic lesion

because of its proliferation index and absence of progression. However, recurrence has occasionally been noted and they may develop in adults with previously normal magnetic resonance imaging scans. Other CNS features include megencephaly (20–70%), heterotopic gray matter, hydrocephalus, mental retardation, and seizures [70].

10.2.5.8 Turcot Syndrome

This is a group of autosomal dominant and possibly autosomal recessive disorders. Diagnostic criteria are coexistence of primary colorectal polyps and tumors and gliomas The gliomas (usually high-grade astrocytomas) almost always occur before age 25 years and are associated with families with hereditary nonpolyposis colorectal cancer (HNPCC) [71]. Other clinical features include café au lait spots in HNPCC and congenital hypertrophic retinal pigmented epithelium. In the Dutch HNPCC registry and in a Finnish study of 50 HNPCC families, the risk of a brain tumor was 4–6 times that of the general population [72, 73]. These tumors may have a more favorable prognosis than sporadic tumors of similar histology.

10.2.5.9 Gardner Syndrome

This is a group of autosomal dominant and possibly autosomal recessive disorders, in which there is coexistence of familial adenomatous polyposis (FAP), associated colonic polyps, and characteristic bone lesions and brain tumors. Most of the brain tumors are medulloblastomas, but gliomas also occur [71]. In the John Hopkins FAP registry, the relative risk for any brain tumor in the first 30 years of life was 23, and the corresponding relative risk for medulloblastoma was 99 [74].

10.2.5.10 Other Conditions with Increased Risk of CNS Tumors

People with Down syndrome have a reduced overall risk of CNS tumors, although the risk of intracranial GCTs is increased [75]. Gorlin syndrome is strongly associated with medulloblastoma, and germ-line mutations in the *INI1* gene are associated with atypical teratoid/rhabdoid tumors, although both of these associations occur almost exclusively in early childhood and are therefore not applicable to the age-focus of this chapter [76–79]. Finally, there are reported medulloblastomas presenting in patients with ataxia-telangiectasia, a syndrome that is characterized by cerebellar degeneration and DNA repair defect and is associated with an increasing number of specific gene mutations within the AT gene complex, making the patient particularly vulnerable to the toxic consequences of radiotherapy [80–93].

10.2.5.11 Familial Aggregation of Brain Tumors

The risk of a brain tumor is approximately doubled in first-degree relatives of brain tumor patients [84]. Relative risks are similar for glioma in first-degree relatives of glioma patients [35] and for meningioma when a first-degree relative also has meningioma [85]; however, the risk of low-grade glioma in first-degree relatives may be considerably higher [85]. The absence of excess risk among spouses of brain tumor patients indicates genetic rather than environmental origins for familial aggregations [86]. Many familial aggregations of CNS tumors are attributable to the aforementioned syndromes, especially NF1, Turcot syndrome, LFS, VHL disease [87], and MEN1. In other instances, however, there is no evidence of a brain tumor predisposition syndrome or germ line TP53 mutation [88] and explanations are, therefore, awaited.

10.3 Presentation, Assessment, Treatment, and Outcome

10.3.1 Clinical Presentation

Prolonged symptom intervals between onset and diagnosis are common in brain tumors in adolescents and young adults. The spectrum of tumors and their common locations in adolescent and young adults, together with the implications of functional anatomy, means that symptomatology is governed by: (1) symptoms of raised intracranial pressure due to obstructive hydrocephalus or large tumor mass with midline shift, and

(2) specific symptoms due to neurological dysfunction of brain regions involved with the tumor, including the primary site of the tumor and areas where metastatic disease exists.

The SEER and CBTRUS databases do not contain anatomical details. However, as a result of the ranked incidence of histological subtypes in this age group (Fig. 10.2), we can predict that midline supratentorial tumors are likely to predominate, followed by posterior fossa tumors due to tailing of childhood tumor pattern distribution, then by meningeal and skull-based tumors, with cortical tumors and spinal cord tumors occurring least frequently.

10.3.2 Symptomatology

Supratentorial midline tumors involve intrasellar/suprasellar regions (craniopharyngioma, GCT), visual pathways (astrocytoma grade 1 ± NF1), the hypothalamus (astrocytoma grade 1 ± NF1, Langerhans cell histiocytosis), the pineal region (GCTs, PNET, astrocytoma grades 2–4, pinealoma/cytoma, retinoblastoma), and the ventricles (choroid plexus tumors, subependymal giant cell astrocytoma, ependymoma). Signs and symptoms at presentation include:

1. Raised intracranial pressure due to mass effect or associated hydrocephalus.
2. Ophthalmic abnormalities: reduced acuity, disordered eye movements, acquired squint, reduced visual field, loss of pupillary reflexes, and fundal abnormalities.
3. Endocrine disturbance: precocious or delayed puberty, wasting syndromes, growth hormone deficiency, diabetes insipidus, hypopituitarism.
4. Disturbances of behavior and sleep: changes in mood, reduced school or work performance, disinhibition, and disturbance of day-night rhythms.
5. Features of associated predisposing syndromes.

Infratentorial tumors involve the cerebellum (astrocytoma grade 1, PNET, ependymoma, AT mutation/RT), or brainstem (astrocytoma grades 1–4, ependymoma, PNET). Signs and symptoms at presentation include:

1. Raised intracranial pressure due to obstructive hydrocephalus: nausea and vomiting, headache, and neck pain as a result of cranial/cervical dural stretching or invasion. Classically these symptoms have a diurnal pattern, although this is not universal.
2. Cerebellar signs and symptoms: gait disturbance, loss of coordination, nystagmus, dysarthria, and deterioration in educational performance.
3. Brainstem signs and symptoms: dysconjugate eye movements, cranial nerve palsies (e.g. 7th nerve palsy, dysarthria, deafness or tinnitus, choking due to swallowing disorder), motor weakness of the limbs, alteration in mood, disturbances of respiratory pattern, altered consciousness, and cardiac arrest.
4. Features of associated predisposing syndromes.

Meningeal, skull, and spine tumors include meningioma, PNET of the bone, Langerhans cell histiocytosis, chordoma, parameningeal tumors (e.g., sarcoma, PNET, lymphoma), astrocytoma, ependymoma, and schwannoma. Signs and symptoms at presentation include:

1. Localized headache.
2. Local bony mass.
3. Cranial nerve palsies.
4. Ophthalmic symptoms including proptosis.
5. Gait disturbance.
6. Spinal cord compression with back pain (particularly at rest), limb weakness, and bladder and bowel disturbance.
7. Nerve root pain.
8. Scoliosis/lordosis/kyphosis.
9. Features of associated predisposing syndromes.

Cerebral cortex tumors include astrocytoma grades 1–4, oligodendroglial tumors, neurocytoma, ependymoma, PNET, dysembryoplastic neuroepithelial tumor, and ganglioglioma arising in any lobe and presenting with:

1. Symptoms of raised intracranial pressure (headache and vomiting) due to mass effect or associated hydrocephalus.
2. Seizures (status epilepticus, focal seizures, or complicated seizures).
3. Behavior disturbance, reduced educational performance, disturbances of mood.
4. Thalamic pain syndromes.
5. Ophthalmic symptoms with reduced acuity and visual field cut.
6. Weakness or sensory changes.
7. Features of associated predisposing syndromes.

10.3.3 Multiprofessional Priorities for Adolescent and Young Adult Centered Care

Adolescent and young adult-centered care for patients with brain tumors must include the following elements: (1) the provision of clear information about the disease and access to appropriate psychosocial and fertility counseling, (2) access to comprehensive rehabilitation services, (3) access to appropriate education and neuropsychological assessment and planning, and (4) access to family support services. These priorities were developed by an experienced, multiprofessional audience at the Teenage Cancer Trust Conference that took place at the Royal College of Physicians, London, in March 2004.

Traditionally, clinical services for the management of severe neurological problems have not been organized with an emphasis on the aforementioned services. However, the adolescent and young adult patient and family confronted with traditional clinical neurosurgical environments is frequently intimidated, frightened, and unable to understand the complex clinical systems and information presented to them as the stages of diagnosis, treatment planning, treatment delivery, rehabilitation, and follow-up evolve. This experience is disempowering and can strongly influence the adolescent and young adults compliance with the complex requirements of therapy and rehabilitation. The family and care providers are as important in this process as the patient because one cannot function effectively without the other. It is helpful to make available the additional resources now provided for adolescent and young adult cancer patients and their families, particularly via the internet [2].

10.3.4 Assessment and Management

10.3.4.1 Neurosurgery

Pediatric and Adult Neurosurgical Services

CNS tumors in adolescence present neurosurgeons with difficulties similar to those found in the pediatric and young adult populations. Clinical management in this age range creates specific patient-management concerns, although tumor management is approached with the same inventory applied to specific tumors in any age range.

Neurosurgery has three roles to play in the management of brain tumors: (1) reduction of raised intracranial pressure, (2) making a diagnosis, and (3) contributing to therapy. These will now be discussed

Management of Raised Intracranial Pressure

Raised intracranial pressure demands surgical intervention to reduce mass effect and brain distortion. Preoperative treatment with high-dose steroids and, in emergencies, mannitol infusions, contributes to the control of raised pressure whilst preparation for surgery is in progress. Surgical treatment is required for large tumors, cysts, and those obstructing cerebrospinal fluid (CSF) pathways. With acute hydrocephalus, CSF diversion may be necessary with external drainage as a temporary measure, or third ventriculostomy or ventriculoperitoneal shunting for a more permanent solution. Although concern exists about the dissemination of malignant cells, it is generally overridden by the need to deal with long-term hydrocephalus. In a posterior fossa PNET there may be a need for temporary external drainage of CSF, but a long-term shunt may be avoided after tumor resection.

Making the Diagnosis

Histological and genetic examination of tumor tissue is an essential part of establishing a tumor diagnosis in the brain, as it is for other sites. On the whole, surgery to biopsy or otherwise achieve tissue diagnosis is straightforward in intracranial lesions. A variety of techniques can be used, including stereotactic, endoscopic, or open biopsy sampling, as well as obtaining tissue at the time of tumor resection. The risks of these techniques vary. Stereotactic biopsy, for instance, has mortality and morbidity rates of less than 1% and less than 5%, respectively, in supratentorial tumors, and a very high positive diagnostic rate.

Midline Supratentorial Tumors

Midline tumors are more common in the adolescent age range than later in life, and present major neurosurgical management difficulties. Their diagnosis may be made by examination of tumor markers [α-fetoprotein (αFP), β-human chorionic gonadotropin (βHCG), and placental-like alkaline phosphatase] in either the blood or CSF, and if these tumor markers are found then diagnostic surgery may be avoided [89]. Surgery may be required for either the management of obstructive hydrocephalus with CSF diversion, or to deal with large masses; the latter is less common. If pineal region tumors present with obstructive hydrocephalus then operative CSF diversion allows the opportunity to take CSF for tumor marker analysis. If, rather than performing a ventricular peritoneal shunt, a third ventriculostomy is considered via a neuroendoscopic procedure, then an opportunity arises to visualize a pineal tumor from the third ventricle and, indeed, perform an endoscopic biopsy procedure. If blood and CSF markers are negative, then it is necessary to obtain a biopsy sample of pineal tumors to determine their histology, which has great influence on their further management. Stereotactic biopsy in the pineal region is not without risk in view of the deep situation of the pineal region and the proximity, in particular, of veins, which together with the chance of lesions "bouncing off" biopsy cannulae, raise the possibility of the procedure failing to provide a tissue diagnosis. These risks are justified by the necessity of making a tissue diagnosis to direct further treatment. Pineal region tumors may, in their own right, cause localized problems and require excision. However, it is more likely that other modalities would be used in their treatment, at least in the initial stages.

Brainstem

The brainstem is not difficult to biopsy with stereotactic techniques, but there is a higher risk of morbidity. Imaging diagnosis has been considered sufficient for typical diffuse pontine gliomas until recently. However, with the introduction of multimodality imaging including diffusion, perfusion, and spectroscopy on magnetic resonance studies, and the need for identifying tissue targets for trial-based therapies, this clinical exclusion from biopsy may be challenged in order to provide more comprehensive information about the tumor [90, 91].

Surgical Therapy

Often tumors will be removed, completely if feasible, or subtotally if in highly eloquent areas. Even large tumors in eloquent brain areas can be removed as long as resection remains within the tumor. Difficulty occurs when attempting to remove all of a tumor with an indistinct edge. Preoperative image guidance with computed tomography or magnetic resonance imaging, intraoperative ultrasound, or even intraoperative magnetic resonance scanning, may be of help. Surgery aimed at resection has a therapeutic role in most tumor types, save perhaps for lymphoma or GCTs. Tumors encountered in adolescence may be a problem increasingly as a result of previous medical interventions such as the use of CNS irradiation for other tumors. Meningiomas and other malignant tumors occur in this age range, presenting particular difficulties. Malignant tumors are difficult to treat in their own right, but benign tumors such as meningiomas are particularly complex because they may be multiple and may occur within previous radiotherapy fields, which not only changes the dura, making complete resection difficult, but limits subsequent radiation doses due to tissue tolerance limits.

Surgery is paramount in dealing with grade 1, pilocytic astrocytomas, which need as complete a resection as possible to give long-term disease control. The management of grade 2 tumors is often determined by their anatomical location. However, the ideal treatment is macroscopic complete resection, which probably produces a better outcome but is limited by the eloquent position of tumors. Subtotal resection is often

employed; although even 90–99% resections will not prevent malignant transformation, bulk reduction does improve progressive symptomatology in the short to medium term.

Surgery for higher-grade astrocytomas has never been subjected to a randomized controlled trial to compare resection versus biopsy sampling, but surgeons generally attempt the most complete resection possible where deemed reasonable. Open surgery also allows for implantation of therapeutic agents such as chemotherapy wafers [92], and gene therapy [93–99].

Following primary surgery there is sometimes a role for a second open operation. A pilocytic astrocytoma or ependymoma in the cerebellum might well be reoperated if a resectable residuum were found on imaging. Recurrent higher-grade tumors are resected more than once depending on their response to adjuvant therapies, patient performance, and overall prognosis. In addition, surgery has a role in symptom control in a palliative setting, the control of raised intracranial pressure, and the resection of symptomatic metastatic tumors in selected cases, as appropriate. Stereotactic radiosurgery may be more appropriate if surgical complications might be reduced by multiple stereotactic procedures.

10.3.4.2 Radiotherapy Techniques

RT is the main adjuvant therapy in CNS tumors where either surgical resection is not possible or incomplete, or in malignant tumors where dissemination or recurrence is predictable. The great advantage of RT is that it can be delivered safely to the whole brain and spinal cord at doses that are known to carry acceptable acute and long-term risks in the vast majority of adolescent and young adult patients.

Balancing the Risk and Benefits of RT in Adolescent and young adult Patients

In pediatric neurooncology, the vulnerability of the growing brain (<7–10 years of age) to the consequences of RT has led to a range of trials attempting to minimize radiation doses and fields by using complementary chemotherapy in order to limit neurocognitive consequences. The endocrine consequences of craniospinal RT (CrSp) in this group are considerable, and include secondary hypothyroidism, growth hormone deficiency, and in girls, either precocious puberty or incomplete pubertal development, as well as risking infertility from irradiation of the hypothalamus, pituitary, and ovaries. Irradiation to the vertebrae will result in failure of these bones to grow during the adolescent growth spurt, causing loss of up to 5 cm in height; this is unresponsive to growth hormone therapy.

The same balance of risks concerning efficacy versus toxicity must be considered for the adolescent and young adult population, even though the neurocognitive toxicity of conventional RT doses at this age is not clear-cut due to the scarcity of good evidence from long-term follow-up studies. There is concern that, although early estimates of neurocognitive function after cranial radiation may be acceptable, long-term survival may reveal progressive accelerated cognitive decline in a proportion of the population, representing a hidden toxicity [100]. The risk of ovarian radiation from spinal fields is an important consideration, worthy of ovarian ultrasound for assessment and consideration of oophoropexy to a location outside the planned radiation fields. These concerns are greatest for those diagnosed in this young age group, as they have the longest time to live and to experience the toxicity. The endocrine consequences of cranial RT are considerable. However, the availability of endocrine replacement therapy, coupled with the more advanced state of skeletal growth in the adolescent and young adult patient prior to diagnosis, means that the growth and development consequences may be less severe than in younger patients. Careful endocrine follow-up of these young adult patients is essential, as the endocrinopathies may develop at a later time. These patients are also at increased risk for malignancies of endocrinological structures that have been irradiated, especially the thyroid. In addition, the late-effects clinic for young adult survivors of childhood cancer, with its specialist, multidisciplinary, cooperative team, should be of help to these patients.

10.3.4.3 Chemotherapy

The outcome for adolescent and young adult patients with brain tumors will depend upon developments in drug therapy aimed at either killing cancer cells or modifying tumor biology. Existing drugs in use are primarily chemotherapeutic agents aimed at attacking the tumor cell during division, leading to cell death. Current experience has identified roles for chemotherapy in most types of brain tumor. As in extracranial malignancies, chemotherapy can assist with multidisciplinary treatment through:

1. Tumor shrinkage to optimize surgical resectability (e.g., GCTs, ependymoma, and low-grade glioma).
2. Adjuvant treatment to complement reduced dose/field RT (e.g., medulloblastoma, ependymoma, low-grade glioma, high-grade glioma, oligodendroglioma, and germinoma).
3. Treatment or prevention of leptomeningeal tumor (e.g. lymphoma, medulloblastoma, and GCT).

However, these roles for chemotherapy are limited in their effectiveness by the difficulties of drug access imposed by the blood brain barrier (BBB). The BBB is located at the endothelial lining of brain capillaries and impairs drug access from blood to brain because the capillaries have:

1. Epithelial-like, high-resistance, tight junctions that fuse the brain capillary endothelia together.
2. A paucity of fenestrations and pinocytic vesicles that restrict transcellular transport.
3. A greater number of mitochondria.
4. A greater number of metabolic enzymes and transporters (e.g., p-glycoprotein multidrug resistance-associated proteins and organic acid transporters).

Access to the interstitial spaces of the brain requires agents to pass through two membranes (luminal and abluminal) and the endothelial cell cytoplasm, which occurs by passive diffusion or facilitated transport. The BBB, as a result, is selectively permeable to lipophilic compounds, which can diffuse through plasma membranes and nutrients, including glucose and amino acids, for which specific transporters facilitate passage. In addition to the BBB there is also the blood-CSF barrier, which has a surface area that is 5,000-fold less than the BBB and is located in the vascular epithelium of periventricular organs (choroid plexus, median eminence, area postrema). These capillaries are porous, allowing small molecules to penetrate the interstitial space of these organs. The composition of the CSF is substantially different from the brain interstitium. The CSF is a product of secretory processes of the choroid plexus, where drug transporter mechanisms also play a role. Finally, the blood-tumor barrier (BTB) restricts drug delivery of systemically administered chemotherapy. There may be factors dictated by the tumor microenvironment that affect BTB permeability, such as the presence of multiple microvessel populations and variations in microvessel density influencing diffusion distances from the blood vessel to the tumor cell. It is known that the BTB merges into the BBB within a few millimeters of the tumor's edge. Taken together, these physical characteristics determine the pharmaceutical qualities required of drugs used to treat brain tumors. For optimal BBB penetration, drugs should: (1) be lipophilic, (2) be buffered to a CSF pH, (3) have low serum protein/tissue binding, and (4) be of small molecular size. Despite these principles, there are several agents that do not meet these requirements but yet have activity against CNS tumors [101]. This subject area therefore remains controversial and worthy of further research.

Optimizing CNS Drug Delivery

Several clinical techniques have been developed and tested to enhance drug delivery, including:

1. BBB disruption including: (1) intra-arterial mannitol, (2) vasoactive compounds (bradykinin analogues – Cereport, RMP-7), (3) local radiation, and (4) inhibition of drug efflux (P-glycoprotein).
2. Targeted drug delivery systems: polymer/nanoparticle drug formulations (liposomal daunorubicin).
3. High-dose systemic chemotherapy (extensively tested but not yet an established treatment, most effective in medulloblastoma, not effective in high-grade glioma, being tested in GCTs at relapse).
4. Regional chemotherapy administration, intrathecal therapy (methotrexate, cytosine arabinoside, and thiotepa are established agents, liposomal cytarabine, diaziquone, 6-mercaptopurine, mafos-

famide, and topotecan are experimental agents) intratumoral (biodegradable polymers, convection enhanced delivery), and intra-arterial (limited application associated with significant risk of toxicity) administration.

Special Considerations for Chemotherapy in CNS Tumors

Drugs that penetrate the BBB have the capacity to produce neurotoxicity as a dose-limiting side effect, which may compound other treatment-related neurotoxicities (e.g., methotrexate and RT). The use of chemotherapy, especially in high doses, in patients with CNS tumors carries additional hazards linked primarily to the infectious risks of ventricular- or lumbar-peritoneal shunts, central venous lines, and frequent episodes of fever, which cause difficulties in discriminating between shunt infections and febrile neutropenia. A recent publication analyzing tolerance of chemotherapy in patients with medulloblastoma showed that patients age 10–20 years were more likely to suffer toxicity and require modifications in treatment than individuals 5–10 years of age [102]. These data suggest that adolescent and young adult patients would benefit from a modification of the aggressive chemotherapy regimens often utilized in children.

Symptom Control

The adolescent and young adult patient with a brain tumor is frequently suffering from both acquired neurological disabilities and side effects of the various treatment modalities. Successful delivery of combined care requires close attention to all aspects of symptom control and integration of rehabilitation both at home and in the hospital. Symptoms of raised intracranial pressure are common at presentation and are treated with corticosteroids preoperatively. However, prolonged postoperative use of steroids leads inevitably to the development of Cushing syndrome and worsening disability due to weight gain, proximal myopathy, personality disorder, metabolic disturbance, striae, acne, and facial and body disfigurement, not to mention the increasing nursing burden for the parents and care providers. If it is not possible to treat the cause of the raised intracranial pressure (e.g., ventricular shunting or ventriculostomy, surgical debulking of the tumor, RT, or chemotherapy), steroids should be used only in short courses of 3–5 days to assess effectiveness while minimizing the risks of severe side effects. Such an approach requires close cooperation by the clinical team, particularly since the transient neurological improvements that occur with short-term steroid use are sometimes grasped by patient, family and doctor alike as a sign of a treatment effect, in otherwise very difficult circumstances [103, 104].

10.3.4.4 Integrated Care

Integrated care, as described, is a major undertaking. It requires great care in communication with adolescents to secure initial and ongoing consent to treatment, rehabilitation, and social and personal development. Furthermore, there are the inevitable risks of reactive depression. Staff with special skills in liaison, counseling, and family support are essential. Access to rehabilitation resources, transportation, educational support, and communication with peers at home can, individually or collectively, make the difference between a young person completing the proposed treatment or rejecting it altogether.

10.3.5 Intracranial GCTs – a Model Tumor of Adolescent and Young Adult Neurooncology Practice

We have elected to discuss the progress made in GCTs as a model adolescent and young adult tumor because their incidence peaks in the age range, the literature reports improved outcomes from multidisciplinary management, and yet there have been no randomized controlled trials for these tumors in this age group.

GCTs are considered to be a heterogeneous group of tumors that arise from primordial germ cells (germinoma) or from germ cells at a later stage of embryonic development (nongerminomatous GCT, NGGCT). They typically arise from midline structures, the pineal gland and suprasellar region being the most common locations. They only rarely arise from other locations (Table 10.4). At the time of diagnosis, 5–10% of GCTs, predominantly germinomas, occur as bifocal disease

located in both the pineal region and the suprasellar region. It is uncertain if this represents simultaneous development of the tumor in two sites or tumor dissemination. GCTs have a propensity for leptomeningeal spread, with 19% of patients showing dissemination of disease at diagnosis in the recent International Society of Pediatric Oncology (SIOP) CNS GCT 96 trial.

10.3.5.1 Epidemiology of CNS GCTs

According to SEER data, CNS GCTs are seen exclusively in individuals between the ages of 0 and 34 years, with a peak incidence at age 15–19 years of age (Fig. 10.8). The incidence of CNS GCTs in males is more than twice that in females (SEER data shows a male:female ratio of 3.6:1), and in the adolescent and young adult group, CNS GCTs are almost exclusively seen in males. SEER data for all subtypes of CNS GCTs at any age show a marked male predominance in the pineal location (male:female of up to 18:1), and no gender predilection for a pituitary location (Table 10.4). The incidence of CNS GCTs is increasing over time; most striking in individuals <15 years of age (Fig. 10.9). Intracranial GCTs are more common in Japan, where the incidence is five- to eightfold greater than that seen

Table 10.4 Anatomic location of CNS germ-cell tumors in patients aged 0–44 years (United States SEER, 1975–1999). NOS Not otherwise specified

	No.	% of Total	Male	Female
Pineal	113	54%	107	6
Pituitary	21	10%	11	10
Ventricle	11	5%	9	2
Cerebrum	10	5%	7	3
Brain overlapping	7	3%	5	2
Brain stem	3	1%	3	0
Cranial nerve	3	1%	1	2
Olfactory nerve	1	0%	1	0
Frontal lobe	1	0%	0	1
Spinal cord	2	1%	0	2
Brain NOS	38	18%	21	17
Total	210			

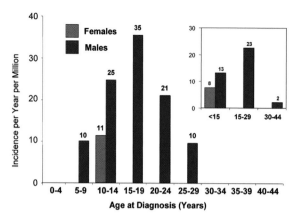

Figure 10.8

Incidence of CNS germ-cell tumors in American children, adolescents and young adults by gender according to age at diagnosis. Data from the United States SEER Program. [1]

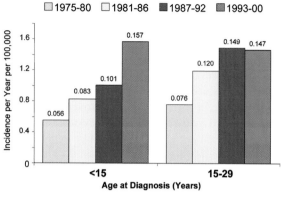

Figure 10.9

Incidence of CNS germ-cell tumors in American children, adolescents and young adults by era according to age at diagnosis. Data from the United States SEER Program. [1]

in the United States. There are no known predisposing conditions.

Intracranial GCTs account for 30% of all GCTs; their histological appearance in the brain is identical to that seen in other anatomical sites. Germinoma is the most common subtype, and according to SEER data, germinomas comprise 82% of CNS GCTs in individuals 15–29 years of age. Germinomas have a syncytiotrophoblastic subtype that secretes low levels of βHCG. NGGCTs comprise 18% of CNS GCTs in the 15–29 year age group [WHO classification: embryonal carcinoma (EC), yolk sac tumor (YST), choriocarcinoma (CC), teratoma (immature, IT; mature, MT), and teratoma with malignant transformation (MalT), and mixed GCTs (MGCT)]. Frequently, NGGCTs will secrete αFP (YST and MGCT) or βHCG (CC and MGCT), which in Europe and the United States has been used to stratify treatment and serve as a marker for persistent or recurrent disease.

10.3.5.2 Tumor Markers and Pathology of CNS GCTs

Histological diagnosis is complicated by difficulties with biopsy and sampling errors of small biopsy spec-

imens from heterogeneous tumors. GGCTs secrete αFP or βHCG in low quantities, whilst the majority of NGGCTs secrete these tumor markers in substantial amounts, embryonal carcinoma being the exception [105–107]. As a result, in Europe and the United States, treatment strategies are now based upon biochemical as well as histological and imaging assessments of the tumor. Serum αFP levels of >25 ng/ml and serum βHCG levels of >50 IU/l define a secreting tumor. In many Japanese studies, more complex interpretations of diagnostic criteria are adopted by different groups. These biochemical markers are also particularly valuable for monitoring disease response [108, 109]. They should be measured at diagnosis both in blood and CSF whenever possible.

10.3.5.3 CNS GCT Literature Review

An extensive literature review identified more than 25 reports over the past 40 years describing results of single-institutional, multi-institutional, and study group retrospective reviews as well as a small number of papers describing tumor response in formal phase 2 and 3 trials and studies of quality of life (QoL) outcomes. The earliest report, by Wara et al. [110], concluded that germinoma was radiocurable, but the metastatic recurrence risk was such that CrSp RT was recommended. Another report, by Jennings et al. [110], reviewed the literature for 399 cases, and concluded that anatomical staging was critical to identify high-risk patients with metastases and suggested that NGGCTs could benefit from additive chemotherapy. In that publication, there was a discussion regarding the biology of GCTs with respect to endogenous surges of sex hormone around puberty as a drive for GCT development [111]. These two very early reports set the scene for two decades of evolution of clinical practice, resulting in current therapies. Primary surgery, followed by combined adjuvant chemotherapy and RT has led to survival rates for GGCTs that exceed 95%, and for NGGCTs that reach nearly 70%. Reports of QoL in survivors, although sparse, have shown substantial improvements over the last two decades.

10.3.5.4 Phase 2 Studies in CNS GCTs

The justification for the use of chemotherapy in intracranial GCTs stems from the early experience of treating advanced testicular cancer in adults. Cisplatin-based regimens were found to be highly effective and were combined with bleomycin and vinblastine, and subsequently etoposide [112, 113]. A case study involving a child with a recurrent suprasellar tumor showed that substantial levels of bleomycin and cisplatin could be detected in the CSF after intravenous administration [114]. Subsequent trials of chemotherapy in relapsed and newly diagnosed patients identified clear evidence of chemosensitivity to cisplatin-based regimens [109, 115–116]. Other phase 2 studies of cyclophosphamide [117] and carboplatin [118] were performed. Taken together, these studies have informed the selection of drugs in current regimens.

10.3.5.5 Retrospective Institutional and Multi-Institutional Reports

Of particular importance in international studies of GCTs are the increasingly collaborative efforts of the Japanese groups to collect and collaborate with an expanding network of surgical units. However, this has not translated into a formal phase 3 trial of therapy and resultant publication of a report. The practice of primary surgical resection became increasingly unfashionable as: (1) diagnostic trials of RT were used to screen pineal region tumors for radiosensitivity [119–122] and (2) cisplatin-based chemotherapy permitted the use of highly effective neoadjuvant treatment, thereby reducing the need for extensive tumor resections in GGCTs initially, and subsequently, NGGCTs [109, 115, 123].

In GGCTs the extension of RT to encompass the whole neuraxis led to high levels of confidence in achieving cure [124] and justified subsequent attempts to introduce chemotherapy aimed at complementing reduced-dose cranial or ventricular RT in nonmetastatic cases. Dose and field selection for the primary site, however, has remained inconsistent and controversial.

The report of Aoyama et al. [125] provides comprehensive guidance with regard to RT techniques, although this single-institution study of 41 patients can only demonstrate tumor response and report a survival rate; it cannot answer scientific questions that might lead to new inquiry. The lack of any formal comparative trials in this regard means that any recommendation for primary tumor dose and volume is vulnerable to conflicting arguments supporting or challenging its validity. The motive to reduce dose and volume was justified articulately using data from CrSp RT in pediatric PNETs, where tumors occurred predominantly in the first 10 years of life. Since the median age of GCTs in these studies is at least 13 years, the difference in age at diagnosis justifies special consideration of late consequences of the different RT regimens.

In NGGCTs, it was not until cisplatin-based therapies were introduced and radiation fields were extended to the neuraxis that cure rates started to rise. The selection of patients by tumor markers and avoidance of primary surgery undoubtedly reduced the toxicity of therapy. There remains controversy as to the relative importance of different histological subtypes and their ability to predict sensitivity to the improved treatment approaches. This will not be addressed until large collaborative trials using consistent staging and treatment approaches are launched

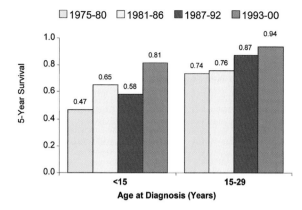

Figure 10.10

Five-year survival rates of American children, adolescents and young adults with CNS germ-cell tumors by era according to age at diagnosis. Data from the United States SEER Program. [1]

and recruit enough patients to study these rare subtypes effectively.

10.3.5.6 Registry Reports

Many registries record all GCTs together, incorporating intracranial tumors along with other extragonadal sites. Childhood cancer study groups similarly plan treatments for all GCTs in single protocols. This organizational arrangement goes against the focus of the intracranial GCT literature that excludes extracranial tumors from their reports because of the special considerations of the neurological requirements for diagnosis, treatment, and follow-up.

SEER survival data for all subtypes of CNS GCTs combined (0–29 years of age) are shown in Fig. 10.10. For individuals 15–29 years of age, the most current 5-year survival rate is excellent at 94%. These survival statistics represent mainly the outcome for germinomas, which comprise 80% of the CNS GCTs in the adolescent and young adult age group. A steady improvement in survival for CNS GCTs has been seen over the last two decades in all age groups <30 years of age.

10.3.5.7 Phase 3 Trials

GGCTs – A United States/ International Approach

The most challenging multinational study performed was one initiated in the United States, proposing chemotherapy-only management of GCTs [126]. The strategy was initiated to test the hypothesis that some GCTs (secreting and nonsecreting) could be cured with chemotherapy alone, with salvage therapy consisting of radiation and further chemotherapy offered to those who relapsed. Four to six courses of carboplatin, etoposide, and bleomycin (PEB) were given according to response; second-look surgery was conducted in a subgroup. Seventy-one patients were enrolled, (45 GGCT and 26 NGGCT). Thirty-nine (57%) achieved a complete response (CR) within 4 cycles of chemotherapy, 16 achieved CR after further chemotherapy or surgical resection; thus, a 78% CR rate was achieved without irradiation (84% for GGCTs and 78% for NGGCTs). Twenty-eight recurred and 7 progressed at a median of 13 months. All but two were salvaged with further therapy and the 2-year survival rate was 84% for GGCTs and 62% for NGGCTs. Seven of the 71 died of predominantly hematological toxicity. The chemotherapy-only strategy was successful as treatment in 41% of survivors and 50% of all patients. The hematological toxicity was significant, with seven toxic deaths during therapy and two thereafter. The authors concluded that the chemotherapy-only approach was less tolerable than historical experience of CrSp RT. All patients who relapsed and underwent further chemotherapy and RT were salvaged; however this was an unacceptable strategy for two patients, who died. Chemotherapy alone has not been demonstrated to be a superior approach when compared to combined-modality approaches.

GGCTs, a European Approach

MAKEI 83/86/89 – German Study Group

The MAKEI studies for nonsecreting, GGCT confirmed that CrSp RT was highly effective [127]. In the MAKEI 83/86 study, CrSp RT for both localized and metastatic tumors was used with a dose of 36 Gy to the whole brain and spine and a boost of 14 Gy to the tumor bed. In the MAKEI 89 study a reduced CrSp RT dose for all to 30 Gy with a tumor boost of 15 Gy was accomplished without loss of efficacy. Survival rates for 60 patients from these 2 studies were 91±3.9% 5-year event-free survival and 93.7±3.6% overall survival. Five patients relapsed, one in the spine 10 months after completing therapy, and four with extracranial disease. Three of the four extracranial relapse patients were salvaged with systemic chemotherapy and the one patient with spinal cord relapse was salvaged with intrathecal chemotherapy and further RT. Two patients died of toxicity.

Societe Francaise d'Oncologie Pediatrique Studies

From 1990 to 1996, the Societe Francaise d'Oncologie Pediatrique (SFOP) initiated a study combining chemotherapy (alternating courses of etoposide-carboplatin and etoposide-ifosfamide for a recommended total of four courses) and 40 Gy local irradiation for patients with localized germinomas [128, 129]. Metastatic patients were allocated to receive CrSp RT (35 Gy). Fifty-seven patients were enrolled, 47 had biopsy-proven germinoma, and 10 did not undergo a biopsy procedure. All but one patient received at least four courses of chemotherapy. Toxicity was mainly hematological or linked to diabetes insipidus ($n=25$). There were no tumor progressions during chemotherapy. Fifty patients received local RT with a median dose of 40 Gy to the initial tumor volume. Six metastatic patients and one patient with localized disease (who had stopped chemotherapy early due to severe toxicity) received CrSp RT. The median follow-up for the group was 42 months, the estimated 3-year survival probability is 98% (confidence interval 86.6–99.7%) and the estimated 3-year event-free survival is 96.4% (confidence interval 86.2–99.1%). Of the four patients who relapsed 9, 10, 38, and 57 months after diagnosis, three achieved second complete remission following salvage treatment with chemotherapy alone or chemo-RT.

SIOP studies: SIOP 96 GGCT – Nonsecreting

Within the GCT strategy of the SIOP, the MAKEI and French TC approaches were recommended and com-

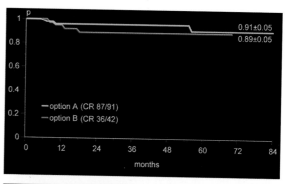

Figure 10.11

Event-free survival of European children and adolescents with CNS germinoma according to the presence of metastases at diagnosis. Data from the Societe Internationale de Oncologie Pediatrique (SIOP) Consortium, 1996 interim analysis [89]. *CR* Complete remission

pared whilst piloting diagnostic processes, data collection, and treatment approaches in the European setting [89]. Strategy A (MAKEI) included CrSp RT with 24 Gy to the neuraxis and a 14-Gy boost to the tumor bed. Strategy B (SFOP) involved two courses of carboplatin PEI (platinum + VP16 + ifosfamide) chemotherapy followed by focal RT of 40 Gy to the tumor bed.

For GGCTs a nonrandomized comparison of the results of the two strategies revealed no difference in event-free survival for both treatments (Fig. 10.11). Review of the registered cases, however, identified noncompliance with diagnostic work-up with respect to performing tumor markers and completing full anatomical and CSF staging before surgery. This meant that patients with secreting tumors were missed and therefore treated inappropriately. There were concerns that three of four relapses were in the combined therapy arm (arm B), raising the possibility that subclinical metastasis at diagnosis may not be controllable by this combination.

Secreting Tumors (NGGCTs)

MAKEI 86 and 89

MAKEI 86 and 89 studies utilized chemotherapy with PVB (cisplatin + vinblastine + bleomycin) after surgery and before CrSp RT (36 Gy CrSp RT with 14 Gy tumor boost), followed by postradiation chemotherapy with etoposide and ifosfamide. Subsequently, MAKEI 89 used preoperative PVB (cisplatin + etoposide + bleomycin) followed by tumor resection, followed by further chemotherapy with PIV (cisplatin + ifosfamide + vinblastine) and RT (30 Gy CrSp, tumor boost of 20 Gy). Twenty-seven patients were treated on these studies. Two died postoperatively; of the 25 remaining who were evaluated, 10 (40%) relapsed locally, of whom 9 died. The most recent event-free survival is 66±6% with a median follow-up of 29 months [130].

The SFOP TC88 protocol was aimed at cure of patients with chemotherapy and no radiotherapy. The chemotherapy regimen involved alternating courses of vinblastine, bleomycin and carboplatin/etoposide and ifosfamide [130]. In the TC 90 protocol, the tumors were treated with six cycles of carboplatin and etoposide, then ifosfamide and etoposide, followed by complete tumor resection of any residue. In both protocols, RT was only used if there was unresectable residual disease. Of 24 evaluable patients, 15 received chemotherapy alone, 14 of whom relapsed. Nine received RT (three CrSp RT) to the primary tumor after chemotherapy. Nine are in first remission, six are in second or third remission after RT and/or high-dose chemotherapy. Eight patients died from disease. The overall survival is about 63%. Twenty-one other follow-up patients were studied, as they were ineligible for the main study. Combining these with the study patients, it was found that cumulative cisplatin dose correlated directly with survival. Cisplatin cumulative dose >400 mg/m^2 doubled event-free survival from 38±17% to 74±5% [130].

The results of these preliminary studies were a marked improvement over previous reports of NGGCTs, where survival was 6% after primary surgery and irradiation. They demonstrated that secreting tumors (NGGCTs) require both chemotherapy and radiotherapy for tumor control. Preoperative chemotherapy has been shown to be effective in facilitating complete resection of large or infiltrating tumors. It would seem that local tumor control is more important for outcome than control of meningeal dissemination [130]. Secreting tumors (NGGCTs) have always had poorer survival rates because of relative insensitiv-

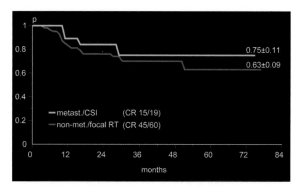

Figure 10.12

Event-free survival of European children and adolescents with nongerminomatous germ-cell tumors according to the presence of metastases at diagnosis. Data from the SIOP Consortium, 1996 interim analysis. [89]

ity to RT and technical difficulties of surgical resection. Large infiltrating tumors are difficult to resect completely, leading to the use of primary chemotherapy to shrink tumors preoperatively. Delayed resections have been shown to be more often complete and technically less difficult. Resected tumors following a course of chemotherapy are frequently histologically benign. [118, 126, 131, 132]

SIOP 96 NGGCTs

This experience stimulated a collaborative approach to NGGCTs between French and German groups and including other European collaborators. The aim was to use markers as diagnostic eligibility criteria (αFP >25 ng/ml and βHCG >50 IU/l), thereby obviating the need for biopsy and to test the combined treatment modality approach using the combination of cisplatin, etoposide, and ifosfamide and involved-field RT. Localized tumors were delivered 54 Gy with 30 Gy CrSp RT, boosting with 24 Gy to metastatic sites. A cohort of 105 patients was recruited, of whom 35 were diagnosed on the basis of tumor markers and were therefore protocol compliant. There were 40 patients who underwent surgery – 26 stereotactic procedures, 43 open procedures of which 10 were biopsies, and 33 attempt-

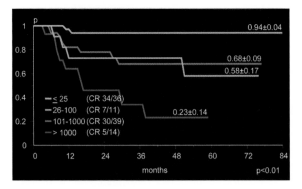

Figure 10.13

Event-free survival of European children and adolescents with nongerminomatous germ-cell tumors as a function of serum alpha-fetoprotein levels at diagnosis. Data from the SIOP Consortium. [89]

ed resections. There were 14 significant surgical complications, including 3 deaths [89].

Survival rates were improved compared to previous experience, with 63% and 75% 5-year survival rates for metastatic and nonmetastatic patients, respectively, indicating that the combined approach negates the adverse impact of metastases at diagnosis (Fig. 10.12). αFP level was shown to predict outcome: the higher the level the worse the outcome (Fig. 10.13). From this study it can be concluded that primary surgery is not beneficial for NGGCT (secreting). Combined chemotherapy and RT have improved the outcome for the majority, but not for those with residual disease or high αFP levels at diagnosis. There is great need to conduct meticulous processes of diagnostic assessment prior to surgery and ensure that staging investigations are thoroughly performed and reviewed before planning any treatment.

10.3.5.8 Late Effects

Endocrine

Tumors in the common GCT regions frequently damage the hypothalamic-pituitary axis, necessitating hormone replacement therapy before initial diagnostic

surgery, where indicated, or during immediate antitumor management. It is unusual for these endocrine deficits to improve after completion of treatment, indeed surgery and RT may make them worse.

Neurological

Focal neurological deficits affecting ophthalmic function at presentation frequently regress with initial steroids and commencement of antitumor treatment. Surgical resection may not improve these symptoms, thus justifying consideration of neoadjuvant chemotherapy or RT.

Cognitive/Health State

Assessment of these measures is becoming increasingly easy now that a battery of generic and specific questionnaire methodologies have been developed for use in children and young people [133, 134]. Adult oncology has already developed this type of measure for evaluating outcomes in order to assist with a selection of preferred palliative drug strategies. Their use in children and adolescent and young adult populations is lagging. Where attempts have been made to measure cognitive and health state outcomes in survivors of GCTs in recent eras, the burden of morbidity has been low, indeed they have compared favorably to normal populations in some cases. This lack of recent evidence of true adverse cognitive outcomes, coupled with the possibility that combined chemotherapy and RT may have a deleterious impact on health state compared to RT alone, further justifies trials of combined treatments aimed at measuring QoL as primary outcome measures.

10.3.5.9 Quality of Life Reports

QoL for survivors is of great importance for this group of patients with increasingly curable tumors. Factors determining adverse QoL outcomes are becoming better understood. Tumor growth and infiltration of brain tissue, particularly in the neurohypophyseal region, causes local neurological damage and may lead to permanent endocrine, visual, and behavioral consequences. Certainly, primary surgery was seen to aggravate these symptoms as well as threaten further neurological

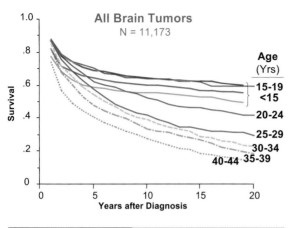

Figure 10.14

Overall survival of American patients with brain tumors who were diagnosed between 1975 and 1998, inclusive, as a function of age at diagnosis. Data from the United States SEER Program [1].

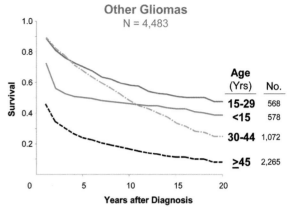

Figure 10.16

Overall survival of American patients with gliomas other than astrocytoma who were diagnosed between 1975 and 1998, inclusive, by age at diagnosis. Data from the United States SEER Program [1].

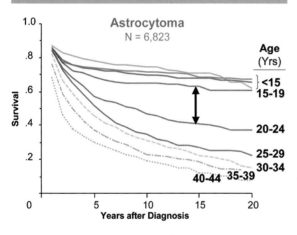

Figure 10.15

Overall survival of American patients with astrocytoma who were diagnosed between 1975 and 1998, inclusive, as a function of age at diagnosis. Data from the United States SEER Program [1].

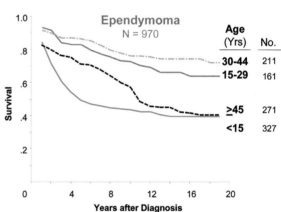

Figure 10.17

Overall survival of American patients with ependymoma who were diagnosed between 1975 and 1998, inclusive, as a function of age at diagnosis. Data from the United States SEER Program [1].

damage and life itself in the early era of this literature review. RT has been widely implicated in causing long-term neurocognitive damage based upon experience in medulloblastoma and leukemia [135]. Chemotherapy, on the other hand, has developed a reputation for min-imal neurotoxicity compared to these other modalities. However, a preliminary report gives results of health state and behavior measurements in survivors of the SIOP PNET3 study at a median of 7 years after completion of treatment, that indicate a lower health state

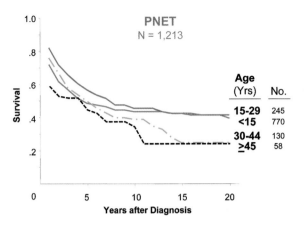

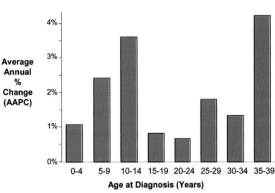

Figure 10.18

Overall survival of American patients with CNS PNETs who were diagnosed between 1975 and 1998, inclusive, as a function of age at diagnosis. Data from the United States SEER Program [1].

Figure 10.19

Average annual percent improvement during the period 1984–1998 in the 5-year survival rate of brain tumors, by 5-year age intervals, in American patients younger than age 40 years. Data from the United States SEER Program[1].

scores for those who received combined chemotherapy and CrSp RT as compared to those treated with CrSp RT alone [135]. The most common long-term complications after diagnosis and treatment of GCTs were endocrine disturbances, especially in patients with suprasellar tumors. Interestingly, most of these endocrinopathies were present at the time of diagnosis or following surgery, although radiation could be implicated in a subset of patients [120, 124, 125, 136]. Other common long-term sequelae include neurocognitive defects, which in most cases were mild [120, 122, 124, 125, 137], and ophthalmologic abnormalities, with Parinaud syndrome seen in pineal region tumors and visual impairment seen in suprasellar tumors. Future trials for GCTs should aim at improving survival while minimizing long-term sequelae of therapy.

10.4 Survival Rates for CNS Tumors; SEER and European Data

There are many reports of survival from CNS tumors in clinical series that include adolescent and young adults, but population-based results are relatively

scarce. International comparisons are complicated by the diversity of age groups and calendar periods, but survival was probably somewhat higher in the United States than in the United Kingdom and southern and central Europe. The especially high survival in the Nordic countries may be an artifact resulting from inclusion of a higher proportion of nonmalignant tumors. Survival in Eastern Europe was somewhat lower than elsewhere. No population-based survival data from developing countries are available for this age group. Five-year survival of children and young adults aged 0–34 years ranged from 9% to 44% in two Chinese and two Thai cancer registries during the 1980s and 1990s [138], indicating substantially lower survival among adolescent and young adults than in developed countries. Survival rates from well-equipped treatment centers in developing countries, however, are comparable with those achieved in developed countries [139, 140].

When reviewing the available SEER survival data for the adolescent and young adult population (Figs. 10.14–10.18), a common theme becomes apparent; Adolescent and young adults with CNS tumors have an intermediate ("astrocytomas") to superior ("other gliomas", PNET/medulloblastoma and ependymoma) survival rate compared to children and older adults, but the improvement in survival in the adolescent and young adult group has lagged behind the other age groups (Fig. 10.19). This lack of progress may be due to the fact that adolescent and young adults are at an "in-between age" and are missing out on enrollment in cooperative trials aimed at either children or adults. These data support the initiative to collaborate nationally and internationally, across the adult and pediatric cooperative groups, to target the adolescent and young adult group for future cooperative trials.

10.5 Conclusions

This chapter has focused on neurooncology as it applies to adolescent and young adults by identifying clinical problems, relevant clinical and scientific data, and how these apply to the emerging subspecialty of neurooncology. Central to this theme is the need to assist the adolescent and young adult patient as he or she moves through the shock of diagnosis and its implications for the future, particularly given the individualized pathway through adolescence and the historical lack of progress in outcomes for this age group. If adolescent and young adult neurooncology teams and trials networks emerge, improved standards of individualized patient care, enhanced recruitment to clinical trials of novel therapies, and improved survival in national statistics will evolve.

Acknowledgments

The authors would like to acknowledge the very capable assistance of Sue Franklin and Jan Watterson Sheaffer in the preparation of this manuscript.

References

1. Bleyer A, O'Leary M, Barr R, Ries LAG (eds) (2006) Cancer Epidemiology in Older Adolescents and Young Adults 15 to 29 Years of Age, Including SEER Incidence and Survival: 1975–2000. National Cancer Institute, NIH Pub. No. 06–5767, Bethesda, MD
2. Capra M, Hargrave D, Bartels U, et al (2003) Central nervous system tumours in adolescents. Eur J Cancer 39:2643–2650
3. IARC (2003) Cancer in Africa: epidemiology and prevention. IARC Press, Lyon, France
4. Parkin DM, Whelen SL, Ferlay J, et al (2002) Cancer Incidence in Five Continents, Vol. VIII. IARC Press, Lyon, France
5. Gurney JG, Wall DA, Jukich PJ, Davis FG (1999) The contribution of nonmalignant tumours to CNS tumour incidence rates among children in the United States. Cancer Causes Control 10:101–105
6. CBTRUS (2004–2005) Statistical report: Primary brain tumours in the United States, 1997–2001. Central Brain Tumour Registry of the United States
7. Birch JM, Alston RD, Quinn M, Kelsey AM (2003) Incidence of malignant disease by morphological type, in young persons aged 12–24 years in England, 1979–1997. Eur J Cancer 39:2622–2631
8. Preston-Martin S, Mack WJ (1996) Neoplasms of the nervous system. In: Schottenfield D, Fraumeni JF (eds) Cancer Epidemiology and Prevention. Oxford University Press, New York, pp 1231–1281
9. Garwicz S, Anderson H, Olsen JH, et al. (2000) Second malignant neoplasms after cancer in childhood and adolescence: a population-based case-control study in the 5 Nordic countries. Int J Cancer 88:672–678
10. Ron E, Modan B, Boice JD, et al. (1988) Tumours of the brain and nervous system after radiotherapy in childhood. N Eng J Med 319:1033–1039
11. Auvinen A, Linet MS, Hatch EE, et al. (2000) Extremely low-frequency magnetic fields and childhood acute lymphoblastic leukemia: an exploratory analysis of alternative exposure metrics. Am J Epidemiol 152:20–31.
12. Hatch EE, Kleinerman RA, Linet MS, et al. (2000) Do confounding or selection factors of residential wiring codes and magnetic fields distort findings of electromagnetic fields studies. Epidemiology 11:189–98.
13. Kheifets LI (2001) Electric and magnetic field exposure and brain cancer: a review. Bioelectromagnetics Suppl 5:S120–S131
14. Kleinerman RA, Kaune WT, Hatch EE, et al. (2000) Are children living near high-voltage power lines at increased risk of acute lymphoblastic leukemia? Am J Epidemiol 151:512–515
15. Little J (1999) Epidemiology of Childhood Cancer. IARC Press, Lyon, France

16. Elwood JM (2003) Epidemiological studies of radio frequency exposures and human cancer. Bioelectromagnetics Suppl 6:S63–S73

17. Huncharek M, Kupelnick B (2004) A meta-analysis of maternal cured meat consumption during pregnancy and the risk of childhood brain tumours. Neuroepidemiology 23:78–84

18. Blot WJ, Henderson BE, Boice JD (1999) Childhood cancer in relation to cured meat intake: review of the epidemiological evidence. Nutr Cancer 34:111–118

19. Huncharek M, Kupelnick B, Wheeler L (2003) Dietary cured meat and the risk of adult glioma: a meta-analysis of nine observational studies. J Environ Pathol Toxicol Oncol 22:129–137

20. Boffetta P, Trédaniel J, Greco A (2000) Risk of childhood cancer and adult lung cancer after childhood exposure to passive smoking: a meta-analysis. Environ Health Perspect 108:73–82

21. Huncharek M, Kupelnick B, Klassen H (2002) Maternal smoking during pregnancy and the risk of childhood brain tumours: a meta-analysis of 6566 subjects from twelve epidemiological studies. J Neurooncol 57:51–57

22. Zahm SH, Ward MH (1998) Pesticides and childhood cancer. Environ Health Perspect 106:893–908

23. Yeni-Komshian H, Holly EA (2000) Childhood brain tumours and exposure to animals and farm life: a review. Paediatr Perinat Epidemiol 14:248–256

24. Ménégoz F, Little J, Colonna M, et al. (2002) Contacts with animals and humans as risk factors for adult brain tumours. An international case-control study. Eur J Cancer 38:696–704

25. Colt JS, Blair A (1998) Parental occupational exposures and risk of childhood cancer. Environ Health Perspect 106:909–925

26. Cordier S, Monfort C, Filippini G, et al. (2004) Parental exposure to polycyclic aromatic hydrocarbons and the risk of childhood brain tumours: the SEARCH International Childhood Brain Tumour Study. Am J Epidemiol 159:1109–1116

27. Cordier S, Mandereau L, Preston-Martin S, et al. (2001) Parental occupations and childhood brain tumours: results of an international case-control study. Cancer Causes Control 12:865–874

28. Carozza SE, Wrensch M, Miike R, et al. (2000) Occupation and adult gliomas. Am J Epidemiol 152:838–846

29. Cocco P, Dosemeci M, Heineman EF (1998) Occupational risk factors for cancer of the central nervous system: a case-control study on death certificates from 24 U.S. states. Am J Ind Med 33:247–255

30. De Roos AJ, Stewart PA, Linet MS, et al. (2003) Occupation and the risk of adult glioma in the United States. Cancer Causes Control 14:139–150

31. Navas-Acién A, Pollán M, Gustavsson P, Plato N (2002) Occupation, exposure to chemicals and risk of gliomas and meningiomas in Sweden. Am J Ind Med 42:214–227

Chapter 10

32. Brenner AV, Linet MS, Fine HA, et al.(2002) History of allergies and autoimmune disease and risk of brain tumours in adults. Int J Cancer 99:252–259

33. Schlehofer B, Blettner M, Preston-Martin S, et al. (1999) Role of medical history in brain tumour development. Results from the international adult brain tumour study. Int J Cancer 82:155–160

34. Wiemels JL, Wiencke JK, Sison JD, et al (2002) History of allergies among adults with glioma and controls. Int J Cancer 98:609–615

35. Wrensch M, Lee M, Miike R, et al (1997) Familial and personal medical history of cancer and nervous system conditions among adults with glioma and controls. Am J Epidemiol 145:581–593

36. Schwartzbaum J, Jonsson F, Ahlbom A, et al. (2003) Cohort studies of association between self-reported allergic conditions, immune-related diagnoses and glioma and meningioma risk. Int J Cancer 106:423–428

37. Wrensch M, Weinberg A, Wiencke J, et al (2001) Prevalence of antibodies to four herpes viruses among adults with glioma and controls. Am J Epidemiol 154:161–165

38. Wrensch M, Weinberg A, Wiencke J, et al. (2005) History of chickenpox and shingles and prevalence of antibodies to varicella-zoster virus and three other herpes viruses among adults with glioma and controls. Am J Epidemiol 161:929–938

39. Franceschi S, Dal Maso L, La Vecchia C (1999) Advances in the epidemiology of HIV-associated non-Hodgkin lymphoma and other lymphoid neoplasms. Int J Cancer 83:481–485

40. Dal Maso L, Rezza G, Zambon P, et al., for the Cancer and Aids Registry linkage (2001) Non-Hodgkin lymphoma among young adults with and without AIDS in Italy. Int J Cancer 93:430–435

41. International Collaboration on HIV and Cancer (2000) Highly active antiretroviral therapy and incidence of cancer in human immunodeficiency virus-infected adults. J Natl Cancer Inst 92:1823–1830

42. Vilchez RA, Kozinetz CA, Arrington AS, et al (2003) Simian Virus 40 in human cancers. Am J Med 114:675–684

43. Engels EA, Sarkar C, Daniel RW, et al. (2002) Absence of Simian virus 40 in human brain tumours from Northern India. Int J Cancer 101:348–352

44. Engels EA, Katki HA, Nielsen NM, et al. (2003) Cancer incidence in Denmark following exposure to poliovirus vaccine contaminated with simian virus 40. J Natl Cancer Inst 95:532–539

45. Sivak-Sears NR, Schwartzbaum JA, Miike R, et al (2004) Case-control study of use of nonsteroidal antiinflammatory drugs and glioblastoma multiforme. Am J Epidemiol 159:1131–1139

46. Friis S, Sorensen HT, McLaughlin JK, et al (2003) A population-based cohort study of the risk of colorectal and other cancers among users of low-dose aspirin. Br J Cancer 88:684–688

47. Gurney JG, Mueller BA, Preston-Martin S, et al. (1997) A study of pediatric brain tumours and their association with epilepsy and anticonvulsant use. Neuroepidemiology 16:248–255

48. Inskip PD, Mellemkjaer L, Gridley G, Olsen JH (1998) Incidence of intracranial tumours following hospitalization for head injuries (Denmark). Cancer Causes Control 9:109–116

49. Wrensch M, Miike R, Lee M, Neuhaus J (2000) Are prior head injuries or diagnostic x-rays associated with glioma in adults? The effects of control selection bias. Neuroepidemiology 19:234–244

50. Preston-Martin S, Pogoda JM, Schlehofer B, et al. (1998) An international case-control study of adult glioma and meningioma: the role of head trauma. Int J Epidemiol 27:579–586

51. Friedman J, Birch P (1997) An association between optic glioma and other tumours of the central nervous system in neurofibromatosis type 1. Neuropediatrics 28:131–132

52. Gutmann DH, Rasmussen SA, Wolkenstein P, et al. (2002) Gliomas presenting after age 10 in individuals with neurofibromatosis type 1 (NF1). Neurology 59:759–761

53. Listernick R, Charrow J, Greenwald MJ, Easterly NB (1989) Optic gliomas in children with neurofibromatosis type 1. J Pediatr 114:788–792

54. Molloy PT, Bilaniuk LT, Vaughan SN, et al. (1995) Brainstem tumours in patients with neurofibromatosis type 1: a distinct clinical entity. Neurology 45:1897–1902

55. Riffaud L, Vinchon M, Ragragui O, et al (2002) Hemispheric cerebral gliomas in children with NF1: arguments for a long term follow up. Childs Nerv Syst 18:43–47

56. Evans DGR, Sainio M, Baser ME (2000) Neurofibromatosis type 2. J Med Genet 37:897–904

57. Maddock IR, Moran A, Maher ER, T et al. (1996) A genetic register for von Hippel-Lindau disease. J Med Genet 33:120–127

58. Roach ES, Smith M, Huttenlocher P, et al (1992) Diagnostic criteria: tuberous sclerosis complex. Report of the Diagnostic Criteria Committee of the National Tuberous Sclerosis Association. J Child Neurol 7:221–224

59. Webb D, Fryer AE, Osborne JP (1996) Morbidity associated with tuberous sclerosis: a population study. Dev Med Child Neurol 38:146–155

60. Corradetti M, Inoki K, Bardeesy N, et al (2004) Regulation of the TSC pathway by LKB1: evidence of a molecular link between tuberous sclerosis complex and Peutz-Jeghers syndrome. Genes Dev 18:1533–1538

61. Inoki K, Zhu T, Guan KL (2003) TSC2 mediates cellular energy response to control cell growth and survival. Cell 115:577–590

62. Kleihues P, Schäuble B, Hausen AZ, et al (1997) Tumours associated with p53 germline mutations. A synopsis of 91 families. Am J Pathol 150:1–13

63. Birch JM, Hartley AL, Blair V, et al. (1990) Cancer in the families of children with soft tissue sarcoma. Cancer 66:2239–2248

64. Garber JE, Goldstein AM, Kantor AF, et al (1991) Follow-up study of twenty-four families with Li-Fraumeni syndrome. Cancer Res 51:6094–6097

65. Li FP, Fraumeni JF Jr, Mulvihill JJ, et al. (1988) A cancer family syndrome in 24 kindreds. Cancer Res 48:5358–5362

66. Varley JM (2003) Germline TP53 mutations and Li-Fraumeni syndrome. Hum Mutat 21:313–320

67. Birch JM, Alston RD, McNally RJQ, et al. (2001) Relative frequency and morphology of cancers in carriers of germline TP53 mutations. Oncogene 20:4621–4628

68. Trump D, Farren B, Wooding C, et al. (1996) Clinical studies of multiple endocrine neoplasia type 1 (MEN1). Q J Med 89:653–669

69. Robinson S, Cohen A (2000) Cowden disease and L'Hermitte-Duclos disease: characterization of a new phakomatosis. Neurosurgery 46:371

70. Kleihues P, Cavenee WK (eds) (2000) Tumours of the Nervous System. World Health Organization Classification of Tumours. Oxford University Press, Lyon, France

71. Paraf F, Jothy S, Van Meir EG (1997) Brain tumour-polyposis syndrome: two genetic diseases? J Clin Oncol 15:2744–2758

72. Aarnio M, Sankila R, Pukkala E, et al. (1999) Cancer risk in mutation carriers of DNA-mismatch-repair genes. Int J Cancer 81:214–218

73. Vasen HFA, Sanders EACM, Taal BG, et al. (1996) The risk of brain tumours in hereditary non-polyposis colorectal cancer (HNPCC). Int J Cancer 65:422–425

74. Hamilton SR, Liu B, Parsons RE, et al. (1995) The molecular basis of Turcot's syndrome. N Eng J Med 332:839–847

75. Hasle H (2001) Pattern of malignant disorders in individuals with Down's syndrome. Lancet Oncol 2:429–436

76. Amlashi SFA, Riffaud L, Brassier G, Morandi X (2003) Nevoid basal cell carcinoma syndrome: relation with desmoplastic medulloblastoma in infancy. A population-based study and review of the literature. Cancer 98:618–624

77. Biegel JA, Zhou J-Y, Rorke LB, et al (1999) Germ-line and acquired mutations of IN11 in atypical teratoid and rhabdoid tumours. Cancer Res 59:74–79

78. Cowan R, Hoban P, Kelsey A, et al (1997) The gene for the naevoid basal cell carcinoma syndrome acts as a tumour-suppressor gene in medulloblastoma. Br J Cancer 76:141–145

79. Stiller C, Bleyer W (2004) Epidemiology. In: Walker D, Perilongo G, Punt J, Taylor R (eds) Brain and Spinal Tumours of Childhood. Arnold, London, pp 35–49

80. Becker Y (1986). Cancer in ataxia-telangiectasia patients: analysis of factors leading to radiation-induced and spontaneous tumours. Anticancer Res 6:1021–1032

81. Chun HH, Gatti RA (2004) Ataxia-telangiectasia, an evolving phenotype. DNA Repair 3:1187–1196

82. Khanna (2000) Cancer risk and the ATM gene: a continuing debate. J Natl Cancer Inst 92:795–802

83. Kuhne M, Riballo E, Rief N, et al (2004) A double-strand break repair defect in ATM-deficient cells contributes to radiosensitivity. Cancer Res 64:500–508

84. Hemminki K, Li X (2004) Association of brain tumours with other neoplasms in families. Eur J Cancer 40:253–259

85. Malmer B, Henriksson, Gronberg H (2002) Different aetiology of familial low-grade and high-grade glioma? A nationwide cohort study of familial glioma. Neuro-epidemiology 21:279–286

86. Malmer B, Henriksson R, Grönberg H (2003) Familial brain tumours – genetics of environment? A nationwide cohort study of cancer risk in spouses and first-degree relatives of brain tumour patients. Int J Cancer 106:260–263

87. Hemminki K, Li X, Collins VP (2001) A population-based study of familial central nervous system hemangioblastomas. Neuroepidemiology 20:257–261

88. Paunu N, Syrjäkoski K, Sankila R, et al. (2001) Analysis of p53 tumour suppressor gene in families with multiple glioma patients. J Neurooncol 55:159–165

89. Nicholson JC, Punt J, Hale J, et al; Germ Cell Tumour Working Groups of the United Kingdom Children's Cancer Study Group (UKCCSG) and International Society of Paediatric Oncology (SIOP) (2002) Neurosurgical management of paediatric germ cell tumours of the central nervous system – a multi-disciplinary team approach for the new millennium. Br J Neurosurg 16:93–95

90. Walker DA, Punt JA, Sokal M (1999) Clinical management of brain stem glioma. Arch Dis Child 80:558–564

91. Walker DA, Punt JAG, Sokal M (2004) Brainstem tumours. In: Walker D, Perilongo G, Punt J Taylor R (eds) Brain and Spinal Tumours of Childhood. Arnold, London, pp 291–313

92. Westphal M, Hilt DC, Bortey E, et al. (2003) A phase 3 trial of local chemotherapy with biodegradable carmustine (BCNU) wafers (Gliadel wafers) in patients with primary malignant glioma. Neuro-oncology 5:79–88

93. Barnett FH, Scharer-Schuksz M, Wood M, et al (2004) Intra-arterial delivery of endostatin gene to brain tumours prolongs survival and alters tumour vessel ultrastructure. Gene Ther 11:1283–1289

94. Chiocca EA, Abbed KM, Tatter S, et al. (2004) A phase 1 open-label, dose-escalation, multi-institutional trial of injection with an E1B-attenuated adenovirus, ONYX-015, into the peritumoural region of recurrent malignant gliomas in the adjuvant setting. Mol Ther 10:958–966

95. Glorioso JC, Fink DJ (2004) Herpes vector-mediated gene transfer in treatment of diseases of the nervous system. Annu Rev Microbiol 58:253–271

96. Immonen A, Vapalahti M, Tyynela K, et al. (2004) AdvHSV-tk gene therapy with intravenous ganciclovir improves survival in human malignant glioma: a randomised controlled study. Mol Ther 10:967–972

97. McKeown SR, Ward C, Robson T (2004). Gene-directed enzyme prodrug therapy: a current assessment. Curr Opin Mol Ther 6:421–435

98. Okada H, Pollack IF (2004) Cytokine gene therapy for malignant glioma. Expert Opin Biol Ther 4:1609–1620

99. Gnekow A, Packer R, Kortmann R (2004) Astrocytic tumours, low-grade: treatment considerations by primary site and tumour dissemination. In: Walker D, Perilongo G, Punt J, Taylor R (eds) Brain and Spinal Tumours of Childhood. Arnold, London, pp 259–276

100. Klein M, Heimans JJ, Aaronson NK, et al. (2002) Effect of radiotherapy and other treatment-related factors on mid-term to long-term cognitive sequelae in low grade gliomas: a comparative study. Lancet 360:1361–1368

101. Balis FM, Poplack DG (1993) Cancer Chemotherapy. In: Nathan DG, Oski FA (eds) Hematology of Infancy and Childhood. WB Saunders, Philadelphia, pp 1207–1238

102. Tabori U, Sung L, Hukin J, et al. (2005) Medulloblastoma in the second decade of life: a specific group with respect to toxicity and management. A Canadian Pediatric Brain Tumor Consortium Study. Cancer 103:1874–1880

103. Glaser AW, Buxton N, Hewitt M, et al (1996) The role of steroids in paediatric central nervous system malignancies. Br J Neurosurg 10:123–124

104. Weissman DE (1988) Glucocorticoid treatment for brain metastases and epidural spinal cord compression: a review. J Clin Oncol 6:543–551

105. Motoyama T, Watanabe H, Yamamoto T, Sekiguchi M (1987) Production of alpha-fetoprotein by human germ cell tumours in vivo and in vitro. Acta Pathol Jpn 37:1263–1277

106. Motoyama T, Watanabe H, Yamamoto T, Sekiguchi M (1988) Production of beta-human chorionic gonadotropin by germ cell tumours in vivo and in vitro. Acta Pathol Jpn 38:577–590

107. Packer RJ, Sutton LN, Rosenstock JG, et al. (1984) Pineal region tumours of childhood. Pediatrics 74:97–102

108. Itoyama Y, Kochi M, Yamamoto H, et al (1990) Clinical study of intracranial nongerminomatous germ cell tumours producing alpha-fetoprotein. Neurosurgery 27:454–460

109. Kida Y, Kobayashi T, Yoshida J, et al (1986) Chemotherapy with cisplatin for αFP-secreting germ-cell tumours of the central nervous system. J Neurosurg 65:470–475

110. Wara WM, Jenkin RD, Evans A, et al. (1979) Tumours of the pineal and suprasellar region: Children's Cancer Study Group treatment results 1960–1975: a report from Children's Cancer Study Group. Cancer 43:698–701

111. Jennings MT, Gelman R, Hochberg F (1985) Intracranial germ-cell tumours: natural history and pathogenesis. J Neurosurg 63:155–167

112. Einhorn LH, Williams SD (1980) Chemotherapy of disseminated testicular cancer. A random prospective study. Cancer 46:1339–1344

113. Williams SD, Stablein DM, Einhorn LH, et al. (1987) Immediate adjuvant chemotherapy versus observation with treatment at relapse in pathological stage II testicular cancer. N Engl J Med 317:1433–1438

114. Kirshner JJ, Ginsberg SJ, Fitzpatrick AV, Comis RL (1981) Treatment of a primary intracranial germ cell tumour with systemic chemotherapy. Med Pediatr Oncol 9:361–365

115. Itoyama Y, Kochi M, Kuratsu J, et al.(1995) Treatment of intracranial non-germinomatous malignant germ cell tumours producing (alpha)-fetoprotein. Neurosurgery 36:459–466

116. Kobayashi T, Yoshida J, Ishiyama J, et al (1989) Combination chemotherapy with cisplatin and etoposide for malignant intracranial germ-cell tumours. An experimental and clinical study. J Neurosurg 70:676–681

117. Allen JC, DaRosso RC, Donahue B, Nirenberg A (1994) A phase II trial of pre-irradiation carboplatin in newly diagnosed germinoma of the central nervous system. Cancer 74:940–944

118. Allen JC, Kim JH, Packer RJ (1987) Neoadjuvant chemotherapy for newly diagnosed germ-cell tumours of the central nervous system. J Neurosurg 67:65–70

119. Shibamoto Y, Abe M, Yamashita J, et al. (1988) Treatment results of intracranial germinoma as a function of the irradiated volume. Int J Radiat Oncol Biol Phys 15:285–290

120. Ogawa K, Shikama N, Toita T, et al. (2004) Long-term results of radiotherapy for intracranial germinoma: a multi-institutional retrospective review of 126 patients. Int J Radiat Oncol Biol Phys 58:705–713

121. Aoyama H, Shirato H, Kakuto Y, et al. (1998) Pathologically-proven intracranial germinoma treated with radiation therapy. Radiother Oncol 47:201–205. Erratum in: Radiother Oncol 1999, 50:241

122. Shirato H, Nishio M, Sawamura Y, et al. (1997) Analysis of long-term treatment of intracranial germinoma. Int J Radiat Oncol Biol Phys 37:511–515

123. Ogawa K, Toita T, Nakamura K, et al. (2003) Treatment and prognosis of patients with intracranial nongerminomatous malignant germ cell tumours: a multiinstitu-tional retrospective analysis of 41 patients. Cancer 98:369–376

124. Kiltie AE, Gattamaneni HR (1995) Survival and quality of life of paediatric intracranial germ cell tumour patients treated at the Christie Hospital, 1972–1993. Med Pediatr Oncol 25:450–456

125. Aoyama H, Shirato H, Ikeda J, et al (2002) Induction chemotherapy followed by low-dose involved-field radiotherapy for intracranial germ cell tumours. J Clin Oncol 20:857–865

126. Balmaceda C, Heller G, Rosenblum M, et al. (1996) Chemotherapy without irradiation – a novel approach for newly diagnosed CNS germ cell tumours: results of an international co-operative trial. The First International Central Nervous System Germ Cell Tumour Study. J Clin Oncol 14:2908–2915

127. Bamberg M, Kortmann RD, Calaminus G, et al. (1999) Radiation therapy for intracranial germinoma: results of the German Co-operative Prospective Trials MAKEI 83/86/89. J Clin Oncol 17:2585–2592

128. Baranzelli MC, Patte C, Boufet E, et al. (1997) Nonmetastatic intracranial germinoma: the experience of the French Society of Pediatric Oncology. Cancer 80:1792–1797

129. Bouffet E, Baranzelli MC, et al. (1999) Combined treatment modality for intracranial germinomas: results of a multicentre SFOP experience. Societe Francaise d'Oncologie Pediatrique. Br J Cancer 79:1199–1204

130. Calaminus G, Bamberg M, Baranzelli MC, et al. (1994). Intracranial germ cell tumours: a comprehensive update of the European data. Neuropediatrics 25:26–32

131. Chang TK, Wong TT, Hwang B (1995) Combination chemotherapy with vinblastine, bleomycin, cisplatin, and etoposide (VBPE) in children with intracranial germ cell tumours. Med Pediatr Oncol 24:368–372

132. Herrman HD, Westphal M, Winkler K, et al (1994) Treatment of non-germinomatous germ-cell tumours of the pineal region. Neurosurgery 34:524–529

133. Eiser C (1997) Children's quality of life measures. Arch Dis Child 77:350–354

134. Glaser AW, Furlong W, Walker DA, et al. (1999) Applicability of the Health Utilities Index to a population of childhood survivors of central nervous system tumours in the United Kingdom. Eur J Cancer 35:256–261

135. Merchant TE, Davis BJ, Sheldon JM, Leibel SA (1998) Radiation therapy for relapsed CNS germinoma after primary chemotherapy. J Clin Oncol 16:204–209

136. Kennedy C, Bull K (2004) Effect of neo-adjuvant chemotherapy on long-term health state and behaviour in the PNET3 RCT of treatment for primitive neuro-ectodermal tumour (PNET). ISPNO, Boston (abstract)

137. Benesch M, Lackner H, Schagerl S, et al (2001) Tumour- and treatment-related side effects after multimodal therapy of childhood intracranial germ cell tumours. Acta Paediatr 90:264–270

138. Sankaranarayanan R, Black RJ, Swaminathan R, Parkin DM (1998) An overview of cancer survival in developing countries. IARC Sci Publ 145:135–173

139. Jenkin D, Shabanah MA, Shail EA, et al.(2000) Prognostic factors for medulloblastoma. Int J Radiat Oncol Biol Phys 47:573–584

140. Liu Y, Zhu Y, Gao L, et al. (2005) Radiation treatment for medulloblastoma: a review of 64 cases at a single institute. Jpn J Clin Oncol 35:111–115

Soft-Tissue Sarcomas

Karen H. Albritton • Andrea Ferrari •
Michela Casanova

Contents

11.1 Introduction

Soft-tissue sarcomas (STSs) are a very heterogeneous group of nonepithelial extraskeletal malignancies that are classified on a histogenic basis according to the mature tissue they most resemble. Different histotypes with different biologies and clinical behaviors are included in this group of tumors. Usually, they are characterized by local aggressiveness and propensity to metastasize, which is correlated to the grade of malignancy. They can arise, generally as an enlarging soft-tissue mass, anywhere in the body (most frequently in the soft tissue of the extremities, and less usually in the trunk or head and neck region). They comprise less than 1% of all malignant tumors but account for 2% of total cancer-related mortality. In addition, they cause a relatively high burden of morbidity, due to deforming surgery, chemotherapy- and radiation-induced complications, and second cancers. They occur at any age, but a shift occurs in adolescence/early adulthood from predominantly rhabdomyosarcoma of childhood to a mixture of several "adult-type" STSs, with some subtypes particularly typical of adolescents and young adults [1–3] Perhaps because it occurs but is rare across all ages, and perhaps because the orthopedic surgeons and radiation oncologists who are often involved treat both children and adults, the field of STS oncology is not "owned" by either pediatric or medical oncology. For this reason too, it seems that STS is an adolescents and young adults cancer.

Across all ages, the survival rate for STSs averages 60%, with substantial differences according to the histotype, the grade of malignancy, and the stage of the disease [1]. The treatment of patients with STSs is complex and necessarily multidisciplinary, requiring adequate expertise. All STS patients, including adolescents and young adults, probably receive better treatment within select experienced institutions that enroll patients into clinical trials; treating patients outside of a referral center has been identified as an independent risk factor for recurrence in STS. Such a suggestion appears more relevant if one considers that the lowest proportion of patients entered onto national clinical treatment trials vs. the number of new cases occurring at age 25–29 years, when it was 0.6% (Fig 11.1). Below age 10 years, it was over 30% and during adolescence it was approximately 12%. Above age 40 years it exceeded 3%. These data have been supposed to partially explain the slower rates of improvement in overall outcome observed (during the last 20-year period) in older adolescents in comparison to the younger [4, 5].

STSs of adolescents and young adults can be separated in two groups. The first includes the highly malignant tumors, characterized morphologically by small round blue cells: rhabdomyosarcoma (RMS), Ewing family of tumors (EFT), and the rare desmoplastic small round cell tumor. EFT [Ewing sarcoma, (ES) and the peripheral primitive neuroectodermal tumor (pPNET), which is cytogenetically the same neoplastic entity as ES but with a different grade of differentiation] is highly aggressive, with a high propensity to metastasize, and is typical of adolescents and young adults. Its natural history and treatment is comparable to that of the more frequent ES arising in the bone, and therefore it will not be described in this chapter, but in Chap. 12. The second group of STSs includes the classic "adult-type" STSs, which are generally characterized by spindle-cell histology and uncertain response to chemotherapy and radiotherapy. Although Kaposi sarcoma is a malignant STS that has historically affected young adults, its relation to the human immunodeficiency virus epidemic makes its epidemiology and management quite different. It will not be considered in this chapter and all comments about STS will pertain to non-EFT, non-Kaposi sarcoma.

11.2 Epidemiology/Etiology

Overall, STSs are rare: with an annual incidence of around 2–3/100,000 persons of all ages. STS incidence increases exponentially with age, but peaks as a percent of all cancers in 5- to 10-year-olds. At a rate of 8.2 cases per million, STS ties as the fifth most common cancer in 15- to 19-year-olds (7.7% of all tumors); in the 20- to 24-year-olds there are 17.9 cases per million – 6.6% of all tumors and the seventh most common. Although rates continue to increase with age and reach 62.3 per million in 25- to 29-year-olds, they start to become a less common proportion of all cancers with age (Fig. 11.2). In the 15–29 years age period, rhabdomyosarcoma (RMS, a tumor predominantly of children and adolescents) and the spindle-cell sarcomas including fibrosarcoma, synovial sarcoma (SS), and malignant peripheral nerve sheath tumor (MPNST), are the most frequent histotypes (Figs. 11.3 and 11.4) [1–3]. Surveillance, Epidemiology and End Results data from the period 1975–1999 finds dermatofibrosarcoma to be the most common non-Kaposi STS among 15- to 29-year-

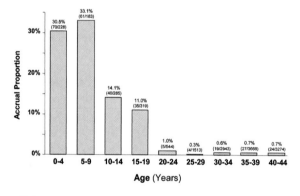

Figure 11.1

Estimated proportion of all patients diagnosed with sarcomas during 1997–2002 who were entered onto United States national treatment trials. Values in the parentheses are the average annual accrual to the trials (numerator) and estimated average number of patients expected to have been diagnosed with the cancer in the United States during the years evaluated (denominator). Accrual data from the Cancer Therapy Evaluation Program, United States National Cancer Institute. Modified from Bleyer et al. [2]

olds, followed by leiomyosarcoma/fibrosarcoma, RMS, SS, and malignant fibrous histiocytoma (Table 11.1).

Arising from immature mesenchymal cells that are committed to skeletal muscle differentiation, RMS is one of the typical cancers of childhood, as it constitutes more than 50% of STSs, with an annual incidence of 4.3 per million children younger than 20 years. On the contrary, it is seen exceedingly infrequently in adults (3% of STSs). The incidence of RMS decreases significantly with increasing age: about three out of four cases occur in children under 10 years, with a peak of incidence between 3 and

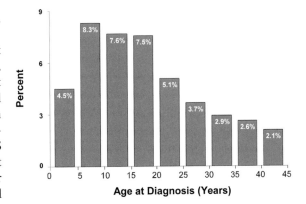

Figure 11.2

Proportion of soft-tissue sarcomas relative to all invasive cancer as a function of age in those diagnosed before age 45 years in the United States. Data from the United States SEER [1]

Table 11.1 Soft-tissue sarcomas by histologic type in 15- to 29-year-olds, 1992–2002. *PNET* Primitive neuroectodermal tumor

Histologic type	% of total
Kaposi Sarcoma	35.3%
Dermatofibrosarcoma, including protuberans	14.9%
Leiomyosarcoma, fibrosarcoma	6.3%
Rhabdomyosarcoma	6.5%
Synovial cell sarcoma	6.0%
Ewing sarcoma/PNET	4.8%
Malignant fibrous histiocytoma	4.3%
Liposarcoma	4.3%
Malignant peripheral nerve sheath tumor	3.8%
Angiomatous/vascular sarcomas	2.3%
Spindle cell sarcoma	1.5%
Epithelioid sarcoma	1.4%
Alveolar soft part sarcoma	1.2%
Clear cell sarcoma	1.0%
Small cell sarcoma	0.6%
Chondrosarcoma (soft tissue)	0.5%
Giant cell sarcoma	0.4%
Desmoplastic small round cell tumor	0.4%
Miscellaneous	4.5%
Total Number	2,812

5 years [6]. A second smaller peak occurs in adolescence [6].

For most STS subtypes, the pathogenesis remains unknown and there are no well-established risk factors. Ionizing radiation clearly causes sarcomas, and chemical carcinogens and oncogenic viruses have been associated with the development of some type of sarcomas, but the etiological relationship remains unclear. A few genetic predispositions are well described, but cause few of all STS: neurofibromatosis type 1 (in particular increases the risk of MPNST) and Li Fraumeni syndrome (which increases the risk of RMS) are the two classic (but not the only) genetic diseases associated with soft-tissue tumors [2–3]. Those with certain genetic conditions are predisposed to have an STS at a younger age, so that the proportion of adolescents and young adults with STSs with a genetic predisposition is probably higher than in older adults.

11.3 Biology/Pathology

The grade of malignancy describes the aggressiveness of the tumor and its natural history. It is determined by a combined assessment of histological features: degree

ADOLESCENTS / YOUNG ADULTS

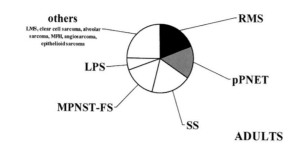

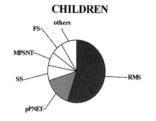

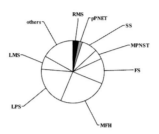

Figure 11.3

Types of relative incidence of soft-tissue sarcomas in adolescents and young adults in comparison to those that occur in children and older adults. *LMS* Leiomyosarcoma, *MFH* malignant fibrous histiocytoma, *LPS* liposarcoma, *MPNST* malignant peripheral nerve sheath tumor, *FS* fibrosarcoma, *SS* synovial sarcoma, *pPNET* peripheral primitive neuroectodermal tumor, *RMS* rhabdomyosarcoma

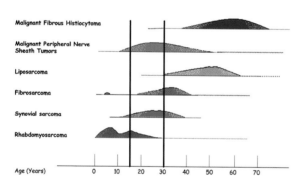

Figure 11.4

Relationship of age to incidence of various types of soft-tissue sarcomas

of cellularity, cellular pleomorphism or anaplasia, mitotic activity, and degree of necrosis. Different histotypes with the same grade of malignancy could display the same clinical behavior. In general, low-grade tumors may have local aggressiveness but a low tendency to metastatic spread. High-grade tumors have a more invasive behavior with a high propensity to metastasize (in particular to the lung). Some histotypes (i.e., RMS, but also SS, alveolar soft parts sarcoma, and angiosarcoma) are usually considered as being high grade inde-

pendently from their mitotic index, necrosis, and cellularity. Different grading systems (generally three-grade systems) have been defined over the years by pediatric and adult oncologists for predicting clinical course and prognosis, and defining a risk-adapted treatment. The most frequently used grading systems for adult sarcomas are the National Cancer Institute (NCI) system and the French Federation of Cancer Centers (FN-CLCC) system. The Pediatric Oncology Group system is similar to the NCI system, but accounts for tumors found exclusively in childhood. Unfortunately, the use of a distinct grading system has made it difficult to compare results in pediatrics to those in adults.

RMS is a distinct entity, clearly different from other STSs typical of adult age. RMS cells can be recognized by the expression of myosin and MyoD protein family antigen. Myoglobin, desmin, and muscle-specific actin are also useful as diagnostic markers. Classically, two histological subtypes of RMS have been distinguished, embryonal and alveolar [7]. The diagnosis of alveolar subtype has to be given if there is any degree of alveolar architecture or cytology. A third form, pleomorphic RMS, needs to be considered separately from other RMS subtypes: it is very rare in both the pediatric population (less than 1%) and in adolescents and young adults, occurring typically at an age older than 45–50 years. It is most common in the deep soft tissues of the extremities, with a predilection for males [1, 6]. Decades ago, pleomorphic RMS was a commonly assigned subtype, then it was regarded as a variant of malignant fibrous histiocytoma and its existence put in doubt. More recently, ultrastructural, immunohistochemical and molecular techniques have refined criteria its for diagnosis. Other data suggest that pleomorphic RMS is probably biologically and clinically closer to high-grade spindle-cell sarcomas of adults than to pediatric RMS.

Cytogenetic and molecular analyses may help in the diagnosis of RMS and in the definition of the subtype. Most alveolar RMSs display a specific translocation t(2;13)(q35;q14), involving the *PAX3* and the *FKHR* genes; a variant, t(1;13)(p36;q14), has been less frequently reported. Embryonal RMS lacks a tumor-specific translocation, but generally exhibits a loss of heterozygosity at chromosome 11p, which may act by inactivating tumor-suppression genes [2, 6].

A pattern of association between histotypes and clinical features has been described (Table 11.2). The alveolar histotype is more frequently localized at the extremities and in the trunk, and it is more typical of adolescents and young adults than of children. The recent International Consensus meeting defined a new International Classification of RMS, based on the relationship between histology and prognosis. Favorable subtypes are two variants of the embryonal type, the botryoid and the spindle-cell (or leiomyomatous) variants. The classic embryonal subtype carries an intermediate prognosis and the alveolar RMS (with the recently described solid variant) has an unfavorable prognosis. Of note, spindle-cell RMS in adults appears to have a different natural history and biology from the morphologically similar spindle-cell RMS of childhood. In adults, it has a propensity to occur in the head and neck area and carries a very poor prognosis.

Besides RMS, there are almost ninety subtypes of STS. Because of their relative rarity in childhood, many pediatric oncologists lump these as "non-RMS STSs" (NRSTS). Medical oncologists find this term amusing, as this describes 98%, not 50% of the tumors they see. The naming and classification of these has been based on the normal tissue the morphology of the cancer most resembles. The classification has undergone wide alteration, and studies suggest a 25% discordance rate between pathologists for classification. However, to date, this has had little impact on clinical therapeutics, as this has been guided more by grade than classification. Clinical trials have "lumped" all STSs together. Recently, more advanced immunohistochemical techniques, cytogenetics (both traditional and targeted hybridization techniques), and even microarray techniques are increasing the precision of the diagnosis. Hopefully, this will allow better prognostication and development of risk-based and targeted therapeutics.

Table 11.2 Translocation and fusion genes in sarcomas. Modified from Borden (2003) [8]

Ewing sarcoma	t(11;22)(q24;q12)	EWS-FLI1
	t(21;22)(q22;q12)	EWS-ERG
Clear cell sarcoma	t(12;22)(q13;q12)	EWS-ATF1
Desmoplastic small round cell tumor	t(11;22)(q13;q12)	EWS-WT1
Extraskeletal myxoid chondrosarcoma	t(9;22)(q22;q12)	EWS-CHN
	t(9;17)(q22;q11)	TAF2N-CHN
Myxoid liposarcoma	t(12;16)(q13;p11)	TLS-CHOP
Angiomatoid fibrous histiocytoma	t(12;16)(q13;p11)	TLS-ATF1
Alveolar rhabdomyosarcoma	t(2;13)(q35;q14)	PAX3-FKHR
	t(1;13)(p36;q14)	PAX7-FKHR
Synovial sarcoma	t(X;18)(p11;q11)	SYT-SSX1,2
Dermatofibrosarcoma protuberans	t(17;22)(q22;q13)	COL1A1-PDGFβ
Congenital fibrosarcoma	t(12;15)(p13;q25)	ETV6-NTRK3
Inflammatory myofibroblastic tumor	t(2p23)	various ALK fusions
Alveolar soft part sarcoma	t(X;17)(p11;q25)	ASPL-TFE3
Endometrial stromal sarcoma	t(7;17)(p15;q21)	JAZF1-JJAZ1

Most pathologists feel that SS needs to be considered as a high-grade tumor, independent of mitotic index, percent of necrosis, and tumor differentiation, given its local invasiveness and propensity for metastatic spread. It is characterized by the presence of epithelial and spindle cells, probably derived from a primitive mesenchymal precursor. There are three histological subtypes: biphasic, monophasic, and poorly differentiated. In the majority of cases, tumor cells (especially the epithelial cells) display immunoreactivity for cytokeratins and epithelial membrane antigen. Immunohistochemistry is essential to differentiate the various spindle-cell sarcomas, but in some cases only the cytogenetic analysis may permit the diagnosis. Several STSs are characterized by specific chromosomal translocations (Table 11.2). The specific translocation t(X;18)(p11.2;q11.2) has been found in more than 90% of SS, with three possible transcripts, SYT-SSX1, SYT-SSX2, and SYT-SSX4 (SYT-SSX2 has recently been associated with better survival) [8].

11.4 Diagnosis/Symptoms and Clinical Signs

The initial signs and symptoms depend on the site of origin and tumor extension. An enlarging painless mass is the most common presentation. In 15- to 29-year olds, about one-third of STS originate in the extremities. RMS can arise anywhere in the body, including sites in which striated muscle tissue is normaly absent. The head and neck region represents the most common location, and the symptoms vary from proptosis, cranial nerve palsy, or nasal obstruction. Hematuria may be present in RMS of the genitourinary tract; ascites and intestinal obstruction can occur with retroperitoneal tumors [2, 3].

In the case of suspected lesions, three diagnostic levels need to be evaluated: (1) the histological diagnosis, for which an incisional biopsy procedure is usually preferred over fine-needle aspiration; (2) the definition of locoregional extension for which magnetic resonance imaging appears to be superior to computed tomography (CT) scan in defining soft-tissue tumor; (3) the staging of the disease for which a chest CT scan and technetium bone scan are usually required. The

value of positron emission tomography scan in staging STS has not yet been determined.

An adequate stratification of the patients is necessary for a risk-adapted therapy. However, as in grading, pediatric and medical oncologists have not used the same systems, making comparison of risk and prognosis difficult. The pediatric Intergroup Rhabdomyosarcoma Study (IRS) postsurgical grouping system [9] supplements the pretreatment clinical tumor-node-metastases (TNM) classification [10], categorizing patients into four groups based on the amount and extent of residual tumor after the initial surgical procedure. Group I includes completely excised tumors with negative microscopic margins; group II indicates grossly resected tumors with microscopic residual disease and/or regional lymph nodal spread; group III includes patients with gross residual disease after incomplete resection or biopsy sampling; group IV encompasses patients with metastases at onset [9]. According to the TNM classification, T1 are those tumors confined to the organ or tissue of origin, while T2 lesions invade contiguous structures; T1 and T2 groups are further classified as A or B depending on whether tumor diameter is $\leq$ or >5 cm, respectively. Regional node involvement is defined as N0 or N1, and the status of distant metastases at onset as M0 or M1 [10].

However, adult oncology groups have generally utilized other systems: the Musculoskeletal Tumor Society Staging System requires the accurate definition of compartmentalization, the American Joint Committee on Cancer Staging System combines TNM definitions and histological grading [11].

11.5 Treatment Management and Outcome

11.5.1 Rhabdomyosarcoma

RMS is a distinct entity and clearly differs from NRSTS in regard to its natural history and its higher sensitivity to chemotherapy and radiotherapy [6].

During the past 30 years the 5-year overall survival (OS) rates of pediatric RMS has improved dramatically from 25–30% to approximately 70% [1, 12–14]. These results are due largely to the development of

Table 11.3 Rhabdomyosarcoma: the histological subtypes and their more frequent characteristics.
RMS Rhabdomyosarcoma

Favorable prognosis	Botryoid RMS	6% of all RMS; mean age 3 ears; polypoid mucosa-associated lesions of genitourinary and head-neck cavities
	Spindle-cell RMS	2%; mean age 7 years; paratesticular regions (leiomyomatous)
Intermediate prognosis	Embryonal RMS	60%; mean age 7 years; all sites, in particular the head-neck regions; Loss of heterozygosity at chromosome 11p15.5
Unfavorable prognosis	Alveolar RMS	30%; older age (10–25 years); deep soft tissue of extremities; t(2;13)(q35;q14) translocation (variant t(1;13)(p36;q14) translocation)
	Pleomorphic RMS	2%; adults older than 45 years; extremities

treatment approaches that are: (1) multidisciplinary (including surgery, radiotherapy, and in particular multiagent effective chemotherapy), (2) risk-adapted (prognostic factors are used to stratify treatment: more intensive therapy improves cure rates in those patients with less favorable disease whereas those with more favorable findings avoid overtreatment and side effects without jeopardizing survival), (3) cooperative multi-institutional trials able to enroll a large number of patients. International cooperative multimodal treatment trials have been carried out by North-American and European groups. Historically, these trials, included subjects up to the age of 18 or 21 years. In 2001, the Children's Oncology Group STS committee raised the upper age limit of all STS protocols to 50 years. In Europe, the opportunity to enroll patients up to 30 years is now in discussion.

Historically, risk stratification and therapy was usually based on the IRS [9] and TNM staging systems [10]. With the recognition of different prognostic factors (i.e., age, histology, tumor site; Table 11.3), the risk assignments has became more complex but also more careful. Table 11.4 shows the risk stratification of the new European pediatric Soft Tissue Sarcoma Study Group (EpSSG) and the Children's Oncology Group protocols for localized RMS, with the estimated survival rates and the proposed treatment for each group [15].

RMS is a markedly chemoresponsive and radiosensitive tumor. Multiagent chemotherapy has a response rate of greater than 80% in the majority of patients. The efficacy of chemotherapy permits partial modification of the aggressive surgical concepts that are essential in the management of adult-type sarcomas of uncertain chemoresponsiveness. Primary resection should be performed only when complete (i.e., histologically free margins) and nonmutilating excision is considered feasible; otherwise biopsy alone is recommended. Tumor size, local invasiveness, and especially tumor site strongly affect the feasibility of surgery, which is also influenced by the surgeon's own judgment and experience. Tumors considered unresectable at diagnosis can be completely resected in a high percentage of cases after tumor shrinkage following primary chemotherapy [16]. Due to the efficacy of adjuvant chemotherapy and radiation, local control can generally be obtained by wide resections (en bloc excisions beyond the reactive zone but within the anatomical compartment with histologically free margins), in contrast to adult NRSTS, which in general should require compartmental resection (en bloc resection of the tumor and the entire compartment of origin).

Table 11.4 Prognostic factors for RMS. *IRS* Intergroup Rhabdomyosarcoma Study

Favorable prognostic factors	Unfavorable prognostic factors
Embryonal histology	Alveolar histology
Initial complete resection (IRS group I)	incomplete resection/unresectability (IRS groups II–III)
Tumor confined to the organ or tissue of origin (T1)	Local invasiveness (T2)
Small tumor size (<5 cm)	Large size (>5 cm)
No regional lymph node involvement (N0)	Nodal involvement (N1)
Localized disease (M0)	Distant metastases at diagnosis (M1)
Age between 1 and 10 years	Age over 10 years (and less than 1 year)

Favorable sites:
    non-parameningeal head-neck (orbital)
    non-bladder/prostate genitourinary (paratesticular, vagina)
	Unfavorable sites:
	    parameningeal region
	    bladder and prostate, abdomen
	    trunk
	    extremities

A large number of different chemotherapeutic regimens have been tested over the years within cooperative trials: today, the VAC regimen (combination of vincristine, actinomycin D, and cyclophosphamide) is still the mainstay of chemotherapy in North America [12, 13, 14], whereas the IVA regimen, which differs in the choice of the alkylating agent (ifosfamide in the place of cyclophosphamide), is the standard therapy in Europe [15, 17, 18]. The different drugs (i.e., cisplatin, etoposide, and melphalan) added over the years to these regimens have not shown clear advantage compared to the standard combinations [13]. Nevertheless, in high-risk patients it is imperative to find out more effective and intensive regimens. In IRS Study V, topotecan is currently administered in patients with less favorable outcome. In EpSSG, as shown in Table 11.5, the role of doxorubicin will be under evaluation within the IVADO regimen, with the concept of administering early the maximum dose intensity of doxorubicin (which is an effective drug, although its role as part of multidrug regimens remains controversial) [19]. In a very selected subset of patients with low-risk characteristics (completely resected small tumor, embryonal histology, paratesticular and vagina sites, age <10 years), a limited chemotherapy without an alkylating agent (VA, vincristine and actinomycin D) has been shown to be enough to maintain excellent results [15]. In adolescents and young adults, given the adverse prognostic significance of age, this regimen should probably not be recommended. At the opposite pattern of risk groups, the outcome of patients with metastatic disease at diagnosis remains poor (about 30% of survivors) despite the use of very intensive treatments, including high-dose chemotherapy followed by reconstitution with peripheral blood stem cells. New drugs are usually evaluated upfront in these patients, even if novel therapeutic approaches are needed (i.e., specific molecular targets for gene therapies).

A quite new noteworthy approach may be the use of maintenance therapy with low-dose continuous chemotherapy (maybe with new antitumor mechanisms, i.e., antiangiogenic); the EpSSG trial (Table 11.5) will randomize patients with localized RMS who are in complete remission after 6 months chemotherapy to receive or not maintenance therapy with oral cyclophosphamide plus vinorelbine (that appears a promising drug in RMS) [20, 21].

If chemotherapy is a keystone in the multimodal treatment, radiotherapy also plays a relevant role because of the high radioresponsiveness of RMS. Con-

Table 11.5 European Pediatric Soft-Tissue Sarcoma Study Group: risk stratification and treatment options for localized RMS. *EFS* Event-free survival, *OS* overall survival, *VA* vincristine-actinomycin D, *IVA* ifosfamide-vincristine-actinomycin D, *IVADO* ifosfamide-vincristine-actinomycinD-doxorubicin, *VNR* vinorelbine, *CTX* cyclophosphamide, *RT* radiotherapy

Risk group		Histology[a]	IRS[b]	N[c]	Site[d]	Size & age[e]	%[f]	EFS – OS[g]	treatment
Low	A	favourable	I	N0	any	favourable	6%	90%–95%	VA, no RT
	B	favourable	I	N0	any	unfavourable	6%	78%–90%	
Standard	C	favourable	II–III	N0	favourable	any	18%	72%–88%	IVA+VA or IVA ± RT
	D	favourable	II–III	N0	unfavourable	favourable	9%	80%–85%	
	E	favourable	II–III	N0	unfavourable	unfavourable	27%	55%–60%	IVADO+IVA vs. IVA + RT
High	F	favourable	II–III	N1	any	any	8%	50%–60%	± maintenance VNR-oral CTX
	G	unfavourable	I–II–III	N0	any	any	20%	50%–60%	
Very High	H	unfavourable	I–II–III	N1	any	any	6%	40%–50%	IVADO+IVA + RT + maintenance chemotherapy

[a] Histology: favorable, embryonal RMS (and variants); not otherwise specified, unfavorable – alveolar RMS

[b] IRS Group: group I, complete resection; group II, microscopic residual disease after initial surgery (or nodal involvement); group III, macroscopic residual tumor after surgery (or biopsy)

[c] N (nodal involvement): N0, no nodal involvement; N1, involvement of regional lymph nodes

[d] Site: favorable, nonparameningeal head-neck (i.e., orbit), nonbladder/prostate genitourinary (i.e., paratesticular, vagina)

[e] Size & age: favorable, tumor size less ≤5 cm AND age between 1 and 10 years

[f] %: estimated percentage of patients

[g] EFS–OS: estimated 5-year event-free survival and overall survival (according to data from the Italian Cooperative Group, ICG)

Table 11.6 Series of 290 patients with RMS treated between 1970 and 1990 at the Memorial Sloan-Kettering Cancer Center, New York.

	Overall series	0–15 years	16–30 years	31–70 years
No. of patients	290	157	89	44
Histology				
% Embryonal	77%	84%	78%	79%
% Alveolar	14%	11%	17%	21%
% Pleomorphic	9%	5%	5%	30%
Sites		33%	18%	18%
% Head-neck	26%	38%	39%	16%
% Genitourinary	35%	20%	25%	52%
% Extremities	27%	8%	18%	6%
% Trunk	13%			
Stage				
% T2	71%	64%	76%	82%
% >5 cm	68%	63%	76%	68%
% N1	28%	27%	33%	20%
% M1	23%	18%	30%	23%

sidering the risk of late radiation damage (together with the effectiveness of systemic treatment), the role of radiotherapy has partially diminished over the years and its indication is now given more carefully. With doses generally ranging between 40 and 55 Gy (depending on age, tumor size and site, response to primary chemotherapy, histology, and extent of residual tumor after surgery), radiotherapy is particularly important in those cases localized in the parameningeal region and in trunk (i.e., the pelvis), and whenever a primary or delayed complete resection is not feasible. Alveolar RMS always requires radiotherapy to improve the local control rate [22, 23].

Radiotherapy must always be administered using megavoltage equipment and allowing wide margins (2–3 cm) around the tumor volume. Careful planning is mandatory, as well as the use of modern techniques such as the three-dimensional conformal radiotherapy, to improve the therapeutic index (high dose of radiation on the tumor with reduction in the dosage to normal tissues), in particular for parameningeal RMS. Although interesting suggestions have derived from hyperfractionated and accelerated schedules, the conventional fractionation scheme currently remains the

standard choice. Interstitial radiotherapy can play a role in specific situations (e.g., small tumors in the head-neck or genitourinary sites) [24].

Debate on the possible different intensities of local therapy, and indications for radiotherapy in particular (e.g., in IRS group III patients who achieve complete remission after chemotherapy, or in group II patients) implicates the concept of the "total burden of therapy" experienced by a given patient and the predicted sequelae; the indication for radiotherapy, in other words, can be given taking into account the probability of OS (rather than disease-free survival) and the "cost" of survival in terms of sequelae [18]. A different philosophy, in fact, was behind previous European studies and North American trials: in the former, the evaluation of "cost" pointed to a lesser use of radiotherapy, which produced higher local relapse rates than those reported elsewhere, but similar OS, since a significant number of locally relapsing patients were cured by salvage treatments; in the meanwhile, a subset of patients were cured without intensive local therapies and therefore without sequelae. This is a matter of debate, and clearly, improvements in risk stratification may lead to more suitable risk-adapted treatment choices [18].

In adolescents and young adults, the frequency of alveolar RMS and of extremity tumor is clearly higher than in younger patients. A study from the Memorial Sloan-Kettering Cancer Center compared the clinical features (and the outcome) of RMS patients of 16–30 years of age, with those of patients less than 16 and older than 30 years [25]. Table 11.6 shows the higher percentage of cases with large, invasive tumors and metastatic tumors in the subset of adolescents and young adults. So, with the increase of age, there is an increase in the presence of adverse prognostic clinical findings. Moreover, as shown in Table 11.3, which lists the main prognostic factors in RMS, age per se has been associated with a less satisfactory outcome (in most pediatric reported studies, the outcome of adolescents was worse than that of children) [26].

The behavior of RMS in adults needs, however, some specific comments. Adult RMS is rare and scanty information is available on its clinical and biological findings; all studies, however, highlight a largely poorer outcome than in children, with OS rates in the range of 20–50%. Apart form pleomorphic subtype, which is probably a completely different tumor, the previous unsatisfactory results raised doubts as to whether adult RMS is biologically the same as childhood RMS, and as to whether chemotherapy should be used at all to treat adults with RMS.

In a recently reported large retrospective study (from the Istituto Nazionale dei Tumori of Milan, Italy, 171 patients >18 years), treatment modalities have been analyzed and patients have been stratified according to the degree to which they had been treated appropriately, based on current treatment guidelines for childhood RMS (assigning a score to each patient) [27]. Although overall results (5-year OS 40%) paralleled those of other published series, in the subset of patients whose treatment was consistent with pediatric trials guidelines, 5-year OS was 61% and increased to 72% for patients with embryonal RMS (Fig. 11.5). A high score for appropriate treatment was assigned to 39% of patients (45% of patients 19–30 years old, and 29% of patients over 30 years). Moreover, the overall response to chemotherapy was 85%, substantially different from that observed in other adult sarcomas (which is definitely less than 50%) and in the same range as the rate for pediatric RMS [27]. In brief, these

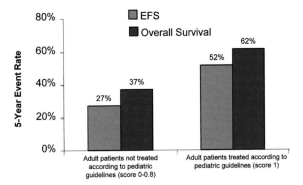

Figure 11.5

Rhabdomyosarcoma in adults: 5-year outcome as a function of "pediatric vs. adult treatment." Data from Ferrari et al. (2003). *EFS* Event-free survival

data suggest that chemotherapy could have the same activity in adult as in childhood RMS, and, when properly employed within a treatment strategy like that adopted for childhood patients, the outcome in adults might also fall in the same range as in children. Of course, other findings might concur with the overall unsatisfactory results of adult RMS, both clinical (i.e., higher proportion of the alveolar subtype and of large and invasive tumors) and biological factors (i.e., more pronounced expression of multidrug resistance proteins). Nevertheless, every effort should be made to improve the number of adults patients with RMS who receive fully adequate treatment: it is known that adults may tolerate intensive treatments to a lesser degree, but also that the adult medical oncologist's attitude toward a tumor so rare in adulthood may be, at least in part, important. Thereafter, young adults with RMS, as well as adolescents, should be treated within pediatric controlled trials, or at least according to the same principles that in recent decades have so dramatically improved prognosis in children.

11.5.2 Adult-Type STS

This group includes a heterogeneous variety of different tumors that are found more frequently in adult age than in childhood and are generally regarded to have uncertain responsiveness to chemotherapy and radiotherapy. These tumors are called non-RMS STS by pediatric oncologists [3, 28–31].

Contrarily to RMS (and extraosseous ES), in which chemotherapy plays a crucial role, standard treatment for localized, adult-type STSs is based on surgery, often complemented by radiation therapy. Surgery remains the mainstay of treatment, but overall treatment strategy has partially changed in recent years [32, 33]. Historically, "radical" interventions in high-grade sarcomas of adult age have been considered: amputations and compartmental resections. Currently, functional wide resection is the goal of surgical approach, complemented by radiotherapy whenever the resection margins are narrow or the tumor is of high grade. Radiotherapy needs to be administered at higher total doses than RMS (60–65 Gy). It is usually planned as a postoperative approach, although various suggestions are in favor of using preoperative irradiation (with or without neoadjuvant chemotherapy) in locally advanced disease, to allow a delayed surgical resection. The theoretical advantages of preoperative radiotherapy are: smaller volume of irradiation with more organ preservation, more efficacy on the nonhypoxic tumor bed, and a lower risk of intraoperative contamination [34, 35].

High-grade sarcomas can recur locally, but also with distant metastases, and despite the relatively good prognosis for grossly resected patients (70–80% survival), it is generally agreed that outcome is good enough for low-grade and small tumors to be treated with surgery alone, but not for high-grade and large tumors. Therefore, in some cases, chemotherapy should be considered as part of the treatment strategy. Actually, the role of chemotherapy in these tumors continues to be controversial. To date, only a minority of the several randomized adjuvant chemotherapy trials performed in adults have shown a significant survival advantage for chemotherapy. Among those, the Italian randomized trial on high-risk patients (high grade, large, deep, extremities site) was stopped early due to evidence at an interim analysis of a significant advantage in EFS and OS for patients who received ifosfamide-doxorubicin chemotherapy versus those treated with local therapy only [36]. Moreover, 14 randomized trials comprising 1,568 adult patients were included in a meta-analysis that demonstrated a reduc-

tion in the risk of local and distant failures in the group treated with intensified doxorubicin-based chemotherapy (advantage of 10% in recurrence-free survival and of 4% in OS) [37]. Recent hints from pediatric series, moreover, suggest that chemotherapy has a more beneficial impact than is generally believed when it is given to high-risk cases, using the more effective combination (full-dose ifosfamide-doxorubicin regimen, as indicated in various adult series) [29]. These two retrospective studies, from the Istituto Nazionale Tumori of Milan [29] and from the Italian and German cooperative group [38], show that the combination of the two variables – high grade and large tumor size – produced a very high risk of metastatic spread (metastatic-free survival in the range of 30–40%), thus suggesting in principle the use of chemotherapy to improve the survival, and that the chances of survival clearly rise in those patients given chemotherapy. In the series from Milan, the response rate to chemotherapy in patients with measurable disease was 39% in terms of complete and partial response, but rose to 58% when minor responses were included [29].

In the absence of standard guidelines, adolescents and young adults could be included in investigational trials, or the issue of adjuvant chemotherapy (still unclear) could be considered suitable for individual clinical use. It is noteworthy that the EpSSG trial for pediatric adult-type sarcomas requires the administration of adjuvant chemotherapy for high-risk cases (G3 tumor, large than 5 cm) [31].

In addition to tumor size and tumor grade, other risk factors have been individuated: the feasibility of a complete resection, the local invasiveness, the proximal sites and deep locations, and obviously the presence of metastases at onset and the recurrent disease. The effect of histopathologic subtype on prognosis is yet unclear, although different findings suggest that some histotypes (e.g., MPNST) are associated with poor outcome, while others (e.g., leiomyosarcoma, fibrosarcoma) have been reported to have a more favorable prognosis in some series, and a poor outcome in others [39].

Different findings suggested that age is also a significant prognostic factors in STS. In various adult series, younger age (generally less than 40 years) is a favorable predictor of survival. Similarly, age has been correlated with clinical features and outcome in childhood series: in the St Jude Children's Research Hospital study (192 patients aged 1 month–22 years), the group of adolescents and young adults, with age over 15 years, had distinctive features [40]. In this age group, SS and MPNST were the most common histotypes. In comparison to younger patients, adolescents and young adults had a higher percentage of tumors that were large and invasive, with high histological grade and with metastases at onset. As a consequence, survival rates were lower (5-year OS 49%, EFS 37%) than for younger children. The tumor characteristics and outcome of this series approach those of the younger patients of adult series [40].

In the case of inoperable locally advanced disease (and moreover in patients with metastases at onset), prognosis is unsatisfactory and all therapeutic resources should be taken into consideration. Chemotherapy, eventually associated with preoperative radiotherapy, is the first option. Adult trials have shown that the combination of ifosfamide and doxorubicin constitutes the regimen with the higher response rate (with a direct relationship between response and doses). In a particular subset of patients, locoregional approaches (i.e., hyperthermic limb perfusion with intra-arterial chemotherapy or immunotherapy) could be considered.

It is evident that every effort should be made to improve the therapeutic arms for advanced tumors. A recent report from the Memorial Sloan-Kettering Cancer Center commented that the outcome of localized extremity STSs has not improved over the last 20 years, suggesting that current therapy has reached the limits of efficacy [41]. New drugs and new approaches are warranted. Some data have suggested a possible role for paclitaxel in the treatment of angiosarcomas and for gemcitabine in leiomyosarcomas. New selective mechanisms, such as that of the antityrosine kinase imatinib mesylate , which dramatically modifies the clinical course of gastrointestinal stromal tumors (GIST: gastrointestinal mesenchymal tumors that are immunohistochemically positive for the product of the c-kit oncogene, CD117), must be explored for novel agents and for other histotypes. The success of imatinib mesylate in the treatment of GIST provides important les-

sons for the development of new therapies designated specifically for targets identified as being critical to the tumor's biology; most of the specific chromosomal translocations present in sarcomas have been cloned (with the identification of fusion genes) and may represent the ideal targets for new molecular therapies [31].

11.5.3 Synovial Sarcoma

SS probably represents the most frequent malignant tumor of soft tissues in adolescents and young adults, accounting for about 15–20% of all cases. The optimal treatment approach to SS remains to be determined. As for other STSs of adult age, the standard treatment for localized disease is surgery. Complete surgical resection of the primary tumor is the unquestionable mainstay of treatment. Extensive surgery with histologically free margins is recommended: compartment resection is the treatment of choice when feasible, otherwise wide excisions may also be accepted.

A general agreement has not yet been achieved regarding the role of adjuvant treatments. Postoperative radiotherapy has a well-defined role to improve local control after less-than-compartmental resection: after wide resection, particularly in the case of a large tumor, but also after marginal and intralesional resection. In the case of locally advanced disease, the radiotherapy sandwich technique (preoperative chemotherapy and radiotherapy, then surgery followed by adjuvant chemotherapy and a possible boost of irradiation) may be useful for shrinking the tumor and making it resectable [31].

More open questions still exist regarding the role of postoperative chemotherapy, given that the rarity of the tumor hinders the adequate accrual for a randomized trial. Over the years, completely different strategies have been worked out in pediatric oncology protocols and as compared to the adult setting. Practically speaking, in European centers, a patient aged 16 years old, enrolled in pediatric trials, was treated very differently from a 22-year-old patient. Pediatricians mutated their approach from the management of RMS: due to the quite good chemotherapy response rate in the pediatric series, SS was considered as an "RMS-like" tumor and was treated with the same protocols designed for RMS, thus giving adjuvant chemotherapy

Table 11.7 Synovial sarcoma series from the Istituto Nazionale Tumori, Milan, Italy. Treatment and results according to the different age groups (from Ferrari et al. 2004)

age	0–16 years	17–30 years	>30 years	Overall
No. of patients	46 patients	83	142	271
Tumor >5 cm	49%	60%	73%	60%
Gross resected disease	41 patients	66	108	215
% Radiotherapy	58%	45%	49%	50%
% Chemotherapy	76%	21%	15%	28%
5-year EFS	66.3%	40.5%	30.9%	40.7%

to the majority of patients, even in cases of completely excised small tumors. On the contrary, adjuvant chemotherapy was employed in adult patients mainly within trials including all histotypes, with a no-therapy control arm: therefore, adjuvant chemotherapy was rarely utilized in adults and only in the recent years has it been routinely proposed for high-risk patients (local invasiveness, large size, deep localization) [42]. What would be the most adequate strategy remains unclear. Published series reported better outcome in pediatric series than in adult studies, but all the known adverse prognostic factors are more frequent in adults (large size, local invasiveness, unresectability, proximal sites), and age per se is probably a prognostic indicator. Nevertheless, the better results obtained within pediatric protocols might also be correlated with the different therapeutic strategies adopted. The most significant pediatric experience is the multicenter analysis coordinated by the University of Texas MD Anderson Cancer Center (which combined the previously published experiences of different research groups) that showed a 5-year OS of 80% and a quite high response rate to chemotherapy (60%). Of the 219 patients, 52% were adolescents (14–20 years) and the risk of event increased 0.06 times for subsequent 1 year increase in age [43]. Concerning the role of adjuvant chemotherapy, this study did not show a clear impact of chemotherapy on survival in resected patients [43].

Conversely, data from the large series of the Istituto Nazionale Tumori of Milan, Italy, showed better out-

comes for patients who received adjuvant chemotherapy (5-year EFS, 55% vs. 35%) [44]. This study compared the clinical findings, the treatment modalities, and the outcome of the different age groups: as shown in Table 11.7, the EFS of grossly resected cases increased with the increase in the use of adjuvant chemotherapy. Far from a demonstration of efficacy of adjuvant chemotherapy in SS, these data would seem suggestive of a role for it [44]. By definition, SS is a high-grade sarcomas, and so this could be consistent with some suggestions regarding high-risk sarcomas coming from adult trials. SS probably stands halfway between the most typical adult STSs and pediatric small round cell sarcomas, and chemotherapy seems to play a greater role in pediatric terms compared to adult sarcomas; roughly, the response rate to chemotherapy could be estimated as around 40% for adult-type STSs, 60% for SS, and 80% for RMS and ES/pPNET. This may imply that the use of chemotherapy in all cases, regardless of prognostic stratification (as developed in previous pediatric European trials) might be considered as overtreatment: a recent pediatric Italian and German review identified a subset of patients (completely resected, tumor <5 cm) treated with adjuvant chemotherapy that showed a very low risk of metastases (48 cases, 4 local relapses, no distant relapse), suggesting that chemotherapy can be omitted in low-risk groups [45]. This will be the indication for the upcoming EpSSG protocol.

Cooperative trials involving pediatric and adults patients with SS could be warranted; moreover, a large accrual of cases could permit investigation of the role of new therapies such as Bcl-2 antisense oligonucleotide, since in most cases of SS the anti-apoptotic protein Bcl-2 (overexpression of Bcl-2 correlates with tumor growth, chemoresistance, and poor outcome in various cancers) is overexpressed.

11.6 Summary and Conclusions

STSs represent about 7% of all malignant tumors in 15- to 29-year-olds. They include a highly heterogeneous group of different histotypes, which are generally characterized by local aggressiveness and propensity to metastasize. Peculiar to childhood, RMS may occur in older age and is characterized by its high responsiveness to chemotherapy and radiotherapy. Multidisciplinary and risk-adapted treatment approaches developed by international cooperative groups have dramatically improved the prognosis of RMS during the past 30 years, improving cure rates from 30% to 70%. Young adults with RMS usually have a less favorable outcome than children, but their prognosis would be improved if fully adequate treatments derived by childhood trials are employed.

Adult-type sarcomas are different tumors with various grades of malignancy, which are generally localized to the extremities. In these tumors, surgery is the mainstay of treatment, and the role of adjuvant therapies remains unclear. In particular, they are regarded to have uncertain responsiveness to chemotherapy, although recent hints would suggest a more significant beneficial impact in high-risk cases than is generally believed. The prognosis is related to the feasibility of surgical resection, and to histological grade, tumor size, local invasiveness and, clearly, the presence of metastases. SSs are typical of adolescents and young adults, and are probably positioned halfway between the pediatric small round cell tumors (such as RMS) and the most typical adult sarcomas with regard to responsiveness to chemotherapy.

In conclusion, this heterogeneous group of tumors includes entities that are not so rare in adolescents and young adults. The treatment of these patients appears particularly complex and necessarily multidisciplinary, and requires adequate expertise. It is very important to emphasize that adolescents and young adults receive better treatments within selected and experienced institutions that enroll patients into clinical trials. Cooperation between pediatric oncologists and adult oncologists is needed to better define the treatment options for adolescents and young adults patients. In particular, histology as well as tumor biology and characteristics appear to be more important than the patients' age. Although age per se may be considered a prognostic factor in STSs, a certain histotype would behave in the same way when arising in children, adolescents, or adults. This leads to the consideration that RMS patients, regardless of their age, would receive the better treatment when following guidelines derived from the large pediatric experience, whereas the treatment of patients with adult-type sarcomas should acquire suggestions from the body of experience gained over the years by adult oncologists.

Cooperative studies are needed to investigate the role of new therapies that are specifically tailored for molecular targets, which might be the several specific chromosomal translocations identified in STSs.

References

1. Bleyer WA, O'Leary M, Barr R, Ries LAG (eds) (2006) Cancer Epidemiology in Older Adolescents and Young Adults 15 to 29 Years of Age, including SEER Incidence and Survival, 1975–2000. National Cancer Institute, NIH Pub. No. 06-5767. Bethesda, MD 2006, pp 220
2. Wexler LH, Meyer WH, Helmann LJ. Rhabdomyosarcoma and the undifferentiated sarcomas. In Pizzo PA, Poplack DC (eds), Principles and Practice of Pediatric Oncology. 5th ed. Lippincott Williams & Wilkins, Philadelphia, pp 971–1001
3. Okcu MF, Hicks J, Merchant TE, et al: Nonrhabdomyosarcomatous soft tissue sarcomas. In Pizzo PA, Poplack DC (eds), Principles and Practice of Pediatric Oncology. 5th ed. Lippincott Williams & Wilkins, Philadelphia, 2006, pp 1033–1073
4. Bleyer WA, Tejeda H, Murphy SB, et al (1997) National cancer clinical trials: children have equal access; adolescents do not. J Adolesc Health 21:366–373
5. Bleyer A, Montello M, Budd T, Saxman S (2005) National survival trends of young adults with sarcoma: lack of progress is associated with lack of clinical trial participation. Cancer 103:1891–1897
6. Pappo AS, Shapiro DN, Crist WM, Maurer HM (1995) Biology and therapy of pediatric rhabdomyosarcoma. J Clin Oncol 13:2123–2139

7. Newton WA, Gehan EA, Webber BL, et al (1995) Classification of rhabdomyosarcomas and related sarcomas. Pathologic aspects and proposal for a new classification – an Intergroup Rhabdomyosarcoma Study. Cancer 70:1073–1085

8. Borden EC, Baker LH, Bell RS, et al (2003) Soft tissue sarcomas of adults: state of the translational science. Clin Cancer Res 9:1941–1956

9. Maurer HM, Beltangady M, Gehan EA, et al: The Intergroup Rhabdomyosarcoma Study I: a final report. Cancer 61:209–220, 1988

10. Harmer MH: TNM Classification of pediatric tumors. Geneva, Switzerland, UICC International Union Against canser, 1982:23–28

11. Wunder JS, Healey JH, Davis AM, Brennan MF. A (2000) comparsion of staging systems for localized extremity soft tissue sarcoma. Cancer 88:2721–2730

12. Crist WM, Anderson JR, Meza JL, et al (2001) Intergroup Rhabdomyosarcoma Study-IV: results for patients with nonmetastatic disease. J Clin Oncol 19:3091–3102

13. Crist WM, Garnsey L, Beltangady MS, et al (1990) Prognosis in children with rhabdomyosarcoma: a report of the Intergroup Rhabdomyosarcoma Studies I and II. J Clin Oncol 8:443–452

14. Raney RB, Anderson JR, Barr FG, et al. Rhabdomyosarcoma and undifferentiated sarcoma in first two decades of life: a selective review of Intergroup Rhabdomyosarcoma Study Group experience and rationale for Intergroup Rhabdomyosarcoma Study V. J. Pediatr Oncol 41:1–6, 2003

15. Ferrari A, Casanova M (2005) Current chemotherapeutic strategies for rhabdomyosarcoma. Expert Rev Anticancer Ther 5:283–294

17. Stevens MC (2005) Treatment for childhood rhabdomyosarcoma: the cost of cure. Lancet Oncol 6:77–84

18. Stevens MC, Rey A, Bouvet N, et al (2005) Treatment of nonmetastatic rhabdomyosarcoma in childhood and adolescence: third study of the International Society of Paediatric Oncology – SIOP Malignant Mesenchymal Tumor 89. J Clin Oncol 23:2618–2628

19. Bisogno G, Ferrari A, Bergeron C, et al (2005) The ifosfamide, vincristine, actinomycin, doxorubicin (IVADo) regimen, an intensified chemotherapy for children with soft tissue sarcoma. A pilot study by the European pediatric Soft Tissue sarcoma Study Group. Cancer 103:1719–1724

20. Casanova M, Ferrari A, Bisogno G, et al (2004) Vinorelbine and low-dose cyclophosphamide in pediatric sarcomas: pilot study for the future European Rhabdomyosarcoma Protocol. Cancer 101:1664–1671

21. Casanova M, Ferrari A, Spreafico F, et al (2002) Vinorelbine in previously treated advanced childhood sarcomas: evidence of activity in rhabdomyosarcoma. Cancer 94:3263–3268

22. Wharam MD, Hanfelt JJ, Tefft MC, et al. (1997) Radiation therapy for rhabdomyosarcoma: local failure risk for Clinical Group III patients on Intergroup Rhabdomyosarcoma Study II. Int J Radiat Oncol Biol Phys 38:797–804

23. Schuck a, Mattke AC, Schmidt B, et al. (2004) Group II rhabdomyosarcoma nad rhabdomyosarcoma like tumors: is radiotherapy necessery? J Clin Oncol 22:143–149

24. Donaldson SS, Asmar l, Breneman J et al. (1995) Hyperfractionated radiation in children with rhabdomyosarcoma--results of an Intergroup Rhabdomyosarcoma Pilot Study.Int J Radiat Oncol Biol Phys 32:903–911

25. La Quaglia MP, Heller G, Ghavimi F, et al (1994) The effect of age at diagnosis on outcome in rhabdomyosarcoma. Cancer 73:109–117

26. Joshi D, Anderson JR, Paidas C. (2004) Age is an independent prognostic factor in rhabdomyosarcoma: a report from the Soft Tissue Sarcoma Committee of the Childre's Oncology Group. Pediatr Blood Cancer 42:64–73

27. Ferrari A, Dileo P, Casanova M, et al (2003) Rhabdomyosarcoma in adults: a retrospective analysis of 171 patients treated at a single institution. Cancer 98:571–580

28. Spunt SL, Poquette CA, Hurt YS, et al (1999) Prognostic factors for children and adolescents with surgically resected nonrhabdomyosarcoma soft tissue sarcoma: an analysis of 121 patients treated at St Jude Children's Research Hospital. J Clin Oncol 17:3697–3705

29. Ferrari A, Casanova M, Collini P, et al (2005) Adult-type soft tissue sarcomas in pediatric age: experience at the Istituto Nazionale Tumori in Milan. J Clin Oncol 23:4021–4030

30. Pappo AS, Devidas M, Jenkins J, et al. (2005) Phase II trial of neoadjuvant vincristine, ifosfamide, and doxorubicin with granulocyte colony-stimulating factor support in children and adolescents with advanced-stage nonrhabdomyosarcoma soft tissue sarcomas: a Pediatric Oncology Group Study. J Clin Oncol 23:4031–4038

31. Ferrari A, Casanova M (2005) New concepts for the treatment of pediatric non-rhabdomyosarcoma soft tissue sarcomas. Expert Rev Anticancer Ther 5:307–318

32. 1. Gronchi a, Casali PG, Mariani L, et al. (2005) Status of surgical margins and prognosis in adult soft tissue sarcomas of the extremities: a series of 911 consecutive patients treated at a single institution. J Clon Oncol 23:96–104

33. Stojadinovic A, Leung DHY, Hoos A et al. (2002) Analysis of the prognostic significance of microscopic margins in 2084 localized primary adult soft tissue sarcomas. Ann Surg, 235:424–443

34. O'Sullivan l. B, Davis AM, Turcotte R, et al. (2002) Preoperative versus postoperative radiotherapy in soft tissue sarcoma of the limbs: a randomized trial. Lancet 359:2235–2241

35. Khanfir K, Alzieu L, Terrier P, et al. (2003) Does adjuvant radiation therapy increases loco-regional control after optimal resection of soft-tissue sarcoma of the extremity? Eur J Cancer 39:1872–1880

36. Frustaci S, Gherlinzoni F, De Paoli A, et al (2001) Adjuvant chemotherapy for adult soft tissue sarcomas of extremities and girdles: results of the Italian randomized cooperative trial. J Clin Oncol 19:1238–1247

37. Thierny JF, for the Sarcoma Meta-analysis Collaboration (1997) Adjuvant chemotherapy for localized resectable soft-tissue sarcoma of adults: meta-analysis of individual data. Lancet 350:1647–1654

38. Ferrari A, Brecht IB, Koscielniak E, et al (2005) Could adjuvant chemotherapy have a role in surgically-resected adult-type soft tissue sarcomas of children and adolescents? Pediatr Blood Cancer 45:128–134

39. Kattan MW, Leung DH, Brennan MF (2002) Postoperative nomogram for 12-year sarcoma-specific death. J Clin Oncol 20:791–796

40. Hayes-Jordan AA, Spunt SL, Poquette CA, et al. (2000) Nonrhabdomyosarcoma soft tissue sarcomas in children: is age at diagnoss an important variable? J Pediatr Surg. 35:948–954

41. Weitz J, Antonescu CR, Brennan MF (2003) Localized extremity soft tissue sarcoma: improved knowledge with unchanged survival over time. J Clin Oncol 21:2719–2725

42. Bergh P, Meis-Kindblom JM, Gherlinzoni F, et al (1999) Synovial sarcoma: identification of low and high risk groups. Cancer 85:2596–2607

43. Okcu MF, Munsell M, Treuner J, et al (2003) Synovial sarcoma of childhood and adolescence: a multicenter, multivariate analysis of outcome. J Clin Oncol 21:1602–1611

44. Ferrari A, Gronchi A, Casanova M, et al (2004) Synovial sarcoma: a retrospective analysis of 271 patients of all ages treated at a single institution. Cancer 101:627–634

45. Brecht IB, Ferrari A, Int-Veen C, et al (2006) Grossly-resected synovial sarcoma treated by the German and Italian Pediatric Soft Tissue Sarcoma Cooperative Groups: discussion on the role of adjuvant therapies. Pediatr Blood Cancer 46:11–17

Bone Sarcomas

Michael S. Isakoff • Michael J. Harris •
Mark C. Gebhardt • Holcombe E. Grier

Contents

12.1 Introduction

Bone tumors, especially osteosarcoma and Ewing sarcoma, are highly aggressive tumors that lead to significant mortality and morbidity amongst adolescents and young adults [1]. A Surveillance, Epidemiology, and End Results (SEER) review of bone tumor incidence reveals a peak in the 10- to 19-year-old age group, with a maximum rate of 19 per million in the United States, and continued prevalence into the young adult age (Fig. 12.1) [1, 2]. The treatment of these tumors requires the skills of a multidisciplinary team that includes surgical orthopedic oncologists, medical oncologists, radiation oncologists, and musculoskeletal pathologists. Close collaboration within this group of physicians has helped to maximize patient care and to decrease the relative morbidity and mortality associated with these cancers. Survival has subsequently improved over each 5-year period since 1975 (Fig. 12.2) [1, 2].

Bone tumors other than Ewing sarcoma and osteosarcoma are extremely rare in early childhood and account for approximately 10% of bone tumors in 10- to 14-year-olds. This fraction rises to 15% in 15- to 19-year-olds, but more than 30% in 20- to 24-year-olds. Most of these tumors are chondrosarcomas, many of which are low-grade tumors (sometimes in the presence of a hereditary enchondroma syndrome), and their management is distinctly surgical. High-grade chondrosarcomas are also treated best by complete excision. No standard chemotherapy has been found to be effective against unresectable or metastatic disease, although many clinicians use agents traditionally effective against osteosarcoma. Chondrosarcoma will not be discussed further in this chapter.

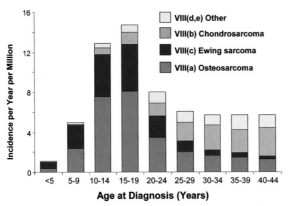

Figure 12.1

Incidence of bone sarcomas in the U.S. by type according to the International Childhood Cancer Classification (ICCC), United States SEER 1975–2000

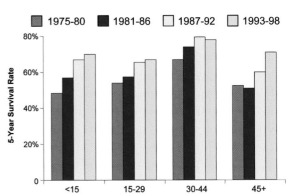

Figure 12.2

5-Year survival rates of bone sarcoma by era, United States SEER 1975–1999

Both osteosarcoma and Ewing sarcoma involving bone are characterized by local destruction, and treatment may require orthopedic surgical intervention, radiation therapy, and chemotherapy. The surgical principle that governs the management of these patients is wide resection of the primary tumor along with a generous cuff of normal tissue. The overall goal of surgical treatment is to completely remove the tumor and then to produce the most functional limb that is reasonably attainable. However, when surgical management is limited by extent or location, then radiation therapy will be used for local therapy in Ewing sarcoma. Radiation is less successful in producing durable local controls in patients with osteosarcoma. Systemic chemotherapy is aimed at treating known or clinically inapparent micrometastatic disease, as well as improving local control of the cancer in conjunction with radiation and/or surgical therapy. The orthopedic, radiation, and chemotherapy advances will be discussed further throughout this chapter.

This chapter will discuss the etiology/biology and epidemiology of two major types of bone sarcoma in the adolescent and young adult age group: osteosarcoma and Ewing sarcoma. For each, the diagnosis, complete management including medical, surgical, and radiation treatment regimens, and late effects are

reviewed. Chondrosarcoma, the third most common bone sarcoma in the age group will not be covered.

12.2 Osteosarcoma

12.2.1 Epidemiology, Etiology, and Biology

Osteosarcoma represents approximately 55% of all primary tumors of bone in each age group under 20 years, and 40% of bone tumors in young adults [1, 2]. Osteosarcoma is slightly more common in males and peaks in incidence at around 16 years of age (Fig. 12.3) [1, 2]. A second peak occurs after age 65 years, and these elderly patients, who certainly have a worse prognosis, probably have a different biology, often arising in the setting of Paget's disease. The adolescent peak happens to correspond to the most rapid rate of osseous growth in the normal child. In addition, the most common locations of osteosarcoma occur in the fastest growing areas of the skeleton: (1) distal femur, (2) proximal tibia, and (3) proximal humerus (Fig. 12.4) [3]. Patients with osteosarcoma are significantly taller than the general population [4]. These tumors do occur in the axial skeleton, but to a lesser extent.

In the pediatric and adolescent patient, most cases of osteosarcoma begin without any identifiable cause.

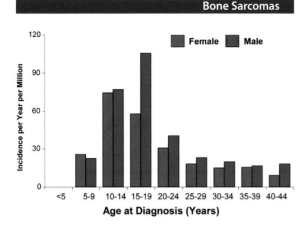

Figure 12.3

Incidence of osteosarcoma by gender, United States SEER, 1975–2000

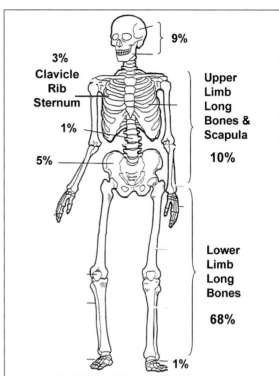

Figure 12.4

Anatomic location of osteosarcoma in 15- to 29-year-olds, United States SEER 1992–2002

However, some studies suggest a multitude of possible inciting factors that may predispose a patient to develop osteosarcoma. Ionizing radiation, which is used to treat cancer, has been linked in a dose-dependent manner to secondary osteosarcoma [5]. Treatment of radiation-induced osteosarcoma may be difficult; however, outcome for these patients can be similar to that of de novo osteosarcoma if surgical resection of the primary is possible [6]. Chemical agents, such as methylcholanthrene, beryllium oxide, and zinc beryllium oxide have been implicated in the pathogenesis of osteosarcoma [7, 8]. Viral infection has also been identified as a cause of osteosarcoma in animal models [9, 10]. In addition, while patients and families often remember trauma to the site of disease, there is no evidence that injury to bone is a predisposing factor. In adults, but not children, cases of osteosarcoma have been reported occurring in the area of bone infarcts [11, 12].

There are specific genetic abnormalities that are known to predispose patients to osteosarcoma. For example, the incidence is increased in patients with germ-line retinoblastoma (*Rb*) gene mutations, thus implicating the *Rb* gene in the development of osteosarcoma [13, 14]. Germ-line derangement of *p53* gene function has also been implicated in the development of osteosarcoma, and is specifically seen in Li-Fraumeni syndrome, in which there is a high rate of malig-

nancy including osteosarcoma [15]. In addition, in vitro studies have shown that p53 is involved in controlling cell-cycle progression in osteosarcoma, thus providing further evidence of its role in the development of this malignancy [16]. Even without evidence of germ-line mutation, analysis of tumor samples frequently detects either *p53* mutations, *Rb* mutations, or both [17].

12.2.2 Pathology/Staging

Osteosarcoma is characterized by malignant spindle cells that produce osteoid or bone. Several histologic variants of osteosarcoma have been described including conventional, telangiectatic, parosteal, periosteal, and small cell osteosarcoma. In children and adoles-

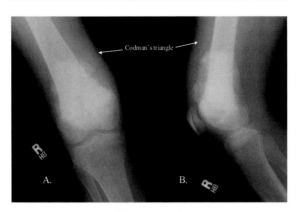

Figure 12.5

Typical presenting radiographic finding of Codman's triangle due to osteosarcoma, epiphysis of distal femur

cents the most common type is conventional osteosarcoma. In this type there is typically a mixture of large, atypical, spindle-shaped cells with large irregular nuclei and abnormal mitotic figures. Telangiectatic osteosarcoma is a rare variant that is typically more vascular and purely lytic in radiographic appearance. The parosteal subtype typically arises from the cortex and forms in bone outside of the periosteum. This subtype typically occurs in the 20- to 29-year-old age group, usually does not form metastases, and has a favorable outcome after wide surgical resection [18]. Similar to parosteal osteosarcoma, the periosteal variant arises on the surface of bone; however the lesion does involve the periosteum. In addition, this lesion has a more intermediate prognosis; it tends to recur locally and may metastasize. These tumors usually require radical surgical resection [19]; the use of adjuvant chemotherapy for periosteal osteosarcoma is controversial. Small-cell osteosarcoma is a rare subtype that must be differentiated from other small cell tumors, such as Ewing sarcoma or lymphoma, to ensure proper therapy [20].

Many oncologists and surgeons use the system devised by Enneking and his group to stage osteosarcoma. Staging is determined by the histological grade (low grade, stage I; high grade, stage II) and whether the lesion is metastatic (stage III). Stage I tumors are rare and include the localized low-grade lesions, such as parosteal osteosarcomas. More common are the high-grade conventional osteosarcomas [21].

12.2.3 Diagnosis

The most common presenting complaint of patients with osteosarcoma is pain in the area of the lesion. The pain initially begins as an intermittent, deep pain. However, this tends to progress and may become unrelenting. Pain at night is a hallmark of malignant bone disease, and may become difficult to manage, even with multiple medications. Other symptoms that may manifest include limping, swelling, a palpable mass, and unusual limitation of daily activities. These changes taken in concert should alert the physician to the possibility of malignancy.

The first step in evaluation of a patient with a possible primary tumor of bone starts with a detailed and careful history and physical examination. Time of presentation, duration of pain, and other associated symptoms are vital clues to making the diagnosis. Questions one should ask include, "Is there pain at night?", "Is it relieved by nonsteroidal anti-inflammatory drugs or other drugs?", and "Is it progressing or has it improved over time?".

The first imaging studies that should be obtained are orthogonal plain radiographs of the area of interest. Osteosarcoma often has distinct radiographic characteristics and may be blastic, lytic, or both. There is often a significant periosteal reaction and possibly the presence of Codman's triangle, an incomplete triangle formed by elevation of the periosteum by the malignant tumor (Fig. 12.5). Sometimes, a soft-tissue mass can be appreciated on plain film.

Magnetic resonance imaging (MRI) of the entire bone allows for evaluation of the accompanying soft-tissue mass, and for the evaluation of neurovascular structures in the vicinity of the tumor. The pretreatment MRI also serves as a baseline from which to evaluate the effectiveness of preoperative chemotherapy: In some cases, the soft-tissue mass decreases in size, and there is often increased necrosis and increased calcification/ossification of the lesion. Finally, the MRI is the major guide for planning the resection, and may help to determine how the osseous deficit is reconstructed (e.g., Can growth plates be preserved? Is an amputation the most feasible procedure?).

In general, computed tomography (CT)-guided core-needle biopsy is sufficient to make a histologic diagnosis of osteosarcoma. If nondiagnostic tissue is obtained, a formal open biopsy procedure should be performed. It is highly recommended that the needle biopsy be performed in consultation with and the open biopsy procedure performed by the treating orthopedic oncologist in order to assure that the subsequent resection and reconstruction are not hindered by a poorly placed biopsy tract.

Approximately 15% of patients with high-grade osteosarcoma present with detectable metastases (including skip lesions, defined as a second lesion within the same bone); 61% of these metastases are isolated to the lung, 7% are isolated skip lesions, 10% are isolated bone metastases, and the rest are combined lung metastases with either skip or bone lesions [22]. The work-up must include a CT scan of the chest and a radionucleotide bone scan to look for metastatic disease. These studies help guide the patient's treatment and allow the clinician to fully educate the patient and family about the prognosis. A complete blood count with differential, electrolytes, creatinine, and an alkaline phosphatase level should be obtained initially to serve as baseline studies to help guide further care once chemotherapy is initiated.

12.2.4 Treatment

Neither population data nor clinical trials have found that age is a significant prognostic factor in the outcome of osteosarcoma under the age of 40 years; therefore, therapy for adolescents and young adults does not differ from that of children. Successful treatment for osteosarcoma requires attention to local control as well as distant metastases, either clinically evident or micrometastatic. A randomized trial comparing neoadjuvant chemotherapy to no chemotherapy revealed only an 11% 6-year survival in those who did not receive chemotherapy compared with a 61% 6-year survival in the group of patients who did receive chemotherapy [23, 24]. Studies such as this indicate that the ideal treatment for patients with clinically localized disease includes surgical resection and chemo-

therapy. If the lesion occurs in an expendable bone (e.g., the fibula), then radical resection is the best option. However, for nonexpendable bones (e.g., the femur, tibia, or weight-bearing portion of the pelvis), the ideal approach consists of wide resection of the lesion leaving a cuff of normal tissue, and then reconstruction of the nonexpendable segment of bone. In the case of a growing child, disarticulation or modified amputation may produce a more functional limb than do attempts at limb salvage. When wide surgical margins are not attainable without sacrificing vital structures (e.g., spinal cord, aorta, or lumbar plexus), neoadjuvant chemotherapy, along with local radiation therapy may be attempted. Studies over the last few years have reported a 45–61% overall survival with chemotherapy and radiation therapy as local control [25, 26]. However, the standard for local treatment remains wide surgical resection of the tumor with negative margins. In addition, radiation to the affected site is very rarely adequate for ridding the primary site of the tumor, and so is rarely used except as described previously.

Surgery is usually performed after an initial period of chemotherapy and outcome does not appear to differ according to whether surgery is performed at diagnosis or later. A Pediatric Oncology Group study assigned patients randomly to an initial resection or neoadjuvant chemotherapy (chemotherapy prior to resection), both followed by adjuvant chemotherapy. The total dose of chemotherapy used in both arms was the same. The overall 5-year event-free survival was 65%, with no statistical difference in the outcome by group [27]. Nearly all pediatric oncologists use neoadjuvant chemotherapy to allow time for planning and discussion regarding surgery.

Historically, chemotherapy for osteosarcoma was used for patients with relapsed or metastatic disease, and included various agents such as high-dose methotrexate (HDMTX) with leucovorin rescue, doxorubicin, cyclophosphamide, and cisplatin. All of these drugs demonstrated activity against this tumor, as evidenced by decreased tumor size. Studies since the early 1980s have demonstrated the effectiveness of adjuvant, and now neoadjuvant, chemotherapy using HDMTX doxorubicin, and cisplatin [22, 23, 27, 28]. This has led to an improvement in 5-year relapse-free survival to 55–65% (Fig. 12.6) [1, 2].

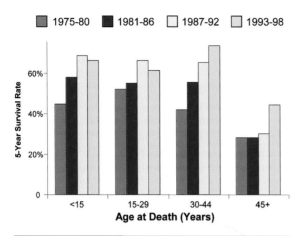

Figure 12.6

5-Year survival rate of osteosarcoma by era, United States SEER 1975–1999

In addition, histologic studies of osteosarcoma specimens following presurgical chemotherapy show a positive correlation of degree of necrosis and outcome. However, trials adjusting postoperative chemotherapy based on the degree of necrosis at surgery have not yet led to an improvement in outcome [29, 30]. For extremity primary tumors in patients without metastases at diagnosis, limb-sparing surgery has become a standard of therapy in those patients with favorable prognostic factors for this procedure [31].

Patients with metastatic osteosarcoma have historically had a dismal outcome, with very few long-term survivors. An analysis of patients who presented with metastatic disease revealed 11% of patients surviving 20 months. Patients in this cohort with unilateral pulmonary metastases had a better survival then those with bilateral disease; there were no survivors with bone or lymph-node metastases [32]. Numerous reports over the last 30 years have shown clearly that aggressive attempts at pulmonary metastatectomy leads to an overall improvement in survival [33, 36]. In addition, a recent study using intensive chemotherapy, including the addition of either ifosfamide alone or in combination with etoposide, has shown some early promise, although more time for follow-up is needed [37]. Unfortunately, other studies using intensified chemotherapy regimens also including the addition of

ifosfamide have not had as promising results for patients presenting with metastases. In a report from the Rizzoli Institute, 36 out of 57 patients had a complete response following surgery and chemotherapy; however, only 7 of those 36 patients who were initially in remission remained disease free, with follow-up times of 2–7 years [38, 39].

The prognosis for patients who relapse following treatment of osteosarcoma is extremely poor. One recent study identified several prognostic factors that influence postrelapse survival. The main factors identified with poor outcome included a short relapse-free interval, greater number of lung metastases, and metastatic lesions in lymph node or bone, when compared to patients with only lung metastases [40].

For patients with a poor prognosis, the goal of treatment is preserving or improving quality of life while attempting to prolong survival. Chemotherapy regimens similar to the treatment of metastatic disease at presentation are utilized frequently, including the use of ifosfamide alone or in combination with etoposide. Without complete surgical resection of metastatic lesions, chemotherapy will rarely lead to a complete response. Newer targeted therapies are starting to enter phase I and II clinical trials, including receptor tyrosine kinase inhibitors, farnasyl transferase inhibitors, and bcl-2 antisense therapy. Unfortunately, the utility of these agents will probably not be clarified for many more years.

12.2.5 Late Effects

Osteosarcoma may not only lead to destruction of bone, but the therapy for this malignancy, including surgery and chemotherapy, may lead to late effects that require lifelong observation. Of great concern is the occurrence of secondary malignancy following therapy for osteosarcoma. Prior to the 1970s there were few survivors and therefore the occurrence rate of secondary malignancy was not known. Since survival has dramatically improved over the last few years it is now clear that patients deserve close observation following therapy.

In 2002, a follow-up study on 509 osteosarcoma patients reported 14 incidents of a variety of secondary tumors. These included four neoplasms of the central nervous system, five cases of either sarcomas or carcinomas, two cases of acute myelogenous leukemia, one case of myelodysplastic syndrome, and one case of non-Hodgkin lymphoma [41].

Long-term care should include routine physical exams along with a periodic complete blood count to evaluate for any evidence of myelodysplastic syndrome or leukemia. Also, since the treatment of osteosarcoma routinely includes therapy with doxorubicin, patients should receive routine surveillance echocardiography and electrocardiograms.

While the studies are not robust, there does not appear to be a marked increase in male or female infertility with the traditional agents of methotrexate, cisplatin, and doxorubicin for osteosarcoma [42]. Oral contraceptive therapy has been used in the past for females in an attempt to prevent postchemotherapy ovarian failure. However, a retrospective analysis revealed no difference in rates of ovarian failure in women who took oral contraceptives versus those who did not [43]. In addition, while azospermia is common while receiving traditional chemotherapy for osteosarcoma, the majority of males recover normal spermatogenesis following therapy [44]. However, ifosfamide has been added to many trials of osteosarcoma, and its use has been associated with a high incidence of male infertility [45]. Investigators should always discuss the option of sperm cryopreservation if ifosfamide is part of the planned therapy.

12.3 Ewing Sarcoma

12.3.1 Epidemiology and Etiology

The Ewing family of tumors, including Ewing sarcoma and the more differentiated counterpart, primitive neuroectodermal tumor (PNET), is the second most common primary malignancy of bone in childhood and adolescence. While this tumor most often originates in bone, approximately 24% arise as a soft-tissue primary (personal communication, L. Granowetter). Ewing sarcoma occurs slightly more commonly in males and has a peak incidence in the 15- to 19-year-old age range; the disease has a slightly earlier peak in females (Fig. 12.7) [1, 2]. In addition, for unknown reasons, these tumors tend to

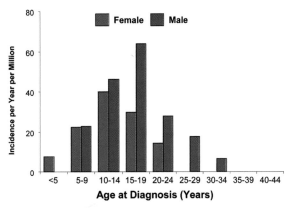

Figure 12.7

Incidence of Ewing sarcoma by gender, United States SEER, 1975–2000

affect those of Caucasian and Hispanic ethnicity and rarely occur in people of African American or Asian descent [46–48].

In spite of these clinical associations, the etiology of Ewing sarcoma continues to elude identification. There does not appear to be an association with familial cancer syndromes, and there are only rare case reports of Ewing sarcoma occurring in siblings [49–51]. Unlike the situation with osteosarcoma, it is quite uncommon for Ewing sarcoma to occur as a secondary cancer following ionizing radiation and chemotherapy [52]. In one retrospective analysis of second tumors following radiation therapy it was noted that 3% of these tumors were Ewing sarcomas, while 69% of secondary tumors following radiation were osteosarcomas. No specific environmental factors have been identified as causal [5].

12.3.2 Biology and Pathology

Ewing sarcoma is a small, round, blue-cell tumor, not dissimilar in appearance from other common solid tumors of children and adolescents, such as rhabdomyosarcoma, non-Hodgkin lymphoma, and neuroblastoma. Thus, pathologic diagnosis of Ewing sarcoma is occasionally very difficult and requires special histological staining and, frequently, molecular diagnostics.

Most cases of Ewing sarcoma have a clonal translocation within the tumor cells. Eighty-five percent of the time this translocation occurs between the long arms of chromosomes 11 and 22 and can be found with standard cytogenetics in 80% of tumors and with reverse-transcriptase polymerase chain reaction (RT-PCR) in up to 95% [53]. This translocation results in a fusion protein containing the amino terminus of the EWS protein joined to the carboxyl terminus of the FLI-1 protein [54]. The FLI-1 protein is a member of the ETS family of transcription factors, which directly bind DNA and either activate or repress transcription. Less is known about the EWS protein, yet some evidence suggests that it has a strong transcriptional activation domain. Researchers have suggested that following DNA binding by FLI-1 within the fusion protein, there is replacement of the weak transcriptional activation domain of FLI-1 with the strong activation domain of EWS [55]. The second most common translocation in Ewing sarcomas also involves the *EWS* gene on chromosome 22, crossed with the *ERG* gene on chromosome 21, also an ETS transcription factor [56]. Other more rare rearrangements are known to occur and also involve the *EWS* gene. The *EWS* gene is also found to be translocated with still different ETS-like oncogenes in other tumors of adolescents and young adults, such as desmoplastic small, round-cell tumor, and clear-cell sarcoma of soft tissue, also called malignant melanoma of soft parts (Table 12.1) [57].

The typical histopathologic characteristics of Ewing sarcoma include sheets of round, moderate-sized cells with scant cytoplasm and round nuclei with few mitotic figures. The cells are usually periodic acid-Schiff (PAS) positive, indicating the presence of glycogen. Immunohistochemistry has been useful to further differentiate Ewing sarcoma from other small, round, blue-cell tumors. A variety of monoclonal antibodies may be used to identify the protein product of the *MIC2* gene, designated as CD99, which is highly expressed on the surface of Ewing sarcoma cells [58]. It is notable, however, that while MIC2 is very sensitive as a marker for Ewing sarcoma, the detection of this protein lacks specificity and can be seen in a variety of other tumors and normal cells (especially in a cytoplasmic staining pattern as opposed to the cell surface pattern usually seen in Ewing sarcomas). Therefore, MIC2 detection is diagnostic only in conjunction with other more specific analyses [59].

The receptor tyrosine kinase c-kit is found to be expressed in 30% of Ewing sarcoma cases. This receptor is found in a handful of sarcomas and its presence may be helpful to immunohistochemically distinguish some sarcomas [60]. C-kit does not appear to have prognostic implications, but may be a potential target of newer targeted therapies [61], as will be discussed later.

PNET is not a separate entity from Ewing sarcoma, but rather a more differentiated form, displaying features of a neural phenotype. It has the same characteristic t(11,22) translocation. Rosettes, positive neuron-specific enolase staining, and neural elements seen under electron microscopy may be present. In addition, PNET tends to have a larger cell size with more cytoplasm and increased mitotic figures [59, 62]. Unfortunately, the term "primitive neurectodermal

Table 12.1 Karyotype abnormalities, fusion proteins, and associated malignancies involving the EWS locus

Gene rearrangement	Fusion protein	Tumor type
t(11;22)(q24;q12)	EWS-FLI1	Ewing sarcoma
t(21;22)(q22;q12)	EWS-ERG	Ewing sarcoma
t(7;22)(p22;q12)	EWS-ETV1	Ewing sarcoma
t(2;21;22)(q33;q22;q12)	EWS-FEV	Ewing sarcoma
t(17;22)(q12;q12)	EWS-E1AF	Ewing sarcoma
t(11;22)(p13;q12)	EWS-WT1	Desmoplastic small round cell tumor
t(12;22)(q13;q12)	EWS-ATF1	Clear cell sarcoma

tumor" is also used for a group of brain tumors, leading some physicians to use the term "peripheral primitive neuroectodermal tumor" when referring to this Ewing tumor variant. Ewing sarcoma/PNET may also present as a soft-tissue mass without any bone involvement. A Children's Oncology Group (COG) study of nonmetastatic Ewing sarcoma/PNET tumor showed that slightly more than 20% of patients had soft-tissue primaries (personal communication, L. Granowetter).

12.3.3 Diagnosis

The most common initial presenting symptoms of Ewing sarcoma include pain, swelling, or both. Ado-

lescents and young adults often attribute this pain to trauma or physical exertion, and may initially disregard these symptoms, leading to a delay in diagnosis. In addition, pelvic or back lesions may cause referred pain at the knee. Thus, evaluation of knee pain should always warrant consideration of referred pain to avoid further delay in the possible diagnosis of hip or back pathology.

Unlike osteosarcoma, individuals who present with Ewing sarcoma may have systemic signs and symptoms including fever, weight loss, malaise, and increased sedimentation rate. These symptoms tend to be present for months prior to medical evaluation and approximately half of patients have symptoms lasting over 6 months prior to diagnosis [63].

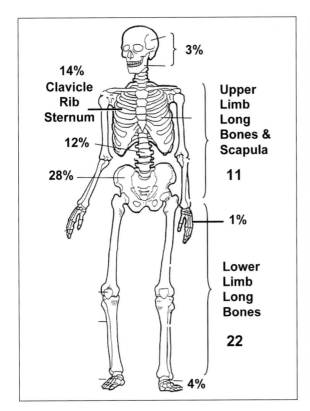

Figure 12.8

Anatomic location of Ewing sarcoma in 15 to 29 year olds, United States SEER 1992–2002

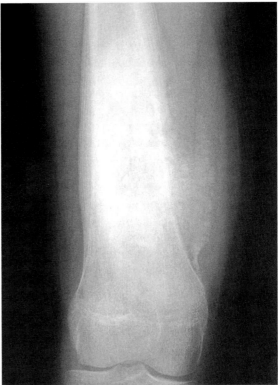

Figure 12.9

Typical presenting radiographic finding of periosteal reaction with "onion skinning" due to Ewing sarcoma, diaphysis of distal femur

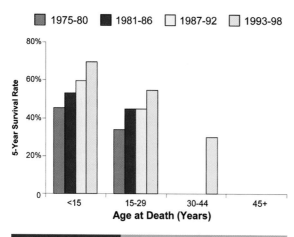

Figure 12.10

5-Year survival rates of Ewing sarcoma by era, U. S. SEER 1975–1999

Ewing sarcoma may occur within any bone, with a slightly increased occurrence in the extremities (Fig. 12.8). The first Intergroup Ewing sarcoma study (IESS) reviewed 303 patients with bone primaries in 1983. They reported that the pelvis was the most common site of Ewing sarcoma, accounting for 20% of tumors. Other common locations include the extremities, with approximately equal proportion of tumors in the proximal and distal long bones [64, 65].

Initial radiographic evaluation should include a plain x-ray of the primary site, which often shows the classic finding of "onion skinning" due to the periosteal reaction surrounding cortical bone tumor (Fig. 12.9). In addition, a more detailed examination with MRI should be done of the primary site to view the extent of disease and to optimally characterize the initial tumor appearance for more accurate follow-up after therapy [66].

It is also imperative to perform a detailed evaluation for metastatic disease. The most common sites include the lungs, bone, and bone marrow. In a cohort of 110 patients with metastases at diagnosis, 35% had isolated lung, 15% had lung plus other sites, 13% had isolated bone, and 7% had isolated bone marrow [67]. Lymph node metastases are rare in bone primaries and the incidence is not yet known for soft-tissue lesions. The prognosis for patients with metastatic disease is

significantly worse, with an approximately 30% 5-year survival if there is lung disease and a less than 10% 5-year survival if there is bone or bone marrow disease [68]. In addition, in a large series of Ewing sarcoma patients, up to 20% with clinically localized disease had bone marrow micrometastasis detected by RT-PCR [69]. These patients were found to have a 2-year disease free survival (DFS) of only 53% compared to those with an 80% DFS in RT-PCR-negative patients [69]. Therefore, a metastatic evaluation should not only include a bone scan and a CT scan of the chest, but should also include a bone marrow examination. Bilateral iliac crest samples are preferable since disease may be sporadically clustered within the marrow space, and should be sent for cytogenetics to evaluate for any occult disease. The clinical role of RT-PCR on bone marrow has yet to be determined. In addition, specific attention to the history and physical exam should be given to any skeletal complaints or findings, other than at the primary tumor site.

Finally, all postpubertal males should be offered cryopreservation of sperm prior to the initiation of chemotherapy, since the alkylating agents used in Ewing sarcoma have a high rate of causing hypo- or azospermia [70].

12.3.4 Treatment

Treatment of Ewing sarcoma historically involved local control with either radiation therapy and/or surgery. With these modalities alone, there was an overall 5-year survival of 22% for patients of all ages with localized disease [63]. This poor overall survival of patients with apparent nonmetastatic disease at presentation indicates a high propensity for micrometastatic disease; therefore treatment has evolved over the last 30 years to include systemic chemotherapy in addition to local control. Following the addition of chemotherapy, the prognosis has greatly improved to close to 70% survival in children <15 years of age, and over 50% in young adults 15–29 years old (Fig. 12.10) [1, 2].

Initial chemotherapy regimens for Ewing sarcoma included combinations of vincristine, actinomycin-D, and cyclophosphamide (VAC). The first Intergroup Ewing Sarcoma Study (IESS) started in 1972 and randomized patients to receive VAC alone, VAC with doxorubicin, or VAC with bilateral pulmonary irradiation. Patients who received doxorubicin had the best outcome, those who received lung radiation therapy had an intermediate outcome; most inferior was VAC alone [71]. The use of ifosfamide with or without etoposide showed promise in patients with relapsed Ewing sarcoma; and therefore, these agents were introduced into clinical trials for patients presenting with nonmetastatic disease. Compared to historical controls, investigators from France found no benefit of ifosfamide [72], while others have showed a benefit from the addition ifosfamide and/or etoposide [73–75]. The cooperative Ewing Sarcoma Study (CESS 86), from the period 1986–1991, incorporated ifosfamide for "high-risk" patients, classified as those with central axis and large tumors, and found a benefit [73]. Most recently, a large randomized comparison by the COG showed significant improvement with the addition of ifosfamide and etoposide for children with Ewing sarcoma. Patients who did not have metastases at presentation received either vincristine, cyclophosphamide, doxorubicin, and actinomycin alone (VACA), or those four drugs alternating with ifosfamide and etoposide. Patients receiving ifosfamide and etoposide had a 69% 5-year survival rate, compared to 54% 5-year survival for patients who received VACA alone [65].

More recently, a COG trial evaluated whether dose intensification of alternating vincristine, doxorubicin, cyclophosphamide with ifosfamide, and etoposide, given every 3 weeks had any effect on outcome, and was tolerable. Preliminary evaluation showed that while there was no increased toxicity for patients treated with the intensified arm, the outcome for the two groups was not significantly different [76].

Unlike osteosarcoma, there does appear to be survival variations for Ewing sarcoma by age that call into question whether we can or should extrapolate the pediatric treatment data to adolescents and young adults. In virtually all retrospective studies and in population data, older adolescents and young adults with Ewing sarcoma do worse than those <15 years of age (Fig. 12.11) [1, 71, 72]. The reason for this disparity may be a variety of influences including premorbid conditions, differences in patient care in pediatric and adult centers, and differences in disease biology. For example, in an analysis of 975 Ewing sarcoma patients

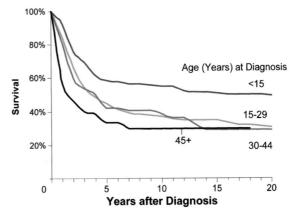

Figure 12.11

Survival of persons with Ewing sarcoma by age, United States SEER, 1975–2000

aged 8 months to 47 years, patients ≥15 years had a significantly higher proportion of pelvic primaries and larger tumor volumes; these older patients also had an inferior 5-year relapse free survival of 52% compared to 63% in those younger than 15 years [77]. In the most recent COG study, young adults older than 18 years had a 5-year survival of only 44%, and the addition of ifosfamide and etoposide did not improve survival in those over age 15 years [65]. Finally, adolescents may fare worse when treated in places other than pediatric institutions. Of the 1,426 patients that were treated on trials CESS81–EICESS92, those registered in pediatric institutions fared better than those in medical or other institutions [79]. This was mainly due to the patients aged >15–20 years, as patients aged above 20 years fared equally (inferiorly) in both institutions. Thus, as yet unexplained differences of care between pediatric and medical oncology institutional settings (perhaps a reflection of experience with the disease), may also contribute to differences in outcome of adolescent and young adult Ewing patients.

Successful treatment of metastatic Ewing sarcoma has been very difficult, and while improvements in outcome have been achieved, the majority of adolescents and adults with metastases at presentation will die of their disease. There is no standard regimen with which to treat metastatic disease. Current trials include a European/COG cooperative study of autologous transplantation for patients with lung metastases and a COG pilot trial of the addition of three times per week vinblastine and daily celecoxib to standard therapy for patients with very-high-risk metastatic disease. Early trials are now underway to investigate the utility of targeted receptor inhibitors, such as imatinab (Gleevec), which has been shown in vitro and in vivo to have activity against Ewing sarcoma [78]. In addition, the presence of a nearly ubiquitous translocation in Ewing sarcoma holds out the hope of exquisitely targeted therapy.

For patients with relapses, various chemotherapy regimens using agents that the patient has not yet received may be attempted. The combination of cyclophosphamide and topotecan has shown activity in patients with relapsed Ewing sarcoma [80, 81], and will be further evaluated by COG in the treatment at presentation of patients with nonmetastatic disease. Patients with a longer duration of disease control may have a good response to retreatment with intensification of chemotherapy agents that they have received previously [82–84]. For patients who relapse on therapy, achieving cure is very difficult, and treatment utilizing new, experimental agents is quite reasonable.

12.3.5 Late Effects

Following therapy patients should continue to have regular follow-ups with their physician to observe for the late effects from treatment or for relapse. Patients who received doxorubicin should have periodic echocardiography and electrocardiograms to screen for cardiac dysfunction. Female patients will probably develop premature menopause as a result of alkylating agents, and need to be counseled regarding this possibility. Secondary malignancy is increased following therapy for Ewing sarcoma. The topoisomerase II inhibition of etoposide and doxorubicin can induce a 11q23-type secondary leukemia, and the alkylating agents used can induce myelodysplastic syndromes and leukemia, typically with monosomy 7. Radiation-induced sarcomas may also occur in patients who receive that modality [85, 86]. In general, all patients should be screened with periodic physical exams and complete blood counts.

12.4 Conclusions

Bone sarcomas, specifically Ewing sarcoma and osteosarcoma, are among the characteristic tumors of adolescence and young adulthood, because they are among the top causes of cancer morbidity and mortality, and because their lifetime incidence peaks in this age group. Therefore, the management of a bone sarcoma is often the management of an adolescent/young adult patient, and the accepted management of bone sarcomas emanates in large part from our experience with adolescents and young adults. Although survival has improved greatly in the last quarter century with the routine use of systemic chemotherapy, much work remains to improve the outlook for patients with metastatic or recurrent disease. Age appears not to be a prognostic factor affecting outcome for osteosarcoma, and management should uniformly include multidisciplinary care, aggressive surgery, and chemotherapy. The prognosis of these tumors is related to the presence of metastases, tumor size and, in the case of osteosarcoma, the ability to surgically resect. For Ewing sarcoma, young adults do have compromised survival compared with younger children, and it can be presumed there are clinical and/or biologic factors for which age is a surrogate. Until it is fully elucidated whether Ewing sarcoma patients should receive stratified care based on age, it is recommended to treat them according to best pediatric practice, including multiagent chemotherapy, and aggressive local control. Adolescent/young adult patients have usually completed their growth and do well with limb salvage for bone sarcomas, and usually tolerate the intensive chemotherapeutic regimens (although compliance with schedule and length of therapy can be problematic). Physicians should be sensitive to the unique psychosocial needs of the adolescent/young-adult-aged bone tumor patient, and assist the patient in ensuring long-term follow-up, especially as secondary malignancies are increased in bone tumor survivors.

The overall outcome for patients with bone sarcomas has improved significantly in the last 30 years. New advances in surgical technique and reconstructive methods have allowed limb salvage to become the surgical standard of care, in lieu of wide or radical amputation of the involved limb, without sacrificing long-term survival. Improvements in chemotherapy and the recognition of early micrometastatic disease, in conjunction with radical surgical resection of the primary tumor or local irradiation, has led to increases in the 5-year survival rates from approximately 30% to approximately 70% [1, 2].

References

1. Bleyer WA, O'Leary M, Barr R, Ries LAG (eds) (2006) Cancer Epidemiology in Older Adolescents and Young Adults 15 to 29 Years of Age, including SEER Incidence and Survival, 1975–2000. National Cancer Institute, NIH Pub. No. 06-5767, Bethesda MD; also available at www.seer.cancer.gov/publications
2. Ries L, Eisner M, Kosary C, et al (2004) SEER Cancer Statistics Review, 1975–2001, National Cancer Institute. Bethesda, MD, http://seer.cancer.gov/csr/1975_2001
3. Dahlin DC, Coventry MB (1967) Osteogenic sarcoma. A study of six hundred cases. J Bone Joint Surg Am 49:101–110
4. Cotterill SJ, Wright CM, Pearce MS, et al (2004) Stature of young people with malignant bone tumors. Pediatr Blood Cancer 42:59–63
5. Tucker MA, D'Angio GJ, Boice JD Jr, et al (1987) Bone sarcomas linked to radiotherapy and chemotherapy in children. N Engl J Med 317:588–593
6. Tabone MD, Terrier P, Pacquement H, et al (1999) Outcome of radiation-related osteosarcoma after treatment of childhood and adolescent cancer: a study of 23 cases. J Clin Oncol 17:2789–95
7. Pritchard DJ, Finkel MP, Reilly CA Jr (1975) The etiology of osteosarcoma. A review of current considerations. Clin Orthop 111:14–22
8. Basombrio MA (1970) Search for common antigenicities among twenty-five sarcomas induced by methylcholanthrene. Cancer Res 30:2458–2462
9. Price CH, Moore M, Jones DB (1972) FBJ virus-induced tumours in mice. A histopathological study of FBJ virus tumours and their relevance to murine and human osteosarcoma arising in bone. Br J Cancer 26:15–27
10. Sekiguchi M, Miyazaki S, Fujikawa K, et al (1996) BK virus-induced osteosarcoma (Os515) as a model of human osteosarcoma. Anticancer Res 16:1835–1842
11. Desai P, Perino G, Present D, et al (1996) Sarcoma in association with bone infarcts. Report of five cases. Arch Pathol Lab Med 120:482–489
12. Resnik CS, Aisner SC, Young JW, et al (1993) Case report 767. Osteosarcoma arising in bone infarction. Skeletal Radiol 22:58–61
13. Hansen MF, Cavenee WK (1987) Retinoblastoma and osteosarcoma: the prototypic cancer family. Acta Paediatr Jpn 29:526–533
14. Hansen MF (1991) Molecular genetic considerations in osteosarcoma. Clin Orthop 270:237–246
15. Malkin D, Jolly KW, Barbier N, et al (1992) Germline mutations of the p53 tumor-suppressor gene in children and young adults with second malignant neoplasms. N Engl J Med 326:1309–1315
16. Diller L, Kassel J, Nelson CE, et al (1990) p53 functions as a cell cycle control protein in osteosarcomas. Mol Cell Biol 10:5772–5781
17. Miller CW, Aslo A, Won A, et al (1996) Alterations of the p53, Rb and MDM2 genes in osteosarcoma. J Cancer Res Clin Oncol 122:559–565
18. Temple HT, Scully SP, O'Keefe RJ, et al (2000) Clinical outcome of 38 patients with juxtacortical osteosarcoma. Clin Orthop 373:208–217
19. Papagelopoulos PJ, Galanis E, Sim FH, et al (1999) Periosteal osteosarcoma. Orthopedics 22:971–974
20. Nakajima H, Sim FH, Bond JR, et al (1997) Small cell osteosarcoma of bone. Review of 72 cases. Cancer 79:2095–2106
21. Wolf RE, Enneking WF (1996) The staging and surgery of musculoskeletal neoplasms. Orthop Clin North Am 27:473–481
22. Kager L, Zoubek A, Potschger U, et al (2003) Primary metastatic osteosarcoma: presentation and outcome of patients treated on neoadjuvant Cooperative Osteosarcoma Study Group protocols. J Clin Oncol 21:2011–2018
23. Link MP, Goorin AM, Miser AW, et al (1986) The effect of adjuvant chemotherapy on relapse-free survival in patients with osteosarcoma of the extremity. N Engl J Med 314:1600–1606
24. Link MP, Goorin AM, Horowitz M, et al (1991) Adjuvant chemotherapy of high-grade osteosarcoma of the extremity. Updated results of the Multi-Institutional Osteosarcoma Study. Clin Orthop 270:8–14
25. Machak GN, Tkachev SI, Solovyev YN, et al (2003) Neoadjuvant chemotherapy and local radiotherapy for high-grade osteosarcoma of the extremities. Mayo Clin Proc 78:147–155
26. Kamada T, Tsujii H, Tsuji H, et al (2002) Efficacy and safety of carbon ion radiotherapy in bone and soft tissue sarcomas. J Clin Oncol 20:4466–4471
27. Goorin AM, Schwartzentruber DJ, Devidas M, et al (2003) Presurgical chemotherapy compared with immediate surgery and adjuvant chemotherapy for nonmetastatic osteosarcoma: Pediatric Oncology Group Study POG-8651. J Clin Oncol 21:1574–1580
28. Edmonson JH, Green SJ, Ivins JC, et al. A controlled pilot study of high-dose methotrexate as postsurgical adjuvant treatment for primary osteosarcoma. J Clin Oncol 2:152–6, 1984
29. Meyers PA, Gorlick R, Heller G, et al (1998) Intensifica-

tion of preoperative chemotherapy for osteogenic sarcoma: results of the Memorial Sloan-Kettering (T12) protocol. J Clin Oncol 16:2452–2458

30. Provisor AJ, Ettinger LJ, Nachman JB, et al (1997) Treatment of nonmetastatic osteosarcoma of the extremity with preoperative and postoperative chemotherapy: a report from the Children's Cancer Group. J Clin Oncol 15:76–84

31. Szendroi M, Antal I, Koos R, et al (2000) Results of limb-saving surgery and prognostic factors in patients with osteosarcoma. Orv Hetil 141:2175–2182

32. Meyers PA, Heller G, Healey JH, et al (1993) Osteogenic sarcoma with clinically detectable metastasis at initial presentation. J Clin Oncol 11:449–453

33. Meyer WH, Schell MJ, Kumar AP, et al (1987) Thoracotomy for pulmonary metastatic osteosarcoma. An analysis of prognostic indicators of survival. Cancer 59:374–379

34. Beattie EJ Jr, Martini N, Rosen G (1975) The management of pulmonary metastases in children with osteogenic sarcoma with surgical resection combined with chemotherapy. Cancer 35:618–621

35. Saeter G, Hoie J, Stenwig AE, et al (1995) Systemic relapse of patients with osteogenic sarcoma. Prognostic factors for long term survival. Cancer 75:1084–1093

36. Karnak I, Emin Senocak M, Kutluk T, et al (2002) Pulmonary metastases in children: an analysis of surgical spectrum. Eur J Pediatr Surg 12:151–158

37. Goorin AM, Harris MB, Bernstein M, et al (2002) Phase II/III trial of etoposide and high-dose ifosfamide in newly diagnosed metastatic osteosarcoma: a pediatric oncology group trial. J Clin Oncol 20:426–433

38. Bacci G, Briccoli A, Ferrari S, et al (2000) Neoadjuvant chemotherapy for osteosarcoma of the extremities with synchronous lung metastases: treatment with cisplatin, adriamycin and high dose of methotrexate and ifosfamide. Oncol Rep 7:339–346

38. Edmonson JH, Green SJ, Ivins JC, et al (1984) A controlled pilot study of high-dose methotrexate as post-surgical adjuvant treatment for primary osteosarcoma. J Clin Oncol 2:152–156

39. Bacci G, Briccoli A, Rocca M, et al (2003) Neoadjuvant chemotherapy for osteosarcoma of the extremities with metastases at presentation: recent experience at the Rizzoli Institute in 57 patients treated with cisplatin, doxorubicin, and a high dose of methotrexate and ifosfamide. Ann Oncol 14:1126–1134

40. Ferrari S, Briccoli A, Mercuri M, et al (2003) Postrelapse survival in osteosarcoma of the extremities: prognostic factors for long-term survival. J Clin Oncol 21:710–715

41. Aung L, Gorlick RG, Shi W, et al (2002) Second malignant neoplasms in long-term survivors of osteosarcoma: Memorial Sloan-Kettering Cancer Center experience. Cancer 95:1728–1734

42. Hosalkar HS, Henderson KM, Weiss A, et al (2004) Chemotherapy for bone sarcoma does not affect fertility rates or childbirth. Clin Orthop Relat Res 428:256–260

43. Longhi A, Pignotti E, Versari M, et al (2003) Effect of oral contraceptive on ovarian function in young females undergoing neoadjuvant chemotherapy treatment for osteosarcoma. Oncol Rep 10:151–155

44. Meistrich ML, Chawla SP, Da Cunha MF, et al (1989) Recovery of sperm production after chemotherapy for osteosarcoma. Cancer 63:2115–2123

45. Bacci G, Ferrari S, Bertoni F, et al (2000) Long-term outcome for patients with nonmetastatic osteosarcoma of the extremity treated at the Istituto Ortopedico Rizzoli according to the Istituto Ortopedico Rizzoli/osteosarcoma-2 protocol: an updated report. J Clin Oncol 18:4016–4027

46. Parkin DM, Stiller CA, Nectoux J (1993) International variations in the incidence of childhood bone tumours. Int J Cancer 53:371–376

47. Li FP, Tu JT, Liu FS, et al (1980) Rarity of Ewing's sarcoma in China. Lancet 1:1255

48. Fraumeni JF Jr, Glass AG (1970) Rarity of Ewing's sarcoma among U.S. Negro children. Lancet 1:366–367

49. Joyce MJ, Harmon DC, Mankin HJ, et al (1984) Ewing's sarcoma in female siblings. A clinical report and review of the literature. Cancer 53:1959–1962

50. Zamora P, Garcia de Paredes ML, Gonzalez Baron M, et al (1986) Ewing's tumor in brothers. An unusual observation. Am J Clin Oncol 9:358–360

51. Hutter RV, Francis KC, Foote FW Jr (1964) Ewing's sarcoma in siblings: report of the second known occurrence. Am J Surg 107:598–603

52. Aparicio J, Segura A, Montalar J, et al (1998) Secondary cancers after Ewing sarcoma and Ewing sarcoma as second malignant neoplasm. Med Pediatr Oncol 30:259–260

53. Delattre O, Zucman J, Melot T, et al (1994) The Ewing family of tumors – a subgroup of small-round-cell tumors defined by specific chimeric transcripts. N Engl J Med 331:294–299

54. Delattre O, Zucman J, Plougastel B, et al (1992) Gene fusion with an ETS DNA-binding domain caused by chromosome translocation in human tumours. Nature 359:162–165

55. Lessnick SL, Braun BS, Denny CT, et al (1995) Multiple domains mediate transformation by the Ewing's sarcoma EWS/FLI-1 fusion gene. Oncogene 10:423–431

56. Sorensen PH, Lessnick SL, Lopez-Terrada D, et al (1994) A second Ewing's sarcoma translocation, t(21;22), fuses the EWS gene to another ETS-family transcription factor, ERG. Nat Genet 6:146–151

57. Arvand A, Denny CT (2001) Biology of EWS/ETS fusions in Ewing's family tumors. Oncogene 20:5747–5754

58. Perlman EJ, Dickman PS, Askin FB, et al (1994) Ewing's sarcoma – routine diagnostic utilization of MIC2 anal-

ysis: a Pediatric Oncology Group/Children's Cancer Group Intergroup Study. Hum Pathol 25:304–307

59. de Alava E, Gerald WL (2000) Molecular biology of the Ewing's sarcoma/primitive neuroectodermal tumor family. J Clin Oncol 18:204–213

60. Smithey BE, Pappo AS, Hill DA (2002) C-kit expression in pediatric solid tumors: a comparative immunohistochemical study. Am J Surg Pathol 26:486–492

61. Scotlandi K, Manara MC, Strammiello R, et al (2003) C-kit receptor expression in Ewing's sarcoma: lack of prognostic value but therapeutic targeting opportunities in appropriate conditions. J Clin Oncol 21:1952–1960

62. Jurgens HF (1994) Ewing's sarcoma and peripheral primitive neuroectodermal tumor. Curr Opin Oncol 6:391–396

63. Pritchard DJ, Dahlin DC, Dauphine RT, et al (1975) Ewing's sarcoma. A clinicopathological and statistical analysis of patients surviving five years or longer. J Bone Joint Surg Am 57:10–16

64. Kissane JM, Askin FB, Foulkes M, et al (1983) Ewing's sarcoma of bone: clinicopathologic aspects of 303 cases from the Intergroup Ewing's Sarcoma Study. Hum Pathol 14:773–779

65. Grier HE, Krailo MD, Tarbell NJ, et al (2003) Addition of ifosfamide and etoposide to standard chemotherapy for Ewing's sarcoma and primitive neuroectodermal tumor of bone. N Engl J Med 348:694–701

66. van der Woude HJ, Bloem JL, Hogendoorn PC (1998) Preoperative evaluation and monitoring chemotherapy in patients with high-grade osteogenic and Ewing's sarcoma: review of current imaging modalities. Skeletal Radiol 27:57–71

67. Bernstein M, Devidas M, Lafreniere D, et al (2006) Intensive Therapy with growth factor support for patients with Ewing tumor metastatic at diagnosis, POG/CCG phase II study 9457: a report from the Children's Oncology Group. J Clin Oncol 24:152–159

68. Miser JS, Krailo MD, Tarbell NJ, et al (2004) Treatment of metastatic Ewing's sarcoma or primitive neuroectodermal tumor of bone: evaluation of combination ifosfamide and etoposide – a Children's Cancer Group and Pediatric Oncology Group study. J Clin Oncol 22:2873–2876

69. Schleiermacher G, Peter M, Oberlin O, et al (2003) Increased risk of systemic relapses associated with bone marrow micrometastasis and circulating tumor cells in localized Ewing tumor. J Clin Oncol 21:85–91

70. Kenney LB, Laufer MR, Grant FD, et al (2001) High risk of infertility and long term gonadal damage in males treated with high dose cyclophosphamide for sarcoma during childhood. Cancer 91:613–621

71. Nesbit ME Jr, Gehan EA, Burgert EO Jr, et al (1990) Multimodal therapy for the management of primary, nonmetastatic Ewing's sarcoma of bone: a long-term follow-up of the First Intergroup study. J Clin Oncol 8:1664–1674

72. Oberlin O, Habrand JL, Zucker JM, et al (1992) No benefit of ifosfamide in Ewing's sarcoma: a nonrandomized study of the French Society of Pediatric Oncology. J Clin Oncol 10:1407–1412

73. Paulussen M, Ahrens S, Dunst J, et al (2001) Localized Ewing tumor of bone: final results of the cooperative Ewing's Sarcoma Study CESS 86. J Clin Oncol 19:1818–1829

74. Rosito P, Mancini AF, Rondelli R, et al (1999) Italian Cooperative Study for the treatment of children and young adults with localized Ewing sarcoma of bone: a preliminary report of 6 years of experience. Cancer 86:421–428

75. Craft A, Cotterill S, Malcolm A, et al (1998) Ifosfamide-containing chemotherapy in Ewing's sarcoma: the Second United Kingdom Children's Cancer Study Group and the Medical Research Council Ewing's Tumor Study. J Clin Oncol 16:3628–3633

76. Granowetter L, Womer R, Devidas M, et al (2001) Comparison of dose intensified and standard dose chemotherapy for the treatment of non-metastatic Ewing sarcoma (ES) and primitive neuroectodermal tumor (PNET) of bone and soft tissue: a Pediatric Oncology Group – Children's Cancer Group phase III trial. Med Pediatr Oncol 37:aO38:172

77. Cotterill SJ, Ahrens S, Paulussen M, et al (2000) Prognostic factors in Ewing's tumor of bone: analysis of 975 patients from the European Intergroup Cooperative Ewing's Sarcoma Study Group. J Clin Oncol 18:3108–3114

78. Merchant MS, Woo CW, Mackall CL, et al (2002) Potential use of imatinib in Ewing's sarcoma: evidence for in vitro and in vivo activity. J Natl Cancer Inst 94:1673–1679

79. Paulussen M, Ahrens S, Juergens HF (2003) Cure rates in Ewing tumor patients aged over 15 years are better in pediatric oncology units. Results of GPOH CESS/EICESS studies. Proc Am Soc Clin Oncol 22:816 (abstract 3279)

80. Saylors RL III, Stine KC, Sullivan J, et al (2001) Cyclophosphamide plus topotecan in children with recurrent or refractory solid tumors: a Pediatric Oncology Group phase II study. J Clin Oncol 19:3463–3469

81. Blaney SM, Needle MN, Gillespie A, et al (1998) Phase II trial of topotecan administered as 72-hour continuous infusion in children with refractory solid tumors: a collaborative Pediatric Branch, National Cancer Institute, and Children's Cancer Group Study. Clin Cancer Res 4:357–360

82. McLean TW, Hertel C, Young ML, et al (1999) Late events in pediatric patients with Ewing sarcoma/primitive neuroectodermal tumor of bone: the Dana-Farber Cancer Institute/Children's Hospital experience. J Pediatr Hematol Oncol 21:486–493

83. Rodriguez-Galindo C, Billups CA, Kun LE, et al (2002) Survival after recurrence of Ewing tumors: the St Jude Children's Research Hospital experience, 1979–1999. Cancer 94:561–569

84. Hayes FA, Thompson EI, Kumar M, et al (1987) Long-term survival in patients with Ewing's sarcoma relapsing after completing therapy. Med Pediatr Oncol 15:254–256

85. Kuttesch JF Jr, Wexler LH, Marcus RB, et al (1996) Second malignancies after Ewing's sarcoma: radiation dose-dependency of secondary sarcomas. J Clin Oncol 14:2818–2825

86. Dunst J, Ahrens S, Paulussen M, et al (1998) Second malignancies after treatment for Ewing's sarcoma: a report of the CESS-studies. Int J Radiat Oncol Biol Phys 42:379–384

Malignancies of the Ovary

Jubilee Brown • Thomas Olson •
Susan Sencer

Contents

13.1 Introduction

Although epithelial ovarian cancers comprise approximately 90% of ovarian malignancies in women [1], the majority of such cancers are nonepithelial in adolescents and young adult women. The most common ovarian tumor in adolescents is of germ-cell origin [2, 3]. In females 15- to 20-years of age, genital tract tumors account for 18% of all invasive cancers [1], which is in distinct contrast to < 2% of cancers being ovarian tumors in females younger than 15 years [4].

Despite their low incidence, ovarian tumors represent a major diagnostic and treatment dilemma for pediatric oncologists. Pediatric general surgeons may be unfamiliar with the current staging recommendations for work-up of these patients, and many patients have therefore undergone unnecessary second surgeries or required an upgrade in therapy. Alternatively, many adolescents with ovarian tumors are treated in adult facilities by gynecologic oncologists, and do not benefit from the age-appropriate, full spectrum of multidisciplinary care provided in a pediatric oncology practice. Adolescents with ovarian tumors are grossly under represented on clinical trials, whether pediatric or adult cooperative group in origin.

Appropriate treatment of ovarian tumors is determined by many factors, including patient age, karyotype, extent of disease, tumor histology, and co-morbid conditions. Conservative surgery to maintain reproductive potential is an important consideration in all adolescents and young adults, and is usually feasible. Appropriate surgical staging and assessment are necessary components in determining the extent of surgery required and the need for postoperative chemotherapy. Pediatric oncologists and surgeons must work closely with gynecologic oncologists to ensure that an appropriate initial evaluation is performed.

Table 13.1 Modified World Health Organization comprehensive classification of ovarian tumors [5]

I.	Common epithelial tumors	
	A.	Mucinous
	B.	Serous
	C.	Endometrioid
	C.	Clear cell
	D.	Brenner
	E.	Transitional
	F.	Small cell
	G.	Malignant mixed mesodermal
	H.	Unclassified
II.	Sex cord-stromal tumors	
	A.	Granulosa stromal cell
	B.	Androblastomas; Sertoli-Leydig cell tumors
	C.	Lipid cell tumors (steroid cell tumors)
	D.	Gynandroblastoma
	E.	Unclassified
III.	Germ cell tumors	
	A.	Dysgerminoma
	B.	Endodermal sinus tumor
	C.	Embryonal carcinoma
	D.	Polyembryoma
	E.	Choriocarcinoma
	F.	Teratomas
	G.	Mixed forms
	H.	Gonadoblastoma
IV.	Soft tissue tumors not specific to the ovary	
V.	Unclassified tumors	
VI.	Metastatic (secondary) tumors	
VII.	Tumor-like conditions	

Clinical behavior, treatment, prognosis, and the potential for maintenance of reproductive capacity are markedly different for nonepithelial and epithelial tumors. The most common non-epithelial tumors are germ-cell tumors (GCTs), sex cord-stromal tumors, and rarer tumor types. Common epithelial tumors are mucinous, serous, and mixed types. Tumors of low malignant potential (LMP), also called borderline tumors, can occur in adolescents and young adults. The classification of ovarian tumors has been formalized by the World Health Organization: an abbreviated version is shown in Table 13.1 [5].

An adolescent or young adult patient will often present with an adnexal mass and undergo exploratory surgery. Precise histology is difficult to determine by frozen section alone. It is important to note that requirements for adjuvant therapy can only be based on final pathology. With close attention to optimal surgical guidelines, the need for re-exploration and more extensive surgery can be minimized and preservation of fertility maximized. This chapter discusses the management of the common ovarian tumors and provides practical guidelines for intra- and post operative management of ovarian neoplasms in adolescents and young adults.

13.2 Epidemiology

Ovarian malignancies are rare in adolescents and young adults; it has been estimated that only 3–17% of ovarian malignancies occur in women younger than 40 years of age, although incidence increases progressively through adult life (Fig. 13.1 and Table 13.2) [1]. There are fewer than 16 cases/million of ovarian cancers diagnosed in girls younger than 15 years of age; this increases to 23.7 cases/million in the age group 15–29 years [1]. While GCTs predominate in girls younger than 15 years (78%) and in those aged 15–19 years (54%), carcinomas predominate in the 20- to 24-year-old group [6]. In a comprehensive review of all pediatric ovarian masses in a 14-year period at Children's Hospital of Philadelphia, 240 cases were identified; 51% were nonneoplastic. Of the 117 neoplastic tumors, 79 were GCTs and 19 were epithelial in nature [7]. Similarly, a Greek study

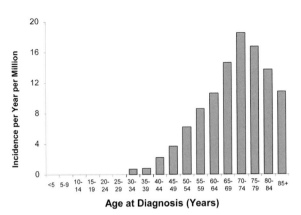

Figure 13.1

Incidence of ovarian malignancies in women, United States SEER registry [1]

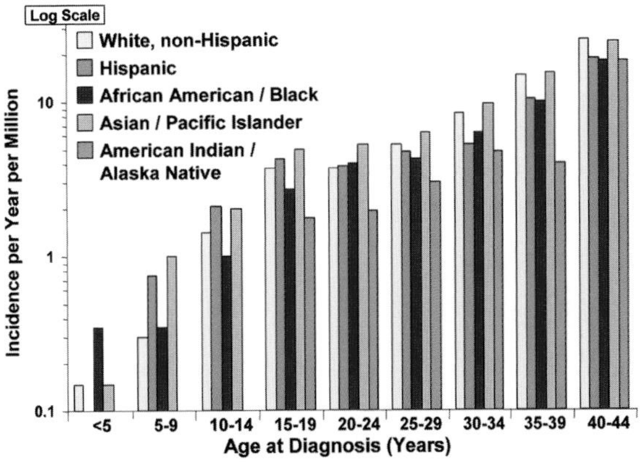

Figure 13.2

Incidence of ovarian malignancies in women as a function of race/ethnicity, United States SEER [1]

showed that GCTs accounted for 61.5% of tumors; 20% were epithelial and 9.5% were sex-cord-stromal tumors [8].

The incidence of ovarian cancer varies with race/ethnicity. Among 15- to 29-year-olds with malignancies of the ovary, Asians/Pacific Islanders have had the highest incidence and American Indians/Alaska Natives the lowest (Fig. 13.2).

13.3 Pathology and Biology

There are multiple tissue types present in the normal ovary, including germ cells, stroma, and surface epithelium. Each of these can give rise to a set of distinctive tumors that can occur in pure or combined forms. The majority of ovarian malignancies found in children involve the germ cells. Epithelial and stromal tumors become more prevalent throughout the adolescent and young adult years.

13.3.1 Germ-Cell Tumors

GCTs arise from germ cells present in the normal ovary. Benign GCTs include mature teratomas and gonadoblastomas. Malignant GCTs include dysgerminomas, mixed GCTs, endodermal sinus tumors, imma-

ture teratomas, choriocarcinomas, embryonal tumors, and polyembryomas.

Malignant GCTs often display heterogeneous histologic differentiation. In adolescent patients, it is not unusual to have GCTs with several histologic patterns in the same tumor. Endodermal sinus tract tumors or yolk sac tumors (YST) are characterized by elevation of alpha fetoprotein (αFP). Choriocarcinomas usually demonstrate an elevation of β-human choriogonadotropin (β-HCG). Both markers may be elevated in embryonal carcinoma. In adolescents and young adults, pure ovarian dysgerminomas may also demonstrate increased β-HCG (Table 13.3) [9].

Table 13.2 Ovarian cancer incidence by age (Surveillance, Epidemiology, and End Results data, 1975–2000 [1]

Age (years)	Incidence
<15	a
15–29	0.237
30–44	1.293
45+	9.868

[a]<16 cases/1,000,000 [1]

Table 13.3 Serum tumor markers in malignant tumors of the ovary [9, 10]. hCG Human chorionic gonadotropin, AFP alpha-fetoprotein, LDH lactate dehydrogenase

Tumor	hCG	AFP	LDH	CA-125
Dysgerminoma	+/-	-	+	
Endodermal sinus tumor	-	+	+/-	
Immature teratoma	-	+/-	+/-	rarely+
Embryonal carcinoma	+	+	+/-	
Choriocarcinoma	+	-	-	
Polyembryoma	+/-	+/-	+/-	
Mixed	+	+	+	
Epithelial				+/-

Table 13.4 Pediatric Intergroup Trial (Pediatric Oncology Group, POG, Children's Cancer Group, CCG) – ovarian germ-cell tumor (GCT) histology [11, 12]. YST Yolk-sac tumor

Histology	Stage I/II		Stage III/IV	
	#	%	#	%
YST	19	33.3%	28	38.9%
Mixed	35	61.4%	17	23.6%
Germinoma	0	0%	25	34.7%
Choriocarcinoma	2	3.5%	1	1.4%
Other	1	1.7%	3	4.2%

From 1990 through 1996, children and adolescents with ovarian GCTs (in addition to other sites of GCT) were enrolled on two Pediatric Intergroup germ-cell protocols; localized (POG9048/CCG8891) and high-risk (POG9049/CCG8882) [11, 12]. Most "mixed" tumors were immature teratomas that contained YST elements. No patient with germinoma was entered onto the localized tumor trial, but germinoma was the second most common histology on the high-risk trial. The high-risk trial included 74 stage III–IV ovarian GCTs. Ages at diagnosis ranged from 2.3 to 20.0 years (median 12.3 years). In girls ≥10 years, 42% presented with dysgerminoma, while 38% had YST (Table 13.4).

Ovarian GCTs bear many histologic and biologic similarities to testicular GCTs (seminomas). However, testicular GCTs in males tend to arise several years after the development of puberty, while ovarian GCTs in females can occur anytime after birth and are much more common in preadolescents. Genetic analysis of ovarian GCTs that present in the second decade of life reveal isochromosome 12p, the characteristic cytogenetic abnormality found in testicular GCT [13–15]. Biologic studies from early co-operative pediatric GCT trials showed that such cytogenetic aberrations were age-dependent. Chromosome I(12p) abnormality has been reported [16] in tumors from pubertal and postpubertal males, but the most common abnormalities in prepubertal females in order of prevalence were gains of 1q, +14, +8, +12, +2, +3, and +7.

Comparative genomic hybridization (CGH), which allows the entire genome to be screened for chromosomal gains or losses, has demonstrated [17] recurrent deletions of 6q and 1p in childhood endodermal sinus tumors. The most common detected region of loss was 6q25-6qter, a finding which is noted in several other human tumors, including ovarian, breast, and hepatocellular carcinoma. Multipotent imprinting analysis showed that gonadal and nongonadal GCTs are derived from primordial germ cells that have lost imprinting of small nuclear ribonucleoprotein N gene (SNRPN) and partial loss of H19 and IGF2 [18]. Cooperative pediatric GCT trials from Pediatric Oncology Group (POG)/Children's Cancer Group (CCG), and Maligne Keimzelltumoren (MAKEI) found that all pure teratomas had normal CGH patterns [19]. Although there were few ovarian GCT specimens in these studies, mono-allelic expression of H19 and IGF2 was seen, suggesting no loss of imprinting. Further studies are needed in adolescents and young adults with ovarian GCTs to identify genes that are important to pathogenesis and therefore potential targets for future treatments.

13.3.2 Sex Cord-Stromal Tumors

Sex cord-stromal tumors originate from the specialized gonadal stromal cells and their precursors. Granulosa cells and Sertoli cells arise from sex cord cells, while theca cells, Leydig cells, lipid cells, and fibroblasts arise from stromal cells and their pluripotential mesenchymal precursors. These tumors can occur as an isolated histologic type or in combination, and together account for 7% of all ovarian malignancies [20], and approximately 5% of ovarian malignancies in women ages 15–24 years [6]. Since these cells are involved in steroid hormone production, physical manifestations of excess estrogen or androgen production can occur at the time of diagnosis. The majorities of these tumors are clinically indolent and have a good long-term prognosis.

13.3.3 Epithelial Tumors

The primary subtypes of epithelial carcinoma in young women are the serous and mucinous types [21]. Adenocarcinoma is found very rarely before the age of 24 years [6]. Little information is available about the biologic issues unique to young women with epithelial ovarian cancer. Certainly women with aberrations of the tumor-susceptibility genes *BRCA1* and *BRCA2* are at increased risk of developing ovarian cancer at a younger age, but there are insufficient data to assess risk in the very young. Women are deemed at high genetic risk of developing ovarian cancer if they carry known *BRCA1/2* mutations, or if they have a strong family history of ovarian and or breast cancer at a young age. Current recommendations are that these women be screened with yearly transvaginal ultrasound and CA125 from the age of 25–30 years, and that they consider prophylactic oophorectomy after completion of childbearing or at the age of 35 years [22]. The cytogenetics of epithelial cancer are often quite complex and may involve a gain of 11p, 12, 18, or 19p, or loss of 17 or X.

13.3.4 Tumors of Low Malignant Potential

LMP tumors represent a category of neoplasms that are distinct from benign cystadenomas and cystadenocarcinomas. First described by Taylor in 1929, they have since been referred to as borderline tumors or atypically proliferating tumors [23, 24]. These tumors arise from the surface epithelium of the ovary and 80–95% are of serous or mucinous histology. LMP tumors of the ovary comprise approximately 15% of all epithelial ovarian tumors [25, 26]. The pathologic criteria for diagnosis of these tumors include the absence of stromal invasion in the ovary and any two of the following characteristics: epithelial "tufting," multilayering of epithelium, mitotic activity, and nuclear atypia. Trisomy 12 has been reported in LMP tumors [27].

13.3.5 Presenting Signs and Symptoms

The most common presenting signs and symptoms of an ovarian tumor are abdominal pain, palpable abdominal mass, increasing abdominal girth, urinary frequency, constipation and dysuria [10, 28]. Some tumors, however, are asymptomatic and only discovered during routine examinations. Abdominal pain is most often chronic, but torsion of the ovary can be associated with acute pain. Since normal sex cord-stromal cells are involved in steroid hormone production, physical manifestations of excess estrogen or androgen production (hirsutism, virilism) should suggest the possibility of a sex cord-stromal tumor, although isosexual precocity may also be seen in mixed malignant GCTs due to tumor production of β-HCG [29]. Teratomas may demonstrate sonographic findings suggestive of dermoids, including sonographic evidence of teeth.

Gynandroblastomas are a separate but rare entity comprised of granulosa cell elements, tubules, and Leydig cells, and can cause premature breast development, hyperestrogenism, or androgenism in adolescents [30, 31].

13.3.6 Diagnostic Work-up

When a patient presents with signs or symptoms suggestive of an ovarian mass, a complete history and physical examination, including abdominal palpation and rectal examination, should be performed. Pelvic examination by a skilled practitioner should be considered, especially in an older adolescent. Laboratory values, including αFP, carcinoembryonic antigen, and β-HCG should be obtained. Other tumor markers, including lactate dehydrogenase (LDH), serum CA-125, estradiol, testosterone, F9 embryoglycan, and inhibin, and Mullerian inhibiting substance may offer further diagnostic or treatment information (Table 13.3) [9, 10].

Imaging studies may include a pelvic ultrasound to delineate the characteristics of the pelvic organs, specifically the ovaries. A computed tomographic (CT) scan of the abdomen and pelvis may be helpful to determine the extent of disease preoperatively. If the ovarian mass is complex or solid, over 8 cm, or has persisted for more than 2 months, surgical exploration is indicated [32].

13.3.7 Surgical Management

Young women who present with ovarian masses generally have many concerns regarding future reproductive potential. Preoperative discussions should occur to review options for maintaining ovarian and/or uterine function based on potential operative findings. In general, effective chemotherapy has allowed the suc-

cessful use of conservative, fertility-sparing surgery in many adolescent and young adult patients with limited disease [33].

13.3.8 General Surgical Guidelines

The absolute diagnosis of an ovarian malignancy can only be made by microscopic pathologic evaluation of a surgically obtained specimen. Detailed surgical approach recommendations are included in the Appendix. The importance of appropriate initial staging cannot be overemphasized, as a small percentage of patients have apparent early-stage disease but have positive lymph nodes on final review. This can then affect the stage, recommended treatment, and overall prognosis.

Although the occasional patient may undergo laparoscopic evaluation for a small solid adnexal mass or complex ovarian cyst, the patient with a large, solid adnexal mass or evidence of hemodynamic instability should undergo laparotomy through a vertical skin incision to ensure appropriate full surgical staging. Upon entering the peritoneal cavity, pelvic washings should be obtained, and hemoperitoneum, if present, evacuated. The site of hemorrhage is most commonly the mass itself, and such that surgical removal of the tumor may be all that is necessary to control the bleeding. A unilateral mass in a patient of any age should be removed by unilateral salpingo-oophorectomy and sent for immediate histologic evaluation. Every attempt should be made to avoid rupture, as this upstages an otherwise stage 1A or 1B carcinoma and may adversely affect survival [34, 35]. For this reason, the tumor should never be morcellated to effect laparoscopic removal.

Occasionally, an ovarian cystectomy is performed in an attempt to preserve ovarian tissue for an apparently benign dermoid cyst. The tumor must be sent for immediate histologic evaluation to confirm its benign nature; in the event of a malignancy the entire ovary should be removed.

If the diagnosis is an epithelial tumor or a malignant GCT of any histologic subtype, excluding the benign mature cystic teratoma, complete surgical staging is indicated. In young patients where fertility is a vital concern, preservation of reproductive potential should be attempted at the time of surgery. The contralateral ovary is inspected and, if normal in appearance, left undisturbed. Due to the low yield from random ovarian biopsy, and the potential for disruption of reproductive potential due to adhesions or trauma, the routine biopsy of a normal-appearing contralateral ovary is not advised [36]. If the contralateral ovary appears to contain a cyst, an ovarian cystectomy should be performed and sent for immediate histologic evaluation. If malignant disease is revealed, bilateral oopho-

Table 13.5 Modified (1987) International Federation of Gynecology and Obstetrics (FIGO) staging system [39, 40]

Stage I:	Growth limited to the ovaries
Stage IA:	Growth limited to one ovary; no malignant cells in ascites or positive peritoneal washings; no tumor on the external surfaces; capsule intact
Stage IB:	Growth limited to both ovaries; no malignant cells in ascites or positive peritoneal washings; no tumor on the external surfaces; capsules intact
Stage IC:	Tumor stage IA or IB but with tumor on the surface of one or both ovaries or with the capsule ruptured or with ascites present containing malignant cells or with positive peritoneal washings
Stage II:	Growth involving one or both ovaries with pelvic extension
Stage IIA:	Extension or metastases to the uterus or tubes
Stage IIB:	Extension to other pelvic tissues
Stage IIC:	Tumor is stage IIA or IIB, but with tumor on the surface of one or both ovaries or with the capsule or capsules ruptured or with ascites containing malignant cells or with positive peritoneal washings
Stage III:	Tumor involving one or both ovaries with peritoneal implants outside the pelvis or positive retroperitoneal or inguinal nodes. Superficial liver metastasis equals stage III. Tumor is limited to the true pelvis but with histologically proved malignant extension to the small bowel or omentum
Stage IIIA:	Tumor grossly limited to the true pelvis with negative nodes but with histologically confirmed microscopic seeding of abdominal peritoneal surfaces
Stage IIIB:	Tumor of one or both ovaries with histologically confirmed implants of abdominal peritoneal surfaces, with none exceeding 2 cm in diameter. Nodes are negative
Stage IIIC:	Abdominal implants greater than 2 cm in diameter or positive retroperitoneal or inguinal nodes
Stage IV:	Growth involving one or both ovaries with distant metastases. If pleural effusion is present, there must be positive cytology to allot a case to stage IV. Parenchymal liver metastasis equals stage IV

Table 13.6 Pediatric Intergroup Trial (POG/CCG) – ovarian GCT staging [11, 12]

I	Limited to ovary, peritoneal washings negative for malignant cells; no clinical, radiologic, or histologic evidence of disease beyond the ovaries (gliomatosis peritonei did not result in upstaging); tumor markers negative after appropriate half-life decline
II	Microscopic residual or positive lymph nodes (<2 cm); peritoneal washings negative for malignant cells (gliomatosis peritonei did not result in upstaging); tumor markers positive or negative
III	Gross residual or biopsy only, tumor positive lymph node(s) >2 cm diameter; contiguous visceral involvement (omentum, intestine, bladder): peritoneal washings positive for malignant cells
IV	Distant metastases that may include liver

rectomy is performed. In 5–10% of malignant GCTs there is an associated contralateral benign mature cystic teratoma, and in these situations the remainder of that ovary can be preserved.

Unless grossly involved with a tumor, the uterus is left in place in the young patient with the desire for continued reproductive potential. The conventional approach of total abdominal hysterectomy with bilateral salpingo-oophorectomy for older patients with epithelial ovarian cancer is not indicated for younger women in view of current assisted reproductive techniques using donor oocytes with hormonal support. Such techniques make conception and childbearing a viable future alternative for such patients with a uterus but no ovaries [36–38].

13.3.9 Staging

Staging of pediatric and adult ovarian tumors of all types is confusing. The International Federation of Gynecology and Obstetrics (FIGO) developed a system for staging ovarian tumors (Table 13.5) [39]. This study provided the basis for the development of several pediatric GCT staging systems [41–43]. Modifications to the FIGO staging by the POG/CCG Intergroup led to a staging system that was similar to other staging systems used in childhood malignancies (Table 13.6). Stage I tumors are those that are completely resected, leaving clear margins. Stage II tumors are those resected with microscopic margins, positive lymph nodes less than 2 cm, or a delay in decline of tumor markers. Stage III disease patients are those with nodes less than 2 cm or visceral involvement, and stage IV patients have distant metastases.

13.3.10 GCTs: Surgical and Staging Considerations

Although 60–70% of malignant GCTs are stage I at diagnosis, 25–30% are stage III, and a proportion of these are advanced in stage due to occult metastases. In the recent pediatric intergroup trial, the distribution of malignant ovarian GCT in girls older than 12 years was: stage I 36%; stage II 8%; stage III 46%; and stage IV 10% [11, 12]. The majority of malignant ovarian GCTs are unilateral and large. One recent review identified a median size of 16 cm, with a range from 7–40 cm [9].

13.3.11 Teratomas: Surgical and Staging Considerations

When an adnexal mass is found to be a mature cystic teratoma, areas of squamous differentiation and small nodules in the wall of the cyst should be evaluated specifically for the presence of malignant elements. If present, the tumor should be treated as a malignant GCT and complete surgical staging attempted. Likewise, if immature elements, typically neural elements, are identified, the tumor is classified and treated as a malignant GCT. If, however, no malignant elements are identified, the neoplasm is benign and can be treated with an ovarian cystectomy alone. The contralateral ovary should be evaluated, as 12% of cases are bilateral. A contralateral cystectomy should be performed in this case, with preservation of as much normal ovarian tissue as possible [44, 45].

13.3.12 Dysgerminoma and Gonadoblastoma: Surgical and Staging Considerations

Patients diagnosed with dysgerminoma on pathologic frozen evaluation present a unique situation. A minority of these tumors have an associated gonadoblastoma and arise in a dysgenetic gonad in a phenotypically normal female with abnormal karyotype. The contralateral dysgenetic or "streak" gonad also carries a high potential for a future malignant GCT. Therefore, in cases of intra-operative diagnosis of dysgerminoma, the pathologist should be asked to carefully evaluate for any residual normal ovary and look for any elements of gonadoblastoma. As the pathologist is evaluating the specimen further, the surgeon should inspect the contralateral adnexa to determine whether a normal ovary or streak gonad is present. Normal ovarian tissue excludes the possibility of dysgenetic gonads, thereby allowing the surgeon to conserve the contralateral ovary and preserve reproductive potential [46]. However, in the event of a "streak" gonad or diagnosis of gonadoblastoma, a bilateral salpingo-oophorectomy should be performed to remove any gonadal tissue, regardless of age [9, 44, 46].

13.3.13 Sex Cord-Stromal Tumors: Surgical and Staging Considerations

A unilateral solid adnexal mass, often yellow and multilobulated in appearance, or hemorrhagic with hemoperitoneum evident, can suggest a granulosa cell tumor or other sex cord-stromal tumor. There is no evidence to recommend ovarian cystectomy in adolescent or reproductive-aged females with sex cord-stromal tumors. Unilateral salpingo-oophorectomy should be performed as the initial step in such patients with apparently limited disease [47]; once the diagnosis of a sex cord-stromal tumor is made, exploration of the entire abdomino-pelvic cavity should be performed, with attention to all peritoneal surfaces and abdomino-pelvic organs. A complete staging procedure should be performed (Appendix). Tumor reductive surgery should be performed for patients with advanced disease to reduce tumor burden as much as possible, preferably leaving the patient with no macroscopic disease [39, 48]. Many of these tumors occur in adolescent and reproductive-aged women, and although the majority are clinically indolent and have a good long-term prognosis, individualized treatment following appropriate guidelines is the key to successful outcomes.

13.3.14 Epithelial Ovarian Cancer: Surgical and Staging Considerations

The recommended surgical procedure for a patient of reproductive age with epithelial ovarian cancer who desires continued fertility, and who has clinically limited disease with no involvement of the contralateral ovary or uterus, includes conservative therapy with unilateral salpingo-oophorectomy and staging. In a review of 36 patients with stage IA disease who underwent conservative fertility-sparing surgery with complete staging, only 3 patients relapsed, 1 of whom had involvement of the residual ovary [49]. The incidence of microscopic disease in the residual ovary at the time of primary surgery is 5–7% [50], and bivalving or biopsy of the normal-appearing contralateral ovary in the patient with true stage I disease may be unwar-

ranted, as this may lead to adhesion formation and decreased fertility. It may be acceptable to preserve a normal-appearing uterus in early-stage disease even if both ovaries are removed, thus preserving the option of donor egg conception. Although these approaches are controversial, fertility-sparing surgery for true early-stage ovarian carcinoma appears to be a viable option if the patient is adequately counseled about fertility preservation and recurrence risk [21]. One exception to this may be for clear-cell histology, which may connote a significantly more aggressive tumor, contra-indicating conservative surgery [50]. In addition, consideration should be given to surgical removal of the contralateral ovary once childbearing is complete [21].

The majority of ovarian epithelial tumors diagnosed in young women are stage I. The rare patient with apparent advanced-stage epithelial disease should undergo cyto-reductive surgery with every attempt made to achieve an optimal tumor reduction (no implant greater than 1 cm) and, when possible, leave no visible tumor. Response to chemotherapy and survival are significantly improved in patients with optimal or complete cytoreduction [51]. Preservation of reproductive capacity in patients with advanced invasive epithelial ovarian cancer cannot be advised; in these patients, the uterus, cervix, tubes, and ovaries should be removed.

Treatment for patients with epithelial tumors who have had inadequate staging is a difficult issue. If the patient has documented large residual disease with a limited initial attempt at tumor reduction, repeat exploration with staging and tumor reductive surgery is indicated. If the patient has had an inadequate exploration, additional studies should be performed, including repeat laparoscopic or open exploration with full surgical staging or, in some circumstances, a post-operative CT, serum inhibin, and serum CA-125 levels.

13.3.15 LMP Tumors: Surgical and Staging Considerations

Although invasive epithelial ovarian cancer is typically a disease of post-menopausal women, LMP tumors tend to occur in younger women, with 71% occurring in pre-menopausal women. The average age at presentation is 40 years, approximately 10 years younger than the average age of women with invasive disease [52].

If the diagnosis of LMP tumor is made post-operatively, the patient may need to undergo repeat exploration for a staging procedure, as up to 24% of patients with apparent stage I or II disease are upstaged on repeat exploration [53], and a percentage of these patients may have invasive metastatic implants [54]. These findings are extremely important since they affect staging and treatment recommendations. Alternatively, close surveillance with periodic history and physical examinations, serum CA-125 levels, and CT scans can be performed.

13.4 Treatment

13.4.1 GCTs: Treatment Issues

The current treatment regimen for all patients with resected early-stage GCTs of the ovary is adjuvant therapy with bleomycin, etoposide, and cisplatin (BEP) [55]. The only exceptions to this schema are patients with stage IA or IB, grade 1 immature teratoma, and stage IA pure dysgerminoma. These patients should not receive adjuvant chemotherapy, but should be closely observed following surgery [56]. In addition, there is also an increasing body of literature supporting no post-surgical treatment (observation only) in patients with any stage I GCT [57, 58]. Future clinical trials should address and resolve this issue. When evaluating a patient, however, caution must be employed in labeling ovarian GCT as stage I. In a localized POG/CCG trial, surgical guidelines were followed in only 1 out of 56 patients. Since all patients subsequently received BEP, surgical attention to guidelines was not essential [12]. However, in trials where low-stage tumors are not treated with adjuvant chemotherapy, adherence to surgical guidelines will be critical.

In a GCT patient with greater than stage I disease, there is seldom a role for repeat laparotomy after an incomplete staging procedure. If it appears that the surgeon performed an adequate initial exploration to exclude gross residual disease, post-operative CT scan of the abdomen and pelvis can be used as confirma-

tion, and adjuvant chemotherapy with BEP should be initiated. If it is not possible to adequately evaluate the extra-pelvic contents and retroperitoneum for residual disease, then a repeat laparotomy with complete surgical staging is indicated.

Patients with gross residual disease or advanced-stage disease after initial surgery should receive BEP as outlined above. These patients should be followed with CT and tumor markers, and a total of three to six courses of BEP should be given [11]. There is no consensus at the present time on the optimal number of treatment cycles. Growth factors should be used to assist recovery of leukocyte counts and to minimize treatment delay for cytopenias [11, 12].

No standard regimen exists for the unusual patient with a recurrent GCT. Regimens that have been useful include EMA-EP; vinblastine, ifosfamide, and cisplatin; and ICE (ifosfamide, carboplatin, and etoposide; unpublished data, Thomas Olson). In selected patients, one should consider consolidation with high-dose chemotherapy and stem-cell rescue, although its role remains unclear.

Second-look surgery is not recommended for most patients with GCTs. The only exception is when the tumor has elements of immature teratoma and no serum markers are positive. In this situation, second-look surgery may be contemplated, but remains controversial [44, 55]. Patients with immature teratoma who have residual disease evident after treatment usually have either benign mature teratoma or gliosis comprising the mass [59]. A CT-guided biopsy to confirm this diagnosis, followed by serial imaging, may be preferable to a second major surgery. Likewise, patients with dysgerminoma who have a mass remaining at the conclusion of chemotherapy usually have only desmoplastic fibrosis [60]. This can be confirmed by CT-guided biopsy and followed with serial imaging.

13.4.2 Dysgerminomas: Treatment Issues

Although patients with dysgerminoma have historically been noted to be sensitive to radiation therapy, chemotherapy with BEP is more effective and less toxic, and it is less likely to adversely affect reproductive potential than is radiation therapy. BEP is therefore the preferred treatment for adjuvant and postoperative therapy. If elevated at diagnosis, LDH levels can be followed to document serologic response and to detect subclinical recurrence. Alternate chemotherapy regimens as outlined above and radiation therapy can be used to treat recurrent disease.

13.4.3 Sex Cord-Stromal Tumors: Treatment Issues

Since these neoplasms are rare, clinical trials designed to determine which regimens are best suited to specific histologic subtypes of sex cord-stromal tumors are not feasible. Most published studies combine most or all sex cord-stromal tumors together. Therefore, the recommendations for treatment of these tumors are based on limited data. The majority of data have been gathered from patients with adult granulosa cell tumors.

Adjuvant treatment for patients with surgically staged stage I disease is not indicated. Patients with stage IC disease may benefit from some adjuvant therapy such as paclitaxel and carboplatin or hormonal therapy with leuprolide acetate. Patients with more advanced disease are typically treated with combination chemotherapy, usually consisting of three to four courses of BEP [61]. A recent evaluation of the utility of taxanes and platinum in this setting has been carried out, but confirmation of equivalent outcomes between these two regimens awaits performance of a larger randomized trial [2, 62]. When patients recur after a long progression-free interval, they are candidates for repeat tumor-reductive surgery. With widespread disease or disease refractory to surgery, chemotherapy and hormonal therapy are options for treatment [63]. Radiation is also occasionally employed in the treatment of localized or symptomatic disease.

13.4.4 Granulosa Cell Tumors: Treatment Issues

Granulosa cell tumors occur in two distinct histologic varieties: juvenile and adult. The patient profile, natural history, and recommended treatment differ between these subtypes. Juvenile granulosa cell tumors present primarily in adolescents. In this patient population, the desire to maintain reproductive capacity without an adverse effect on survival is of paramount impor-

tance [47]. Survival of patients with early-stage tumors is above 95%, but accurate surgical staging is (therefore) imperative. Advanced-stage disease is typically more aggressive and less responsive to therapy. The adult type of granulosa cell tumor is rarely seen in younger women.

Any patient with greater than stage IA disease should receive platinum-based chemotherapy, usually in the form of BEP. When juvenile granulosa cell tumor recurs, it usually does so with a shorter progression-free interval than the adult type. For patients with recurrent disease there are many approaches to treatment, including surgical cytoreduction, radiation therapy, and chemotherapy. Despite aggressive treatment, however, few sustained responses have been noted. Hormonal therapy with leuprolide acetate has resulted in several cases of stable disease [63]. Although adult granulosa cell tumors are indolent lesions, they can recur many years, even decades, following the initial diagnosis and treatment. Patients should be followed at gradually increasing intervals with physical examinations and with serum inhibin and CA-125 levels.

13.4.5 Sertoli-Leydig Cell Tumors: Treatment Issues

This classification of tumors includes tumors comprised of Sertoli cells only, as well as tumors containing both Sertoli and Leydig cells. Tumors composed of Sertoli cells only are uniformly stage I, and only one death has been reported [64]. Sertoli-Leydig cell tumors, also called arrhenoblastomas, are rare, accounting for less than 0.2% of all ovarian tumors, and usually present in adolescents and young adults. Since stage is the most important predictor of outcome, these patients should be accurately staged (Table 13.5). Over 95% of these tumors are confined to one ovary at the time of diagnosis; therefore, a normal-appearing uterus and contralateral ovary can usually be preserved. Patients with disease greater than IB, with poorly differentiated tumors, or with heterologous elements present should be treated with BEP [65] or paclitaxel and carboplatin. Patients can be followed with physical examinations and with serum αFP, inhibin, and testosterone levels. Of the 18% of patients who recur, two-thirds do so within the 1st year after

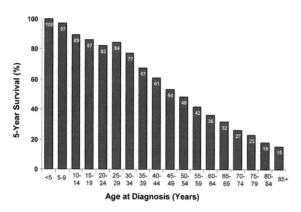

Figure 13.3

Five-year survival rates of females with ovarian malignancies, United States SEER [1]

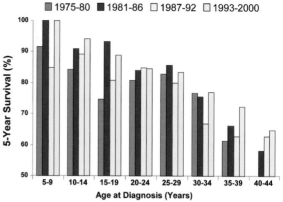

Figure 13.4

Five-year survival rates of females with ovarian malignancies as a function of era, United States SEER [1]

diagnosis. Additional platinum-based chemotherapy is the mainstay of treatment for recurrent disease.

A subgroup of the sex-cord tumor grouping is the ovarian sex-cord tumor with annular tubules. The biologic behavior of this lesion is thought to be intermediate between granulosa cell tumors and Sertoli cell tumors, and is associated with Peutz-Jeghers Syndrome [30, 31]. Surgical treatment recommendations are similar to those for other sex-cord stromal tumors, but patients should be carefully screened for adenoma malignum of the cervix, as 15% of patients harbor an occult lesion. For such patients, hysterectomy must be strongly considered [66].

Steroid cell tumors not otherwise specified are a distinct category of steroid cell tumor that can be malignant and aggressive; when diagnosed intraoperatively, these patients should be staged and aggressively cyto-reduced [67, 68]. Lipid cell tumors with pleomorphism, increased mitotic count, large size, or advanced stage should receive additional post-operative platinum-based therapy [68].

13.4.6 Epithelial Tumors: Treatment Issues

Patients with stage IA or IB, grade 1 epithelial tumors can be treated with surgery alone, although some would argue that patients with clear-cell histology should receive adjuvant chemotherapy regardless of stage [49, 50]. At the current time, patients with stage II and higher disease receive six courses of paclitaxel and platinum therapy. Consideration is given to consolidation chemotherapy thereafter, but this is not standard. Some debate exists over the optimal management of patients with stage IA or IB, grade 2 or 3 cancers, and stage IC cancers [50]. Most practitioners administer three to six courses of the aforementioned regimen, but the optimal number of courses in this situation is currently being investigated in a Gynecologic Oncology Group trial.

13.4.7 Ovarian Tumors of LMP: Treatment Issues

Multiple regimens of chemotherapy have been investigated for the treatment of advanced-stage LMP tumors, but no benefit in disease-free or overall survival (OS) has been demonstrated for any regimen at any stage. Therefore, chemotherapy is not administered to patients with LMP tumors of the ovary.

A minority of patients with LMP tumors of the ovary will have invasive implants on staging biopsies. These patients have a worse prognosis and a higher recurrence rate than patients with non-invasive implants [69]. Since these invasive implants represent small foci of invasive carcinoma, treatment recommendations are similar to those for women with epithelial ovarian carcinoma.

13.5 Outcomes

Survival of women with cancer of the ovary has been inversely proportional to age (Fig. 13.3). Progress in the 5-year survival rate over the past quarter century has been less in 15- to 29-year-olds than in younger or older women (Fig. 13.4).

13.5.1 Germ-Cell Tumors

Historically, patients with malignant ovarian GCTs treated with surgery alone had a poor survival rate. Prior to the consistent use of chemotherapy, the outcome for patients with ovarian non-germinomatous tumors was poor, with survival rates of 15–20% [70]. Patients with germinomatous tumors could be cured with surgery alone [71, 72] or with surgery combined with chemotherapy [73, 74].

In the POG/CCG Intergroup studies, patients were assigned treatment based on tumor histology (immature teratoma) and clinical (surgical) staging. Patients (n=44) with ovarian immature teratomas were treated successfully with surgery and observation [56]. Despite the presence of yolk sac elements in resected specimens (13/44), only 1 patient relapsed and was salvaged with chemotherapy.

In the POG/CCG study, all stage I/II ovarian GCTs were treated with four cycles of BEP, but only received 33% of the adult bleomycin dose, due to concerns about pulmonary toxicity. Even at the reduced dose, there was a 6-year event-free survival (EFS) of 93% and 6-year OS of 94% in this group of patients [12]. Recent adult and pediatric studies suggest that patients with stage I ovarian GCTs can be managed with surgery and observation [41, 75]. In a report on 15 patients with ovarian stage I GCT (9 immature teratoma and 6 endodermal sinus tumors) treated with surveillance, only 3 relapsed (20%), two of whom were salvaged successfully with chemotherapy. Salvage chemotherapy [59] might be reserved for patients with progressive tumors or for those whose markers do not decline appropriately and normalize [76]. Several European studies have similarly shown that resected stage I tumors can be treated with observation alone, with a 20–50% relapse rate; most, however, can subsequently be salvaged with chemotherapy [42, 43, 75].

Between 1990 and 1996, 299 eligible pediatric patients with stage III/IV gonadal and stage I–IV extragonadal GCTs were randomized on POG9049/CCG8882 to standard BEP or high-dose BEP (HDBEP), with high-dose cisplatin (40 mg/m2/day × 5). HDBEP resulted in a significantly improved 6-year EFS (89.6±3.6% vs BEP 80.5±4.8%; p=0.0284). There was no difference in OS (HDPEB 91.7±3.3% vs BEP 86.0±4.1%). Although the study was not designed to have sufficient power to test for differences within each smaller susbset (testicular, ovarian, extragonadal), there was a trend toward improved EFS and OS for each subset. The trend was most pronounced for extragonadal GCT. However, severe ototoxicity (grade 3/4, resulting in the need for hearing aids) was a consequence of HDBEP (67% vs BEP 10.5%) [11]. The treatment results for high-risk ovarian GCTs are shown in Table 13.7. Few patients had stage IV ovarian GCT; the ten treated with HDBEP all survived. Two of six who were treated with BEP recurred, although one was salvaged. Both patients were under 10 years of age. These small numbers make conclusions difficult. The results for all ovarian GCT patients on both POG/CCG trials are shown in Table 13.8.

13.5.2 Sex Cord-Stromal Tumors

In a study of 72 patients with sex cord-stromal tumors registered at the German Pediatric Tumor Registry, EFS was 88% at 10 years. Refractory tumors in this group were characterized by high proliferative activity [77].

13.5.3 Epithelial Tumors

The prognosis for young women with epithelial ovarian cancer appears to be independent of age [21]. Surveillance after treatment may consist of a CT scan at the completion of therapy, followed by physical examinations and serum CA-125 levels every 3 months for the 1st year, every 4 months for the next year, every

Table 13.7 POG/CCG high-risk trial – ovarian GCT [11, 12]. *EFS* Event-free survival, *OS* overall survival

Stage and age	N	6-year EFS (%) ± SE	6-year OS (%) ± SE
Stage III <10 years	18	94.4 ± 8.4	100
Stage III >10 years	40	97.5 ± 3.5	97.5 ± 3.5
Stage IV <10 years	6	66.7 ± 22.2	83.3 ± 17
Stage IV >10 years	10	100	100

Table 13.8 Treatment of ovarian GCT – Pediatric Intergroup Trials [11, 12]

Stage	N	6-year EFS (%)	6-year OS (%)
I	41	95.1	95.1
II	16	87.5	93.8
III	58	96.6	98.3
IV	16	86.7	93.3

6 months for the ensuing 3 years, and annually thereafter. CT surveillance is recommended only for patients with symptoms, physical findings, or elevated serum CA-125 levels. In one review of 19 patients diagnosed before the age of 21 years, 15 (79%) had stage I disease and 4 (21%) had stage III disease. There were two deaths in this series, both from small-cell anaplastic carcinoma, which is rare in this age group [78].

13.5.4 Tumors of LMP

The indolent nature of LMP tumors is best demonstrated by the 95% 5-year survival and 80% 20-year survival for all stages. Although the recurrence rate is between 7 and 30%, these tumors usually recur as LMP tumors and not invasive malignancies. Thus, they are amenable to repeat surgical resection. In one study of 12 patients <40 years of age with early-stage disease who were treated with fertility-sparing surgery, there was 100% survival and up to 50% subsequent conception [79].

13.6 Conclusions

Ovarian tumors are rare in children, adolescents, and young adults. As a result, relatively little information exists about incidence rates, treatment, and outcomes for specific ovarian tumors for these age groups. This chapter is designed as a guide for the evaluation and treatment of ovarian tumors in adolescents and young adults, with the goal of engendering interest in studies aimed specifically at this patient population.

Ovarian neoplasms represent a diagnostic and therapeutic dilemma because of the desire to maintain fertility in this young age group. Thankfully, the majority of neoplasms present at an early stage with generally good long-term survival. Further work is necessary to delineate appropriate screening for young women at risk for ovarian cancers. Advances in assisted reproductive medicine will probably impact the management of this group of patients in the future.

Although the vast majority of ovarian cancers in adult women are epithelial in origin, 60–70% of ovarian malignancies in children and adolescents are non-epithelial, consisting primarily of germ-cell and sex cord-stromal tumors [80]. Hence, the adolescent and young adult years are a time of transition in tumor type, as the incidence of non-epithelial tumors gradually decreases and epithelial tumors become more common. Surgery, chemotherapy, radiation, and hormonal therapy are all components of treatment, but specific management recommendations are dependent on many factors, including patient age, tumor histology, karyotype, and extent of disease. Conservative surgery to maintain reproductive potential is an important consideration in the treatment of all adolescents and young adults with ovarian tumors.

Appropriate surgical staging and assessment are necessary components in determining the extent of surgery required and the need for post-operative chemotherapy. With the advent of modern surgical and post-surgical techniques, response rates and survival have improved dramatically and are excellent for most tumor types.

Acknowledgments

The authors wish to thank Jan Watterson for her assistance in the preparation of this manuscript and the Pine Tree Apple Tennis Classic Oncology Research Fund for their support.

Appendix: Surgical Guidelines for the Adolescent with an Ovarian Tumor

Surgery should be preceded by a thorough bowel preparation. The patient should be placed in the dorsal lithotomy position in the operating room, and a vertical midline incision is made. Ascites, if present, is aspirated and sent for permanent cytologic examination. If no ascites is present, the pelvis should be irrigated with 100–200 ml of normal saline, which should be aspirated and sent for permanent cytologic examination. The abdomen and pelvis should then be thoroughly examined by visualization and palpation, with attention directed to all peritoneal surfaces, the liver and sub-hepatic region, diaphragm, retroperitoneal structures, omentum, colon, small bowel, mesentery, and all pelvic contents, including both adnexae, the uterus, and all peritoneal surfaces. The enlarged ovary or pelvic mass should be removed and sent to pathology for immediate evaluation.

If the unequivocal diagnosis of invasive ovarian cancer is made, a gynecologic oncologist should be consulted immediately for intra-operative assistance. The surgeon must determine the extent of disease. If there is extra-ovarian disease, the surgeon must first determine if the disease can be resected to less than 1 cm of residual disease. This concept of a maximal cyto-reductive surgical effort is imperative for a successful outcome. Every attempt should be made to remove all visible disease, as patients with no macroscopic disease at the completion of the surgical procedure have the best prognosis. If the largest residual focus of disease after tumor-reductive surgery is 1 cm or less, this is referred to as "optimal cyto-reduction" and connotes a significant survival benefit. If the tumor is unresectable to this extent, leaving residual disease greater than 1 cm in any one location, this is considered "sub-optimal," and the patient should have appropriate surgery to relieve symptoms and the procedure should then be terminated. That is, if an impending bowel obstruction exists, a bowel resection and re-anastomosis should be performed; if the patient has a large amount of ascites with an omental cake, an omentectomy should be performed. However, there is no justification for performing extensive tumor-reductive surgery if a focus of disease greater than 1 cm will remain at the completion of the surgery.

In the patient with no gross evidence of extra-ovarian disease, a full staging procedure should be performed. This consists of cytology of each hemi-diaphragm, infra-colic omentectomy, and peritoneal biopsy specimens from each paracolic gutter, the vesico-uterine fold, and the pouch of Douglas. In addition, any suspicious areas should be sampled. Pelvic and para-aortic lymph node sampling are recommended for full staging, as a small percentage of patients will have apparent early-stage disease but have positive lymph nodes on final review, thereby changing the stage, recommended treatment, and prognosis. The bowel should be inspected from the ileocecal valve to the ligament of Treitz, specifically evaluating for tumor implants and sites of obstruction. Approximately 30% of patients with apparent limited disease are upstaged at the time of staging. This significantly impacts treatment recommendations and prognosis.

It should be noted that the majority of adolescents and young adults with ovarian cancers will have non-epithelial histology. These patients can usually be treated with fertility-sparing surgery, as the tumor generally impacts only one adnexa. Therefore, in the absence of a grossly abnormal contra-lateral ovary or uterus, a unilateral salpingo-oophorectomy can be performed with a complete staging procedure and tumor-reductive surgery as outlined above, preserving the contralateral ovary and tube and the uterus.

References

1. Bleyer WA O'Leary M, Barr R, Ries LAG (eds) (2006) Cancer Epidemiology in Older Adolescents and Young Adults 15 to 29 Years of Age, including SEER Incidence and Survival, 1975–2000. National Cancer Institute, NIH Pub. No. 06-5767, Bethesda MD; also available at www.seer.cancer.gov/publications

2. Brown J, Shvartsman HS, Deavers MT, et al (2004b) The activity of taxanes in the treatment of sex cord-stromal ovarian tumors. J Clin Oncol 22:3517–3523

3. Raney RB Jr, Sinclair L, Uri A, et al (1987) Malignant ovarian tumors in children and adolescents. Cancer 59:1214–1220

4. Bernstein L, Smith MA, Liu L, et al (1999) Germ cell, trophoblastic and other gonadal neoplasms ICCC X. In: Ries AG, Smith MA, Gurney JG, et al (eds) Cancer incidence and survival among children and adolescents: United States SEER Program 1975–1995. NIH Pub. No. 99-4649. Bethesda: National Cancer Institute, SEER Program, pp 139–147

5. Serov SF, Scully RE, Robin IH (1973) Histological Typing of Ovarian Tumors: International Histological Classification of Tumors, World Health Organization, Geneva, No. 9

6. Young JL Jr, Wu XC, Roffers SD, et al (2003) Ovarian cancer in children and young adults in the United States, 1992–1997. Cancer 97: 2694–2700

7. Morowitz M, Huff D, von Allmen D (2003) Epithelial ovarian tumors in children: a retrospective analysis. J Pediatr Surg 38:331–335

8. Fotiou SK (1997) Ovarian malignancies in adolescence. Ann NY Acad Sci 816:338–346

9. Williams SD, Gershenson DM, Horowitz CJ, et al (2000) Ovarian GCT. In: Hoskins WJ, Perez CA, Young RC (eds) Principles and Practice of Gynecologic Oncology (3rd edn). Lippincott Williams and Wilkins, Philadelphia, pp 1059–1073

10. Emans SJH, Laufer MF, Goldstein DP (eds) (1998) Pediatric and Adolescent Gynecology (4th edn). Lippincott-Raven, Philadelphia, p 562

11. Cushing B, Giller R, Cullen JW, et al (2004) Randomized comparison of combination chemotherapy with etoposide, bleomycin, and either high-dose or standard-dose cisplatin in children and adolescents with high-risk malignant germ cell tumors: a pediatric intergroup study – Pediatric Oncology Group 9049 and Children's Cancer Group 8882. J Clin Oncol 22:2691–2700

12. Rogers PC, Olson TA, Cullen JW, et al (2004) Treatment of children and adolescents with stage II testicular and stages I and II ovarian malignant germ cell tumors: a Pediatric Intergroup Study – Pediatric Oncology Group 9048 and Children's Cancer Group 8891. J Clin Oncol 22:3563–3569

13. Castedo SM, de Jong B, Oosterhuis JW, et al (1989) Chromosomal changes in human primary testicular nonseminomatous germ cell tumors. Cancer Res 49:5696–5701

14. Riopel MA, Spellerberg A, Griffin CA, et al (1998) Genetic analysis of ovarian germ cell tumors by comparative genomic hybridization. Cancer Res 58:3105–3110

15. Samaniego F, Rodriguez E, Houldsworth J, et al (1990) Cytogenetic and molecular analysis of human male germ cell tumors: chromosome 12 abnormalities and gene amplification. Genes Chromosomes Cancer 1:289–300

16. Bussey KJ, Lawce HJ, Olson SB, et al (1999) Chromosome abnormalities of eighty-one pediatric germ cell tumors: sex-, age-, site-, and histopathology-related differences – a Children's Cancer Group study. Genes Chromosomes Cancer 25:134–146

17. Perlman EJ, Hu J, Ho D, et al (2000) Genetic analysis of childhood endodermal sinus tumors by comparative genomic hybridization. J Pediatr Hematol Oncol 22:100–105

18. Schneider DT, Schuster AE, Fritsch MK, et al (2001) Multipotent imprinting analysis indicates a common precursor cell for gonadal and nongonadal pediatric germ cell tumors. Cancer Res 61:7268–7276

19. Schneider DT, Schuster AE, Fritsch MK, et al (2001) Genetic analysis of childhood germ cell tumors with comparative genomic hybridization. Klin Padiatr 213:204–211

20. Koonings PP, Campbell K, Mishell DR Jr, et al (1989) Relative frequency of primary ovarian neoplasms: a 10-year review. Obstet Gynecol 74:921–926

21. Duska LR, Chang Y, Flynn CE (1999) Epithelial ovarian cancer in the reproductive age group. Cancer 85:2623–2629

22. Hogg R, Friedlander M (2004) Biology of epithelial ovarian cancer: implications for screening women at high genetic risk. J Clin Oncol 22:1315–1327

23. Taylor HC (1929) Malignant and semimalignant tumors of the ovary. Surg Gynecol Obstet 48:204–230

24. Lawrence WD (1995) The borderland between benign and malignant surface epithelial ovarian tumors. Current controversy over the nature and nomenclature of 'borderline' ovarian tumors. Cancer 76:2138–2142

25. Katsube Y, Berg JW, Silverberg SG (1982) Epidemiologic pathology of ovarian tumors: a histopathologic review of primary ovarian neoplasms diagnosed in the Denver Standard Metropolitan Statistical Area 1 July–31 December 1969 and 1 July–31 December 1979. Int J Gynecol Pathol 1:3–16

26. Scully RE (1982) Common epithelial tumors of borderline malignancy. Bull Cancer (Paris) 69:228–238

27. Kohlberger PD, Kieback DG, Mian C, et al (1997) Numerical chromosomal aberrations in borderline,

benign, and malignant epithelial tumors of the ovary: correlation with p53 protein overexpression and Ki-67. J Soc Gynecol Invest 4:262–264

28. Gribbon, M, Ein SH, Mancer K (1992) Pediatric malignant ovarian tumors: a 43-year review. J Pediatr Surg 27:480–484

29. Lacson AG, Gillis DA, Shawwa A (1988) Malignant mixed germ-cell-sex cord-stromal tumors of the ovary associated with isosexual precocious puberty. Cancer 61:2122–2133

30. Scully RE (1970) Sex cord tumor with annular tubules: a distinctive ovarian tumor of the Peutz-Jeghers syndrome. Cancer 25:1107–1121

31. Young RH, Welch WR, Dickersin GR, Scully RE (1982) Ovarian sex cord tumor with annular tubules: review of 74 cases including 27 with Peutz-Jeghers syndrome and four with adenoma malignum of the cervix. Cancer 50:1384–1402

32. Berek JS, Hacker NF (eds) (1994) Nonepithelial ovarian and fallopian tube cancers. In: Practical Gynecologic Oncology (2nd edn). Williams and Wilkins, Baltimore, pp 380–381

33. Tewari K, Cappuccini F, Disaia PJ, et al (2000) Malignant germ cell tumors of the ovary. Obstet Gynecol 95:128–133

34. Bjorkholm E, Silfversward C (1981) Prognostic factors in granulosa-cell tumors. Gynecol Oncol 11:261–274

35. Vergote I, De Brabanter J, Fyles A, et al (2001) Prognostic importance of degree of differentiation and cyst rupture in stage I invasive epithelial ovarian carcinoma. Lancet 357:176–182

36. Billmire D, Vinocur C, Rescorla F, et al (2004) Outcome and staging evaluation in malignant germ cell tumors of the ovary in children and adolescents: an intergroup study. J Pediatr Surg 39:424–429

37. Abu-Rustum NR, Aghajanian C (1998) Management of malignant germ cell tumors of the ovary. Semin Oncol 25:235–242

38. Gershenson DM (1994) Management of early ovarian cancer: germ cell and sex cord-stromal tumors. Gynecol Oncol 55:S62–72

39. Cannistra SA (1993) Cancer of the ovary. N Engl J Med 329:1550–1559

40. International Federation of Gynecology and Obstetrics (1987) Changes in definitions of clinical staging for carcinoma of the cervix and ovary. Am J Obstet Gynecol 156:263–264

41. Baranzelli MC, Flamant F, De Lumley L, et al (1993) Treatment of non-metastatic, non-seminomatous malignant germ-cell tumours in childhood: experience of the "Societe Francaise d'Ongologie Pediatrique" MGCT 1985–1989 study. Med Pediatr Oncol 21:395–401

42. Gobel U, Calaminus G, Haas RJ, et al (1989) Combination chemotherapy in malignant non-seminomatous germ-cell tumors: results of a cooperative study of the German Society of Pediatric Oncology (MAKEI 83). Cancer Chemother Pharmacol 24:34–39

43. Mann JR, Raafat T, Robinson K, et al (2000) The United Kingdom Children's Cancer Study Group's second germ cell tumor study: carboplatin, etoposide, and bleomycin are effective treatment for children with malignant extracranial germ cell tumors, with acceptable toxicity. J Clin Oncol. 18:3809–3818

44. Gershenson DM (1994) Editorial: The obsolescence of second-look laparotomy in the management of malignant ovarian germ cell tumors. Gynecol Oncol 52:283–285

45. Disaia PJ, Creasman WT (eds) (2002) Germ cell, stromal, and other ovarian tumors. In: Clinical Gynecologic Oncology (6th edn). Mosby, St. Louis, MO, pp 362–363

46. Brewer M, Gershenson DM, Herzog CE, et al (1999) Outcome and reproductive function after chemotherapy for ovarian dysgerminoma. J Clin Oncol 17:2670–2675

47. Schumer ST, Cannistra SA (2003) Granulosa cell tumor of the ovary. J Clin Oncol 21:1180–1189

48. Pfleiderer A (1993) Therapy of ovarian malignant germ cell tumors and granulosa tumors. Int J Gynecol Pathol 12:162–165

49. Colombo N, Chiari S, Maggioni A, et al (1994) Controversial issues in the management of early epithelial ovarian cancer: conservative surgery and role of adjuvant therapy. Gynecol Oncol 55:S47–S51

50. Le T, Krepart GV, Lotocki RJ, Heywood MS (1999) Clinically apparent early stage invasive epithelial ovarian carcinoma: should all be treated similarly? Gynecol Oncol 74:252–254

51. Hoskins WJ (1994) Epithelial ovarian carcinoma: principles of primary surgery. Gynecol Oncol 55:S91–96

52. Lin PS, Gershenson DM, Bevers MW, et al (1999) The current status of surgical staging of ovarian serous borderline tumors. Cancer 85:905–911

53. Yazigi R, Sandstad J, Munoz AK (1988) Primary staging in ovarian tumors of low malignant potential. Gynecol Oncol 31:402–408

54. Gershenson DM, Silva EG, Levy L, et al (1998) Ovarian serous borderline tumors with invasive peritoneal implants. Cancer 82:1096–1103

55. Williams S, Blessing JA, Liao S-Y, et al (1994) Adjuvant therapy of ovarian GCT with cisplatin, etoposide, and bleomycin: a trial of the Gynecologic Oncology Group. J Clin Oncol 12:701–706

56. Marina NM, Cushing B, Giller R, et al (1999) Complete surgical excision is effective treatment for children with immature teratomas with or without malignant elements: a Pediatric Oncology Group/Children's Cancer Group Intergroup Study. J Clin Oncol 17:2137–2143

57. Dark GG, Bower M, Newlands ES, et al (1997) Surveillance policy for stage I ovarian germ cell tumors. J Clin Oncol 15:620–624

58. Gobel U, Calaminus G, Haas RJ, et al (2000) Germ-cell tumors in childhood and adolescence. GPOH MAKEI and the MAHO study groups. Ann Oncol 11:263–271

59. Gershenson DM, Copeland LJ, del Junco, et al (1986) Second-look laparotomy in the management of malignant germ cell tumors of the ovary. Cancer 67:789–793

60. Munkarah A, Gershenson DM, Levenback C, et al (1994) Salvage surgery for chemorefractory ovarian germ cell tumors. Gynecol Oncol 55:217–223

61. Homesley HD, Bundy BN, Hurteau JA, et al (1999) Bleomycin, etoposide, and cisplatin combination therapy of ovarian granulosa cell tumors and other stromal malignancies: a Gynecologic Oncology Group study. Gynecol Oncol 72:131–137

62. Brown J, Shvartsman HS, Deavers MT, et al (2004) Taxane-based chemotherapy compared with bleomycin, etoposide, and cisplatin for the treatment of sex cord-stromal ovarian tumors. Gynecol Oncol 92:402

63. Fishman A, Kudelka AP, Tresukosol D, et al (1996) Leuprolide acetate for treating refractory or persistent ovarian granulosa cell tumor. J Reprod Med 41:393–396

64. Young RH, Scully RE (1984) Ovarian Sertoli cell tumors: a report of 10 cases. Int J Gynecol Pathol 2:349–363

65. Gershenson DM, Morris M, Burke TW, et al (1996) Treatment of poor-prognosis sex cord-stromal tumors of the ovary with the combination of bleomycin, etoposide, and cisplatin. Obstet Gynecol 87:527–531

66. Srivatsa PJ, Keeney GL, Podratz KC (1994) Disseminated cervical adenoma malignum and bilateral ovarian sex cord tumors with annular tubules associated with Peutz-Jeghers syndrome. Gynecol Oncol 53:256–264

67. Gershenson DM, Copeland LJ, Kavanagh JJ, et al (1987) Treatment of metastatic stromal tumors of the ovary with cisplatin, doxorubicin, and cyclophosphamide. Obstet Gynecol 70:765–769

68. Hartmann LC, Young RH, Podratz KC. (2000) Ovarian sex cord-stromal tumors. In: Hoskins WJ, Perez CA, Young RC (eds) Principles and Practice of Gynecologic Oncology (3rd edn). Lippincott Williams and Wilkins, Philadelphia, pp 1075–1097

69. Deavers MT, Gershenson DM, Tortolero-Luna G, et al (2002) Micropapillary and cribiform patterns in ovarian serous tumors of low malignant potential: a study of 99 advanced stage cases. Am J Surg Pathol 26:1129–1141

70. Kurman RJ, Norris HJ (1976) Endodermal sinus tumor of the ovary: A clinical and pathologic analysis of 71 cases. Cancer 38:2404–2419

71. Marina N, Fontanesi J, Jun L, et al (1992) Treatment of childhood germ cell tumors: review of the St. Jude experience from 1979–1988. Cancer 70:2568–2575

72. Susnerwala SS, Pande SC, Shrivastava SK, Dinshaw KA (1991) Dysgerminoma of the ovary: review of 27 cases. J Surg Oncol 46:43–47

73. Gershenson DM, Morris M, Cangir A, et al (1990) Treatment of malignant GCT of the ovary with bleomycin, etoposide, and cisplatin. J Clin Oncol 8:715–720

74. La Polla JP, Brenda J, Vigliotti AP, Anderson B (1987) Dysgerminoma of the ovary. Obstet Gynecol 69:859–864

75. Baranzelli MC, Bouffet E, Quintana E, et al (2000) Nonseminomatous ovarian germ cell tumours in children. Eur J Cancer 36:376–383

76. Murphy BA, Motzer RJ, Mazumdar M, et al (1994) Serum tumor marker decline is an early predictor of treatment outcome in germ cell tumor patients treated with cisplatin and ifosfamide salvage chemotherapy. Cancer 73:2520–2526

77. Schneider DT, Janig M, Calaminus, et al (2003) Ovarian sex-cord stromal tumors – a clinicopathological study of 72 cases from the Kiel Pediatric Tumor Registry. Virchows Arch 443:549–560

78. Tsai JY, Saigo PE, Brown C, La Quaglia MP (2001) Diagnosis, pathology, staging, treatment, and outcome of epithelial ovarian neoplasia in patients age < 21 years. Cancer 91:2065–2070

79. Demeter A, Csapo Z, Szantho A, et al (2002) A retrospective study of 27 ovarian tumors of low malignant potential. Eur J Gynaecol Oncol XXIII:415–418

80. DeCherney AH, Nathan L (2003) Current Obstetric and Gynecologic Diagnosis and Treatment (9th edn). Lange Medical Books/McGraw-Hill, New York, p 612

81. Plante M (2000) Fertility preservation in the management of gynecologic cancers. Curr Opin Oncol 12:497–507

Testicular Tumors

John W. Cullen • Robert Fallon

Contents

14.1 Introduction

Cancer of the testis is the most common solid tumor diagnosis in males aged 15–29 years [1]. During the past quarter century in the United States, it increased in incidence among all age groups between 15 and 30 years and was the third most rapidly increasing cancer in males 25 to 40 years of age [1]. Advances in the treatment of testicular cancer, especially platinum-based combination chemotherapy over the last 25 years, have resulted in survival figures of 80–90%. Despite these achievements, challenges remain in understanding the biological and molecular mechanisms of aggressive and resistant tumors, and in delivering curative therapy to the adolescent and young adult population. This chapter describes the pathology, incidence, and treatment of testicular cancer, highlighting where possible the special considerations applicable to the adolescent and young adult population.

14.2 Epidemiology and Etiology

Testicular cancer is the most common solid-tumor neoplasm in males aged 15–29 years, accounting for 21.4% of cancers in this age group and reaching a peak incidence between 30 and 35 years of age (Fig. 14.1) [1]. This contrasts sharply with the incidence of testicular cancer in individuals aged 0–14 years, in whom it represents 2% of all cancers, and in the 30- to 45-year age group, in whom it comprises 7% of cancer diagnoses. Approximately 2,088 cases of testicular cancer were diagnosed in the United States in adolescent and

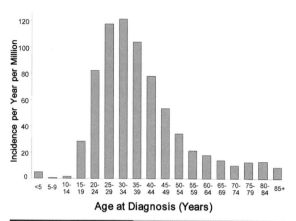

Figure 14.1

Incidence of testicular cancer, United States SEER 1975–2000 [1]

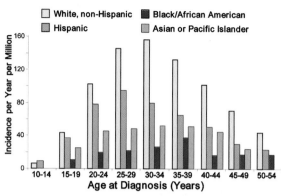

Figure 14.2

Incidence of testicular cancer by ethnicity, United States SEER 1975–2000 [1]

young adult men, aged 15–29 years, during 2000, according to recent Surveillance, Epidemiology, and End Results (SEER) data [1, 2]. The incidence of testicular cancer varies dramatically with race/ethnicity in the following order from most to least common: non-Hispanic whites, Hispanics/Latinos, Asian/Pacific Islanders, African Americans/blacks (Fig. 14.2).

The incidence of testicular cancer has increased in all age groups during the past quarter century (Fig. 14.3), and this increase appears to be worldwide. However, considerable variation in incidence has been observed between countries. Denmark, for example, has an incidence of 92 cases per million, while neighboring Finland's rate is only 25 per million. Ethnic and racial factors have a profound effect on testicular cancer incidence. In the United States, for example, white men are diagnosed at a rate 4–5 times that of black men, although the incidence rates for both are increasing.

Cryptorchidism is a proven risk factor for testicular cancer, both on the ipsilateral and the contralateral side. The risk of developing cancer in an undescended testis is increased by a factor of 2.5- to 11-fold. Other environmental and genetic causative factors have been proposed but not proven. Klinefelter's syndrome is associated with mediastinal germ-cell tumor, but not with increased risk of testicular cancer. Assessment of several environmental or hormonal factors has failed

to show a convincing association with testicular cancer (hernia, trauma, x-ray exposure, viral infection, positive family history, or high maternal hormone levels).

14.3 Biology and Pathology

The primordial germ cells arise in the yolk sac during the 4th week of gestation and then migrate to the gonadal ridge. During this migration, the stromal sex cords form from celomic epithelium and will develop into the seminiferous tubules and supportive structures of the testicle, including Sertoli cells. Differentiation into the testes begins in the 6th week of gestation, under the influence of the Y chromosome. Further migration to the iliac fossa and, finally, the scrotum should occur by the 8th month of gestation. Failure in the processes of differentiation and migration, at the varying steps, accounts for the pathological variety in testicular germ-cell tumors.

The expression of c-kit receptor has been demonstrated in fetal and infantile gonocytes and carcinoma in situ, but not in normal adult testes. Its persistence may indicate the presence of an unstable fetal phenotype or lack of adult-type differentiation and raises the question of whether c-kit contributes to invasive germ-cell tumors.

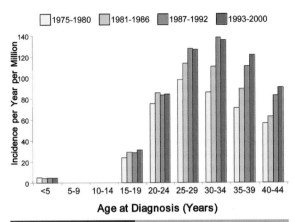

☐ 1975-1980 ☐ 1981-1986 ▨ 1987-1992 ■ 1993-2000

Figure 14.3

Incidence of testicular cancer by era, United States SEER 1992–2000 [1]

Yolk sac endodermal sinus tumors arise as a result of lack of differentiation. They are the most common testicular tumor in prepubertal boys, accounting for more than 90% of all germ-cell tumors in this group, but are virtually non-existent in adults. Genetically, these tumors are commonly diploid or tetraploid, whereas adolescent and adult germ-cell tumors are aneuploid. In addition, the chromosomal abnormalities found in testicular tumors vary between pre-pubertal and pubertal or post-pubertal males. Pubertal and post-pubertal males with germ-cell tumors express the isochromosome 12p, and in some cases, multiple copies may be present [3]. In pre-pubertal boys, gains of 21, 7, and 1q and deletions of 1p have been demonstrated [4].

Germ-cell tumors usually produce one or more substances that may be measured to assist in diagnosis, assign stage, determine prognosis, assess tumor response to therapy, and monitor for recurrence. Alpha-fetoprotein (AFP) is produced by cells of yolk sac origin, (i.e., yolk sac tumors: endodermal sinus tumor, Teilum's tumor), embryonal carcinoma, and teratocarcinoma (mixed nonseminomatous germ-cell tumors), whereas AFP is not produced by a pure seminoma or a pure choriocarcinoma. Thus, even when a diagnosis of pure seminoma is made, in the presence of an elevated AFP, the tumor must be considered mixed and should be treated as a non-seminomatous

tumor. The half-life of AFP is generally considered to be 4–5 days in adults. The initial level may assist in prognosis and the rate of fall with treatment may predict response. Elevated AFP levels can be monitored in stage I patients, in the surgery and observation strategy. Failure of AFP to normalize or elevations following normalization are indications for institution of chemotherapy. However, while AFP is an excellent tumor marker for germ-cell tumor it is not pathognomonic, with elevations of AFP first reported in hepatocellular carcinomas. Other malignancies, including hepatoblastoma, gastric, pancreatic, and pulmonary tumors, have been associated with elevations of AFP. AFP is also elevated in ataxia telangectasia, tyrosinemia, pregnancy, and benign liver diseases. For this reason, the Children's Oncology Group (COG) requires a level greater than five times the upper limit of normal for a diagnosis of recurrence in the absence of histological proof of relapse.

Human chorionic gonadotropin (hCG) is secreted by syncytiotrophoblasts and consists of alpha (α) and beta (ß) subunits. The α subunit is closely related to the α subunit of follicle stimulating hormone, luteinizing hormone (LH), and thyroid stimulating hormone. The ß subunit, however, is structurally distinct and can be measured. The half-life is 16–24 h, and it is elevated in 40–60% of all germ-cell tumors, 100% of choriocarcinomas, and 80% of embryonal carcinomas. In addition, it is elevated in 10–25% of seminomas. hCG can be used in a manner similar to AFP when elevations are present at diagnosis. Occasionally, the ß subunit of LH may interfere or crossreact in immunoassays for ß-hCG. Similar to AFP, elevated hCG levels may be seen in a variety of other malignancies as well as in pregnancy and some gestational disorders.

Lactate dehydrogenase (LDH) has been incorporated into the TNM (tumor-node-metastases) staging system and the International Germ Cell Consensus Classification Group (IGCCCG) prognostic classification for metastatic testicular germ-cell tumors. It is a very non-specific marker and may be elevated in many common conditions. It is not associated with specific histologic types of germ-cell tumor. It is not helpful in diagnosis, but may be used as a marker for response and recurrence. It is not currently employed by the

COG for prognostication, nor in the formulation of treatment decisions.

Germ-cell tumors account for 75% of testicular tumors in childhood and 90% of adult testicular tumors. However, in the adolescent and young adult patient groups, non-seminomatous tumors predominate. In the 15- to 21-year-old population, mixed non-seminomatous tumors (teratocarcinoma) with various combinations of embryonal carcinoma, yolk sac tumor, choriocarcinoma, and teratoma are most common. The peak age for seminomas occurs at age 30 years. When all ages of adults are considered, pure seminomas constitute 40%, non-seminomatous tumors 35%, and mixed seminoma non-seminomatous tumors 15%.

14.4 Clinical Symptoms and Evaluation

Testicular tumors most commonly present as a firm to hard painless mass. Occasionally, scrotal swelling and acute pain (10%) may be present. The presence of acute pain increases the likelihood of infection, trauma, torsion, and infarction, but does not rule out tumor or tumor in addition to another diagnosis. A history of trauma is present in 30% of cases. Carcinoma in situ most commonly presents in patients being evaluated for infertility. Germ-cell tumors present more commonly in patients with a history of cryptorchidism and testicular atrophy. Patients with either condition should have both testicles carefully evaluated periodically. Carcinoma in situ occurs in 5% of testes corrected for non-descent and in 5% of the contra-lateral testes in patients with a primary testicular germ-cell tumor. In children, up to 20% of cases are associated with hernia or hydrocele. Tran-silumination will assist with diagnosis of the hydrocele, but does not rule out the co-existence of tumor.

Patients with small or even occult primary testicular tumors may present with symptoms of large metastases (10%). These most commonly occur in the retroperitoneum and may cause low-back pain, small bowel or ureteral obstruction, and even compression of the inferior vena cava. Anterior mediastinal tumors may be extra-gonadal primaries and may present with superior vena cava syndrome and associated testicular

atrophy and Klinefelter's syndrome. Enlarged, firm, non-tender supraclavicular lymph nodes in an adolescent or young adult male should also prompt a thorough evaluation of the testes.

Radiographic evaluation of the testicle has improved the pre-operative diagnosis rates for these tumors. Such evaluation allows for the accurate determination of the correct surgical approach and procedure. Ultrasound may be used to evaluate scrotal masses, the contralateral testes when a tumor has been detected, and both testes when determining whether an extra-gonadal germ cell tumor is a primary or metastatic lesion from an occult testicular primary.

Abdominal computed tomography (CT) scan is currently the gold standard for evaluation of the abdomen and retroperitoneum, the most common site for metastases. CT scan of the chest should be performed in the staging of all patients. Magnetic resonance imaging (MRI) of the brain should be performed when symptoms indicate. Bone metastases are usually painful and may be evaluated with plain radiographs, bone scan, or MRI.

The role for positron emission tomography (PET) scan has yet to be determined, but may be most useful in the evaluation of residual masses. Germ-cell tumors actively take up 18-fluoro-2-deoxyglucose and, thus, PET scanning deserves further evaluation to determine its ultimate usefulness in these diseases.

14.5 Staging and Risk Stratification

The COG uses a staging system based on extent of disease and surgical intervention (Table 14.1). Based on this system and results of the pediatric intergroup trials Pediatric Oncology Group (POG) 9048/CCG 8891 and POG 9049/CCG 8882, a risk stratification system was developed. For testicular primaries, stage I patients are considered to have a good prognosis and are treated with surgery for the primary tumor followed by observation. This approach resulted in 82% event-free survival (EFS) and 100% survival at 7 years, with all patients who recurred being treated successfully with low-dose bleomycin (15 u/M^2 on day 1 of each course), standard-dose etoposide (500 mg/M^2/course), and cisplatin (100 mg/M^2/course) given at 21-day intervals

Table 14.1 Children's Oncology Group staging system for testicular germ cell tumors [5]. *CT* Computed tomography

Stage	Extent of disease
I	Limited to testis (testes), completely resected by orchiectomy; no clinical, radiographic, or histologic evidence of disease beyond the testes. Patients with normal or unknown tumor markers at diagnosis must have a negative ipsilateral retroperitoneal node sampling to confirm stage I disease. Radiographic studies demonstrate lymph nodes <2 cm
II	Transscrotal biopsy, microscopic disease in scrotum or high in spermatic cord (≤5 cm from proximal end)
III	Retroperitoneal lymph node involvement, but no visceral or extra-abdominal involvement. Lymph nodes >4 cm by CT or >2 cm and <4 cm with biopsy proof
IV	Distant metastases, including liver

for four cycles. Within COG, stage II–IV testicular patients are considered intermediate risk, with survival rates in excess of 90% at 6 years (in the COG staging system, only extragonadal stage III–IV germ cell patients are considered high-risk, with survival rates of 83.4±4.4% at 6 years) [6, 7].

In adult testicular tumors, the TNM (S) staging system is employed (see Table 14.2). In this system, the S denotes serum tumor marker status as follows: S_x not available; S_0 all markers normal; S_1 LDH < 1.5 × upper limit of normal, hCG < 5000 IU/l and AFP < 1000 ng/ml; S_2 LDH 1.5–10 × upper limit of normal, hCG 5000–50,000 IU/l, and AFP 1000–10,000 ng/ml; and S_3 LDH > 10 × upper limit of normal, hCG > 50,000 IU/l, and AFP > 10,000 ng/ml [8]. As in the pediatric studies cited above, the staging system was used to develop a risk-stratification system and subsequent treatment guidelines. The IGCCCG analyzed patients with metastatic disease (all stage III) from numerous studies with a combined enrollment of more than 5,000 patients. The analysis allowed division of the patients into three prognostic groups, as detailed in Table 14.3 [9, 10].

14.6 Treatment

The correct surgical approach is assured when a testicular tumor is suspected pre-operatively. Orchiectomy via an inguinal incision with high ligation of the spermatic cord is the recommended procedure. In the past, a scrotal incision was considered a violation of the scrotum and a hemi-scrotectomy was recommended but

this is no longer considered necessary unless actual contamination of the scrotum has occurred.

The need for retroperitoneal lymph-node dissection (RPLND) in localized tumors is controversial. This procedure has undergone major advancements

Table 14.2 American Joint Committee on cancer staging for testicular germ cell tumors [6]. *TNM* Tumor, node, metastasis

TNM Stage	Criteria
0	pTis, N0, M0, S0
I	pT1–4, N0, M0, SX
IA	pT1, N0, M0, S0
IB	PT2–4, N0, M0, S0
IS	Any T, N0, M0, S1–3
II	Any T, N1–3, M0, SX
IIA	Any T, N1, M0, S0–1
IIB	Any T, N2, M0, S0–1
IIC	Any T, N3, M0, S0–1
III	Any T, any N, M1, SX
IIIA	Any T, any N, M1a, S0–1
IIIB	Any T, N1–3, M0, S2
IIIB	Any T, any N, M1a, S2
IIIC	Any T, N1–3, M0, S3
IIIC	Any T, any N, M1a, S3
IIIC	Any T, any N, M1b, any S

Table 14.3 International germ cell consensus classification for metastatic germ-cell testicular cancer [9, 10]. *AFP* α-Feto-protein, *hCG* human chorionic gonadotrophin, *LDH* lactate dehydrogenase, *PFS* problem-free survival, *norm* normal

Good prognosis	
Non-seminoma	**Seminoma**
Testis/retroperitoneal primary	Any primary site
and	*and*
No non-pulmonary and visceral metastases	No non-pulmonary visceral metastases
and	*and*
Good markers – all of	Normal AFP, any hCG, any LDH
AFP < 1000 ng/ml and	
hCG < 5000 IU/l and	
LDH < 1.5 × upper limit of norm	
56% of non-seminomas	90% of seminomas
5-year PFS 89%	5-year PFS 82%
5-year survival 92%	5-year survival 86%

Intermediate prognosis	
Non-seminoma	**Seminoma**
Testis/retroperitoneal primary	Any primary site
and	*and*
No non-pulmonary visceral metastases	Non-pulmonary visceral metastases
and	*and*
Intermediate markers – any of	Normal AFP, any hCG, any LDH
AFP ≥ 1000 and ≤ 10,000 ng/ml or	
hCG ≥ 5000 IU/l and ≤ 50,000 IU/l or	
LDH ≥ 1.5× norm and ≤ 10 × norm	
28% of non-seminomas	10% of seminomas
5-year PFS 75%	5-year PFS 67%
5-year survival 80%	5-year survival 72%

Poor prognosis	
Non-seminoma	**Seminoma**
Mediastinal primary	
or	
Non-pulmonary visceral metastases	
or	
Poor markers – any of	
AFP > 10,000 ng/ml or	
hCG > 50,000 IU/l (10,000 ng/ml) or	
LDH > 10 × upper limit of norm	No patients classified as poor prognosis
16% of non-seminomas	
5-year PFS 41%	
5-year survival 48%	

from the en bloc procedure that led to a high incidence of emission failure and retrograde ejaculation. Dissection of the major vessels and sympathetic nerves, along with a directed approach, is now employed. As the pattern of metastasis is usually on the ipsilateral side (95%), lymph node dissection with sparing of the contralateral sympathetic nerves can be employed. The pattern of metastasis becomes less certain with bulky disease and the procedure is less valuable in such patients. As a staging procedure, RPLND is more accurate than CT scan (false negative rate 15–20%, false positive rate 15–23%). However, since 80–85% of patients with a negative CT scan will not have disease and those who recur are highly curable with chemotherapy, to operate on 100 patients to potentially help 15–20 may not be the best approach for the majority of stage I patients. In an effort to improve the chances that RPLND may be helpful, risk factors for metastasis have been identified. These include the presence of lymphatic invasion in the primary tumor (19%), vascular invasion (50%), absence of yolk sac elements (32%), and presence of embryonal carcinoma (87%) [11]. The presence of three of the four cited risk factors is associated with a 46% relapse rate; two of the four factors present with a 21% relapse rate and only one of the risk factors with a 16% relapse rate. The total relapse rate, in a meta-analysis of 29 studies, was 28%, but the overall survival was still 98% [10]. Forty-six percent of relapses occurred only in the retroperitoneum. In addition, markers were elevated in 68% of relapses, facilitating early detection. Finally, the cure rate for patients with recurrence who had not previously received chemotherapy exceeds 90%. Hence, RPLND should not be performed in all low-stage patients, either for staging or curative purposes, but, depending on risk factors, it remains an option for selected cases. In the pediatric intergroup study (POG 9048/CCG 8891), stage I patients treated with surgery and surveillance, had a 6-year EFS of 78.5% (±7%) and an overall survival of 100% [12]. Currently, COG protocols do not employ this approach routinely with lymph-node sampling reserved for patients with indeterminate lymph nodes of >2 cm but <4 cm. by CT scan evaluation. Lymph nodes >4 cm are considered to be involved with the tumor, and such patients are treated with chemotherapy. Lymph nodes <2 cm are considered negative and treated with surgery for the primary tumor and a surveillance protocol.

The use of surgery and a surveillance program for stage I non-seminomatous germ-cell tumors is well established. Although irradiation therapy to the retroperitoneum decreased the rate of relapse in these patients, 11% of patients still relapsed outside of the treatment field and the only 2 deaths among 156 patients in a study conducted in Denmark occurred in the radiation treatment arm of the study [13]. Likewise, the toxicity and costs of chemotherapy make it contraindicated, even using single-agent therapy.

The major problem with the strategy of surgery and observation is compliance. This is especially true for adolescents and young adults, who are more spontaneous, move frequently, and have a higher un-insured rate. In addition, the optimal frequency, extent, and duration of the surveillance program are yet to be determined. Combining eight previously reported studies, patients with adequate follow-up (N=1169) demonstrated that 95.5% of all relapses occurred in the first 2 years following diagnosis [10]. Another 1.8% of relapses occurred in the 3rd year. Only 2.7% (N=9) of all relapses occurred beyond 3 years postdiagnosis. Tumor markers were elevated in 68% of all relapses. This would support the concept of tumor marker assessment at gradually decreasing frequency for as long as 7–10 years. Omitting CT scans after 3 years would, however, potentially allow three cases of relapse (33% of nine) to go undetected for a longer period. The impact on chance of survival for these patients is unknown. With current surveillance, 19% of patients relapse as TNM stage III and overall survival remains >90%. The cost-effectiveness of continuing radiographic follow-up must be questioned.

The role of RPLND for radiographically TNM stage II patients differs from stage I. Due to the false-positive rate of CT scan, a non-confirmatory lymph-node dissection may obviate un-necessary chemotherapy. Conversely, confirmation and resection of nodal involvement may be curative and eliminate the need for chemotherapy. RPLND is not performed in pediatric protocols in the United States and all patients with nodal involvement would receive chemotherapy. In the COG trials, four cycles at 21-day intervals of 5-day bleomycin, etoposide, and cisplatin (BEP) is the standard therapy. Bleomycin is administered at 15 u/M^2 once every 3 weeks. Doses of etoposide (500 mg/M^2/course) and cisplatin (100 mg/M^2/course) are administered over 5 days. Patients who are partial responders after four cycles receive two additional cycles of therapy. This represents an approximately 67% decrease in exposure to bleomycin, compared to the weekly dosing on the standard Einhorn regimen. This dose of bleomycin was successful in the pediatric intergroup trials POG 9048/CCG 8891 and POG 9049/CCG 8882. The 6-year EFS for testicular tumors, stage II–IV, was 93.3% [5].

Studies of adult germ-cell tumors have also focused on modifications to the Einhorn regimen in an effort to decrease late effects in this group of patients with good prognosis. Attempts to decrease the dose of etoposide per cycle to 360 mg/M^2 failed to demonstrate efficacy when compared with the 500 mg/M^2 dosing schedule [14]. However, decreasing the number of treatment cycles, from four to three, given at 21-day intervals, did not adversely affect outcome [15]. In addition, three cycles of BEP were equally efficacious when compared with four cycles of etoposide and cisplatin (EP) [16]. A study reported by the Medical Research Council/European Organization for the Research and Treatment of Cancer (EORTC) demonstrated that administering the same total doses of etoposide and cisplatin over 3 days instead of 5 days was equally efficacious when only three cycles of therapy were given [15], with a slight increase in acute nausea and vomiting being the only differences noted. Thus, the current recommendation in adult testicular cancer is to use three cycles of 3-day BEP (with bleomycin 30 units weekly) unless there is a contraindication to the administration of bleomycin (e.g., underlying respiratory disease, older age, and prior allergic reaction), in which case, four cycles of EP can be employed.

The role of surgery in patients with radiographic pulmonary or visceral metastasis requires judgment. Occasionally, benign granulomas of the pulmonary parenchyma cannot be distinguished from lung metastases. If the presence or absence of malignancy within these lesions would make the difference between TNM stage I and III or COG stage I and IV, an excisional biopsy procedure should be performed.

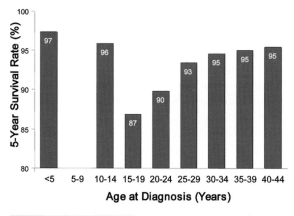

Figure 14.4

Five-year survival rates of testicular cancer, United States SEER 1975–2000 [1]

In patients with residual masses following chemotherapy, surgical evaluation remains important. When tumor markers remain elevated, the residual mass is most likely malignant and resection may be curative. When the tumor markers are negative, the residual mass is usually benign. Of particular note, when the primary tumor contains teratoma, surgery is the treatment of choice since the teratoma will not be chemosensitive. Likewise, suspected recurrences should be histologically proven except in the presence of recurrent elevations of one or more tumor markers.

In adult patients with poor-prognosis metastatic disease, the standard therapy remains four cycles of 5-day BEP at 21-day intervals with doses as follows: bleomycin 30 weekly; etoposide 500 g/M^2/course; and cisplatin 100 g/M^2/course. Studies evaluating autologous peripheral blood stem-ell transplantation in the initial treatment of poor prognosis patients are currently in progress. The addition of cyclophosphamide or ifosfamide to etoposide and cisplatin is also being evaluated in this context as well as for previously treated relapsed patients.

Seminoma differs from non-seminoma in its marked response to radiation therapy. Hence, this modality has been incorporated in treatment of stage I and II disease. In stage I seminoma of the testis, the low recurrence rate after combined surgery and irradiation (5%) coupled with a reported incidence of late

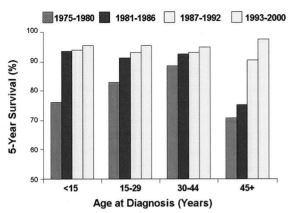

Figure 14.5

Five-year survival rates of testicular cancer by era, United States SEER 1975–2000 [1]

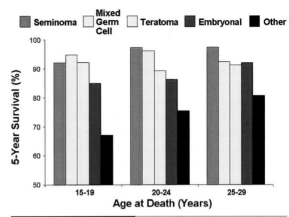

Figure 14.6

Five-year survival rates of testicular cancer by histologic type, United States SEER 1975–2000 [1]

recurrences (>5 years) in non-irradiated patients has argued against a treatment policy of observation alone following surgery. Front-line chemotherapy, in place of irradiation therapy for younger adolescents with stage I and II nonbulky seminoma, is controversial. The morbidity of irradiation therapy in specialized centers is low [17, 18].

Selected patients with seminoma should be treated with chemotherapy. These include patients with bulky abdominal nodal involvement, supra-diaphragmatic metastases, or with extra-nodal metastases above or below the diaphragm. The volume of abdominal-nodal metastases requiring treatment with chemotherapy varies from center to center. In the IGCCCG review of 637 patients treated for advanced seminoma, the 3-year survival rate was 82% [9]. In patients with only nodal or pulmonary metastases, the 5-year survival was 86%, while patients with non-pulmonary visceral metastases had a 5-year survival of 72%. Protocols using cisplatin and etoposide yield 80–90% disease-free survival rates, with three cycles being sufficient for advanced seminoma [19, 20].

Non-germ-cell-derived testicular tumors are rare, with an incidence of 5% or less in most series. The tumors seen may be functional steroid-secreting (some Leydig cell tumors, Sertoli cell tumors, and granulosa cell tumors) or non-functional (sarcomas, primarily paratesticular rhabdomyosarcoma, gonadoblastoma,

adenocarcinoma, mesothelioma, and lymphoma). Sarcomas and lymphomas are treated according to guidelines for these tumors in other sites, while the other histologies require radical inguinal orchiectomy. Retroperitoneal metastases are rare but may be amenable to resection and cure. Unresectable and recurrent metastatic disease in these tumor types is poorly responsive to chemotherapy and radiation.

14.7 Outcome

The survival of patients with testicular cancer has improved substantially over the last 25 years. This is due primarily to improvements in chemotherapy and to the education of oncologists in new treatment approaches. The 5-year survival rates for older adolescents and young adults with testicular cancer from 1975 to 1999 are shown in Fig. 14.4. Survival of 91% was observed in the 15- to 29-year age group. When examined by 5-year age intervals (Fig. 14.4), the 15- to 19-year and 20- to 24-year age groups had the lowest survival rates, at 87% and 90%, respectively.

The trends in testicular cancer survival during the years 1975–2000 are presented in Fig. 14.5. All age groups experienced improvements in survival during this observation period. Individuals in the age groups 15–19 and 20–24 years demonstrated the largest increases in 5-year survival rates between 1975–1980 and 1993–2000. Furthermore, the relatively poor survival rates in the age groups 15–19 and 20–24 years reflect in large part the results reported from the period 1975–1980.

The histology of testicular cancer has a profound effect on 5-year survival rates (Fig. 14.6). This was observed across all three adolescent and young adult 5-year age intervals presented (Fig. 14.6), and varied from 66% for non-seminomatous tumors (e.g., choriocarcinoma and yolk sac) in 15- to 19-year-olds, to greater than 95% for 25- to 29-year-old individuals with seminoma.

14.8 Late Effects

Given the high cure rates for testicular cancer, the long-term impact of surviving cancer and its treatment has gained importance. While undergoing treatment, fear of cancer, sleep disturbances, and cognitive dysfunction occur frequently ([21]. After therapy, a minority of patients (10–15%) report continued fear of cancer, sleep disturbances, and inability to concentrate, complete tasks, or think clearly. Symptoms of anxiety or depression persist in 30% of survivors at an average of 9 years after therapy compared to 5% of controls [22]. Conversely, other investigators have found no difference in the level of psychological functioning of long-term survivors versus normal controls [23]. Some have even reported improvement in areas such as personal optimism, family relationships, perceived quality of life, and self respect [24].

Sexual function has been studied extensively in survivors. During treatment and soon thereafter, approximately one-third of survivors report sexual dysfunction and/or dissatisfaction with level of sexual activity. However, this effect does not seem to be permanent in the majority of cases and studies indicate the level of dysfunction returns to baseline by 3 years after completion of therapy. The sexual dysfunction of some patients at the time of diagnosis, due to testicular atrophy and to the presence of disease, must be taken into account. The complications of RPLND and ejaculation have been well documented and have decreased with improved surgical techniques.

Late or prolonged toxicities of chemotherapy are agent- and dose-specific. Early studies showed high rates of bleomycin-induced pulmonary toxicity ranging from 34 to 46%. In a recent EORTC study, BEP induced a 20% decrease in carbon monoxide diffusing capacity versus 2% in the EP group [25]. Efforts to reduce this toxicity by decreasing the dose of bleomycin (three cycles vs. four) or administering bleomycin only on the 1st day of each cycle rather than weekly (decreasing the total dose by 66.6%) may ameliorate this toxicity without decreasing survival in selected patients.

Cisplatin causes proximal renal tubule defects with hypomagnesemia, hypokalemia, and hypocalcemia. Acute decreases in glomerular filtration also occur. Some studies report persistence of these abnormalities, while others report gradual improvement. The late occurrence of hypertension has also been reported.

Ototoxicity is related to the total dose of cisplatin, is permanent, and occurs in 20–40% of patients. It begins as a high-frequency loss and progresses to involve frequencies in the speech range with continued exposure to the drug. The concurrent exposure to ototoxic environmental factors (e.g., rock concerts, airplanes, jack hammers) by adolescents and young adults may increase their risk of hearing loss. Appropriate anticipatory guidance and monitoring of audiograms may lessen the impact of ototoxicity. The delivery of only three cycles of cisplatin, when appropriate, will decrease the incidence of severe toxicity.

Peripheral neurotoxicity is characterized by paresthesias and dysesthesias. It is induced in 30–40% of patients who receive cisplatin and persists over time [26, 27]. Vascular toxicities reported with cisplatin include Raynaud's phenomenon, venous thrombosis, and myocardial infarctions.

An increased risk of second malignant neoplasms has been reported for survivors of testicular tumors. Cancer in the contralateral testis is the most common finding and is probably not treatment related. Patients who receive irradiation therapy have an increased risk of stomach cancer (van Leeuwen et al. 1993). Leukemia and myelodysplasia also occur in testicular tumor patients. These complications are usually associated with total doses of etoposide in excess of 2 g/M^2 and are often characterized by an 11q23 or 21q22 translocation [28]. Some secondary leukemias appear to be related to the germ-cell tumor and not the treatment.

14.9 Conclusions

Testicular cancer is the most common solid tumor in male adolescents and young adults and is increasing in frequency. The differences between age groups in incidence, frequency of histological types, biologic markers, and tumor cytogenetics have been identified. Tumor markers assist in the diagnosis, prediction of prognosis, evaluation of response, and surveillance for relapse. Ultrasonography is the preferred modality for evaluation of the primary tumor and the contralateral testis, with CT scan used for radiographic staging. Inguinal orchiectomy with high ligation of the spermatic cord is the initial treatment of choice. The role of retroperitoneal lymph node dissection in stage I and II tumors is discussed. The importance of surgery in evaluating and treating residual masses as well as recurrences is emphasized. Five-year survival exceeds 80%. Chemotherapy can be avoided in 80% of patients with localized tumors. The preferred chemotherapy, for those requiring it, remains bleomycin, etoposide, and cisplatin. Refinements in the number of cycles, drug doses, and treatment days are discussed herein in detail. Minimizing the late effects of testicular cancer and its treatment on long-term survivors remains a challenge. Changes in therapy may now have an impact for the next 60 years for these survivors.

In summary, the development of a paradigm for the treatment of germ-cell tumors of the testicle should be viewed as a model of success and demonstrates the importance of a multidisciplinary approach in the diagnosis, treatment, and long-term follow-up of these patients. Cure rates approach 90% for most patients. Only high-risk metastatic patients and patients who relapse continue to have unsatisfactory outcomes. Much still needs to be learned about the biology of these tumors. Clinical studies should continue to focus on limiting long-term toxicities and risks for these patients, who might otherwise live for another 60 years.

References

1. Bleyer WA, OLeary M, Barr R, Ries LAG (eds) (2006) Cancer Epidemiology in Older Adolescents and Young Adults 15 to 29 Years of Age, including SEER Incidence and Survival, 1975–2000. National Cancer Institute, NIH Pub. No. 06-5767, Bethesda MD, June 2006; also available at www.seer.cancer.gov/publications
2. Ries LAG, Eisner MP, Kosary CL, et al (2002) SEER cancer statistics review, 1973–1999. National Cancer Institute, Bethesda, MD
3. Chaganti RS, Rodriguez E, Bosl GJ (1993) Cytogenetics of male germ cell tumors. Urol Clin North Am 20:55–66
4. Bussey KJ, Lawce HJ, Olsen SB, et al (1999) Chromosome abnormalities of 81 pediatric germ cell tumors: Sex-, age-, site-, and histopathology-related differences: a Children's Cancer Group study. Genes Chromosomes Cancer 25:134–146
5. Cullen JW, Olson TA, Giller R, et al (2002) Low dose bleomycin every three weeks with cisplatin and etoposide results in excellent EFS and survival rates for children and adolescents with gonadal germ cell tumors (MGCT): a POG/CCG intergroup report. In: Harden P, Joffe JK, Jones WG (eds) Germ Cell Tumors V. Springer-Verlag, London
6. Cushing B, Giller R, Cullen JW, et al (2004) Randomized comparison of combination chemotherapy with etoposide, bleomycin, and either high-dose or standard-dose cisplatin in children and adolescents with high-risk malignant germ cell tumors: a pediatric intergroup study – Pediatric Oncology Group 9049 and Children's Cancer Group 8882. J Clin Oncol 22:2691–2700
7. Rogers PC, Olson TA, Cullen JW, et al (2004) Treatment of children and adolescents with stage II testicular and stages I and II ovarian malignant germ cell tumors: a pediatric intergroup study – Pediatric Oncology Group 9048 and Children Cancer Group 8891. J Clin Oncol 22:3563–3569
8. Green FL, Balch CM, Page DL, et al (eds) (2002) American Joint Commission on Cancer (AJCC) Cancer Staging Manual (6th edn). Springer-Verlag, New York, pp 77–87
9. International Germ Cell Cancer Collaborative Group (1997) International germ cell consensus classification: a prognostic factor-based staging system for metastatic germ cell cancers. J Clin Oncol 15:594–603
10. Daugaard G, Rorth M (2003) Active surveillance for stage I nonseminomatous germ cell tumors. In: Raghavan D (ed) American Cancer Society Atlas of Clinical Oncology: Germ Cell Tumors. Decker, London, p 132
11. Freedman LS, Parkinson MC, Jones WG, et al (1987) Histopathology in the prediction of relapse in patients with stage I testicular teratoma treated by orchidectomy alone. Lancet 2:294–298

12. Schlatter M, Resorla F, Giller R, et al (2003) Excellent outcome in patients with stage I germ cell tumors of the testes: a study of the Children's Cancer Group/Pediatric Oncology Group. J Pediatric Surg 38:319–324

13. Rorth M, Jacobsen GK, von der Maase H, et al (1991) Surveillance alone versus radiotherapy after orchidectomy for clinical stage I nonseminomatous testicular cancer. J Clin Oncol 9:1543–1548

14. Toner GC, Stockler MR, Boyer MJ, et al (2001) Comparison of two standard chemotherapy regimens for good-prognosis germ-cell tumours: a randomized trial of the Australian and New Zealand Germ Cell Trial Group. Lancet 357: 739–745

15. de Wit R, Roberts JT, Wilkinson PM, et al (2001) Equivalence of three or four cycles of bleomycin, etoposide, and cisplatin chemotherapy and of a 3- or 5-day schedule in good-prognosis germ cell cancer: a randomized study of the European Organization for Research and Treatment of Cancer Genitourinary Tract Cancer Cooperative Group and the Medical Research Council. J Clin Oncol 19:1629–1640

16. Culine S, Kerbrat P, Bouzy J, et al (1999) Are 3 cycles of bleomycin, etoposide, and cisplatin (3BEP) or 4 cycles of etoposide and cisplatin (4EP) equivalent regimens for patients with good-risk metastatic non seminomatous germ cell tumours? Preliminary results of a randomized trial. Proc Am Soc Clin Oncol 18:A1188

17. van Leeuwen F, Stigglebout A, Canden Belt-Dusebout A (1993) Second cancer risk following testicular cancer: a follow-up study of 1909 patients. J Clin Oncol 11:415–424

18. Wanderas EH, Fossa SD, Tretli S (1997) Risk of subsequent non-germ-cell cancer after treatment of germ cell cancer in 2006 Norwegian male patients. J Clin Oncol 11:253–259

19. Arranz Arija JA, Garcia del Muro X, Guma J, et al (2001) E400P in advanced seminoma of good prognosis according to the International Germ Cell Cancer Collaborative Group (IGCCCG) classification: the Spanish Germ Cell Cancer Group experience. Ann Oncol 12:487–491

20. Horwich A, Oliver RTD, Wilkinson PM, et al (2000) A Medical Research Council randomized trial of single agent carboplatin versus etoposide and cisplatin for advanced metastatic seminoma. Br J Cancer 83:1623–1629

21. Gritz ER, Wellisch DK, Wang HJ, et al (1989) Long-term effects of testicular cancer on sexual functioning in married couples. Cancer 64:1560–1567

22. Gritz ER, Wellisch DK, Landsverk JA (1988) Psychosocial sequelae in long-term survivors of testicular cancer. J Psychosoc Oncol 6:41–63

23. Joly F, Heron JF, Kalusinski L, et al (2002) Quality of life in long-term survivors of testicular cancer: a population-based case-control study. J Clin Oncol 20:73–80

24. Rieker PP, Edbril SD, Garnick MB (1985) Curative testis cancer therapy: psychosocial sequelae. J Clin Oncol 3:1117–1126

25. de Wit R, Stoter G, Kaye SB, et al (1997) Importance of bleomycin in combination chemotherapy for good-prognosis testicular nonseminoma: a randomized study of the European Organization for Research and Treatment of Cancer Genitourinary Tract Cancer Cooperative Group. J Clin Oncol 15:1837–1843

26. Boyer MJ, Raghavan D, Harris PJ, et al (1990) Lack of late toxicity in patients treated with cisplatin-containing combination chemotherapy for metastatic testicular cancer. J Clin Oncol 8:21–26

27. Hansen SW, Olsen N (1989) Raynaud's phenomenon in patients treated with cisplatin, vinblastine, and bleomycin fpr germ cell cancer: measurement of vasoconstrictor response to cold. J Clin Oncol 7:940–942

28. Pedersen-Bjergaard J, Philip P, Larsen SO, et al (1993) Therapy-related myelodysplasia and acute myeloid leukemia. Cytogenetic characteristics of 115 consecutive cases and risk in seven cohorts of patients treated intensively for malignant diseases in the Copenhagen series. Leukemia 7:1975–1986

Non-Germ-Cell Genitourinary Tract Tumors

Michael Leahy • W. Archie Bleyer

Contents

15.1 Introduction

Unlike most of the other chapters in this book, which essentially deal with single disease entities, this chapter covers several completely distinct conditions. Each of these entities present much more commonly in other age groups. For example, Wilms' tumor (nephroblastoma) usually presents in childhood, while renal cell carcinoma (RCC), transitional cell carcinoma (TCC) of the urothelium, adenocarcinoma of the prostate, and carcinoma of the Fallopian tubes, endometrium, and uterus (including cervical carcinoma), present much more frequently in later adult life. It is not possible within the scope of this chapter to describe each or any of these tumors in detail and the reader is referred to standard texts or recent reviews in the literature for further reading. However, when reading those texts, it must be remembered that they apply primarily to a different age group. This chapter will therefore concentrate principally on comparing and contrasting the available evidence regarding these tumors in the teenager and young adult with their more common age group, in an attempt to guide treatment if one of these tumors is diagnosed in a teenager or young adult.

The tumors described in this chapter are mostly epithelial tumors, which are seen more frequently in much later life. All of these are associated with good outcomes if diagnosed and radically resected before metastatic spread has occurred. Unfortunately, many patients are diagnosed with metastatic disease or relapse after initial surgery. In these cases, systemic therapy is of generally modest use in the adult setting in providing temporary and partial tumor control as part of palliative therapy.

15.2 Epidemiology and Etiology

Individually, these tumors are so rare in the 15- to 20-year-old age range that several of them do not merit attention in the Surveillance, Epidemiology, and End Results pediatric monograph [1, 2]. Most adult epithelial malignancies are thought to arise as a result of cumulative chronic genotoxic exposure [3]. Cigarette smoking accounts for a high proportion of attributable risk in many cancers, including TCC of the urothelium, which will be discussed herein. In contrast, the diagnosis of one of these tumors in a teenager should prompt consideration of genetic predisposition to cancer. Several well-characterized inherited syndromes are associated with an increased risk of malignancy (e.g., von Hippel Lindau syndrome and RCC). Furthermore, it is increasingly recognized that polymorphisms in genes that regulate DNA repair and the metabolism of carcinogens may be associated with a general increased risk of developing cancer. The most well known of these is the Li-Fraumeni syndrome, which is caused by a germ-line p53 mutation, but it seems likely that combinations of polymorphisms of much lower penetrance may account for a higher degree of attributable risk age group. The cancers that arise in those affected in these families characteristically appear at a younger age than usual.

15.3 Biology and Pathology

In the adult setting, each organ site is usually affected by one predominant histological type of cancer (e.g., in the kidney, RCC; in the bladder, TCC; in the prostate, adenocarcinoma). However, other histological types are also diagnosed, although less commonly: small-cell carcinoma may occur in the bladder, cervix, and prostate; collecting-duct tumors may occur in the kidney; lymphomas and sarcomas are also infrequently diagnosed. The pattern of histologies seen in the adult setting is presumably in part due to the result of exposure to prevalent carcinogenic agents and one would therefore predict that a different profile of histologies might be seen in teenagers and young adults. This is difficult to confirm given the very small numbers in any of the reported series, but there is a general impression that a wider or more even spectrum of histology is seen in the very young adults with cancer in the genitourinary system.

Histological tumor grade is a very important indicator of prognosis in adult cancers. While grade progression (i.e., low grade to higher grade) is seen in some cancers (e.g., superficial, well-differentiated TCC progressing to muscle invasive disease), it is not common. Where this does occur, however, one might predict that younger patients would present with lower-

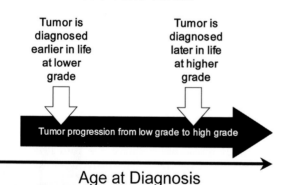

Figure 15.1

Theoretical relationship between lead-time bias and tumor grade associated with increasing patient age

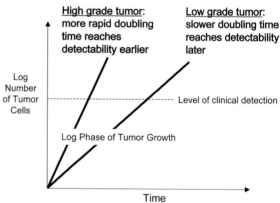

Figure 15.2

Theoretical relationship between tumor doubling time during log phase of growth and tumor grade at patient age at diagnosis

grade disease as a result of "lead-time effect" (Fig. 15.1). However, the opposite might apply if high-grade cancer has a shorter doubling time and therefore a shorter time after malignant initiation before the tumor becomes clinically apparent (Fig. 15.2). There is some evidence that both of these effects are seen (in different tumors) in those described here, as will be discussed.

15.4 Clinical Presentations and Diagnosis

Diagnosis of these tumors in this age group is challenging. The classic triad of local symptoms of the primary malignant tumor – bleeding, a mass and pain – may be absent or appear late. Metastatic disease may present with local symptoms from metastatic sites or with generalized symptoms of weight loss, cachexia, fevers, and sweats. Symptoms are thus non-specific and clinical examination is relatively insensitive at detecting a small tumor and, in view of the rarity of a malignant diagnosis in this age group, clinical examination may not be appropriately directed. The differential diagnosis is likely to be dominated by non-malignant conditions. Inevitably this contributes to a delay in diagnosis for many patients. For example, hematuria in this age group is usually due to urinary tract infection. In older patients, in whom malignant disease is more likely, hematuria is routinely a trigger for full investigation to exclude malignant disease by imaging, cytology, and endoscopy. However, in the younger patient, empiric treatment with a suitable antibiotic is reasonable for the first episode, although assessment should include microbiological examina-

tion of the urine. For patients with recurrent or persistent hematuria, especially when no infective agent is identified, they should be referred for further investigation including a pelvic examination, intravenous urography, and/or renal tract ultrasound, urine cytology, and cystoscopy.

15.5 Treatment

Apart from Wilms' tumor, the tumors described here are not so sensitive to systemic agents that they can be reliably cured by such use, and their management is centered on good surgical technique. Complete surgical removal at the earliest possible occasion remains the approach most likely to lead to a full recovery. In the older-adult setting, radical radiotherapy may be an appropriate alternative to surgery for organ-confined disease; however, the doses used are high and this would argue against its use in a young patient who would have a much longer time at risk after treatment to develop late effects. In particular, secondary malignancy would be a concern.

In none of these tumors has adjuvant treatment with radiotherapy to reduce the risk of local relapse, or with systemic therapy to reduce the risk of metastatic relapse, or neo-adjuvant therapy prior to surgery been shown to improve outcomes significantly. Such evidence has been hard to obtain even in the adult setting for various reasons, and where randomized clinical trials exist they have usually, to date, been too small to detect the order of clinical benefit that can be expected from adjuvant treatment.

Table 15.1 Relative roles of adjuvant chemotherapy, neo-adjuvant chemotherapy, and adjuvant radiotherapy in renal cell carcinoma (*RCC*), transitional-cell carcinoma (*TCC*) of the bladder, and adenocarcinoma of the prostate

Tumor	Neo-adjuvant systemic therapy	Adjuvant systemic therapy	Adjuvant radiotherapy
RCC	Not tested	No benefit, not well tested	No benefit, not well tested
TCC of bladder	Small survival benefit in meta-analysis	No benefit, not well tested	No benefit, not well tested
Adenocarcinoma of the prostate	No benefit	Benefit in node-positive patients	Controversial results

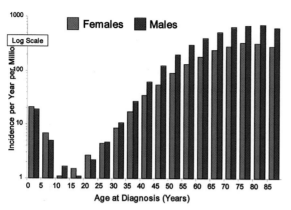

Figure 15.3

Incidence of renal cancer by gender, United States SEER 1975–2000 [1]

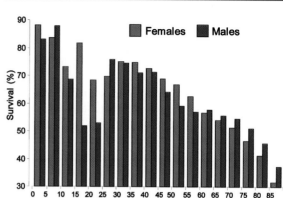

Figure 15.4

Five-year relative survival, renal cancer, by age and gender, United States SEER 1975–1999 [1]

Table 15.1 reviews the place of adjuvant and neo-adjuvant therapy in the standard management of these tumors in the adult setting.

15.6 Specific Tumors

Each non-germ cell genitourinary tract cancer type is reviewed below, with the available tumor-specific data on epidemiology, etiology, biology and pathology, diagnostic work-up, and standard of care for management.

15.6.1 Kidney tumors

The incidence of renal cancer has an early-childhood peak and a late-adulthood peak, with a nadir between 15 and 20 years of age (Fig. 15.3). Above age 25 years, the incidence is greater in males than females, whereas in children it predominates among females (Fig. 15.3).

The survival of patients with renal cancer had a lower rate for 15- to 30-year-olds diagnosed between 1975 and 2000 than either younger or older patients, and particularly for males (Fig. 15.4). Survival has improved in all age groups below 45 years, albeit the relatively small number of patients in the 15- to 24-year age category limits this conclusion with regard to patients in this age group (Fig. 15.5).

In the United States, African Americans/blacks had the highest mortality rate at all ages up to at least 45 years, and Asians/Pacific Islanders the lowest (Fig. 15.6).

About 5% of cases of Wilms' tumor are diagnosed in patients older than 15 years [4]. This presumably includes cases in which diagnosis was delayed significantly for various reasons. In contrast, the diagnosis of RCC is nearly twice as common in the 15- to 19-year-olds, and incidence rises thereafter [4]. The average annual age-adjusted incidence rate for kidney tumors in the 15- to 19-year-old age range is 0.4 per million for Wilms' tumor and 0.7 per million for RCC [4].

In the UKW3 trial for patients with Wilms' tumor, increasing age is a poor prognostic factor (although the age categories studied were less than 2 years, 2–4 years, and greater than 4 years, and very few, if any, patients were older than 15 years) [5]. The tumor is very sensitive to chemotherapy and children presenting with metastatic disease are curable, with long-term survival over 70% [6]. The possibility that chemo-sensitivity may reduce with age is supported by case reports of older patients who failed to respond to treatment [7, 8], but aggressive poly-chemotherapy is indicated and successful in some cases [8, 9]. In the largest series in the literature of adult Wilms' tumor, 3 out of 5 patients with metastatic disease died, and the overall survival of 17 patients was 67% [10]. Cytogenetic stud-

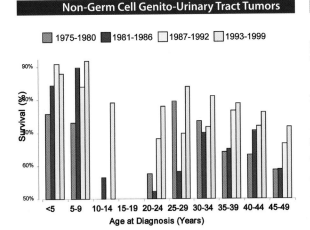

Figure 15.5

Five-year relative survival, renal cancer, by era, United States SEER 1975–1999 [1]

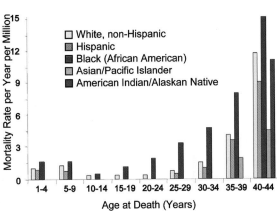

Figure 15.6

Mortality rate of renal cancer by race/ethnicity, United States SEER 1992–2002 [1]

ies of a single case suggest that there may be different molecular lesions in adult cases [11].

Staging and work-up of patients with kidney tumors should include computed tomography (CT) scan of the chest, abdomen, and pelvis. The lung is the most common site of metastatic spread. Pelvic imaging is usually negative in the absence of symptoms of concern. Primary treatment should be a radical nephrectomy. The value of ipsi-lateral adrenalectomy and lymph-node dissection is unknown and probably does not affect outcome, although these may contribute to prognostic information. The laparoscopy technique is being used increasingly for this operation. Large tumors are often extremely friable and immediate preoperative embolization reduces intraoperative blood loss. Partial nephrectomy is possible for peripheral tumors and may be indicated if there is reduced renal function for any other reason. No adjuvant therapy has been found to reduce the risk of local or metastatic relapse and patients are routinely offered follow-up with surveillance for pulmonary relapse with chest x-ray [12].

In the adult, treatment of metastatic RCC using conventional cytotoxic chemotherapy has not been associated with clear evidence of significant benefit. Research has focused largely on biological therapies, with tantalizing results in small series that suggest that the disease is amenable to manipulations of the immune system with cytokines such as interferon and interleukins, and vaccines. However, few of these have been tested in large randomized phase III trials. Both interleukin-2 and interferon have shown a small benefit over supportive care with steroids and could be considered a standard of care. Surgery may also be useful even in the face of metastatic disease and two randomized clinical trials have shown a survival advantage for nephrectomy in patients with metastatic disease who subsequently received immunotherapy [13]. Furthermore, selected patients may benefit from metastasectomy of the lung and even the brain.

15.6.2 Urothelial and Bladder Tumors

The incidence of bladder cancer is similar to that for renal cancer, with a nadir between 15 and 20 years of age and a prominence in males from age 15 years upward (Fig. 15.7).

In contrast to renal cancer, however, 15- to 29-year-olds with bladder cancer had a better 5-year relative survival rate than younger or older patients (Fig. 15.8).

In the adult population, the commonest cancer of the bladder is TCC of the urothelium, which may also present in the urothelium of the renal pelvis and ureter. Clearly, this reflects the fact that this tissue is exposed to carcinogens in the urine. Polymorphism with regard to key protective pathways may account

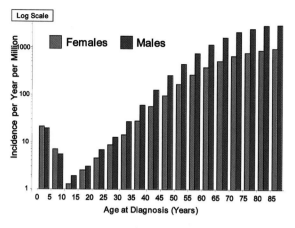

Figure 15.7

Incidence of bladder cancer by gender, United States SEER 1975–2000 [1]

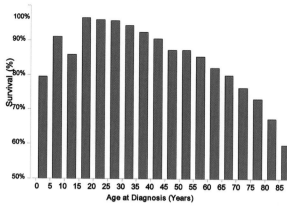

Figure 15.8

Five-year relative survival, bladder cancer, by age, United States SEER 1975–1999 [1]

for increased risk [14] and may be implicated in patients with a very young age at diagnosis. Normal urinary physiology is also protective, and young patients who require bladder augmentation due to neurological disorders are at a higher risk of developing TCC [15]. Excess incidence of urinary cancer, including very young patients, has been detected in studies of areas affected by heavy pollution [16]. Rare histological variants are also found in adults, and one might expect these tumors to account for a higher proportion of cases in the much younger patient population [17].

A lead-time effect, with regard to the pattern of tumor grade at presentation, is perhaps seen in this tumor. In one of the few published series of adolescent patients diagnosed with bladder cancer, all of the patients had well-differentiated and low-stage tumors [18]. This hypothesis is also supported by a very large epidemiological study from the National Cancer Database, which demonstrated an association between young age and low stage [19].

Bladder tumors are usually diagnosed as a result of investigation of hematuria. Diagnostic work-up should then include endoscopic biopsy of the tumor itself and mapping biopsies of the rest of the bladder to look for carcinoma in situ. Bi-manual examination under anesthetic remains a critical part of assessing tumor stage.

Patients with invasive tumors should have staging cross-sectional imaging of the chest, abdomen and pelvis, and imaging of the upper urinary tracts. Bone scanning is advised increasingly in view of the high incidence of asymptomatic bone metastases. Other investigations will be determined by the patient's clinical symptoms and signs.

Tumors of pTa and pT1 are usually managed by endoscopic extirpation with a single post-resection instillation of epirubicin, mitomycin-C, or BCG (Bacillus Calmette-Guerin) into the bladder. Surveillance for local relapse is mandatory and can be performed by flexible cystoscopy. Urine cytology is of potential benefit in follow-up.

Invasive tumors (pT2–pT3) are usually managed by radical cystectomy (or nephro-ureterectomy in the case of upper-tract tumors) with lymph-node dissection. Recent data, from re-analysis of a systematic meta-analysis of randomized clinical trials of neoadjuvant chemotherapy with platinum-containing combination regimens such as MVAC (methotrexate, vinblastine, adriamycin, and cisplatin), suggests a small improvement in overall survival of approximately 6% at 5 years [20]. Patients who are unfit for radical surgery (common in the usual elderly adult population but unlikely in the teenager or young adult presenting with this disease) may be managed with radical radiotherapy, although this would only really be appropriate in the young patient for those who are clearly beyond treatment of curative intent.

Metastatic TCC of the urothelium is sensitive to both radiotherapy and cytotoxic chemotherapy, and patients with metastatic or inoperable local disease should be managed with a multi-modal treatment plan to optimize their survival and quality of life. This will result in a small number of long-term survivors among selected patients who have received aggressive combination chemotherapy based on cisplatin, had good performance status at the start of treatment, and have metastases restricted to lymph node sites [21]. In the adult, cisplatin is the drug associated with the highest single-agent activity, and randomized controlled trials have shown that combination therapy is superior to single-agent treatment. Doxorubicin, methotrexate, vinblastine, gemcitabine, and the taxanes all have demonstrable activity. Several well-tested combinations exist: MVAC, CMV (cisplatin, methotrexate, and vinblastine), and GC (gemcitabine and cisplatin), and many new doublets and triplets have been tested in small series.

15.6.3 Prostate Cancer

Prostate cancer in teenagers is so rare that almost no epidemiological data have been published and the literature is confined to case reports [22]. Studies of early-onset prostate cancer (defined as diagnosed under the age of 55 years) generally only contain cases aged down to the mid 30s, but reveal associations with inherited polymorphisms of critical genes [23–26].

The impression gained from the few case reports of prostate cancer in the under-25 years age group is of tumors that are different biologically to those seen in the normal age range of elderly men. The tumors are usually undifferentiated, metastasize early, have lytic rather than sclerotic bone metastases, and respond poorly to hormonal therapies [22]. This is the opposite of what has been observed in bladder cancer.

Patients may present with pelvic pain, dysuria, poor urinary stream, and possibly hematuria. Digital rectal examination may reveal clues to the diagnosis, but is relatively insensitive. Pelvic imaging by MRI, CT scan, or trans-rectal ultrasound may also sometimes miss a diffuse tumor of the prostate, and biopsy procedures

(transrectal ultrasound-guided Tru-cut biopsy procedures) are therefore often performed to a template to ensure coverage of the gland.

Staging should include screening for bone metastases by whole-body radionucleotide bone scintigraphy as well as cross-sectional imaging to exclude soft-tissue and visceral metastases. Various serum markers are used routinely in the adult population, particularly prostate-specific antigen, and this can be a very useful marker of disease activity and response to treatment.

In the rare patient with clinically organ-confined disease, radical prostatectomy is offered increasingly over the alternatives based on radiotherapy (radical external beam radiotherapy and brachytherapy). In view of the comments above, surgery may be preferred to radiotherapy in the very young patient being treated with curative intent. Nerve-sparing techniques to preserve continence and sexual function are possible without sacrificing outcome if the tumor is very small. Neo-adjuvant treatment with hormonal therapy is of unproven benefit and is not advised outside the context of a clinical trail. Post-operative hormonal treatment may have a small impact in patients with node-positive disease.

In the adult, metastatic adenocarcinoma of the prostate is sensitive to a variety of hormone manipulations. First-line therapy is usually with gonadotrophin-releasing hormone analogues such as goserelin or leuprolide. These agents suppress androgen production by the testis and have largely replaced orchidectomy, which was used routinely in the past. Second-line therapy typically involves attempting to ensure that even peripheral and hepatic testosterone production is blocked; this is achieved by adding an anti-androgen to the luteinizing hormone-releasing hormone analogue. Stilboestrol fell out of favor in view of an excess of thromboembolic events, but may still have a role in third-line therapy in selected patients. Hormone therapy has dominated the management of the elderly adult with prostate carcinoma, and cytotoxic therapies are reserved for the final hormone-refractory phase in selected patients. However, recent evidence showing a small survival advantage with docetaxel-based therapy has demonstrated that cytotoxic chemotherapy may have an important role to play in the treatment of prostate carcinoma [27]. Given the suggestion that

Table 15.2 Five-year age-standardized, stage-specific survival of RCC, TCC of the bladder, and adenocarcinoma of the prostate [28]

Tumor	Stage I/localized	Stage II, III/regional	Stage IV/distant
RCC of kidney	91.1%	59.1%	9.3%
TCC of bladder	94.1%	48.8%	5.5%
Adenocarcinoma of prostate	100%	98%	33.5%

hormonal therapies are ineffective in the very young patient with prostate cancer, and that some success in partial response and palliation may be obtained with cytotoxic chemotherapy, it would be reasonable to select younger patients for this modality of therapy early in their treatment. Bisphosphonate treatment has also been shown to be of some benefit in maintaining quality of life in the adult population by reducing the risk of skeletal events.

15.7 Comparative Survival Rates

For patients who present with non-localized disease at diagnosis, both RCC and TCC of the bladder have a much worse long-term survival rate than prostate carcinoma (Table 15.2). For localized presentations, the results are comparable.

15.8 Conclusions

There are significant challenges in managing teenage and young adult patients with the conditions described in this chapter. Diagnosis is difficult and may be delayed, but as soon as a malignant diagnosis is confirmed the patient and their family should be referred without delay to an institution that can provide both the highly specialized tumor-specific multi-disciplinary team to deliver treatment and, ideally, one where age-specific support services are available.

Confirmation of the diagnosis is the first crucial step. Expert histopathologic review should be preformed on all tumors, since the chance of an unusual histology in this age group is high. Treatment planning should involve surgical, radiation

oncology, and medical oncology input. To optimize outcomes, patients should be managed by tumor-specific multi-disciplinary teams in conjunction with specialist services to provide age-specific psychosocial support. Treatment guidelines developed for the management of adult patients should be assessed carefully before extrapolating them to a different age group, but in the absence of good data to support different approaches, these are still the best recommendations for care in many cases. More research is required into the etiology (in which genetic susceptibility may play a greater part), natural history, and response to therapy in the unusually young patient with theses forms of cancer.

In general, existing tumor-specific treatment strategies have been defined in patients in a different age group, and there is concern that this may mean that these strategies may not be the best for adolescent and young adult patients because of the different biology of the host and possibly the different biology of the disease. Nevertheless, in the absence of better data, these strategies may be the best to apply, with caution, while at the same time encouraging and supporting research to clarify these issues.

References

1. Bleyer WA, OLeary M, Barr R, Ries LAG (eds) (2006) Cancer Epidemiology in Older Adolescents and Young Adults 15 to 29 Years of Age, including SEER Incidence and Survival, 1975–2000. National Cancer Institute, NIH Pub. No. 06-5767, Bethesda MD; also available at www.seer.cancer.gov/publications.
2. Ries LAG, Smith MA, Gurney IG, et al (eds) (1999) Cancer Incidence and Survival among Children and Adolescents: United States SEER Program 1975–1995. National Cancer Institute, SEER Program, NIH Pub.

No. 99-4649. Bethesda, MD

3. World Health Organization (2003) The causes of cancer. In: Stewart BW, Kleihues P (eds) World Cancer Report. IARC Press, Lyon pp 22–28

4. Bernstein L, Linet M, Smith MA, Olshan AF, et al (1999) Renal tumors. In: Ries LAG, Smith MA, Gurney JG, Linet M, Tamra T, Young JL, Bunin GR (eds) Cancer Incidence and Survival among Children and Adolescents: United States SEER Program 1975–1995. National Cancer Institute, SEER Program, NIH Pub. No. 99-4649. Bethesda, MD, pp 79–90

5. Pritchard-Jones K, Kelsey A, Vujanic G, et al (2003) Older age is an adverse prognostic factor in stage I, favorable histology Wilms' tumor treated with vincristine monochemotherapy: a study by the United Kingdom Children's Cancer Study Group, Wilms' Tumor Working Group. J Clin Oncol 21:3269–3275

6. Pritchard-Jones K (2002) Controversies and advances in the management of Wilms' tumour. Arch Dis Child 87:241–244

7. Dawson NA, Klein MA, Taylor HG (1988) Salvage therapy in metastatic adult Wilms' tumor. Cancer 62:1017–1021

8. Adolphs HD, Knopfle G, Vogel, Hartlapp J, et al (1983) Wilms' tumor in the adolescent and adult. Eur Urol 9:281–287

9. Tawil A, Cox N, Roth AD, et al (1999) Wilms' tumor in the adult – report of a case and review of the literature. Pathol Res Pract 195:105–111; discussion 113–114

10. Terenziani M, Spreafico F, Collini P, et al (2004) Adult Wilms' tumor: a monoinstitutional experience and a review of the literature. Cancer 101:289–293

11. Li P, Perle MA, Scholes V, et al (2002) Wilms' tumor in adults: aspiration cytology and cytogenetics. Diagn Cytopathol 26:99–103

12. Sene AP, Hunt L, Mc Mahon RF, Carroll RN, (1992) Renal carcinoma in patients undergoing nephrectomy: analysis of survival and prognostic factors. Br J Urol 70:125–134

13. Flanigan RC, Mickisch G, Sylvester R, et al (2004) Cytoreductive nephrectomy in patients with metastatic renal cancer: a combined analysis. J Urol 171:1071–1076

14. Lin J, Spitz MR, Wang Y, et al (2004) Polymorphisms of folate metabolic genes and susceptibility to bladder cancer: a case-control study. Carcinogenesis 25:1639–1647

15. Soergel TM, Cain MP, Missen R, et al (2004) Transitional cell carcinoma of the bladder following augmentation cystoplasty for the neuropathic bladder. J Urol 172:1649–1651; discussion 1651–1652

16. Pan BJ, Hong YJ, Chang GC, et al (1994) Excess cancer mortality among children and adolescents in residential districts polluted by petrochemical manufacturing plants in Taiwan. J Toxicol Environ Health 43:117–129

17. Richter ER, Dean RC (2004) Leiomyosarcoma of the urinary bladder in a teenage male. Mil Med 169:155–156

18. Kawaguchi T, Hashimoto Y, Kobayashi H, et al (1999) [A clinical study of bladder cancer in adolescent patients]. Nippon Hinyokika Gakkai Zasshi 90:614–618

19. Fleshner NE, Herr HW, Stewart AK, et al (1996) The National Cancer Data Base report on bladder carcinoma. The American College of Surgeons Commission on Cancer and the American Cancer Society. Cancer 78:1505–1513

20. Advanced Bladder Cancer Meta-analysis Collaboration (2003) Neoadjuvant chemotherapy in invasive bladder cancer: a systematic review and meta-analysis. Lancet 361:1927–1934

21. Bajorin DF, Dodd PM, Mazumdar M, et al (1999) Long-term survival in metastatic transitional-cell carcinoma and prognostic factors predicting outcome of therapy. J Clin Oncol 17:3173–3181

22. Sandhu DP, Munson KW, Benghiat A, Hopper IP, et al (1992) Natural history and prognosis of prostate carcinoma in adolescents and men under 35 years of age. Br J Urol 69:525–529

23. Camp NJ, Swensen J, Horne BD, et al (2005) Characterization of linkage disequilibrium structure, mutation history, and tagging SNPs, and their use in association analyses: ELAC2 and familial early-onset prostate cancer. Genet Epidemiol 28:232–243

24. Edwards SM, Kote-Jarai Z, Meitz J, et al (2003) Two percent of men with early-onset prostate cancer harbor germline mutations in the BRCA2 gene. Am J Hum Genet 72:1–12

25. Oakley-Girvan I, Feedman D, Ecceshall TR, et al (2004) Risk of early-onset prostate cancer in relation to germ line polymorphisms of the vitamin D receptor. Cancer Epidemiol Biomarkers Prev 13:1325–1330

26. Kotsis SV, Spencer SL, Peyser PA, et al (2002) Early onset prostate cancer: predictors of clinical grade. J Urol 167:1659–1663

27. Tannock IF, De Wit R, Berry WR, et al (2004) Docetaxel plus prednisone or mitoxantrone plus prednisone for advanced prostate cancer. N Engl J Med 351:1502–1512

28. Ries LAG, Eisner MP, Kosary CL, et al. (eds) (2004) SEER Cancer Statistics Review, 1975–2001. National Cancer Institute, Bethesda, MD

Thyroid Cancer

Steven G. Waguespack • Samuel A. Wells

Contents

16.1 Introduction

In adolescents and young adults, thyroid carcinoma represents approximately 7.5% of all malignancies in the 15- to 19-year-old age group and 10.6% of all cancers in patients 20–24 years old [1, 2]. In children younger than 15 years of age, it is a much rarer malignancy. Fortunately, in young patients diagnosed with thyroid carcinoma, the overall 5-year survival rate is 98–100% [3], assuring an excellent long-term prognosis in most cases. Because of the small number of cases in children each year and because of the extended follow up necessary to perform prospective clinical studies, pediatric thyroid carcinoma remains a poorly studied disease, with most treatment recommendations based upon the experience treating adults. Although this is adequate in most cases, there are potentially significant differences in the biology of pediatric thyroid carcinomas that need to be appreciated by the clinician who is providing care to this group of patients. Furthermore, as with any rare disorder, optimal treatment for pediatric thyroid carcinoma is best accomplished at a center with familiarity and multi-specialty expertise in treating this disease.

Pediatric thyroid malignancies arise typically from one of two normal thyroid cell populations, either the thyroid follicular epithelium or the parafollicular C cell, which has a distinct embryologic origin. Differentiated thyroid carcinoma (DTC) – including papillary thyroid carcinoma (PTC), follicular thyroid carcinoma (FTC), and their variants – arises from the former, whereas medullary thyroid carcinoma (MTC) arises from the latter. Appreciating this major histologic distinction is fundamental to understanding the differences in the biologic behavior and treatment applicable to these very different thyroid cancers. Although poorly differentiated and frankly anaplastic thyroid carcinomas can occur in the adolescent and young adult population, they are exceedingly rare. Therefore, the current chapter will focus only on DTC and MTC.

16.2 Epidemiology

The incidence of thyroid cancer peaks between 40 and 70 years of age, with an earlier peak in females than males (Fig. 16.1) [1]. At all ages it is more common in females, with the female:male ratio highest in older adolescents and young adults (Fig. 16.2). At all ages, thyroid cancer in the United States is most common among non-Hispanic whites and Asian/Pacific Islanders, and least common blacks/African-Americans (Fig. 16.3)

16.3 Differentiated Thyroid Carcinoma

16.3.1 Epidemiology

In childhood, thyroid carcinoma is more a disease of teenagers, with the approximate median age of diagnosis being 15 years [4]. The incidence of DTC varies from 0.5–1.5 cases/million/year in children less than 15 years of age to 14.6, 36.1, and 53.2 cases per million per year in the 15–19, 20–24, and 25–29 year age groups, respectively [2, 5]. DTC is more common in females, and the female:male incidence is greater than 5:1 in adolescents and young adults [1, 2]. This sex difference is not pronounced in children younger than 10 years. Although a definite increase in thyroid cancer cases has been identified in females age 20–40 years between the years 1975 and 2000, the same has not been found in males or in females less than age 20 years [2].

DTC is among the most curable of malignancies, particularly if identified early and treated appropriately. The overall prognosis of pediatric DTC is favorable even for patients with disseminated disease at diagnosis [6, 7]. However, some of these individuals may succumb to their disease or die from treatment-related complications decades after diagnosis, which under-

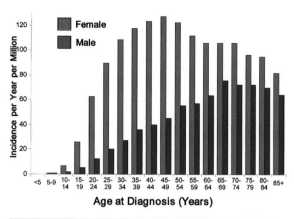

Figure 16.1

Incidence of thyroid cancer among males (*blue*) and females (*pink*) as a function of age at diagnosis. United States SEER 1975–2000 [1]

scores the importance of life-long follow up in these cases [6]. Children diagnosed prior to age 10 years may have a higher chance of dying from their disease, albeit still many years to decades after diagnosis [5, 78].

Although several prognostic scoring systems have been described for thyroid carcinoma, a thorough discussion of these is beyond the scope of the current chapter. The pathological tumor-node-metastasis (TNM) classification is used as the international reference staging system and may be superior, given that it takes into account the prognostic effects of lymph node metastases at presentation [9]. By definition, however, the highest TNM stage that anyone less than age 45 years can achieve is stage II, even with distant metastases. Therefore, utilizing the TNM staging system as an indicator of prognosis or how aggressive treatment should be is not very useful in managing children and young adults with DTC.

16.3.2 Etiology/Pathology

DTC is the most commonly encountered thyroid cancer in childhood, with PTC representing about 80% and FTC being roughly 20% of malignancies that arise from the follicular epithelium [5, 10, 11]. The diagnosis of PTC and FTC is based upon unique histopathological features, and there are subtypes of each, includ-

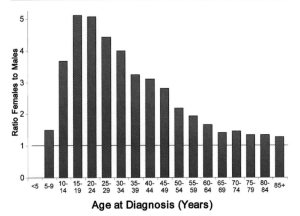

Figure 16.2

Relative prevalence of thyroid cancer among males and females (shown as the ratio of females to males as a function of age at diagnosis). United States SEER 1975–2000 [1]

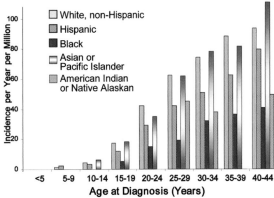

Figure 16.3

Incidence of thyroid cancer in the United States as a function of race/ethnicity. United States SEER 1975–2000 [1]

ing follicular cell, tall cell, diffuse sclerosing, columnar cell, and encapsulated variants in PTC. Variants of FTC include Hürthle-cell (oncocytic), clear cell, and insular carcinoma. Certain tumor subtypes, such as the follicular and diffuse sclerosing variants of PTC, are more common in children and young adults as compared to older individuals [12]. Furthermore, as compared to the classical type found in older individuals, childhood PTC, particularly in patients less than 10 years of age: (1) may be unencapsulated and widely invasive throughout the gland and (2) may have a follicular and solid architecture with unique nuclear features and abundant psammoma bodies [5, 7].

Despite the fact that PTC and FTC are both derived from the follicular epithelium and are treated in a similar fashion, there are some key differences in clinical behavior, specifically the risk and pattern of metastases. PTC is more likely to metastasize through lymphatic channels to regional neck lymph nodes. Hematogenous metastases, primarily to the lung, occur less frequently and typically only when locally metastatic disease is also present. FTC, on the other hand, is more prone to hematogenous metastases (affecting predominantly the lungs and bones); they metastasize less often to regional lymph nodes. Furthermore, PTC is more likely to be multifocal and bilateral [13]; FTC, in contrast, is usually a unifocal tumor.

The major established environmental risk factor for the development of benign and malignant thyroid neoplasms, particularly PTC, is radiation exposure to the head and neck [14, 15]. Children, particularly those less than age 5 years, are much more sensitive to the tumorigenic effects of irradiation [4, 15]; this may in part be due to the higher rate of thyroid cell replication in children as compared to adults [12, 16, 17]. Since children are no longer treated with radiation for benign conditions, such as thymic enlargement, tonsillar hypertrophy, or acne, there are now fewer thyroid cancer patients with this well-established risk factor; however, the use of external-beam radiotherapy to treat malignancies (especially Hodgkin disease) remains a significant risk for the development of thyroid carcinoma, even many years after therapy is complete [18]. Although there are some conflicting data, it appears that cases of radiation-induced thyroid carcinoma are not significantly different in clinical behavior as compared to sporadic non-radiation-induced tumors [18, 19].

Internal ionizing radiation, such as that which occurred with the large environmental exposure to radioactive iodine from the Chernobyl nuclear accident, is another well-documented risk for the development of PTC, particularly in children less than 10 years of age at the time of exposure [20, 21]. Recent evidence suggests that the thyroid gland in younger children is better equipped to transport iodine as compared to older children [17]. Assuming that the mean radiation exposure per gram of thyroid tissue is inversely related to the age of the individual at exposure, it would make sense why the youngest children are most at risk for developing PTC after accidents such as Chernobyl. Fortunately, the doses of radioactive iodine used in diagnostic studies and the treatment of hyperthyroidism appear to be below the threshold needed for tumorigenesis [14].

Researchers are beginning to unravel the molecular and genetic basis of the differentiated thyroid carcinomas. One of the major early somatic events that is associated with the development of papillary thyroid carcinoma is a chromosomal rearrangement linking the promoter region of an unrelated gene(s) (named *PTC*) to the carboxyl terminus of the *RET* (rearranged during transfection) proto-oncogene [12, 16, 21]. This occurs either because of a simple inversion of a segment of chromosome 10 (where *RET* resides) or a translocation of *RET* to a different chromosome. The *RET/PTC* rearrangement produces a chimeric oncogene, resulting in a constitutively activated form of the *RET* receptor tyrosine kinase (i.e., activation in the absence of ligand), thereby promoting tumorigenesis. Although it is believed that *RET/PTC* rearrangements may be critical for the development of pediatric and radiation-induced PTC [22–28], some recent reports have challenged these conclusions [29].

Other important genes and gene products implicated in thyroid tumorigenesis and biological behavior include *RAS* and *B-RAF* (important for intracellular signaling pathways; *B-RAF* is implicated in PTC only), rearrangement of the *TRK* proto-oncogene (akin to *RET*, but found in only a minority of PTCs), *MET* overexpression (mostly in PTCs), the *p53* tumor suppressor gene (specifically involved in anaplastic thyroid cancer), and *Pax8-PPARγ1* translocations (follicular adenomas and follicular thyroid carcinomas only) [12, 16, 30, 31].

Approximately 3–5% of patients with PTC have a family history of the disease [12, 32]. Having a positive family history may portend a worse prognosis, given that these cases appear to have more aggressive disease and shorter disease-free intervals after initial treatment [32, 33]. As of yet, the genetic basis for dominantly inherited non-MTC has not been elucidated. Other familial tumor syndromes in which there is an increased risk of DTC include familial adenomatous polyposis (Gardner syndrome), Cowden disease, and the Carney complex [12].

16.3.3 Diagnosis and Clinical Presentation

In childhood, DTC usually presents as an asymptomatic neck mass [34, 35]. Occasionally, the diagnosis may be made incidentally after the discovery of pulmonary nodules on a chest radiograph. In any individual younger than 20 years of age presenting with a solitary thyroid nodule, there is a higher likelihood of malignancy [10, 36]. The overall prevalence of thyroid carcinoma is about 20–25% of thyroid nodules in children, compared to 5% in adults [10, 12, 37, 38]. Symptomatic thyroid cancers (i.e., those associated with hoarseness, dysphagia, or cough, thus suggesting more locally advanced disease) are rare in young individuals. Uncommonly, thyroid carcinoma arises ectopically in a thyroglossal duct remnant or cyst. Arguably, this would be an unusual presentation of childhood thyroid carcinoma, but it must be kept in mind for patients presenting with a midline mass in the region of the hyoid. Finally, although most patients are euthyroid at the time of diagnosis, rare cases of differentiated follicular thyroid carcinomas can present as a functioning nodule associated with a suppressed thyroid stimulating hormone (TSH) or frank thyrotoxicosis.

In children and young adults, it is not unusual for thyroid carcinoma to present only with cervical lymphadenopathy, and locally metastatic disease is indeed present at diagnosis in the majority of pediatric PTC cases [67, 35, 39, 40]. In addition, children more often have disseminated disease at diagnosis, with lung metastases identified in up to 20% of cases [7, 39–41]. Metastases to other sites, such as bone and brain, are rare.

In a patient presenting with a painless thyroid nodule, the first procedure should be a high-quality neck ultrasound (US; together with fine-needle aspiration, FNA), which assists greatly with surgical planning [42]. US is useful in determining the size and appearance of the lesion, assessing for other nodules, ensuring the accuracy of FNA, and looking for evidence of metastatic lymphadenopathy. For these reasons, US should be considered even when the diagnosis of thyroid carcinoma is already known. However, it should not be understated that the utility of ultrasound is greatly dependent upon the expertise of the ultrasonographer, particularly when it comes to identifying metastatic lymphadenopathy. Baseline thyroid function tests should also be obtained at presentation. Nuclear imaging studies using radioactive iodine or technetium pertechnetate are not very useful in the initial evaluation of these patients, except in those with a low TSH, because even benign thyroid nodules will be "cold" on nuclear imaging. In DTC, tumor cells typically retain the ability to produce the thyroid-specific glycoprotein, thyroglobulin (TG). Measuring TG is not routinely recommended in the initial evaluation of a thyroid neoplasm, because elevated TG levels are identified in a variety of benign thyroid processes, thereby lowering the specificity of this diagnostic test. Once a diagnosis of thyroid carcinoma is established, however, a baseline TG may be useful for follow up. A chest x-ray or chest computed tomography without contrast to assess for pulmonary metastases should also be considered at diagnosis, noting that many individuals with lung metastases may not have abnormalities visualized on plain radiographs [40].

There remains some controversy about the definitive management of thyroid nodules in children. For example, biopsy (often using US guidance) is the recommended initial procedure in adults and can easily be accomplished in mature adolescents and young adults [38, 43–46]. Although FNA can also be easily performed in younger children, conscious sedation may be required. On the other hand, many experts feel that the initial diagnostic step should be surgery (i.e., lobectomy and isthmusectomy), given the higher likelihood that a thyroid nodule in a child, particularly when accompanied by palpable lymphadenopathy, is a carcinoma. Although this is a reasonable approach, it is our feeling that a preoperative FNA (and subsequent pathologic diagnosis) allows for better operative planning and minimizes the need for a second surgery, particularly in children who present with a single thyroid nodule only.

16.3.4 Management

The initial care of children and young adults with DTC is fairly algorithmic in nature, and consensus guidelines exist that can help the practitioner manage these patients [46]. However, it cannot be emphasized enough that established recommendations always need to be individualized for each patient. Therefore, they provide only a framework in which to practice. Finally, it is imperative to note that no prospective clinical trials have been undertaken in children to determine the optimal therapeutic approach.

Assuming that a diagnosis of PTC is made preoperatively, the initial procedure of choice is a total thyroidectomy with care to preserve the parathyroid glands and the laryngeal nerves [47, 48]. Total thyroidectomy, compared to lesser procedures, is associated with a higher incidence of surgical complications, particularly hypoparathyroidism. It cannot be emphasized enough that the thyroidectomy be done by a surgeon who has great experience performing the procedure. Lobectomy and isthmusectomy may suffice in the older teenager and young adult with a small unifocal PTC, but a total thyroidectomy (to facilitate ^{131}I therapy) is usually recommended for children less than 15 years of age because of the greater risk of disease recurrence and the higher likelihood of metastatic disease in this age group [4, 34, 40, 41, 46, 49]. Typically, a selective dissection of visibly enlarged or palpable lymph nodes is performed at the initial surgery. However, a complete neck dissection is indicated in patients with extensive involvement of the cervical nodes. In children with known distant metastases to the lungs, a total thyroidectomy and neck dissection is still required to facilitate subsequent radioactive iodine (RAI) therapy.

A diagnosis of FTC is typically made only after pathologic review of a resected thyroid nodule, since the characteristics of FTC (capsular and/or vascular invasion) cannot be seen on an FNA specimen, which is usually read as a "follicular neoplasm" or "follicular lesion." Although the prognosis of FTC may not be as dependent on the extent of the initial surgery (unlike PTC), a total thyroidectomy facilitates the use of ^{131}I therapy to ablate the normal thyroid remnant, which permits an increased sensitivity to detect disease recurrence, thus improving the outcome for patients with FTC [50].

Following total or completion thyroidectomy (if the initial surgery entailed only a lobectomy), the patient is rendered hypothyroid with plans to administer RAI therapy 4–6 weeks later. This treatment is based upon studies in adults that demonstrate a lower recurrence rate and subsequent lower cancer-related mortality rate in patients treated with [131]I [51]. Although RAI therapy in low-risk patients is controversial, it is generally recommended that all patients less than 15 years who have been treated surgically for PTC or FTC receive additional therapy with ^{131}I, both to ablate the normal thyroid gland remnant (hence making long-term follow up easier) and to treat any remaining thyroid cancer or metastases [52].

Although short-term triiodothyronine therapy (Cytomel 1–2 µg/kg/day divided twice daily to three times daily) is used frequently in adolescents and young adults, younger children are often quite tolerant of hypothyroidism. Therefore, it is also reasonable to give no thyroid hormone therapy and have them return about 4 weeks after surgery, when the TSH should be well above the desired range of 25–30 µU/ml. A low-iodine diet is also followed for 2 weeks prior to scanning with ^{131}I to facilitate RAI uptake by any remaining thyroid tissues. A discussion of the necessity and type (^{123}I vs ^{131}I) of a pretherapy thyroid scan (i.e., a diagnostic scan) is beyond the scope of the current chapter, although most centers routinely obtain this to help determine the appropriate treatment dose of [131]I. There are no standard recommendations for the dose of ^{131}I to be administered to children, and most experts determine the dose based on a weight (or body surface area) adjustment of the typical adult dose used in that situation [48]. Alternatively, dosimetry studies can be used in select cases to estimate the appropriate dose of RAI. Finally, in any female patient, pregnancy should be ruled out prior to the administration of any radioiodine.

After the initial therapies of surgery and RAI ablation, the long-term management of DTC includes replacing thyroid hormone with a brand-name levothyroxine product, appreciating that thyroid hormone requirements are higher in childhood and understanding that thyroid function tests often have to be monitored regularly (every 3–6 months) to keep pace with a growing child. Mildly supra-physiologic dosing is administered so that the TSH is kept below the lower limits of normal to prevent TSH-stimulated thyroid carcinoma growth. Thyroglobulin serves as an excellent tumor marker, and it is expected that TG levels will become undetectable after successful therapy. If TG does not become undetectable with TSH-suppressive therapy, the possibility of residual disease must be entertained and appropriate diagnostic studies should be ordered. TG samples should also be screened routinely for the presence of TG autoantibodies, which occurs in up to 25% of thyroid cancer patients. In any individual with positive antibodies, the TG cannot be interpreted due to assay interference and a likely false-negative result. In these cases, the antibody titer can be followed, since many patients cured of their disease will ultimately reach levels of zero, albeit several years after diagnosis [53].

Unlike other childhood cancers, DTC in children and young adults is not treated routinely with chemotherapy or external-beam radiation therapy. Chemotherapy has not been shown to be effective in thyroid cancer, although it may be tried as a last resort in patients who have rapidly progressive disease, despite maximized surgical and RAI therapies. External-beam radiation therapy is not offered routinely to patients who are younger than 45 years of age, although the rare case of a pathologically unfavorable thyroid carcinoma with known residual neck disease may warrant such an aggressive approach.

Children and young adults with DTC require lifelong surveillance, both to identify delayed recurrences and to assess for any late treatment effects. This is accomplished through TG measurements and appropriate radiologic studies, such as intermittent neck US and RAI scans as indicated. If a patient is identified to have a local recurrence, surgery is the treatment of choice. If the recurrence is not amenable to surgical therapy or if distant metastases are identified, assessment and treatment with RAI is appropriate, assuming that the disease readily concentrates the isotope on diagnostic imaging.

16.3.5 Late Effects

One of the unique aspects of DTC is the use of RAI in the evaluation and treatment of patients with this disease. Therapy with ^{131}I is generally well tolerated and safe. Early and usually transient side effects of ^{131}I may include nausea, vomiting, sialoadenitis, xerostomia, loss of taste, thyroiditis (if a sizable thyroid remnant remains after surgery), and, rarely, bone marrow suppression (leukopenia and thrombocytopenia) [54]. Some of these early side effects may be minimized by having the patient drink lots of water after therapy and suck on tart candies, such as lemon drops, to promote salivary flow. The long-term consequences of ^{131}I therapy in children remain an area of concern, particularly in individuals who receive high cumulative doses in early childhood. Much remains to be learned about possible late effects, which can include infertility (particularly in men), permanent damage to the salivary glands resulting in chronic xerostomia or salivary duct stones, excessive dental caries, reduced taste, pulmonary fibrosis (in those with diffuse pulmonary metastases), and the possibility of the development of other cancers (stomach, bladder, colon, salivary gland, breast, and leukemia) after very high cumulative doses of ^{131}I [54]. Therefore, caution should be exercised when giving multiple repeat doses of ^{131}I to children and young adults, particularly in those patients whose disease is more indolent and does not require such aggressive therapy.

16.4 Medullary Thyroid Carcinoma

16.4.1 Epidemiology

In children and young adults, MTC is an uncommon disease with an incidence of less than 1 case/million/year [2]. It accounts for approximately 7–10% of all thyroid malignancies. As compared to DTC, there is no clear gender predilection, as would be expected for a malignancy that is largely a dominantly inherited disease when diagnosed at a young age (see below). Five-year survival rates for MTC are between 90 and 95% in the pediatric and young adult population [2]. In patients not diagnosed early, incurable yet indolent disease is often the norm.

16.4.2 Etiology/Pathology

Even though MTC is a unique endocrine neoplasm with several distinguishing features, it was not recog-

nized as a distinct clinical entity until 1959 [55]. During embryogenesis, progenitor C cells stream from the neural crest and populate several endocrine organs, including the pituitary, the thyroid, the pancreatic islet cells, the adrenal medulla, and the enterochromaffin system of the gut. In mammals, the neural-crest-derived C cells become entrapped in the upper portion of the lateral thyroid complex as it develops during embryogenesis. The greatest concentration of these parafollicular C cells is at the intersection between the upper one-third and lower two-thirds of the thyroid cephalad–caudal central axis. It is these cells that give rise to MTC. Therefore, although MTC is recognized as a thyroid tumor, it is more properly characterized as a malignancy of neural crest origin.

Sporadic MTC rarely occurs in children and young adults. Therefore, it is more appropriately characterized as a genetic disease when it affects this age group. Almost all children with MTC are afflicted with one of three hereditary cancer syndromes: multiple endocrine neoplasia type 2a (MEN2A) or type 2b (MEN2B), and familial MTC (FMTC). In addition to MTC, 50% of patients with MEN2A and MEN2B develop pheochromocytomas, and up to 20% of MEN2A patients develop hyperparathyroidism [56]. Patients with MEN2A may also develop a pruritic cutaneous lesion on the upper back, termed "cutaneous lichen amyloidosis" [57], and some kindreds can have associated Hirschsprung's disease [58]. All patients with MEN2B develop a generalized ganglioneuromatosis, manifested most obviously by the presence of oral mucosal neuromas, and a characteristic facial appearance and Marfanoid body habitus. Patients with FMTC only develop MTC.

MTC occurs in virtually all patients with these familial endocrinopathies, and it is the most common cause of death in affected individuals. The development of MTC in this setting is particularly relevant in children because, with current methods of diagnosis and treatment, MTC is one of the few malignancies that can be prevented or cured before it becomes clinically relevant.

Over 10 years ago, it was found that characteristic mis-sense mutations in the *RET* proto-oncogene caused MEN2A, MEN2B, and FMTC [59–61]. *RET* encodes for a tyrosine kinase receptor that is important for the differentiation of neural-crest-derived tissues. These point mutations cause activation of intracellular signaling pathways in the absence of ligand. In patients with MEN2A, mutations are located mostly in the extracellular cysteine-rich domain of the *RET* proto-oncogene, usually in exon 10 (codons 609, 611, 618, or 620) or exon 11 (codon 634). In almost all cases, there is a family history of MEN2A-associated neoplasms. In patients with MEN2B, which occurs as a de novo mutation in over half the cases, the mutation is almost exclusively in exon 16 (a change from methionine to threonine at codon 918), located in the intracellular tyrosine kinase domain of the gene. In patients with FMTC, the *RET* mutations are found in codons similar to MEN2A, or less often, in exon 13 (codons 768, 790, and 791), exon 14 (codon 804), or exon 15 (codon 891). There is a correlation between genotype and phenotype in that patients with MTC, pheochromocytomas, and hyperparathyroidism almost always have mutations in codon 634, whereas patients with MTC and pheochromocytomas, but not hyperparathyroidism, most often have mutations in codons 618, 620, or 634.

The exact etiology of sporadic MTC is unknown. However, after the discovery that familial forms of MTC are associated with germ-line mutations in the *RET* proto-oncogene, it was discovered that somatic mutations in *RET*, namely in codon 918, can be identified in over 40% of sporadic cases of MTC [62]. Due to the rarity of sporadic MTC in the population less than 20 years of age, no comparative analysis can be made between the tumor in young and old patients.

On gross examination, MTC is whitish tan and located in the upper pole(s) of the thyroid lobe. Larger tumors often become calcified. In patients with sporadic tumors, only one thyroid lobe is involved. In patients with heritable disease, the MTC is virtually always bilateral, multicentric and located at the junction of the upper one-third and lower two-thirds of the thyroid lobes. Therefore, the finding of a multifocal MTC in any patient should raise concern for an underlying *RET* mutation. On microscopic examination the tumor cells have a spindle-shape appearance, and with special staining, one sees material with histological properties of amyloid. Also, in patients with the familial forms of MTC, clusters of C cells (C-cell hyperplasia) are also routinely identified pathologically. This C-cell hyperplasia is believed to be one of the initial stages in the development and progression of MTC [63].

The biological aggressiveness of MTC depends on the hereditary setting in which it develops. In patients with MEN2B, the MTC progresses rapidly and thyroidectomy, regardless of the age at which it is performed, is rarely curative. In patients with FMTC, however, the MTC progresses slowly, and it is uncommon for patients to die from this malignancy. In patients with MEN2A, the MTC is somewhat capricious; it usually follows an indolent course, but in some patients, it may progress rapidly. The reasons for this variable biological behavior of MTC in these various clinical entities are unknown. It is also difficult to assess the behavior of MTC in sporadic compared to familial cases. It is known that the MTC has a biological behavior that is more aggressive than PTC or FTC but less aggressive than anaplastic or poorly differentiated thyroid carcinomas.

16.4.3 Diagnosis and Clinical Presentation

The MTC cells have great biosynthetic activity and secrete calcitonin (CTN) and carcinoembryonic antigen (CEA), both of which are excellent tumor markers for the disease. CTN, in particular, provides a high degree of diagnostic sensitivity, specifically in the long-term follow up of MTC. Occasionally, MTC can lose its ability to produce CTN, which is usually indicative of a more aggressive tumor and hence a poorer prognosis. Intravenous calcium and pentagastrin are potent CTN secretagogues that stimulate production of the hormone within minutes of injection. Measurement of basal and stimulated plasma CTN levels is especially useful in the evaluation of patients following thyroidectomy. Elevated levels post-operatively indicate the presence of metastatic MTC, even though it may not be evident clinically. Furthermore, a pre-operative diagnosis can also be made by measuring basal or stimulated levels of plasma CTN. Considering the rarity of MTC and the possibility of false-positive results, preoperative measurement of CTN in children presenting with nodular thyroid disease is not performed routinely . However, in kindred members of MEN2A, MEN2B, or FMTC families who present with a thyroid nodule, the diagnosis of MTC must be excluded, and measuring plasma CTN levels in this setting may be useful.

Similar to DTC, MTC usually presents as a firm, painless neck mass without associated abnormalities. However, in those who have very high plasma CTN levels, diarrhea and/or flushing may be present. The tumor has spread usually beyond the thyroid gland by the time it becomes clinically apparent. Therefore, most patients presenting with a palpable MTC already have metastases to regional cervical nodes at diagnosis [58]. The overall approach to the evaluation of a child suspected to have MTC is similar to the assessment of PTC and FTC, including the use of US and FNA. One major difference, however, rests in our ability to diagnose MTC (in the context of a positive family history and a known *RET* mutation) in advance of clinical disease (i.e., a palpable thyroid nodule). As genetic testing becomes more widely utilized in families with MEN2A and FMTC, more children and young adults are presenting with C-cell hyperplasia or microscopic MTC that is detected early only because genetic testing was undertaken.

16.4.4 Management

The identification of *RET* proto-oncogene mutations as the cause for hereditary MTC has provided the opportunity for direct DNA analysis in clinically normal individuals at risk for having inherited a mutated allele, thus permitting identification at a young age of those destined to develop MTC. This technology has revolutionized the surgical management in this group of patients, since these children can now have prophylactic thyroidectomy before they develop a thyroid malignancy [64].

Any child or young adult diagnosed with MTC should have a total thyroidectomy with resection of lymph nodes in the central zone of the neck (an anatomical region bounded above and below by the hyoid bone and the sternal notch, and laterally by the carotid arteries). If nodal metastases are evident grossly, the lymph node dissection should be extended to the lateral neck(s). Children from kindreds with MEN2A, MEN2B, or FMTC found by direct DNA screening to have inherited a mutated *RET* allele should also have a

total thyroidectomy. Resection of lymph nodes in the central zone of the neck is required in MEN2B patients, but can be performed selectively in MEN2A and FMTC patients, specifically those undergoing prophylactic thyroidectomy, as long as the pre-operative evaluation is favorable.

The timing of prophylactic thyroidectomy remains an area of debate, and recommendations are based upon the earliest ages at which children with a particular mutation present with clinically relevant disease. Currently, *RET* proto-oncogene mutations are stratified into one of three levels [56]. It is the usual practice in MEN2A kindreds (level 2) to perform total thyroidectomy by 5 years of age, whereas in MEN2B patients (level 3), surgery is recommended within the first 6–12 months of life. Children with level 1 mutations (codons 609, 768, 790, 791, 804, and 891) have the lowest risk for the development of aggressive MTC, and the timing of thyroidectomy in these cases remains controversial [56].

In patients with MTC and/or MEN2, it is critically important that the presence of a pheochromocytoma be excluded prior to thyroidectomy, since severe complications and even death due to excessive catecholamine release may occur during anesthetic induction or during the operative procedure. The most useful way to screen for this is via plasma metanephrines, particularly in young children in whom timed urine collections may be difficult. If identified, the pheochromocytoma(s) should be resected, usually laparoscopically, prior to thyroidectomy. As with any case of pheochromocytoma, surgery should proceed only after appropriate alpha (and beta) blockade.

In patients with sporadic or heritable MTC and no evidence of hyperparathyroidism, every effort should be made to preserve parathyroid gland function at the time of thyroidectomy. If there is any question about parathyroid gland viability during the procedure, parathyroid tissue is typically grafted into a sternocleidomastoid muscle. If this procedure is performed carefully, it virtually assures that the patient will have normal parathyroid function in the post-operative period. In patients with MEN2A and hyperparathyroidism, a total parathyroidectomy with autotransplantation of parathyroid gland tissue to the non-dominant forearm is the procedure of choice. Some surgeons prefer to perform a radical subtotal 3½-gland parathyroid-ectomy in these cases. However, in combination with a total thyroidectomy, this procedure is associated with a greater risk of permanent post-operative hypoparathyroidism. If there is no evidence of hyperparathyroidism and the patient has a *RET* codon 634 mutation, which is commonly associated with hyperparathyroidism, parathyroid tissue is grafted to the non-dominant forearm. It is critically important that parathyroid function be preserved in all of these patients, especially in young children, since permanent hypoparathyroidism can be a difficult problem to manage.

Children who have thyroidectomy performed prior to the time that the disease is evident clinically have an excellent chance of being cured. Patients are cured infrequently if the disease progresses beyond the thyroid gland. In these cases, patients may have microscopic disease (detectable only via tumor markers) and be asymptomatic for years. However, the tumors tend to grow progressively and can metastasize to mediastinal lymph nodes, lung, liver, and/or bone. Metastases are often vascular, and hepatic metastases may be confused with hemangiomas on imaging studies. The management of patients with metastatic disease presents a major challenge because the tumors are not sensitive to standard chemotherapeutic regimens, which usually incorporate the agent dacarbazine (DTIC), nor are they very sensitive to conventional doses of external-beam radiotherapy. Unlike DTC, the use of RAI in MTC is not beneficial or indicated.

The long-term follow up of children and young adults diagnosed with MTC involves monitoring CTN and CEA levels, obtaining US and other imaging studies as indicated by tumor markers, and screening routinely for the other endocrine manifestations of MEN2A and MEN2B, noting that these typically have their onset in adulthood. The life-long management of heritable MTC also includes appropriate genetic counseling, and it is ideal to involve a genetic counselor at the outset to assist these children and their families in understanding this dominantly inherited disease.

16.4.5 Late Effects

If the initial surgical procedure is successful, patients are cured of MTC and have normal serum calcium lev-els and phonation. If the recurrent laryngeal nerves or the external branches of the superior laryngeal nerve are damaged, patients may be hoarse following surgery and require reconstruction procedures of the vocal cords. Patients who develop permanent hypoparathyroidism will require life-long vitamin D and oral calcium preparations to maintain eucalcemia.

16.5 Conclusions

Thyroid carcinoma in childhood is a rare clinical entity that can usually be treated successfully, particularly if the disease is diagnosed at an early stage. The adolescent or young adult diagnosed with a thyroid malignancy becomes part of a larger group of individuals dealing with an uncommon and sometimes chronic disease that requires life-long follow up, even if it is just to adjust thyroid hormone replacement. The future is often uncertain for young patients, specifically for those with metastatic disease, given the paucity of prospective clinical studies.

Acknowledgments

We would like to express our sincere appreciation to Drs. Rena Vas-Sellin and Nicholas Sarlis for their thoughtful review of this manuscript.

References

1. Bleyer WA, OLeary M, Barr R, Ries LAG (eds) (2006) Cancer Epidemiology in Older Adolescents and Young Adults 15 to 29 Years of Age, including SEER Incidence and Survival, 1975–2000. National Cancer Institute, NIH Pub. No. 06-5767, Bethesda MD; also available at www.seer.cancer.gov/publications
2. Wu XC, Chen VW, Steele B, et al (2003) Cancer incidence in adolescents and young adults in the United States, 1992–1997. J Adolesc Health 32:405–415
3. Ries LAG, Eisner MP, Kosary CL, et al (2003) SEER Cancer Statistics Review, 1975–2000. National Cancer Institute, Bethesda, MD
4. Sklar CA, La Quaglia MP (2003) Thyroid cancer in children and adolescents. In: Radovick S, MacGillivray MH (eds) Pediatric Endocrinology: A Practical Clinical Guide. Humana Press, Totowa, NJ, pp 327–339
5. Harach HR, Williams ED (1995) Childhood thyroid cancer in England and Wales. Br J Cancer 72:777–783

6. Vassilopoulou-Sellin R, Goepfert H, Raney B, Schultz PN (1998) Differentiated thyroid cancer in children and adolescents: clinical outcome and mortality after long-term follow-up. Head Neck 20:549–555

7. Zimmerman D, Hay ID, Gough IR, et al (1988) Papillary thyroid carcinoma in children and adults: long-term follow-up of 1039 patients conservatively treated at one institution during three decades. Surgery 104:1157–1166

8. Travagli JP, Schlumberger M, De Vathaire F, et al (1995) Differentiated thyroid carcinoma in childhood. J Endocrinol Invest 18:161–164

9. Voutilainen PE, Siironen P, Franssila KO, et al (2003) AMES, MACIS and TNM prognostic classifications in papillary thyroid carcinoma. Anticancer Res 23:4283–4288

10. Raab SS, Silverman JF, Elsheikh TM, et al (1995) Pediatric thyroid nodules: disease demographics and clinical management as determined by fine needle aspiration biopsy. Pediatrics 95:46–49

11. Hung W (1992) Nodular thyroid disease and thyroid carcinoma. Pediatr Ann 21:50–57

12. Schlumberger M, Pacini F (2003) Thyroid Tumors. Nucleon, Paris

13. Katoh R, Sasaki J, Kurihara H, et al (1992) Multiple thyroid involvement (intraglandular metastasis) in papillary thyroid carcinoma. A clinicopathologic study of 105 consecutive patients. Cancer 70:1585–1590

14. Schneider AB (2003) Radiation-induced thyroid cancer: UpToDate Online 11:3

15. Boice JD Jr (1996) Cancer following irradiation in childhood and adolescence. Med Pediatr Oncol Suppl 1:29–34

16. Alberti L, Carniti C, Miranda C, et al (2003) RET and NTRK1 proto-oncogenes in human diseases. J Cell Physiol 195:168–186

17. Faggiano A, Coulot J, Bellon N, et al (2004) Age-dependent variation of follicular size and expression of iodine transporters in human thyroid tissue. J Nucl Med 45:232–237

18. Acharya S, Sarafoglou K, LaQuaglia M, et al (2003) Thyroid neoplasms after therapeutic radiation for malignancies during childhood or adolescence. Cancer 97:2397–2403

19. Samaan NA, Schultz PN, Ordonez NG, et al (1987) A comparison of thyroid carcinoma in those who have and have not had head and neck irradiation in childhood. J Clin Endocrinol Metab 64:219–223

20. Shibata Y, Yamashita S, Masyakin VB, et al (2001) 15 years after Chernobyl: new evidence of thyroid cancer. Lancet 358:1965–1966

21. Williams D (2002) Cancer after nuclear fallout: lessons from the Chernobyl accident. Nat Rev Cancer 2:543–549

22. Ito T, Seyama T, Iwamoto KS, et al (1993) In vitro irradiation is able to cause RET oncogene rearrangement. Cancer Res 53:2940–2943

23. Nikiforov YE (2002) RET/PTC rearrangement in thyroid tumors. Endocr Pathol 13:3–16

24. Fenton CL, Lukes Y, Nicholson D, et al (2000) The ret/PTC mutations are common in sporadic papillary thyroid carcinoma of children and young adults. J Clin Endocrinol Metab 85:1170–1175

25. Fugazzola L, Pilotti S, Pinchera A, et al (1995) Oncogenic rearrangements of the RET proto-oncogene in papillary thyroid carcinomas from children exposed to the Chernobyl nuclear accident. Cancer Res 55:5617–5620

26. Klugbauer S, Lengfelder E, Demidchik EP, Rabes HM (1995) High prevalence of RET rearrangement in thyroid tumors of children from Belarus after the Chernobyl reactor accident. Oncogene 11:2459–2467

27. Nikiforov YE, Rowland JM, Bove KE, et al (1997) Distinct pattern of ret oncogene rearrangements in morphological variants of radiation-induced and sporadic thyroid papillary carcinomas in children. Cancer Res 57:1690–1694

28. Bounacer A, Wicker R, Caillou B, et al (1997) High prevalence of activating ret proto-oncogene rearrangements, in thyroid tumors from patients who had received external radiation. Oncogene 15:1263–1273

29. Elisei R, Romei C, Vorontsova T, et al (2001) RET/PTC rearrangements in thyroid nodules: studies in irradiated and not irradiated, malignant and benign thyroid lesions in children and adults. J Clin Endocrinol Metab 86:3211–3216

30. Sarlis NJ (2000) Expression patterns of cellular growth-controlling genes in non-medullary thyroid cancer: basic aspects. Rev Endocr Metab Disord 1:183–196

31. Kimura ET, Nikiforova MN, Zhu Z, et al (2003) High prevalence of BRAF mutations in thyroid cancer: genetic evidence for constitutive activation of the RET/PTC-RAS-BRAF signaling pathway in papillary thyroid carcinoma. Cancer Res 63:1454–1457

32. Malchoff CD, Malchoff DM (1999) Familial nonmedullary thyroid carcinoma. Semin Surg Oncol 16:16–18

33. Alsanea O, Wada N, Ain K, et al (2000) Is familial non-medullary thyroid carcinoma more aggressive than sporadic thyroid cancer? A multicenter series. Surgery 128:1043–1050; discussion 1050–1051

34. Feinmesser R, Lubin E, Segal K, Noyek A (1997) Carcinoma of the thyroid in children – a review. J Pediatr Endocrinol Metab 10:561–568

35. Frankenthaler RA, Sellin RV, Cangir A, Goepfert H (1990) Lymph node metastasis from papillary-follicular thyroid carcinoma in young patients. Am J Surg 160:341–343

36. Schlumberger MJ (1998) Papillary and follicular thyroid carcinoma. N Engl J Med 338:297–306

37. Hung W (1999) Solitary thyroid nodules in 93 children and adolescents. a 35-years experience. Horm Res 52:15–18

38. Khurana KK, Labrador E, Izquierdo R, et al (1999) The role of fine-needle aspiration biopsy in the management of thyroid nodules in children, adolescents, and young adults: a multi-institutional study. Thyroid 9:383–386

39. Samuel AM, Sharma SM (1991) Differentiated thyroid carcinomas in children and adolescents. Cancer 67:2186–2190

40. Vassilopoulou-Sellin R, Klein MJ, Smith TH, et al (1993) Pulmonary metastases in children and young adults with differentiated thyroid cancer. Cancer 71:1348–1352

41. Schlumberger M, De Vathaire F, Travagli JP, et al (1987) Differentiated thyroid carcinoma in childhood: long term follow-up of 72 patients. J Clin Endocrinol Metab 65:1088–1094

42. Kouvaraki MA, Shapiro SE, Fornage BD, et al (2003) Role of preoperative ultrasonography in the surgical management of patients with thyroid cancer. Surgery 134:946–954; discussion 954–95

43. Corrias A, Einaudi S, Chiorboli E, et al (2001) Accuracy of fine needle aspiration biopsy of thyroid nodules in detecting malignancy in childhood: comparison with conventional clinical, laboratory, and imaging approaches. J Clin Endocrinol Metab 86:4644–4648

44. Arda IS, Yildirim S, Demirhan B, Firat S (2001) Fine needle aspiration biopsy of thyroid nodules. Arch Dis Child 85:313–317

45. Al-Shaikh A, Ngan B, Daneman A, Daneman D (2001) Fine-needle aspiration biopsy in the management of thyroid nodules in children and adolescents. J Pediatr 138:140–142

46. Sherman SI (2002) Clinical Practice Guidelines in Oncology: Thyroid Carcinoma version 1. 2002: National Comprehensive Cancer Network

47. La Quaglia MP, Black T, Holcomb GW III, et al (2000) Differentiated thyroid cancer: clinical characteristics, treatment, and outcome in patients under 21 years of age who present with distant metastases. A report from the Surgical Discipline Committee of the Children's Cancer Group. J Pediatr Surg 35:955–959; discussion 960

48. Hung W, Sarlis NJ (2002) Current controversies in the management of pediatric patients with well-differentiated nonmedullary thyroid cancer: a review. Thyroid 12:683–702

49. Welch Dinauer CA, Tuttle RM, Robie DK, et al (1999) Extensive surgery improves recurrence-free survival for children and young patients with class I papillary thyroid carcinoma. J Pediatr Surg 34:1799–1804

50. Taylor T, Specker B, Robbins J, et al (1998) Outcome after treatment of high-risk papillary and non-Hurthle-cell follicular thyroid carcinoma. Ann Intern Med 129:622–627

51. Mazzaferri EL, Jhiang SM (1994) Long-term impact of initial surgical and medical therapy on papillary and follicular thyroid cancer. Am J Med 97:418–428

52. Yeh SD, La Quaglia MP (1997) 131I therapy for pediatric thyroid cancer. Semin Pediatr Surg 6:128–133

53. Chiovato L, Latrofa F, Braverman LE, et al (2003) Disappearance of humoral thyroid autoimmunity after complete removal of thyroid antigens. Ann Intern Med 139:346–351

54. Meier DA, Brill DR, Becker DV, et al (2002) Procedure guideline for therapy of thyroid disease with (131)iodine. J Nucl Med 43:856–861

55. Hazard JB, Hawk WA, Crile G Jr (1959) Medullary (solid) carcinoma of the thyroid; a clinicopathologic entity. J Clin Endocrinol Metab 19:152–161

56. Brandi ML, Gagel RF, Angeli A, et al (2001) Guidelines for diagnosis and therapy of MEN type 1 and type 2. J Clin Endocrinol Metab 86:5658–5671

57. Gagel RF, Levy ML, Donovan DT, et al (1989) Multiple endocrine neoplasia type 2a associated with cutaneous lichen amyloidosis. Ann Intern Med 111:802–806

58. Moley JF, DeBenedetti MK (1999) Patterns of nodal metastases in palpable medullary thyroid carcinoma: recommendations for extent of node dissection. Ann Surg 229:880–887; discussion 887–888

59. Donis-Keller H, Dou S, Chi D, et al (1993) Mutations in the RET proto-oncogene are associated with MEN 2A and FMTC. Hum Mol Genet 2:851–856

60. Mulligan LM, Kwok JB, Healey CS, et al (1993) Germline mutations of the RET proto-oncogene in multiple endocrine neoplasia type 2A. Nature 363:458–460

61. Carlson KM, Dou S, Chi D, et al (1994) Single missense mutation in the tyrosine kinase catalytic domain of the RET protooncogene is associated with multiple endocrine neoplasia type 2B. Proc Natl Acad Sci U S A 91:1579–1583

62. Romei C, Elisei R, Pinchera A, et al (1996) Somatic mutations of the ret protooncogene in sporadic medullary thyroid carcinoma are not restricted to exon 16 and are associated with tumor recurrence. J Clin Endocrinol Metab 81:1619–1622

63. Machens A (2004) Early malignant progression of hereditary medullary thyroid cancer. N Engl J Med 350:943

64. Wells SA Jr, Chi DD, Toshima K, et al (1994) Predictive DNA testing and prophylactic thyroidectomy in patients at risk for multiple endocrine neoplasia type 2A. Ann Surg 220:237–247; discussion 247–250

Malignant Melanoma

Cynthia E. Herzog • Archie Bleyer •
Alberto S. Pappo

Contents

17.1 Introduction

Malignant melanoma is one of the most common cancers in young adults and its incidence has increased dramatically over the past decade in fair-skinned individuals. Despite its relatively good prognosis, the increased health-care burden and the fact that it is largely preventable render melanoma one of the most important malignances in the age group. As with most cancers that are considered preventable, the most effective preventive strategies are those that are applied early in life. As such, melanoma has a special role in pediatric and young adult oncology. This chapter will examine the epidemiology, etiologies, risk factors, clinical presentations, diagnostic and staging evaluation, treatment, and late effects of the disease and its therapies, with special emphasis on incidence trends and early detection.

17.2 Epidemiology

17.2.1 Incidence Trends

The incidence of melanoma has increased steadily in the United States (Figs. 17.1 and 17.2) and in many other countries with a predominantly white population. For the period 1975–2000, the incidence rate among 15- to 29-year-olds increased at a statistically significant average annual rate of 1.3% for females (Fig. 17.1), or more than triple in the last quarter century [1]. The increase in young men was slower, but for men and women over the same interval, 20- to 25-year-olds had a peak increase of >1.2% per year (Fig. 17.2), also a tripling. The current rates for whites are 18.3 per 100,000 for males, and 13 per 100,000 for females [2]. In New Zealand and Australia, the two countries with the highest incidence of melanoma in the world, the age-standardized rates for melanoma are 562 and 289 per year per million, respectively [1]. The age-standardized incidence of melanoma in Scotland for men and women rose from 35 and 70 per year per million, respectively, in 1979, to 106 and 131 per year per million, respectively, in 1998. This translates to an increase of 303% for men and 187% for women over a 19-year period [4].

In the United States, melanoma has become the fifth most common cancer among men, and the sixth most common cancer in women, accounting for 3.5% of all malignancies [5]. Furthermore, melanoma is the ninth most commonly diagnosed cancer among 15- to 19-year-olds, the fourth most common among 20- to 24-year-olds, and the most common cancer in females aged 25–29 years.

Melanoma preferentially affects white individuals in the third and fourth decade of life, and its incidence

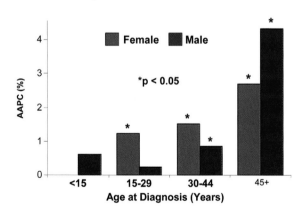

Figure 17.1

Average annual percent change (AAPC) in incidence of malignant melanoma by gender, United States SEER 1975–2000 [1]

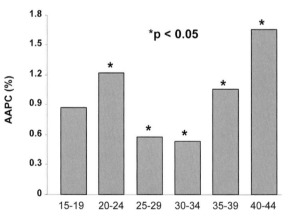

Figure 17.2

Average annual percent change (AAPC) in incidence melanoma, 1975–2000, by 5-year age intervals from 15 to 44, United States SEER 1975–2000 [1]

Table 17.1 Incidence, incidence trends and number of cases of malignant melanoma in the United States by age up to 30 years (Surveillance, Epidemiology, and End Results, SEER). *na* Not available

Age at diagnosis (years)	<5	5–9	10–14	15–19	20–24	25–29
United States population, year 2000 census	19,175,798	20,549,505	20,528,072	20,219,890	18,964,001	19,381,336
Average incidence, 1975–2000, per million	0.7	0.9	2.8	14.0	38.9	69.4
Average annual increase, 1975–2000, SEER	na	na	na	0.87	1.23	0.58
Estimated incidence, year 2000, per million	na	na	4.0	15.5	44.4	73.8
Number of persons diagnosed with malignant melanoma, year 2000, United States	13	19	81	314	841	1,431

is linked closely to geographical location (higher rates are seen in countries whose latitudes are closer to the equator), pigmentary traits, and sun exposure patterns. The incidence rates for melanoma appear to be stabilizing or even decreasing in many countries, including the United States. This trend is most noticeable among the birth cohort of males and females born in the United States between 1945 and 1950 (Fig. 17.1) [5]. Despite this trend, the Surveillance Epidemiology, and End Results (SEER) section of the National Cancer Institute (NCI) estimates that in the United States there were 54,200 cases of melanoma and 7,600 deaths from melanoma in 2003, and it is likely that an increased trend will continue for several years. Based on these findings, melanoma must continue to be viewed as a threat to public health.

Melanoma is rare during the first two decades of life, particularly among pre-pubertal patients. As described in Fig. 17.3 and Table 17.1, the incidence of melanoma increases rapidly with age, with a nearly 100-fold incidence difference between children younger than 5 years of age and young adults aged

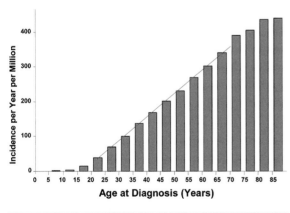

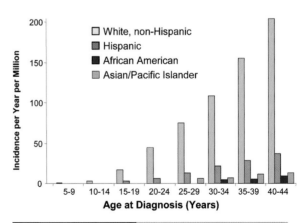

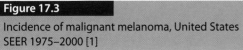

Figure 17.3

Incidence of malignant melanoma, United States SEER 1975–2000 [1]

Figure 17.4

Incidence of malignant melanoma ba race/ethnicity, 1975–2000, United States SEER 1975–2000 [1]

25–29 years. When the incidence of melanoma relative to the incidence of all cancers is compared by age, melanoma accounts for less than 1% of malignancies in patients under the age of 10 years, while it accounts for 7.1% of cancers in the 15–19 year age group and for more than 12% of cancers in those 20–29 years of age. Approximately 427 new cases of melanoma were predicted to be diagnosed in 2000 in the United States in patients under 20 years of age; 74% of these cases were predicted to be in patients 15–19 years of age. These findings are of significant importance since the adolescent and young adult population has been grossly under-represented in NCI-sponsored clinical trials. In a linkage study of consolidated files of invasive cancer between 1992 and 1997, the age-specific and age-adjusted registration rates for patients aged 15–19 years was only 24% when compared to 74.3% for patients younger than 5 years of age. Furthermore, the registration rates for carcinomas (melanoma is coded under carcinomas in the SEER registries) for 15- to 19-year-olds was only 6.3% [6].

17.2.2 Race/Ethnic Differences in Incidence

Melanoma affects predominantly white, non-Hispanic persons, as a fair-skinned population, including those of adolescent and young adult age (Fig. 17.4). Hispanics/Latinos have the second highest rates among adolescents and young adults, albeit their rates are a dis-tant second. African Americans/blacks are essentially unaffected by this cancer, at least among those aged below 30 years.

17.2.3 Gender Differences in Incidence

Overall, in the United States, males have higher incidence rates of melanoma than females [4]. As shown in Fig. 17.5, melanoma in adolescents and young adults has a female predominance, in contrast to the male predominance seen after age 45 years. The male:female ratio (Fig. 17.6) varies more for this cancer than for any other.

17.2.4 Incidence by Anatomic Location

In the United States, age-adjusted rates for invasive melanoma have increased for the trunk as well as lower and upper limbs in men and for the trunk and lower limbs in females [4]. The incidence of melanoma tends to be higher in anatomic areas that have been intermittently exposed to sun (trunk and limbs) in patients younger than 50 years of age, whereas chronically sun-exposed areas such as the head and neck predominate in older patients [4]. Figure 17.7 demonstrates that in the 15- to 29-year age group, females have a higher incidence than males of melanoma of both the lower and upper limbs and trunk. Only the incidence of head and neck melanoma is higher in males in this age group.

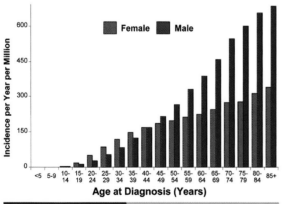

Figure 17.5

Incidence of malignant melanoma by gender, United States SEER 1975–2000 [1]

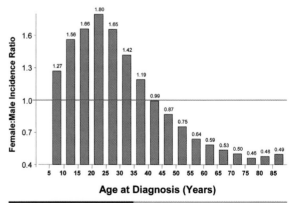

Figure 17.6

Female:male ratio of malignant melanoma as function of age at diagnosis, United States SEER 1975–2000 [1]

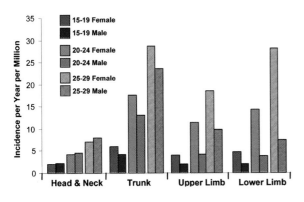

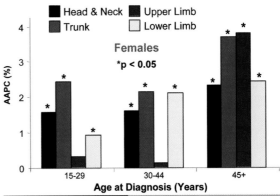

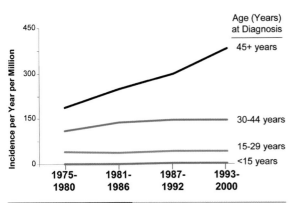

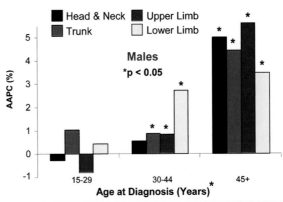

17.2.5 Incidence Trends by Anatomic Location

The rising incidence of melanoma over time has been well established (Figs. 17.1 and 17.2); however, as shown in Fig. 17.8, this increase has been slowing in age groups younger than 45 years. Although the overall incidence trend in younger patients appears unchanged during the past decade (Fig. 17.8), the incidence of melanoma for 15- to 29-year-old females had been increasing in all age groups at all of the anatomic locations evaluated except the upper extremity (Fig. 17.9). In males younger than age 30 years, there has been no statistically significant change in the incidence of melanoma during the past quarter century at any of the anatomic sites evaluated (Fig. 17.10). Some of the increase in melanoma at specific anatomic sites may be explained by better reporting.

17.2.6 Stage and Thickness Trends in Incidence

The majority of invasive melanomas (86.4%) in the United States are localized and only 4% have distant metastases at the time of initial diagnosis. Over the last 15 years there has been a shift toward an increased number of in situ melanomas, with the percentage increasing from 3.6% in 1973 to 35.3% in 1998. In the United States, between 1973 and 1997, the rate of melanoma for each stage, as well as the estimated annual percentage change in each tumor stage was higher for males than for females [7]. During the same time period, rates for patients under age 40 years decreased for each tumor stage in males, while in females only rates for metastatic disease decreased. However, the rates increased statistically for regional disease among females. For patients aged 40–59 years, the rates for localized disease increased only among males and for those 60 years of age or older, statistically significant upward trends were evident for localized and regional disease among males and for localized disease among females.

17.3 Etiology and Risk Factors

Pre-pubertal melanoma is rare, accounting for less than 1% of cases of melanoma and for 0.9% of all malignancies in patients younger than 15 years of age. Richardson et al. have defined pre-pubertal melanoma as a melanoma that has been diagnosed unequivocally by histologic examination before sexual maturity [8]. The authors have further divided this entity into three categories based on the age at which melanoma was diagnosed: congenital (in utero to birth), infantile (birth to 1 year), and childhood (1 year to puberty). Among 23 cases of infantile and congenital melanoma identified in the literature by the authors, 11 were present at birth and 12 developed during the 1st year of life. The disease arose from intermediate and large-sized nevi in 57% of cases, and from smaller cutaneous nevi in 26% of cases. Only one child had a true de novo malignancy and three had transplacentally acquired disease. The latter phenomenon has been reviewed recently [9]. In this report, 6 of 15 cases of transplacentally acquired fetal malignancy were due to melanoma (40%), and prematurity was a common presenting feature. Five of the affected infants died within the first 10.5 months of life and the disease became evident in the affected infant anywhere from 11 days of life to 8 months of life.

The authors recommend that placentas of all women with suspected metastatic melanoma during pregnancy should be closely evaluated by gross and microscopic examination including immunohistochemical staining for melanoma, and that unaffected newborns be followed for up to 24 months postpartum.

17.3.1 Xeroderma Pigmentosum

Xeroderma pigmentosum is a rare autosomal recessive disorder characterized by increased cutaneous light sensitivity and a greater than a 1,000-fold increase in the frequency of sunlight-induced cancers. Neurological abnormalities are present in approximately 20–30% of these patients. In patients with xeroderma pigmentosum, the median age at diagnosis of skin tumors is approximately 8 years; however, the median age at diagnosis of melanoma, which occurs in 5% of these patients, is 19 years. Melanomas in this population more commonly affect the head and neck. Avoiding sun exposure is the mainstay of prevention, but administration of retinoids has been found to decrease the incidence of cutaneous neoplasms [10, 11].

17.3.2 Immunosuppression

Patients with inherited immune deficiencies have an increased risk of developing melanoma [12]. Organ transplant recipients have a 1.6- to 4-fold increased risk of developing melanoma when compared to the general population. In this population, melanomas tend to affect patients with a light complexion, a tendency to freckle, and light eyes and hair. Melanoma accounts for 6.2% of cancers after organ transplantation in adults and for 15% in children [13].

A five-fold increased risk of melanoma has been described following the use of conditioning regimens that incorporate total body radiation prior to allogenic bone marrow transplantation. The relative risk of developing melanoma is 8.2 after higher doses of total-body irradiation (>10 Gy per single dose, or >13 Gy for fractionated dosing) and a relative risk of 4.5 was described for patients who received T-cell-depleted donor marrows [14].

More recently, the administration of local radiotherapy at doses of >15 Gy and the administration of alkylating agents and spindle cell inhibitors have also been reported to increase the risk of melanoma. Interestingly, children treated for gonadal tumors had an increased risk of developing melanoma [15]. The latter observation has recently been confirmed by Avril et al. [16], suggesting that the relationship between germ-cell tumors and melanoma needs to be explored further.

There have been a variety of reports documenting the association between melanoma and an increased number of nevi that measure less than 5 mm in patients who are affected with human immunodeficiency virus [17–19]. Survivors of childhood leukemia are also at increased risk for developing melanoma. These children have been shown to have higher counts of nevi, higher nevus densities, and a large number of melanocytic nevi more than 6 mm in size when compared to the general population [20, 21]. These findings emphasize the importance of host immunity in the developmental of melanoma and should reinforce the need for cautious follow up of these patients.

17.3.3 Familial Melanoma

A family history of melanoma in first- or second-degree relatives of patients with melanoma can be elicited in up to 10% of cases. Germ-line inactivating mutations of the CDKN2A gene have been documented in 25–40% of families with three or more affected individuals, and in up to 15% of individuals with multiple primary melanomas [22, 23]. CDKN2A encodes two tumor-suppressor proteins: p16 and ARF, which are known to negatively regulate the retinoblastoma and p53 pathways, respectively. Their loss has been documented to predispose to the development of melanoma. Mutations of the CDKN2A gene that affect p16 are much more common than those that affect the p14 gene. The estimated frequency of a mutated p16 gene in the general population is 0.01%, and the incidence of mutations in sporadic melanoma cases is only 0.2% [22, 24]. Similarly, the incidence of germ-line CDKN2A mutations in patients with early-onset disease, a population that would resemble a familial cancer syndrome, is also exceedingly low (1.6%) [25].

It is estimated that in patients with germ-line CDKN2A mutations, the overall cumulative risk of developing melanoma by age 50 years is 0.3, and by age 80 years is 0.67 [26]. However, the penetrance of the gene can be modified by the geographical location and the degree of ultraviolet exposure of the population. For example, by age 80 years, the age-specific penetrance estimate in Europe was 0.58, whereas the estimates for patients in the United States and Australia were 0.76 and 0.91, respectively [26]. Among subsets of families with germ-line CDKN2A mutations there also appears to be an increased risk for the development of pancreatic cancer and oral squamous cell carcinomas [5, 22]. Further collaborative efforts from the Melanoma Genetics Consortium are underway to help clarify these complex cancer associations. ARF mutations, although very rare, have also recently been demonstrated to predispose to the development of melanoma, as well as nervous system tumors [22].

Activating mutations of the CDK4 gene, which negatively regulates the pRb pathway, have been described in three families. All mutations have been clustered within codon 24 and the clinical characteristics of these patients are similar to those seen in patients with CDKN2A mutations [22, 27].

The melanocortin receptor 1 gene (MC1R) is a key determinant of the pigmentary process. In humans, three variants of the MC1R gene have been associated with the red hair phenotype (RHC), which includes red hair, fair complexion, inability to tan, and a tendency to freckle [28]. Patients with one or more of the variants of the MC1R gene have a compromised capability of inducing the switch from pheomelanin to eumelanin and therefore have a compromised ability to respond to damage by ultraviolet light. The presence of one or more MC1R variants has been associated with the red hair phenotype and an increased penetrance of mutations in CDKN2A-melanoma-prone families [29, 30].

Other recently described low-penetrance genes that are associated with increased melanoma risk include the rare alleles at the C500G and C540T polymorphisms of the CDKN2A gene, and null GSTM1 (glutathione S-tranferase gene) phenotype [22, 31, 32].

Finally, activating somatic BRAF mutations have been identified in approximately two-thirds of malignant melanomas and in common benign and dysplastic nevi. However, germ-line BRAF mutations are extremely rare (0.29%), suggesting that the BRAF gene is an important initiating factor in the transformation of melanocytic neoplasia, but that it does not contribute significantly to melanoma susceptibility [33, 34].

17.3.4 Nevus Phenotype and Environmental Factors

The potential for malignant transformation of small congenital nevi, which affect up to 1% of all newborn infants, continues be a source of debate. A study by Mackie et al. revealed that melanoma develops in a small nevus that was present either at birth or during early childhood, in 44% of patients under the age of 30 years [35]. However, two recent studies do not support the view of an increased risk of melanoma in patients with small or medium-sized congenital nevi [36, 37].

Patients with large congenital melanocytic nevi (defined as those that exceed 20 cm in diameter during adulthood) have approximately a 5–15% lifetime risk of developing melanoma, and the risk is greatest in the first decade of life [38]. The risk of cutaneous melanoma in these patients appears to be confined to those with axial lesions, and an equal risk of extra-cutaneous involvement has recently been documented [39]. Patients with symptomatic neuro-cutaneous melanosis have an increased risk of developing melanoma. Most of these patients have large congenital nevi in the scalp or posterior axial location, and the prognosis is poor [40, 41]. The non-symptomatic form of neuro-cutaneous melanosis has recently been described and is characterized by the presence of focal magnetic resonance imaging signal abnormalities in the brain in up to 25% of patients with large congenital nevi, and the large majority of these patients have not developed melanoma [42].

A two- to fourfold increased risk of melanoma has been consistently documented with increasing number of acquired nevi [43]. Given the close association between the presence of acquired nevi and melanoma, multiple epidemiologic studies have been performed examining the association between environmental and constitutional factors and the development of nevi and melanoma in various populations. In a study of over 3,000 Italian school children age 13–14 years, patients who burned easily following their first sun exposure and those with an ability to tan had an increased number of nevi. The nevus density was directly related to recurrent episodes of sunburn, and large nevi size was closely associated with the presence of a lighter pigmentary trait and a propensity to sunburn easily. In another study from Queensland, 111 schoolchildren aged 13–14 years who were followed for up to 5 years, the degree of shoulder freckling and habitual sun exposure were the most important determinant of melanocytic nevi in adolescents in a area of high sun exposure [44]. In another study of 61 children from Queensland diagnosed with melanoma at 13 and 14 years of age, the presence of multiple large nevi, sun-sensitive phenotype, and inability to tan strongly, predicted the risk of melanoma development in this population [45]. In this study, a family history of melanoma was present in nearly one-third of cases and was associated with an increased risk of developing melanoma, suggesting that heredity plays an important role in the predisposition to childhood melanoma. In a study of 250 eligible cases of melanoma in patients aged 15–19 years, the strongest predictor of melanoma development was the presence of more than 100 nevi 2 mm or more in diameter. Other risk factors included pigmentary traits that are commonly associated with the development of melanoma, such as, red hair, blue eyes, inability to tan after prolonged exposure, heavy facial freckling, and a family history of melanoma. Only 2 of 147 cases tested had a CDKN2A mutation. A slightly higher number of cases reported more than ten episodes of peeling sunburn, and a statistically significant increased risk of melanoma was documented with increasing number of peeling or blistering sunburns [46].

Dysplastic nevi or clinically atypical moles affect approximately 5% of the United States population and are known to confer an increased risk of melanoma. In 1 study of 716 patients with melanoma, the presence of 1 dysplastic nevus was associated with a 2-fold risk of melanoma, whereas 10 or more nevi conferred a 12-fold risk [43]. In a study of 33 families with two or more members with invasive melanoma, comprising a total of 844 subjects, the authors identified 86 cases of melanoma in 37 individuals over a follow-up period of 2–25 years. Of these melanomas, 51 were found to have a precursor lesion and 32 met the criteria for dysplastic nevi. In an earlier study, 37% of children in melanoma-prone families had dysplastic nevi, and cases of pediatric melanoma only occurred in those individuals with these nevi [47].

17.3.5 The Sun and Other Ultraviolet Exposures

The sun and other ultraviolet exposures are a major risk factor for the development of melanoma. Analyses of 29 case control studies demonstrated a positive association between intermittent sun exposure and melanoma with an odds ratio of developing melanoma of 1.71. In this study there was also a twofold increase of melanoma following sunburns at any age [48]. The current data are consistent with cumulative exposure being important whether acquired as a adult or as a child, and ultraviolet exposure is important in all stages of melanoma development.

Whether sunscreens protect or enhance the risk of developing melanoma continues to be a source of debate. A meta-analysis of 20 studies of sunscreen use and melanoma in humans did not support a positive association between the use of sunscreen and melanoma development [49]. Among adolescents in Australia, the lack or rare use of sunscreen under the age of 5 years doubled the risk of melanoma [46]. In another trial the use of sunscreen decreased the number of new nevi in children [5]. This could indicate that sunscreens might protect against melanoma, since the number of nevi is directly correlated with the risk of developing melanoma.

The use of tanning beds has been popular only since the 1970s, thus there is limited information regarding its effects on the risk of developing melanoma. However, in the United States the use of tanning devices has been associated with an increased risk for squamous- and basal-cell carcinomas. In a population study from Sweden, a significantly increased risk was found for developing melanoma with regular exposure to sun beds after adjusting for hair color, race, nevi, skin type, and number of sunburns [4].

17.4 Clinical Presentation

An increased risk of melanoma at an early age is known to occur in the setting of large congenital nevus, xeroderma pigmentosum, and dysplastic nevi. However

the majority of melanomas in adolescent and young adult patients occur in patients with none of these risk factors. The patient often does not consider the possibility of melanoma and presents late. More often the physician fails to consider the diagnosis of melanoma in younger patients, and therefore delays removal of the lesion. Failure to consider the possibility of melanoma in the adolescent and young adult population can delay the diagnosis. In two reports on melanoma in pediatric and adolescent patients, delays in diagnosis were reported in about half of the patients [50, 51].

In the SEER data, 6,112 cases of cutaneous melanoma have been reported in patients age 15–29 years. Melanoma in this population has a female predominance, in contrast to the male predominance seen with older adults (male to female ratio of 1:1.7) [52]. The most common primary site was the trunk, followed by the upper and lower limbs. The lowest incidence was in head and neck tumors, and this is the only site where there was a slight male predominance.

As in older adults, changes in the appearance of a pigmented lesion should alert the physician to the possibility of melanoma in younger patients. The most common clinical presentation includes increasing size, color change, bleeding, itching, or palpable adenopathy. The initial approach for a suspected melanoma is a biopsy procedure. This can be a punch or excisional biopsy, to confirm the diagnosis and determine pathologic criteria that will then dictate further surgical management.

17.5 Pathology

Melanomas in adolescents and young adults are pathologically similar to those in older adults. However, this age group has a higher incidence of Spitz nevus, which must be distinguished from melanoma.

17.5.1 Primary Skin Tumor

All suspicious skin lesions should be removed and sent for pathologic review. The revised American Joint Committee on Cancer (AJCC) melanoma staging criteria [53] provides a reproducible model that reflects the natural history of melanoma and incorporates important prognostic variables that are predictive of

Table 17.2 Tumor-Nodes-Metastasis (TNM) classification

Tumor	Thickness	Ulceration
T1	≤1.0 mm	a: no ulceration, II/III b: ulceration or IV/V
T2	1.01–2.0	a: no ulceration b: ulceration
T3	2.01–4.0	a: no ulceration b: ulceration
T4	>4.0	a: no ulceration b: ulceration
Nodes	**Number of positive nodes**	**Ulceration**
N1	1	a: micro b: macro
N2	2–3	a: micro b: macro c: in transit, satellite with negative nodes
N3	≥4, or matted, or in transit, satellite with positive nodes	

Table 17.3 Tumor staging

Clinical staging				Pathologic staging			
0	Tis	N0	M0	0	Tis	N0	M0
1A	T1a	N0	M0	1A	T1a	N0	M0
1B	T1b T2a	N0	M0	1B	T1b T2a	N0	M0
IIA	T2b T3a	N0	M0	IIA	T2b T3a	N0	M0
IIB	T3b T4a	N0	M0	IIB	T3b T4a	N0	M0
IIC	T4b	N0	M0	IIC	T4b	N0	M0
III	Any	N+	Mo	IIIA	T1–4a T1–4a	N1a N2a	M0
				IIIB	T1–4b T1–4b T1–4a T1–4a T1–4a	N1a N2a N1b N2b N2c	M0
				IIIC	T1–4b T1–4b T1–4b Any T	N1b N2b N2c N3	M0
IV	Any	Any	Any	IV	Any	Any	Any

clinical outcome (Tables 17.2 and 17.3). The pathology report for primary cutaneous melanoma should incorporate these prognostic variables, including tumor thickness, level of invasion, presence of ulceration, presence of perineural, venous or lymphatic invasion, presence of lymphocytes, presence of regression, and mitotic index [54]. In the revised AJCC melanoma staging criteria, the most important prognostic factors for the primary tumor were thickness and ulceration. Level of invasion was only of prognostic value in melanomas <1 mm in thickness [53].

The distinction between Spitz nevus and melanoma, particularly among younger patients, can be controversial and difficult. Some authors advocate the term atypical Spitz tumor to describe controversial melanocytic lesions that resemble Spitz nevi, but raise the diagnostic possibility of melanoma [55]. Furthermore, these lesions may be classified as being at "high risk" for aggressive behavior based on presence of ulceration, large size, asymmetry, deep extension, hypercellularity, cytologic atypia, and prominent and atypical mitosis [55].

17.5.2 Sentinel Node

Sentinel-node biopsy allows for the careful pathologic assessment of a limited number of lymph nodes. The analysis of the sentinel node(s) has evolved over time. Initial analyses consisted of routine hematoxylin and eosin (H&E) staining of the bisected node. This method has been shown to under-estimate the presence of disease. Serial sections and immunohistochemistry (IHC) increases the sensitivity for detecting microscopic lymph node metastases. Retrospective evaluation of lymph nodes using serial sections and IHC has been performed for patients with a false-negative sentinel lymph node (SLN) biopsy. These patients had nodal recurrences in the lymph node basin for which the SLN was initially reported to be negative. More detailed analysis of the SLN has revealed the presence of sentinel-node tumor in 80% [56] and 31% [57]. IHC staining can be performed with a variety of melanoma-specific antibodies, including those for detection of S100, tyrosinase, gp100 (HMB-45), and melan-A (melanoma antigen recognized by T cells-1, MART-1).

More recently reverse transcriptase-polymerase chain reaction (RT-PCR) has been evaluated as a tool for the detection of occult metastases in SLNs and found to further increase the percentage of positive nodes detected [58]. Kuo et al. have shown that RT-PCR can be done using archival tissue, thus eliminating the need for additional, immediate processing to obtain fresh tissue for RT-PCR [59]. Using four markers (tyrosinase, MART-1, and tyrosinase-related protein 1 and 2, TRP-1 and TRP-2, respectively) to evaluate paraffin-embedded specimens, they were able to upstage 25% of negative SLNs based on two or more positive markers by RT-PCR. Of the ten patients whose disease was upstaged by RT-PCR, eight developed recurrence, while two have not.

Although RT-PCR increases the percentage of positive nodes, part of this increase may be due to false positives. Cook et al. reported a 7.2% false-positive rate due to the detection of capsular or trabecular nevus cells by RT-PCR [60]. Based on these findings, the European Organization for Research and Treatment of Cancer has adopted a protocol for evaluating SLNs using serial sectioning and IHC, without the use of RT-PCR.

17.5.3 Lymph Node Dissection

When patients undergo lymph node dissection (LND), all lymph nodes should be submitted in their entirety with each node evaluated. The total number of nodes evaluated, as well as the number that are positive for tumor should be reported. The involvement of more than one node is predictive of a worse outcome [61].

17.6 Surgery

Early detection and surgical removal of any suspicious pigmented lesion is the mainstay of therapy for melanoma. The extent of surgery is determined by clinical and pathologic findings. The patient should be evaluated clinically for evidence of regional disease, including satellite lesions, in transit lesions, or lymph node metastasis. Patients should also be evaluated clinically for evidence of distant metastases. With thicker melanomas or evidence of regional or distant metastases, patients should be evaluated for metastases using imaging studies.

17.6.1 Treatment of the Primary Tumor

There are no specific guidelines for the surgical treatment of melanoma in adolescent and young adult patients. Thus, recommended guidelines for resection of primary melanomas in adolescent and young adult patients should follow the same principles as those published for adult melanoma. The margins of excision are determined by the thickness and site of the primary tumor. Generally, the margins employed are 0.5 cm for in situ lesions, 1 cm for lesions less than 1 mm [62, 63], and 2 cm for lesions 2–4 mm [64]. The margins of excision for tumors 1–2 mm are more controversial, with recommendation for margins of 1–2 cm [62, 64]. For lesions greater than 4 mm, a margin of at least 2 cm is recommended, but there have been no prospective trials. More conservative margins are often employed in anatomically restricted areas such as the face.

17.6.2 Lymph Node Mapping

SLN biopsy has become a standard staging procedure in adult melanoma and should be incorporated into the surgical management of younger patients. Prior to the introduction of SLN biopsy, the alternative for patients with intermediate-thickness melanoma, who were at risk of developing regional disease, was either an elective LND (ELND) or observation. ELND was an unappealing alternative due to the facts that only 15–20% of patients were ultimately found to have evidence of lymph node involvement and ELND is associated with a high incidence of morbidity, including seroma formation, infection, and edema. Morton et al. reported the first use of SLN biopsy in melanoma in 1992 [65]. An SLN was identified in 82% of patients, with tumor identified by H&E in 12% of the nodes, and by IHC in 9% of the nodes. Subsequent evaluation of the remainder of the lymph nodes, after a complete LND revealed only 1% of the non-sentinel nodes were positive for tumor.

As with the pathologic evaluation of the SLN, the technique used for identification of the SLN(s) has evolved over time. In the initial study, isosulfan blue or patent blue-V was injected around the primary melanoma to enable identification of a blue sentinel node in 82% of patients [65]. Subsequent use of intra-operative lymphoscintigraphy with intra-dermal injection of ^{99m}Tc-sulfur colloid or ^{99m}Tc-human serum albumin improved the identification of the SLN. The intra-operative use of both isosulfan blue and ^{99m}Tc-sulfur colloid with the use of a hand-held gamma counter results in the identification of a SLN in almost 100% of cases [56, 58]. The false negative rate, that is patients who are reported to have a negative SLN but subsequently relapse in the nodal region from which the SLN was taken, is less than 10% with experienced surgeons [56, 66].

Lymphoscintigraphy can identify the lymph node basin(s) at risk in cases where the primary melanoma is located on the trunk or in the head and neck area where one or more of several lymph node basins can be involved. Lymphoscintigraphy also allows for detection of abnormal lymph node drainage sites in 5–7% of patients [67–70]. However, use of the hand-held gamma counter intra-operatively appears to be more sensitive for the detection of ^{99m}Tc-sulfur colloid in unusual locations. SLNs were identified in unusual sites in 7–12% of melanomas on the trunk, 0–6% of head and neck melanomas, and 4–7% and 1–2% of melanomas of the upper or lower limbs, respectively. The unusual site may be the only site of lymph nodes identified as harboring occult disease.

The morbidity of SLN biopsy is low. A report from the Sunbelt Melanoma Trial gave a 4.6% incidence of complications after SLN biopsy, in comparison to an incidence of 23.2% after SLN biopsy and complete LNDs. Complications for both procedures were more common in the groin than in the axilla [71].

A positive SLN is the single most important prognostic factor in patients that have clinical stage I or II melanomas. Because of this prognostic significance, as well as the fact SLN biopsy sampling is both sensitive and specific, and has a low morbidity, the recently revised AJCC Staging for Cutaneous Melanoma recommends SLN biopsy for patients with melanomas >1 mm in thickness without evidence of regional or distant metastases on exam (T2-4N0M0) [53].

The indication for lymph node mapping and SLN biopsy in patient with thin melanomas (<1 mm thick) needs further evaluation. Using the new AJCC staging, patients with thin melanomas, but with ulceration or level IV or V invasion (T1b) have a worse outcome than patients with thin melanomas without these features [61]. At the MD Anderson Cancer Center, patients with T1b melanomas routinely undergo SLN biopsy. A positive SLN has been found in 4.7 % of these cases [72]. Bleicher et al. identified a positive SLN in 1.7% of 118 patients with melanoma ≤0.75 mm in thickness, in 3.9% of 154 patients with 0.76–1 mm tumors, and 7.1% of 240 patients with 1.01–1.5 mm tumors [73]. There was evidence in the Bleicher study that the incidence of SLN involvement in thin melanomas was higher in patients under age 44 years. Although lymph node mapping and SLN biopsy is not routinely recommended in older adults with thin melanomas, it should be considered in adolescent and young adult patients.

17.6.3 Lymph Node Dissection

When melanoma is detected clinically or microscopically in any lymph nodes, further treatment with LND is recommended. Whether selective LND (SLND) improves survival is not yet documented [66, 74]. In a retrospective study of stage III patients, when survival was measured from the time of the LND procedure, those who had SLND did better than those who had clinical LND. However, no benefit was seen for SLND in comparison to clinical LND when survival was measured from the time of primary tumor resection [75]. This suggests that while SLND may be of prognostic value, it does not impact ultimate outcome.

17.6.4 Surgical Treatment of Spitz Nevus

Spitz nevi can be difficult to distinguish from melanoma histologically, and are more likely to occur in adolescent and young adult patients than in older adults. In cases where melanoma cannot be ruled out as a possibility, the patient should undergo both wide local excision and SLN biopsy. In a survey of dermatologists in the United States, over 90% of the responding dermatologists stated that they would biopsy sample a lesion suspected of being a Spitz nevus, and 43% favored a complete excision. Most respondents selected a 1- to 2-mm margin of excision and 69% recommended complete reexcision in cases where the lesion was initially incompletely excised. In this survey, only 8% of respondents recalled ever seeing cases of metastatic melanoma arising from lesions designated as Spitz nevus [76].

The role of SLN biopsy sampling in controversial melanocytic lesions such as Spitz nevus remains to be established. Involvement of the SLN in these cases can further suggest a diagnosis of melanoma; however, isolated regional-node metastases have been reported in patients with Spitz nevus with no subsequent distant metastases. Nevertheless, the "benign" nature of Spitz nevus with regional metastases is questionable [77].

Two studies have been reported on the evaluation of SLN in patients with atypical Spitz nevi in which a diagnosis of malignant melanoma could not be definitively excluded [78, 79]. In the first report, five out of ten patients had a positive SLN. All are without evidence of disease at a mean follow-up of 34 months [79]. In the second report, 8 out of 18 patients (44%) had a positive SLN and all were without evidence of disease at a mean follow-up of 12 months [78]. It is clear that further evaluation is needed to determine the natural history of these controversial melanocytic lesions.

17.7 Staging

The revised staging system developed by the AJCC [53] incorporates pathological and clinical factors that are predictive of clinical outcome. For localized disease, there are new thresholds for melanoma thickness and recognition that the presence of ulceration is an important predictor of outcome. The results of SLN biopsy have also been incorporated to account for the reported differences in outcomes between pathologically and clinically involved nodes. For patients with nodal spread, the new system recognizes the importance of the number of lymph nodes involved, as well as the prognostic significance of ulceration and in-transit or satellite metastases. For patients with metastatic disease, the new staging system incorporates a description of sites of metastases and the diagnostic value of serum lactic dehydrogenase (LDH). It is vital that trials for melanoma in adolescent and young adult patients incorporate this staging system in order to facilitate the interpretation of results from different institutions and patient populations.

Given the scarce literature describing the use of SNL biopsy for pediatric melanoma [80, 81] and the suggestion that younger patients have a higher incidence of positive SLN biopsy specimens with thin melanoma [73], future trials must mandate the routine use of SLN biopsy sampling in order to determine the prognostic and therapeutic value of this procedure in adolescent and young adult patients and to compare these results with those in the older adults.

For patients with localized disease, a complete blood count, serum chemistries including liver function tests, and a chest radiograph are sufficient to screen for metastatic disease. For patients with thicker melanomas or evidence of regional or distant metastases, further workup with cross-sectional imaging is indicated.

17.7.1 Blood Tests

There is no good blood test to screen melanoma patients for metastatic disease, although LDH and alkaline phosphatase have long been used. Recently, several markers have been evaluated for their ability to improve staging and prediction for outcome in patients with melanoma. Tyrosinase, an enzyme involved in melanin synthesis, has been one of the most widely studied. Other markers include S-100β, melanoma-inhibiting activity (MIA), and MART-1.

Elevated LDH is included in the new AJCC staging criteria as a variable for staging patients with metastatic disease [53]. Patients with stage IV disease and elevated LDH levels have been shown to have a worse outcome, with no additional prognostic information added by the evaluation of S-100β or MIA in these patients [82].

The value of serum markers in stage I–III disease is less clear. Detection of circulating melanoma cells by multimarker RT-PCR at the time of diagnosis did not increase the ability to predict progression-free survival when evaluated by multivariant analysis including stage [83]. Others have suggested that monitoring serum markers in patients with melanoma allows for the earlier detection of recurrence [84, 85]. Prospective studies are needed to determine the role of tumor marker analysis in the follow-up of melanoma patients.

17.7.2 Imaging Studies

A baseline chest x-ray to evaluate for metastases is indicated for all patients except those with thin melanoma. Data regarding which patients need further imaging studies and, indeed, the most appropriate imaging studies continues to evolve.

17.7.2.1 Ultrasound

Ultrasound is useful for the evaluation of clinically suspicious lymph nodes and can be used to guide fine-needle aspiration for the pathologic evaluation of suspicious nodes. It can also be used to evaluate liver metastases, but is not as sensitive as computed tomography (CT) or magnetic resonance imaging (MRI).

17.7.2.2 Computed Tomography

Buzaid et al. [86] looked at 89 patients with locoregional disease who were asymptomatic and had a normal LDH and chest x-ray. Further imaging revealed true positive findings in 6 cases and false positives in 20 cases. They therefore recommended only chest x-ray and CT scan of the abdomen as baseline exams. For patients with recurrence below the waist, a CT of the abdomen is recommended, and, with recurrence in the head and neck region, a CT of the neck. However, a study at St. Jude Children's Hospital identified clinically undetectable metastases in 25% of pediatric patients with thick localized melanomas or melanomas arising at an unknown primary site [87], suggesting that younger patients have a higher risk of clinically undetectable metastases. This should be further evaluated in pediatric, and adolescent and young adult patients.

17.7.2.3 Magnetic Resonance Imaging

MRI, rather than CT, should be done to look for brain metastases. However, in the absence of symptoms, the routine use of MRI to assess the brain is not recommended.

17.7.2.4 Positron Emission Tomography

Positron emission tomography (PET) scanning has been approved for the evaluation of melanoma. PET is not as sensitive as SLN biopsy sampling in detecting subclinical regional lymph node involvement [88], but is more sensitive than CT in detecting distant metastases, except for pulmonary metastases [89] In patients with known recurrence of melanoma, PET imaging can identify additional unsuspected sites of disease in up to 20% of cases when compared to CT scanning [90, 91].

Pediatric patients frequently have reactive lymph nodes that raise concerns about metastatic disease. In these cases, PET may be helpful in differentiating reactive nodes from metastatic nodes. To date, there are no published studies using PET imaging to stage pediatric melanoma.

17.8 Non-surgical Therapy

17.8.1 Adjuvant therapy

17.8.1.1 Interferon

The role of interferon in the treatment of melanoma remains under study. The Eastern Cooperative Oncology Group (ECOG) has performed several trials with interferon. In the first trial (1684) patients were randomized to either observation or high-dose interferon (HDI) [92]. HDI consisted of interferon α-2b 20 MU/m^2/day given intravenously 5 days a week for 4 weeks, followed by 10 MU/m^2/day given subcutaneously 3 days a week for 48 weeks. The first trial enrolled 287 patients with melanomas >4 mm or with regional lymph node involvement. At a median follow-up of 7 years, a significant improvement in relapse-free survival (RFS) and overall survival (OS) was seen in patients who received HDI. The benefit of HDI was most marked in patients with clinically detectable lymph node metastases.

A subsequent trial (1690) compared HDI, low-dose interferon (LDI), and observation [93]. In an attempt to lower the rate of interferon-associated toxicity, LDI was given at a dose of 3 MU/m^2/day given subcutaneously 3 days a week for 2 years. With 608 patients enrolled and a median follow up of 52 months, a significant improvement in RFS was observed with HDI, but there was no significant difference in OS. Several differences between these two trials may account for the differences in outcome. There was higher proportion of patients on 1684 with lymph node involvement and a higher proportion with regional recurrence. The outcome on the later trial was better in comparison to the former trial for both the observation arm and the HDI arm, suggesting an impact of improvement of surgical staging and treatment. In addition, a substantial number of patients on the observation arm who relapsed were treated with salvage HDI therapy, thus potentially prolonging the OS in this group.

A third trial (1694) compared HDI to GM2-KLH/QS-21 vaccine therapy [94]. A total of 880 patients were randomized, prior to early termination of the trial due to a significantly better RFS and OS with HDI. The greatest difference was seen in node-negative patients. There was no observation arm in this study, but vaccine therapy did not appear to negatively impact outcome and may have provided some benefit.

The Sunbelt melanoma trial [95] is currently ongoing. This is a prospective, randomized trial that was designed to evaluate the role of interferon in patients with lymph node metastases detected only by histology, IHC, or RT-PCR.

Despite the evidence that adjuvant HDI is effective in patients with high-risk melanoma, the use of HDI is associated with significant toxicity, including anorexia and weight loss, neuro-psychiatric symptoms, myelo-suppression, and hepatotoxicity [92–94]. There are limited data on the use of this interferon regimen in patients under age 18 years. At the MD Anderson Cancer Center, 11 patients under aged 18 years have been treated with HDI, 1 patient was lost to follow-up after completion of the IV interferon (age 4 years), 6 completed the regimen with no problems (ages 9–16 years), and 4 had therapy discontinued early due to toxicity, 2 liver (age 6 and 11 years), 1 each neuro-cognitive (age 5 years) and pancreatic (age 2 years). At St. Jude Children's Hospital, 11 patients have been treated with HDI. It was well tolerated during induction, with only two grade 4 hematologic events and one grade 4 liver event (WL Furman, personal communication).

Adolescent and young adult patients without measurable disease, but with higher-stage disease, and therefore at increased risk of recurrence, should be considered for adjuvant therapy. Since interferon can be associated with significant toxicity, it is best to use it in the setting of a clinical trial. Although melanoma trials have in the past excluded patients under the age of 18 years, ECOG studies have recently opened to include younger patients with melanoma. This should allow for evaluation of the benefit and toxicity of the HDI regimen in younger patients.

17.8.1.2 Radiotherapy

Radiotherapy should be considered in patients with high-risk head and neck melanomas, defined as cervical lymph nodes, with any of the following: (1) extracapsular extension, (2) node greater than or equal to 3 cm, (3) involvement of four or more lymph nodes, or (4) recurrence. Ballo et al. reported on 160 adult patients with cervical lymph node metastases, all but 43 of whom had at least 1 of these high-risk features [96]. These patients, who were at high risk for recurrence, had a 10-year regional control rate of 94% when treated with radiation at a median dose of 30 Gy given at 6 Gy twice weekly.

17.8.2 Treatment of Measurable Disease

The majority of adolescent and young adult patients present with localized or local regional disease that will be treated with surgery and, possibly, adjuvant treatment. However, for patients with metastatic disease either at presentation or subsequently, effective treatment options are limited.

17.8.2.1 Biotherapy

Interleukin-2 (IL-2) has been used extensively in adult melanoma with response rates of approximately 17% [97].

17.8.2.2 Bio-chemotherapy

The use of bio-chemotherapy has been shown to have response rates of 40–60% in patients with measurable disease [86, 98]. Although the exact regimen varies between studies, bio-chemotherapy generally consists of cisplatin-based chemotherapy in combination with interferon and IL-2. The activity of chemotherapy is augmented by the addition of biologic response modifiers [99]. The response rate, complete response rate, and median time to progression were 48%, 6%, and 4.9 months, respectively, for bio-chemotherapy, as compared to 25%, 2%, and 2.4 months, respectively, for chemotherapy alone. This increase in activity is at the cost of significant increase in toxicity. Atkins et al. reported a randomized phase III study comparing chemotherapy to bio-chemotherapy performed in patients with metastatic disease [100]. Biochemotherapy was associated with higher response rate and higher toxicity, but no difference was seen in OS.

17.8.2.3 Chemotherapy

Recently, temozolomide has shown promise in the treatment of melanoma [101, 102]. Danson et al. evaluated 181 patients with metastatic melanoma [101]. Treatment with temozolomide alone resulted in response or stabilization in 20%, with a median survival of 5.3 months. In combination with interferon, the results were 26% and 7.7 months, respectively, while combination with thalidomide resulted in 24% disease response or stabilization and a median survival of 7.3 months. Hwu et al. reported a 32% response rate with temozolomide and thalidomide [102].

17.8.2.4 Vaccine Therapy

Numerous vaccine approaches have been attempted in melanoma [103], including cell-based, peptides, recombinant viruses, DNA, and dendritic cell vaccines. To date, this approach has not had a significant impact on patients with melanoma. Vaccine trials have generally not been open to patients under 18 years of age.

17.9 Prognosis

Most adolescent and young adult patients with melanoma have an excellent prognosis due to the high incidence of lower-stage disease in these patients. Examination of SEER data shows that adolescent and young adult patients have a 5-year OS rate of about 90%, similar to that seen in the 30- to 44-year age group. Both age groups have a better outcome than patients older than age 44 years. In all age groups, females have a better outcome than males. Despite the higher incidence of melanoma in adolescent and young adult females, the mortality from melanoma is higher in adolescent and young adult males (16% vs 6%) [52].

Prognosis is based on clinicopathologic staging. There is very little data on the stage, treatment, and outcome of patients under age 18 years. SEER data from 1988–1999 include 431 patients <20 years of age and 2,823 age 20–29 years. In the <20 years age group, 23% had in situ lesions, 73% had localized disease, and 4% had regional disease. Stage at diagnosis was similar for 20- to 29-year-olds, 19% in situ lesions, 75% localized disease, 5% regional disease, and 1% with metastases. Survival rates were also similar for both age groups, 99–100% for in situ lesions, 96–97% for localized disease and 60–62% for regional disease.

Balch et al. [61] looked at survival for stage I and II patients and showed 5-year and 10-year survival rates of 85–87% and 75–81%, respectively, for each age decade between 10 and 50 years. After age 50 years survival decreased with increasing age. For all ages survival for stage I and II disease decreased with increasing tumor thickness and the presence of ulceration. The outcome for patients with stage III disease is impacted by the number of involved nodes and whether the nodes were microscopically or macroscopically involved; 5-year survival was 61% with a single microscopic nodule, but decreased to 35% with four or more microscopic nodes, and to 46% with a single macroscopic node. The presence of four or more macroscopically involved nodes was associated with a 24% 5-year survival. Ulceration was also associated with a worse outcome.

For patients with stage IV disease, the outcome is very poor. Patients with skin, subcutaneous, or distant lymph node metastases have a better survival than patients with visceral metastases, with a 5-year survival of 19% and 10%, respectively [53]. Patients with lung metastases have a better short-term survival than those with involvement of other visceral sites, but the survival at 2 years is the same [53, 61].

17.10 Conclusions

Melanoma makes up a significant proportion of the cancer seen in the adolescent and young adult population, and sun exposure appears to be leading to increased incidence. There are no data to indicate that melanoma in this age group is biologically different than melanoma in older patients. Therefore, adolescent and young adult patients with melanoma should be treated according to the guidelines established for older adults. The mainstay of treatment is surgical, including wide local excision of the primary tumor with lymph node mapping, and if indicated by nodal disease, LND. Patients with stage IIIB or greater disease should be offered systemic therapy, consisting of immunotherapy and/or chemotherapy.

References

1. Bleyer WA, O'Leary M, Barr R, Ries LAG (eds) (2006) Cancer Epidemiology in Older Adolescents and Young Adults 15 to 29 Years of Age, including SEER Incidence and Survival, 1975–2000. National Cancer Institute, NIH Pub. No. 06-5767, Bethesda MD; also available at www.seer.cancer.gov/publications
2. Bevona C, Sober A (2002) Melanoma incidence trends. Dermatol Clin 20:589–595
3. Desmond R, Soong S-J (2003) Epidemiology of malignant melanoma. Surg Clin North Am 83:1–29
4. Mackie RM, Bray CA, Hole DJ (2002) Incidence of and survival from malignant melanoma in Scotland: an epidemiological study. Lancet 360:587–591
5. Tucker MA, Goldstein AM (2003) Melanoma etiology: where are we? Oncogene 22:3042–3052
6. Liu L, Krailo M, Reaman GH, Bernstein L (2003) Childhood cancer patients' access to cooperative group cancer programs: a population-based study. Cancer 97:1339–1345
7. Jemal A, Devesa SS, Hartge P, Tucker MA (2001) Recent trends in cutaneous melanoma incidence among whites in the United states. J Natl Cancer Inst 93:678–683
8. Richardson SK, Tannous ZS, Mihm MC Jr (2002) Congenital and infantile melanoma: review of the literature and report of an uncommon variant, pigment-synthesizing melanoma. J Am Acad Dermatol 47:77–90
9. Alexander A, Samlowski WE, Grossman D (2003) Metastatic melanoma in pregnancy: risk of transplacental metastases in the infant. J Clin Oncol 21:2179–2186
10. Lambert WC, Kuo HR, Lambert MW (1995) Xeroderma pigmentosum. Clin Dermatol 13:169–209

11. Kraemer KH, Lee MM, Scotto J (1987) Xeroderma pigmentosum. Cutaneous, ocular and neurologic abnormalities in 830 published cases. Arch Dermatol 123:241–250

12. Ceballos PJ, Ruiz-Maldanado R, Mihm MC (1995) Melanoma in children. N Engl J Med 332:656–662

13. Euvrard S, Kanitakis J, Claudy A (2003) Skin cancers after organ transplantation. N Engl J Med 348:1681–1691

14. Curtis RE, Rowlings PA, Deeg HJ (1997) Solid cancers after bone marrow transplantation. N Engl J Med 336:897–904

15. Guerin S, Dupuy A, Anderson H (2003) Radiation dose as a risk factor for malignant melanoma following childhood cancer. Eur J Cancer 39:2379–2386

16. Hamre MR, Chuba P, Bakhshi S, Thomas R, Severson RK (2002) Cutaneous melanoma in childhood and adolescence. Pediatr Hematol Oncol 19:309–317

17. Duvic M, Lowe L, Rapini RP, et al (1989) Eruptive dysplastic nevi associated with human immunodeficiency virus infection. Arch Dermatol 125:397–401

18. Grob JJ, Bastuji-Garin S, Vaillant L (1996) Excess of nevi related to immunodeficiency: a study in HIV-infected patients and renal transplant recipients. J Invest Dermatol 107:694–697

19. Calista KD (2001) Five cases of melanoma in HIV positive patients. Eur J Dermatol 11:446–449

20. Baird EA, McHenry PM, Mackie RM (1992) Effects of maintenance chemotherapy in childhood on numbers of melanocytic naevi. BMJ 305:799–801

21. de Wit PE, de Vaan GA, de Boo TM, et al (1990) Prevalence of naevocytic naevi after chemotherapy for childhood cancer. Med Pediatr Oncol 18:336–338

22. Hayward N (2003) Genetics of melanoma predisposition. Oncogene 22:3053–3062

23. Monzon J, Liu L (1998) CDKN2A mutations in multiple primary melanomas. N Engl J Med 338:879–887

24. Bataille V (2003) Genetic epidemiology of melanoma. Eur J Cancer 39:1341–1347

25. Pappo AS (2003) Melanoma in children and adolescents. Eur J Cancer 39:2651–3661

26. Bishop DT, Demenais F, Goldstein AM (2002) Geographical variation in the penetrance of CDKN2A mutations for melanoma. J Natl Cancer Inst 94:894–903

27. Goldstein AM, Struewing JP, Chidambaram A, et al (2000) Genotype-phenotype relationships in U.S. melanoma-prone families with CDKN2A and CDK4 mutations. J Natl Cancer Inst 92:1006–1010

28. Valverde P, Healy E, Jackson I, et al (1995) Variants of the melanocytes-stimulating hormone receptor gene are associated with red hair and fair skin in humans. Nat Genet 11:328–330

29. van der Velden PA, Sandkuijl LA, Bergman W (2001) Melanocortin-1 receptor variant R151C modifies melanoma risk in Dutch families with melanoma. Am J Hum Genet 69:774–779

30. Palmer JS, Duffy DL, Box NF (2000) Melanocortin-1 receptor polymorphisms and risk of melanoma: is the association explained solely by pigmentation phenotype? Am J Hum Genet 66:176–186

31. Aitken J, Welch J, Duffy DL (1999) CDKN2A variants in a population-based sample of Queensland families with melanoma. J Natl Cancer Inst 91:446–452

32. Kumar AP, Smeds J, Berggren P (2001) A single nucleotide polymorphism in the 3' untranslated region of the CDKN2A gene is common in sporadic primary melanomas but mutations in the CDKN2B, CDKN2C, CDK4 and p53 genes are rare. Int J Cancer 95:388–393

33. Casula M, Colombino M, Satta MP, et al; Italian Melanoma Intergroup Study (2004) BRAF gene is somatically mutated but does not make a major contribution to malignant melanoma susceptibility: the Italian Melanoma Intergroup Study. J Clin Oncol 22:286–292

34. Pollock PM, Harper UL, Hansen KS (2003) High frequency of BRAF mutations in nevi. Nat Genet 33:19–20

35. Mackie RM, Watt D, Doherty V, Aitchison T (1991) Malignant melanoma occurring in those aged under 30 in the west of Scotland 1979–1986: a study of incidence, clinical features, pathological features and survival. Br J Dermatol 124:560–564

36. Swerdlow AJ, English JS, Qiao Z (1995) The risk of melanoma in patients with congenital nevi: a cohort study. J Am Acad Dermatol 32:595–599

37. Sahin S, Levin L, Kopf AW (1998) Risk of melanoma in medium-sized congenital melanocytic nevi: a follow-up study. J Am Acad Dermatol 39:428–433

38. Makkar HS, Frieden IJ (2002) Congenital melanocytic nevi: an update for the pediatrician. Curr Opin Pediatr 14:397–403

39. Bittencourt FV, Marghoob AA, Kopf AW, et al (2000) Large congenital melanocytic nevi and the risk for development of malignant melanoma and neurocutaneous melanocytosis. Pediatrics 106:736–741

40. Kadonaga JN, Frieden IJ (1991) Neurocutaneous melanosis: definition and review of the literature. J Am Acad Dermatol 24:747–755

41. DeDavid M, Orlow SJ, Provost N (1996) Neurocutaneous melanosis: clinical features of large congenital melanocytic nevi in patients with manifest central nervous system melanosis. J Am Acad Dermatol 35:529–538

42. Foster RD, Williams ML, Baryonic AJ, et al (2001) Giant congenital melanocytic nevi: the significance of neurocutaneous melanosis in neurologically asymptomatic children. Plats Reconstruct Surge 107:933–941

43. Tucker MA, Helper A, Holly EA (2001) Clinically recognized dysplastic nevi. A central risk factor for cutaneous melanoma. JAMA 277:1439–1444

44. Darlington S, Siskind V, Green L, Green A (2002) Longitudinal study of melanocytic nevi in adolescents. J Am Acad Dermatol 46:715–722

45. Whiteman DC, Valery P, McWhirter W, Green AC (1997) Risk factors for childhood melanoma in Queensland, Australia. Int J Cancer 70:26–31

46. Youl P, Aitken J, Hayward N, et al (2002) Melanoma in adolescents: a case-control study of risk factors in Queensland, Australia. Int J Cancer 98:92–98

47. Goldstein AM, Fraser MC, Clark WH Jr, Tucker MA (1994) Age at diagnosis and transmission of invasive melanoma in 23 families with cutaneous malignant melanoma/dysplastic nevi. J Natl Cancer Inst 86:1385–1390

48. Elwood JM, Jopson J (1997) Melanoma and sun exposure: an overview of published studies. Int J Cancer 73:198–203

49. Dennis LK Beane Freeman LE, VanBeek MJ (2003) Sunscreen use and the risk for melanoma: a quantitative review. Ann Intern Med 139:966–978

50. Saenz N, Saenz-Badillos J, Busam K, et al (1999) Childhood melanoma survival. Cancer 85:750–754

51. Melnik MK, Urdaneta LF, Jurf AS, et al (1986) Malignant melanoma in childhood and adolescence. Am Surg 52:142–147

52. Herzog C, Pappo A, Bondy M, et al (2006) Malignant melanoma. In: Bleyer A, O'Leary M, Barr R, Ries LAG (eds) Cancer Epidemiology in Older Adolescents and Young Adults 15 to 29 Years of Age, Including SEER Incidence and Survival: 1975–2000. National Cancer Institute, NIH Pub. No. 06-5767, Bethesda, MD, pp 53–64

53. Balch CM, Buzaid AC, Soong S-J, et al (2001) Final version of the American Joint Committee on Cancer Staging System for Cutaneous Melanoma. J Clin Oncol 19:3635–3648

54. Compton CC, Barnhill R, Wick MR, Balch CM (2003) Protocol for the examination of specimens from patients with melanoma of the skin. Arch Pathol Lab Med 127:1253–1262

55. Barnhill RL, Flotte TJ, Fleischli M, Perez-Atayde A (1995) Cutaneous melanoma and atypical Spitz tumors in childhood. Cancer 76:1833–1845

56. Gershenwald JE, Colome MI, Lee JE, et al (1998) Patterns of recurrence following a negative sentinel lymph node biopsy in 243 patients with stage I or II melanoma. J Clin Oncol 16:2253–2260

57. Li BM Ling-Xi L, Scolyer RA, et al (2003) Pathologic review of negative sentinel lymph nodes in melanoma patients with regional recurrence. Am J Surg Pathol 27:1197–1202

58. Reintgen DS, Albertini J, Berman C, et al (1995) Accurate nodal staging of malignant melanoma. Cancer Control 2:405–414

59. Kuo CT, Hoon DSB, Takeuchi H, et al (2003) Prediction of disease outcome in melanoma patients by molecular analysis of paraffin-embedded sentinel lymph nodes. J Clin Oncol 21:3566–3572

60. Cook MG, Green MA, Anderson B, et al, EORTC Melanoma Group (2003) The development of optimal pathological assessment of sentinel lymph nodes for melanoma. J Pathol 200:314–319

61. Balch CM, Soong S-J, Gershenwald JE, et al (2001) Prognostic factors analysis of 17,600 melanoma patients: validation of the American Joint Committee on Cancer Melanoma Staging System. J Clin Oncol 19:3622–3634

62. Veronesi U, Cascinelli, N, Adamus J, et al (1988) Thin stage I primary cutaneous malignant melanoma. Comparison of excision with margins of 1 or 3 cm. N Engl J Med 318:1159–1162

63. Veronesi U, Cascinelli N (1991) Narrow excision (1-cm margin). A safe procedure for thin cutaneous melanoma. Arch Surg 126:438–441

64. Balch CM, Urist M, Karakousis CP, et al (1993) Efficacy of 2-cm surgical margins for intermediate-thickness melanomas (1–4 mm). Results of a multi-institutional randomized surgical trial. Ann Surg 218:262–269

65. Morton DL, Wen D-R, Wong JH, et al (1992) Technical details of intraoperative lymphatic mapping for early stage melanoma. Arch Surg 127:392–399

66. Vuylsteke RJ, Leeuwen PA, Statius Muller MG, et al (2003) Clinical outcome of stage i/ii melanoma patients after selective sentinel lymph node dissection: long-term follow-up results. J Clin Oncol 21:1057–1065

67. Sumner WE, Ross MI, Mansfield PF, et al (2002) Implications of lymphatic drainage to unusual sentinel lymph node sites in patients with primary cutaneous melanoma. Cancer 95:354–360

68. Uren RF, Howman-Giles R, Thompson JF, et al (2000) Interval nodes: the forgotten sentinel nodes in patients with melanoma. Arch Surg 135:1168–1172

69. Uren RF, Thompson JF, Howman-Giles R (2000) Sentinel nodes. Interval nodes, lymphatic lakes, and accurate sentinel node identification. Clin Nucl Med 25:234–236

70. Roozendaal GK, de Vries JDH, Jansen L, et al (2001) Sentinel nodes outside lymph node basins in patients with melanoma. Br J Surg 88:305–308

71. Wrightson WR, Wong SL, Edwards MJ, et al (2003) Complications associated with sentinel lymph node biopsy for melanoma. Ann Surg Oncol 10:676–680

72. Gershenwald JE, Thompson W, Mansfield PF, et al (1999) Multi-institutional melanoma lymphatic mapping experience: the prognostic value of sentinel lymph node status in 612 stage I or II melanoma patients. J Clin Oncol 17:976–983

73. Bleicher RJ, Essner R, Foshag LJ, et al (2003) Role of sentinel lymphadenectomy in thin invasive cutaneous melanomas. J Clin Oncol 21:1326–1331

74. Morton DL, Hoon DSB, Cochran AJ, et al (2003) Lymphatic mapping and sentinel lymphadenectomy for early-stage melanoma: therapeutic utility and implications of nodal microanatomy and molecular staging for improving the accuracy of detection of nodal micrometastases. Ann Surg 238:538–550

75. Rutkowski P, Nowecki ZI, Naierowska-Guttmejert A, Ruka W (2003) Lymph node status and survival in cutaneous malignant melanoma – sentinel lymph node biopsy impact. Eur J Surg Oncol 29:611–618

76. Gelbard SN, Tripp JM, Marghoob AA, et al (2002) Management of Spitz nevi: a survey of dermatologists in the United States. J Am Acad Dermatol 47:224–230

77. Barnhill RL (1998) Childhood melanoma. Semin Diagn Pathol 15:189–194

78. Su LD, Fullen DR, Sondak VK, et al (2003) Sentinel lymph node biopsy for patients with problematic Spitzoid melanocytic lesions. Cancer 97:499–507

79. Lohmann CM, Coit DG, Brady MS, et al (2002) Sentinel lymph node biopsy in patients with diagnostically controversial Spitzoid melanocytic tumors. Am J Surg Pathol 26:47–55

80. Neville HL, Andrassy RJ, Lally KP, et al (2000) Lymphatic mapping with sentinel node biopsy in pediatric patients. J Pediatr Surg 35:961–964

81. Kogut KA, Fleming M, Pappo AS, Schropp KP (2000) Sentinel lymph node biopsy for melanoma in young children. J Pediatr Surg 35:965–966

82. Deichmann M, Benner A, Bock M, et al (1999) S100-Beta, melanoma-inhibiting activity, and lactate dehydrogenase discriminate progressive from nonprogressive American Joint Committee on Cancer Stage IV melanoma. J Clin Oncol 17:1891–1896

83. Palmieri G, Ascierto PA, Perrone F, et al (2003) Prognostic value of circulating melanoma cells detected by reverse transcriptase-polymerase chain reaction. J Clin Oncol 21:767–773

84. Garbe C, Leiter U, Ellwanger U, et al (2003) Diagnostic value and prognostic significance of protein S-100 B, melanoma-inhibitory activity, and tyrosinase/MART-1 reverse transcription-polymerase chain reaction in the follow-up of high-risk melanoma patients. Cancer 97:1737–1745-

85. Wascher RA, Morton DL, Kuo C, et al (2003) Molecular tumor markers in the blood: early prediction of disease outcome in melanoma patients treated with a melanoma vaccine. J Clin Oncol 21:2558–2563

86. Buzaid AC, Tinoco L, Ross MI, et al (1995) Role of computed tomography in the staging of patients with local-regional metastases of melanoma. J Clin Oncol 13:2104–2108

87. Kaste SC, Pappo AS, Jenkins JJ III, Pratt CB (1996) Malignant melanoma in children: imaging spectrum. Pediatr Radiol 26:800–805

88. Ackland KM, Healy C, Calonje E, et al (2001) Comparison of positron emission tomography scanning and sentinel node biopsy in the detection of micrometastases of primary cutaneous malignant melanoma. J Clin Oncol 19:2674–2678

89. Rinne D, Baum RP, Hor G, Kaufmann R (1997) Primary staging and follow-up of high risk melanoma patients with whole-body ^{18}F-Fluorodeoxyglucose positron. Cancer 82:1664–1671

90. Cobben DC, Koopal S, Tiebosch AT, et al (2002) New diagnostic techniques in staging in the surgical treatment of cutaneous malignant melanoma. Eur J Surg Oncol 28:692–700

91. Longo MI, Lazaro P, Carreras JL, Montz R (2003) Fluorodeoxyglucose-positron emission tomography imaging versus sentinel node biopsy in the primary staging of melanoma patients. Dermatol Surg 29:245–248

92. Kirkwood JM, Strawderman MH, Ernstoff MS, et al (1996) Interferon alfa-2b adjuvant therapy of high-risk resected cutaneous melanoma: The Eastern Cooperative Oncology Group trial EST 1684. J Clin Oncol 14:7–17

93. Kirkwood JM, Ibrahim JG, Sondak VK, et al (2000) High- and low-dose interferon alfa-2b in high-risk melanoma: first analysis of intergroup trial E1690/S9111/C9190. J Clin Oncol 18:2444–2458

94. Kirkwood JM, Ibrahim JG, Sosman JA, et al (2001) High-dose interferon alfa-2b significantly prolongs relapse-free and overall survival compared with the GM2-KLH/QS-21 vaccine in patients with resected stage IIB–III melanoma: results of Intergroup Trial E1694/S9512/C509801. J Clin Oncol 19:2370–2380

95. McMasters KM (2001) The sunbelt melanoma trial. Ann Surg Oncol 8:41–43

96. Ballo MT, Bonnen MD, Garden AG, et al (2003) Adjuvant irradiation for cervical lymph node metastases from melanoma. Cancer 97:1789–1796

97. Rosenberg SA, Yang JC, Topalian SL, et al (1994) Treatment of 283 consecutive patients with metastatic melanoma or renal cell cancer using high-dose bolus Interleukin 2. JAMA 271:907–913

98. Buzaid AC, Atkins MB (2001) Practical guidelines for the management of biochemotherapy-related toxicity in melanoma. Clin Cancer Rese 7:2611–2619

99. Eton O, Legha SS, Bedikian AY, et al (2002) Sequential biochemotherapy versus chemotherapy for metastatic melanoma: results from a phase III randomized trial. J Clin Oncol 20:2045–2052

100. Atkins MB, Lee S, Flaherty LE, et al (2003) A prospective randomized phase III trial of concurrent biochemotherapy (BCT) with cisplatin, vinblastine, dacarbazine (CVD), IL-2 and interferon alpha-2b (IFN) versus CVD alone in patients with metastatic melanoma (E3695): an ECOG-coordinated intergroup trial. Proc Am Soc Clin Oncol 22:708

101. Danson S, Lorigan P, Arance A, et al (2003) Randomized phase ii study of temozolomide given every 8 hours or daily with either interferon Alfa2b or thalidomide in metastatic malignant melanoma. J Clin Oncol 21:2551–2557

102. Hwu W-J, Krown SE, Menell JH, et al (2003) Phase II study of temozolomide plus thalidomide for the treatment of metastatic melanoma. J Clin Oncol 21:3351–3356

103. Minev BR (2002) Melanoma vaccines. Semin Oncol 29:479–493

Breast Cancer

Marianne Phillips • Banu Arun •
Archie Bleyer

Contents

18.1 Introduction

Breast cancer in adolescence and early adulthood is a rare condition. Data from the National Cancer Institute Surveillance, Epidemiology, and End Results (SEER) database in the United States demonstrates that less than 1% of breast cancers occur in patients younger than 30 years and 2.7% occur in those younger than 35 years, with an estimated incidence of less than 0.1 per 100,000 women below the age of 20 years, 1.4 for women 20–24 years, 8.1 for women 25–29 years, and 24.8 for women 30–34 years old [1, 2].

Breast cancer accounts for less than 1% of childhood cancers, and less than 0.1% of all breast cancers occur in childhood [3, 4]. The most common type of breast cancer in childhood is secretory carcinoma, formerly known as juvenile carcinoma [5, 6], a morphologically distinct type of breast carcinoma with highly indolent clinical behavior. Management is with wide local excision and axillary lymph node dissection; distant metastases are extremely rare. The prognosis is favorable, but patients require long-term follow-up in view of the potential risk of late recurrence.

Invasive ductal carcinoma in adolescents and young women has a more aggressive biological behavior and a worse prognosis than breast cancer in older premenopausal women Age is an independent prognostic factor, with the youngest patients having the poorest survival [7–9]. Tumors in younger women tend to be less well differentiated, and have a higher proliferating fraction and more lymphovascular invasion than those in older patients [10–13]. As a group, women younger than 35 years of age have more advanced disease at diagnosis and worse 5-year survival than older, premenopausal patients [11, 14–17]. Consensus statements recommend that all women under the age of 35 receive adjuvant therapy, regardless of stage [18, 19], due to their worse outcome and an increased risk of loco-regional recurrence with breast-conserving surgery compared with older pre-menopausal patients.

Optimal management of young women and adolescents requires consideration of the long-term physical and psychological consequences of all treatments. Several special issues require consideration for young women presenting with a diagnosis of breast cancer, including the risk of treatment-induced impaired fertility and potential premature menopause. In addition, there is evidence that young women are more vulnerable to emotional distress and have a higher risk of psychosocial problems [20–24].

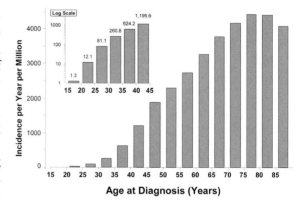

Figure 18.1

Incidence of breast cancer in women, United States SEER 1975–2000 [1]

18.2 Epidemiology

18.2.1 Incidence

The SEER incidence data in this section were collected between 1975 and 2000. Less than 1% of all breast cancer cases occurred in women under the age of 30 years. Breast cancer incidence rose steadily with age, stabilized, and then dropped slightly after 80 years of age (Fig. 18. 1).

In the United States, there was an increase in average incidence of breast cancer per million females per year between the age groups, from 1.3 in 15- to 19-year-olds, to 12.1 in 20- to 24-year-olds, to 81.1 in 25- to 29-year-olds (Table 18.1). However, there was no

annual increase apparent within each age group over the same time period.

At diagnosis, women younger that age 30 years presented with less advanced disease (smaller proportion with distant metastases) than those older than 30 years (Fig. 18.2), and yet as a group have had a worse outcome than older women, as is reviewed below.

18.2.1.1 Ethnic Differences in Incidence

From 1992 to 2001, in the United States, African Americans/blacks were more likely than any other race/ethnicity to develop breast cancer at age 10–49 years (Fig. 18.3). Above 50 years of age, non-His-

Table 18.1 Incidence of breast cancer in the United States (U.S.) in persons younger than 30 years of age. *SEER* Surveillance, Epidemiology, and End Results Program

Age at diagnosis (years)	15–19	20–24	25–29
U.S. population, year 2000 census (in millions), females	10.11	9.48	9.69
Average incidence per million, 1975–2000, SEER	1.3	12.1	81.1
Average annual % change in incidence, 1975–2000, SEER	0	0	0
Estimated incidence per million, year 2000, U.S.	1.3	12.1	81.1
Estimated number persons diagnosed, year 2000, U.S.	26	229	1,571

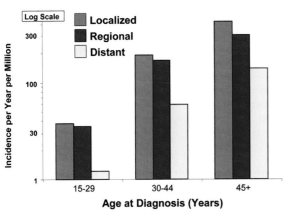

Figure 18.2

Incidence of breast cancer in women by stage of disease at diagnosis; United States SEER 1975–2000 [1]

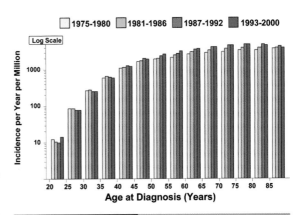

Figure 18.4

Incidence of breast cancer in women by era; United States SEER 1975–2000 [1]

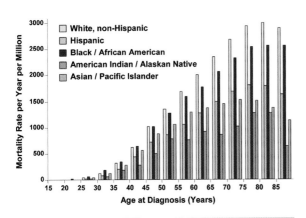

Figure 18.3

Incidence of breast cancer in women by race/ethnicity; United States SEER 1992–2001 [1]

panic white women had the highest incidence in all older age groups. American Indians/Alaska Natives had a lower incidence of breast cancer at all ages.

18.2.1.2 Trends in Incidence

The incidence of breast cancer in young women has remained relatively stable over the period 1975–2000 (Fig. 18.4).

18.3 Diagnosis

Breast cancers diagnosed in adolescents and young adults tend to be larger and to have a longer history of a palpable mass than tumors diagnosed in older women [25]. There are several reasons for this, many as a consequence of the recognized, statistical improbability of breast cancer occurring in this age group. There are low rates of routine screening by mammography and only a small percentage of women under 40 years report performing regular self-examination. The accuracy of clinical physical examination in detecting malignant tumors is lower in very young women as they often have dense or nodular breast tissue that is subject to cyclical hormonal changes. Even once a mass is clinically palpable, there is a low clinical suspicion of malignancy, as most discrete breast masses in this age group are fibroadenomas. In a study of 30 women under the age of 30 years with breast cancer, clinical examination correctly identified a palpable mass to be malignant in only 37% of cases, reinforcing the need for a tissue diagnosis in all young women presenting with a non-cystic breast mass [25]. In a young woman with an asymptomatic palpable mass, it may be reasonable to repeat the examination after the next menstrual period with advice regarding avoidance of caffeine in the interval. The role of magnetic resonance imaging (MRI) in the management of very young women remains to be clarified. Certainly MRI has lower specificity in young women as benign fibroadenomas in this age group share more features in common with malignancy than do fibroadenomas in older women [26].

The accuracy of mammography is inferior in young women due to their denser breast tissue [27] and only 55% of mammograms in young women with breast cancer demonstrated definite malignant changes [25]. Ultrasound demonstrates malignant features in only 58% and is interpreted as benign in 30% of cases. The greatest accuracy of diagnosis is provided by fine-needle aspiration cytology of suspicious lesions, with 78% samples obtained definitely malignant and a further 15% suspicious of malignancy.

18.4 Prognostic Characteristics

Published studies compare the stage and pathological characteristics of breast tumors occurring in young women with those occurring in older pre-menopausal women. In 1,703 patients treated at Institute Curie between 1981 and 1985, young age predicted for poorer survival [9]. The relationship between risk and age was a log-linear function, demonstrating a 4% decrease in the risk of recurrence and 2% decrease in the risk of death for every year of age. In multivariate analysis for survival and disease-free interval, young age was of independent prognostic significance when tumor size, nodal status, grade, hormone receptor status, loco-regional treatment, and adjuvant systemic therapy were all evaluated.

Among 1,837 pre-menopausal women treated at the European Institute of Oncology between April 1997 and August 2000, 185 were aged less than 35 years at diagnosis. Young women were found to be more likely to have tumors that were estrogen receptor (ER)-negative (38.8 vs. 21.6%; p<0.001), and grade 3 (61.9% vs. 37.4%; p<0.001) compared to older, premenopausal women. Young women were also more likely to have lymphovascular invasion. No difference was found in the proportion of tumors that overexpressed HER2/neu [28]. Again, in multivariate analyses, age younger than 35 years remained a significant predictor for

shorter disease-free interval, shorter time to distant recurrence, and increased overall mortality.

A retrospective analysis of 885 pre-menopausal patients confirmed that age <35 years was an independent prognostic factor in multivariate analyses for recurrence-free survival (RFS) and overall survival (OS), and is the second most powerful risk factor after lymph node involvement [29]. The survival of 15 women aged under 25 years was not significantly different from that of women aged 26–35 years, but the survival of all women aged ≤35 years was significantly worse than that of women aged 36–65 years (p<0.001) [30].

In a Danish population study of 10,356 premenopausal women with breast cancer, the negative prognostic effect of young age was identified almost exclusively in women <35 years with low-risk disease who did not receive adjuvant chemotherapy or radiotherapy [17]. Young women with node-negative disease had a significantly increased risk of dying compared to women aged 45 to 49 years who had also not received adjuvant therapy. However, the effect of age was not seen in patients who did receive adjuvant chemotherapy.

Poor outcomes for women <30 years with stage I disease who did not receive adjuvant treatment has also been identified by others [31]. Young women had a 5-year RFS and OS of 46% and 87%, respectively, compared with the population-based estimate of 97% 5-year RFS observed in older pre-menopausal patients with stage I disease (National Cancer Database data).

Data from multiple organizations and studies have shown worse outcomes for younger women with ER-positive tumors treated with adjuvant chemotherapy alone [28, 32, 33]. A retrospective review of 3,700 pre-menopausal women in the International Breast Cancer Study Group (IBCSG) trials I, II, V, and VI identified 314 patients younger than 35 years at the time of diagnosis. The distribution of tumor size and number of involved nodes was similar in the younger and older pre-menopausal women, but the proportion of ER-positive tumors was lower in the younger age group (51% vs 63%). Younger women had significantly worse 10-year disease-free survival (DFS) and OS compared with older pre-menopausal women (35% vs. 47%; p<0.001 and 49% vs. 62%; p<0.001, respectively). Contrary to the pattern seen in older women, young women with ER-positive tumors had a poorer prognosis than young women with ER-negative tumors (10-year DFS 25% vs. 47%; p=0.014; 10-year OS 39% vs. 56%; p=0.12), a finding that is thought to be due to the insufficient endocrine effect of chemotherapy in younger women and the absence of any adjuvant endocrine therapy in these studies [34].

At the Royal Marsden Hospital, among 1,161 women who received adjuvant chemotherapy for early breast cancer between 1990 and 2001, 104 were aged less than 35 years. Younger patients had significantly poorer 5-year DFS compared with older women (48% vs. 74%; p<0.001). The effect of age on DFS was limited to the subset of women with ER-positive disease, despite 82% of the patients aged <35 years with ER-positive tumors receiving adjuvant endocrine therapy (5-year DFS 54% vs. 79%; p=0.02) [35].

At the University of Texas MD Anderson Cancer Center, 452 women were diagnosed to have breast cancer before age 36 years; 69% of the tumors had nuclear grade 3, 52% were ER-positive, and 48% were progesterone-receptor positive. HER-2/neu status was evaluable for 60% of the tumors: 34% were HER-2/neu positive. RFS was significantly shorter in patients who reported a family history of ovarian cancer (p<0.0001) and those who had hormone-receptor-negative tumors (p=0.001). OS was significantly shorter in patients who reported a family history of ovarian cancer (p=0.001) and those who had hormone-receptor-negative tumors (p<0.0001) or nuclear grade 3 tumors (p=0.005) [36].

18.5 Treatment and Management

The principles of managing invasive breast carcinoma in very young women are the same as for all older women, but there are several additional issues that require special consideration.

18.5.1 Surgery

Breast-conserving surgery is obviously desirable for most young women. The two principal considerations when deciding between breast-conserving surgery and mastectomy are the risk of local recurrence and the overall cosmetic result. The most important risk factors for local recurrence after breast-conserving sur-

gery are young age (<35 years) [36–43], infiltrating tumor with an extensive intraductal component [37, 43–46], vascular invasion [47], and microscopic involvement at the excision margins [42, 48–50]. In an analysis of two large trials of mastectomy versus conservative surgery and radiotherapy, patients aged <35 years at the time of surgery were found to have a nine times higher risk of local recurrence after conservative surgery than patients over 60 years at the time of surgery [39]. However, young patients treated with mastectomy did not have an increased risk of local recurrence compared to older patients. Similarly, women aged less than 40 years treated conservatively had a fivefold greater risk of local recurrence compared to older patients, but the effect of young age on the risk of local recurrence was not seen in women treated with mastectomy [38]. No studies have demonstrated that conservative surgery in young women has a negative impact on survival. Young women should be aware of the increase in the risk of local recurrence associated with conservative surgery in this age group, but this should not preclude breast conservation.

18.5.2 Adjuvant Therapies

Patients under the age of 35 years are regarded as having an average/high risk of recurrence and warrant recommendation of adjuvant therapies [18, 19]. Certainly, consensus panels of the National Institutes of Health and the St. Gallen conference recommend adjuvant therapy be given to all patients aged under 35 years based on the evidence that they have a poorer prognosis. However, the use of adjuvant therapies in young women raises significant issues of long-term side effects including the induction of an early menopause, fertility impairment, and adverse effects on bone mineral density and cognition [18, 19].

The current choices of adjuvant therapy for premenopausal patients include cytotoxic chemotherapy, ovarian ablation (by surgery, irradiation, or chemical ovarian suppression), anti-estrogen therapy or any combination of these modalities. Adjuvant chemotherapy for early breast cancer in patients under 50 years old reduces the relative risk of recurrence by 35% and death by 27%, and for patients with ER-negative tumors, adjuvant chemotherapy alone is appropriate [51]. However, patients with ER-positive tumors require either chemotherapy and endocrine therapy or endocrine therapy alone. Five years of adjuvant tamoxifen has been shown to reduce the relative risk of recurrence by 54% in women with ER-positive disease diagnosed prior to age 40 years [52].

18.5.3 Adjuvant Chemotherapy

In the Danish and MD Anderson studies, women under 30 years with early-stage disease and not given adjuvant chemotherapy had particularly poor RFS [17, 32]. Anthracycline-containing regimens were found to be more effective than CMF (cyclophosphamide, methotrexate, 5-fluorouracil), with the use of an anthracycline resulting in a 2.7% absolute survival benefit at 5 years of follow-up [51]. A Canadian study comparing CEF (cyclophosphamide, epirubicin, 5-fluorouracil) with CMF showed improvement in outcome for the anthracycline-containing combination, with women receiving CEF demonstrating significantly improved 5-year RFS and OS (63% vs. 53%; $p<0.001$; 77% vs. 70%; $p=0.03$, respectively) [53].

At the current time, anthracycline-containing combinations remain the standard of care for adjuvant chemotherapy; however, the optimal chemotherapy for young women remains controversial, particularly with the advent of studies examining the role of taxanes and dose-intensive adjuvant therapies.

The CALGB 9344 trial randomized 3,121 patients with node-positive early breast cancer to 4 cycles of doxorubicin, cyclophosphamide (AC) or 4 cycles of AC followed by 4 cycles of paclitaxel [54]. Patients who received paclitaxel had a 17% reduction in the risk of recurrence and an 18% reduction in the risk of death. Results from the National Surgical Adjuvant Breast and Bowel Project (NSABP)-28 trial also showed a 17% reduction in the risk of recurrence by the addition of 4 cycles of paclitaxel, although no significant OS benefit has yet been observed [55]. The Breast Cancer International Research Group (BCIRG) 001 trial compared six cycles of docetaxel, doxorubicin, and cyclophosphamide (TAC) with 5-fluorouracil, doxorubicin and cyclophosphamide (FAC) and showed that, at a median follow-up of 33 months, there was a significant improvement in

both DFS and OS for patients with one to three positive lymph nodes treated on the TAC arm [56].

Recently published results of the Cancer and Leukemia Group B (CALGB) 9741 trial show a survival advantage for a dose-intense regimen of AC followed by paclitaxel given every 2 weeks with growth factor support; 2,005 women were randomized on this study. At a median follow-up of 36 months, there was a 26% reduction in the risk of relapse ($p=0.01$) and a 31% reduction in the risk of death ($p=0.013$) associated with the dose-intensive arms, but no significant differences between schedules giving paclitaxel sequentially or concurrently with chemotherapy [57].

18.5.4 Adjuvant Endocrine Therapy

Amenorrhea may be important in the action of chemotherapeutic agents for pre-menopausal patients, with pre-menopausal women experiencing chemotherapy-induced amenorrhea demonstrating a better prognosis than those retaining their menstrual cycle [58–61]. RFS and OS appears to be improved by the induction of amenorrhea, but the optimal duration of the amenorrhea is unknown. The likelihood of becoming amenorrheic following adjuvant chemotherapy is dependent on age, with younger women less likely to become amenorrheic and, therefore, less likely to maximize on the benefits of the endocrine effect of adjuvant chemotherapy [62]. Suppression of ovarian functional, however, creates significant problems for very young women, including menopausal symptoms, psychological distress, and the need to adjust personal and family plans.

As described, cytotoxic chemotherapy for young women with ER-negative tumors is the only useful adjuvant therapy. However, the situation for young women with ER-positive tumors is more complex. A retrospective review of four IBCSG trials showed that women aged less than 35 years with ER-positive tumors had a worse outcome than young women with ER-negative tumors [34], although no patients in these studies received adjuvant endocrine therapy.

Published studies have compared adjuvant CMF chemotherapy with endocrine therapy in premenopausal women. There were no differences in DFS or OS between the two groups: patients receiving six

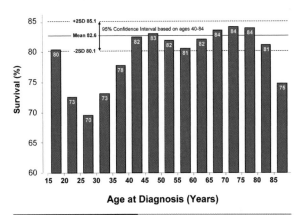

Figure 18.5

Five-year relative survival rate, breast cancer in women; United States SEER 1975–2000 [1]

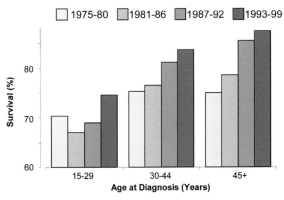

Figure 18.6

Five-year relative survival rates, breast cancer in women, by era and age at diagnosis; United States SEER [1]

cycles of oral CMF compared with the combination of tamoxifen and ovarian suppression in patients with ER-positive early breast cancer [63]. Two-thirds of patients randomized to CMF became amenorrheic as a result of their chemotherapy, and there was a significant difference in OS in favor of these patients (p=0.05). In another study comparing 3 years of goserelin plus 5 years of tamoxifen to six cycles of intravenous CMF, at a median follow-up of 5 years the group that received adjuvant endocrine therapy had a significant improvement in RFS (81% versus 76%; p=0.037), but there were no differences in OS and only 7% of patients in this trial were aged less than 35 years [64]. Two years of goserelin has been compared with 6 cycles of either oral or intravenous CMF in 1,640 patients with node-positive early breast cancer unselected for ER status [65]. For patients with ER-positive disease, 2 years of goserelin was equivalent to CMF chemotherapy for DFS and OS, whereas in ER-negative or receptor-status-unknown patients, CMF chemotherapy was superior to goserelin. However, in all three of these trials a chemotherapy arm was used that would now be considered sub-optimal and the proportion of very young women (<35 years) in these trials was small.

In the 1998 Early Breast Cancer Trialists' Collaborative Group overview there were only 177 premenopausal women with ER-positive disease randomized to adju-

vant chemotherapy or a combination of chemotherapy and tamoxifen [51]. More recently, a trial comparing cyclophosphamide, doxorubicin, 5-fluorouracil (CAF), with CAF plus goserelin or CAF followed by tamoxifen and goserelin has been analyzed. The addition of goserelin to CAF failed to improve DFS, whereas tamoxifen added to CAF and goserelin significantly improved the outcome (5-year DFS 67% versus 78%) [66].

Further trials are required to better evaluate the potential benefit of the addition of optimal endocrine therapy to optimal adjuvant chemotherapy in very young women.

18.6 Outcome

18.6.1 Survival

Five-year survival rates for breast cancer, by age, revealed that survival was lowest for those in the adolescent and young adult age group. Within that group, 25- to 29-year-old women had the lowest survival rates. Females in the 20- to 39-year age range had statistically significantly lower rates than those aged 40–84 years at diagnosis (Fig. 18.5). A recent study of more than 45,500 cases of breast cancer has suggested that 10-year survival rates in women with stage I disease are determined more by age at diagnosis than

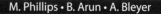

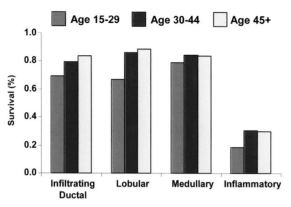

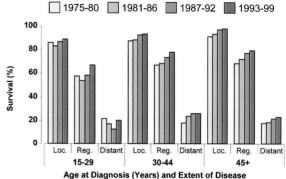

Figure 18.7

Five-year relative survival rates, breast cancer in women, by histologic type and age at diagnosis; United States SEER 1975–1998 [1]

Figure 18.8

Five-year relative survival rates, breast cancer in women, by era, stage of disease at diagnosis, and age at diagnosis; United States SEER [1]

tumor size, tumor location, number of examined lymph nodes, histology, grade, hormone receptor status, marital status, race, registry area, year of diagnosis, type of surgery, and radiotherapy [24]. In this analysis, breast-cancer-specific mortality increased 5% per each year younger than 45 years ($p=0.0001$).

The lower survival rate for young women may be due to several factors: breast cancer in young women is typically invasive, more aggressive, and is associated with a worse prognosis than in older women, detection rates are lower due to lack of suspicion in the general population and medical community, and breast tissue in younger women is commonly more dense than in older women, resulting in mammography results that may be inconclusive.

Five-year survival rates, by 6-year eras, reveal that although survival rates for the adolescent and young adult population remained relatively stable over time, a slight improvement was seen for each age cohort in the most recent era (Fig. 18.6).

Breast cancer survival is consistently lower for adolescent and young adult women than for other age groups, regardless of histologic type. Five-year survival is limited for women with inflammatory disease for all age groups (Fig. 18.7). Lower survival rates reflect the aggressive biologic and pathologic characteristics tumors specific to this age group and the fact that rou-

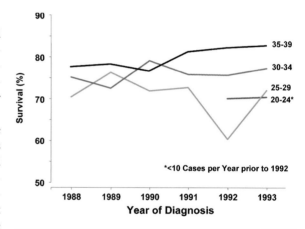

Figure 18.9

Five-year relative survival rates, breast cancer in women, by age at diagnosis and year of at diagnosis, age less than 40 years, United States SEER 1988–1993 [1]

tine screening for breast cancer is not the standard of care for adolescents and young adults. Although treatment modalities have improved considerably over the last 30 years, improvements in survival of breast cancer patients in the U. S. have not been observed in adolescents and young adults to the extent seen for older females.

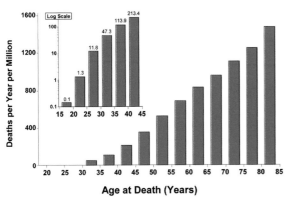

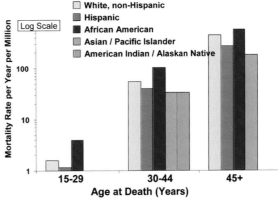

Figure 18.10

National breast cancer mortality rate by era; United States SEER 1975–2000 [1]

Figure 18.12

National breast cancer mortality rate by race/ethnicity; United States SEER 1992–2001 [1]

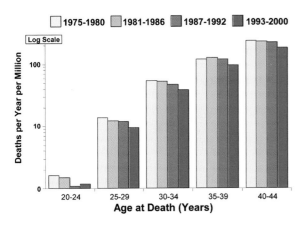

Figure 18.11

National breast cancer mortality rate in women; United States SEER 1975–2000 [1]. The inset is a semilogarithmic representation of the rates for women younger than age 45 years

had high survival rates, although rates were relatively high for all ages (Fig. 18.8). For regional and distant disease, survival rates increased with age (Fig. 18.8).

It may be that with all of the diagnostic and therapeutic advances that have occurred during the past decade, survival in young women may have improved since 1998, the latest era for which is able to provide 5-year survival data. It is more difficult to be certain of survival outcomes when not all patients have been followed for at least as long as the survival end-point being evaluated. Nonetheless, there is little evidence that survival rates among those less than 30 years of age at diagnosis have improved during the most recent, evaluable era: 1998–2003 (Fig. 18.9).

18.6.2 Mortality

During 1975–2000 in the United States, breast cancer mortality rates rose steadily with age, reflecting an increasing breast cancer incidence (Fig. 18.10). Mortality for all age groups remained stable or dropped after 1981. The decrease in mortality was more pronounced for those over 30 years of age, particularly in the most recent era of 1993–2000 (Fig. 18.11), and is likely to reflect the introduction of screening programs, improved diagnostic techniques, and adjuvant chemo- and radiation therapies. There was a more significant improvement in mortality over time for older age groups.

As expected, 5-year survival rates for all women were best for those with localized disease, followed by those with regional disease. Survival was poor for all women with distant disease. However, 5-year survival rates were consistently low for 20- to 24-year-old women, regardless of extent of disease at diagnosis. For localized disease, women in the age groups 20 to 24 and 40 to 44 years

18.6.3 Race/Ethnic Differences in Mortality

In the United States, for women younger than 45 years of age, the mortality for African Americans/blacks was nearly twice as high as that for other racial/ethnic groups (Fig. 18.12). The death rate for African Americans/blacks was disproportionately high despite the increased incidence of breast cancer in these women compared to other ethnic groups. African American/black patients have been reported to present with higher-stage or more advanced disease [23]. White women were significantly more likely to be older and to have smaller tumors, less lymph node involvement, and to have ER-positive tumors compared with Hispanic or African American/black women [23].

An additional analysis of treatment modalities used for women under 35 years of age with invasive breast cancer revealed that African American/black women – and some Hispanic females – received less aggressive initial therapy than white, non-Hispanic women, despite similar prognostic variables. These analyses were multivariate and adjusted for stage, grade, lymph node status, and treatment. Overall, 9% of the women in this study were registered on clinical trials, although African American/black women were less likely to be included in this group. African American/black and Hispanic women had worse outcomes and a higher mortality rate than white, non-Hispanic women [23].

18.6.4 Trends in Mortality

In the United States, a reduction in breast cancer mortality occurred over time, and was significant for each age group. This improvement has been considerable in more recent years (Fig. 18.13). The average annual percent change in mortality for whites compared to African Americans/blacks reveals a significant discrepancy between the two racial groups. Whites experienced substantial improvements in survival in all age groups in the period 1975–2000, whereas similar improvements were not observed in the African American/black population. Decreases in mortality during this time period were three times greater for whites than for African Americans/blacks (Fig. 18.14).

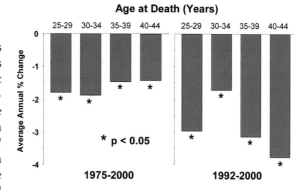

Age at Death (Years)

Figure 18.13

Average annual percent change in the national breast cancer mortality rate; United States SEER [1]. The left panel depicts the change over the last quarter century; the panel on the right displays a more recent, era: the last decade

18.7 Special Considerations

18.7.1 Fertility Issues

Young women are especially likely to have concerns regarding the potential effects of chemo- and endocrine therapy on their fertility. In patients with ER-positive tumors it is unclear whether there is any advantage to permanent menopause compared with reversible hormonal manipulation. Of patients aged less than 40 years treated with goserelin for 2 years at randomization, 90% had a return of menstrual function, and this did not adversely affect their outcome [65].

Chemotherapy can be cytotoxic to the ovaries and a proportion of pre-menopausal women receiving chemotherapy for early breast cancer will develop menstrual abnormalities and premature menopause, although younger women require higher cumulative doses of chemotherapy to develop gonadal failure [67]. The histological effect of chemotherapy is fibrosis and atrophy, resulting in a dose-related progressive and permanent depletion of primordial follicles [67, 68]. Increasing age at chemotherapy exposure is correlated with increasing ovarian failure rate [62, 67–70]. Alkylating agents (e.g., cyclophosphamide) appear to be the most gonadotoxic, but there is limited information con-

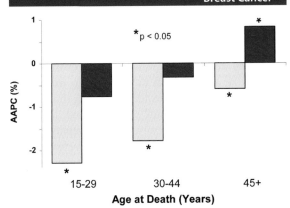

Figure 18.14

Average annual percent change (AAPC) in the national breast cancer mortality rate, by race (*cream bars* whites, *brown bars* African American/blacks); United States SEER 1975–2000 [1]

cerning newer agents including taxanes [70]. In addition, for young women, chemotherapy-related amenorrhea may be reversible in 22–56% of patients [67].

Most data addressing the risk of becoming amenorrheic with adjuvant chemotherapy for early breast cancer is derived from women receiving CMF, and results may not be comparable for anthracycline-based chemotherapy regimens. In the MD Anderson series, no patient under 30 years of age treated with a doxorubicin-containing regimen ceased menstruation, compared with 33% of patients aged 30–39 years and 96% of those aged 40–49 years [36].

Chapter 18

Current fertility preservation options for women commencing adjuvant chemotherapy are limited. The option of submitting to a cycle of ovarian hyperstimulation and egg harvest raises concerns over the safety of ovarian hyperstimulation in the breast cancer setting. The possibility of ovarian cryopreservation requires further progress in in-vitro maturation of thawed primordial follicles, their fertilization, and subsequent embryo transfer. Attempts to reduce the gonadotoxic effect of chemotherapy have been tried with co-treatment with a gonadotropin-releasing hormone (GnRH) agonist analogue. In 13 breast cancer patients aged between 26 and 39 years given leuprolide during their adjuvant chemotherapy; all patients resumed spontaneous menstruation within 1 year of completion of therapy [71]. In addition, in 64 patients who received goserelin, 3.6 mg monthly in combination with their adjuvant chemotherapy with a median follow-up of 55 months, 86% of patients resumed normal menses and one patient achieved a successful pregnancy [72].

18.7.2 Breast Cancer During Pregnancy

Between 0.02 and 0.1% of all pregnancies are complicated by cancer [73]. A high index of suspicion is required to diagnose breast cancer during pregnancy due to the anatomic and physiologic changes occurring in the breast during this period, and studies have found an average delay of 5 months between first symptoms and the diagnosis [74]. Pregnant women have a 2.5-fold higher risk of presenting with metastatic disease

Table 18.2 Features associated with a high risk of breast cancer

Three or more women diagnosed with breast or ovarian cancer on the same side of the family
Women diagnosed with breast cancer under 40 years of age
Women with bilateral breast cancer
Women with ovarian cancer under 50 years of age
Women with breast and ovarian cancer
Male relative with breast cancer
Ashkenazi Jewish ancestry
Demonstrated germ-line mutation in a high-risk breast cancer-associated gene

and a decreased chance of stage I disease, and delay in diagnosis may contribute to the more advanced stage of presentation in such women [75]. The pathology of pregnancy-associated breast cancer is almost identical to that occurring in non-pregnant women but with a higher incidence of ER-negative tumors, probably reflecting the young age of the patient cohort [76, 77].

Treatment of pregnancy-associated breast cancer should follow the same principles as in non-pregnant women. Early termination of pregnancy has not been shown to improve outcome [78]. Modified radical mastectomy is the standard surgical treatment, as radiotherapy during pregnancy would deliver high doses of radiation to the developing fetus. Breast conservation is an alternative if radiotherapy is scheduled for after the delivery of the baby. Recommendations for adjuvant chemotherapy should be based on the stage, age, and pathological findings as for non-pregnant women, although chemotherapy should be delayed until the second trimester to minimize exposure of the fetus to cytotoxics during organogenesis and as administration of chemotherapy in the second and third trimesters does not appear to carry an increased risk of teratogenesis [79].

With appropriate management, pregnant women have similar actuarial survival and RFS to non-pregnant women [75, 80–81]. For breast cancer survivors, despite the theoretical risk that the hormonal effects of a pregnancy after breast cancer may cause relapse, there is no evidence to support this [82].

18.7.3 Risk Reduction in Women with Inherited Predisposition to Breast Cancer

The management of young women at an increased risk of developing breast cancer at a young age requires consideration. These include women who have germline mutations in *BRCA1*, *BRCA2*, *p53* (Li Fraumeni syndrome), or *PTEN* (Cowden's syndrome). Factors that define women at potentially high risk of developing breast cancer are summarized in Table 18.2. For example, clinical disease may develop in about 50% by age 50 years and 80% by age 70 years in women with a mutated *BRCA1* gene.

Li Fraumeni syndrome is a rare, dominantly inherited condition caused by germ-line mutation in the Tp53 gene on chromosome 17 [83]. Affected patients have a 50% risk of developing cancer by age 35 years and a 90% lifetime risk. The syndrome is characterized by pediatric bone or soft tissue sarcoma, early-onset breast cancer, and other cancers including those affecting the brain, lung, and adrenals, and leukemia. Cowden's syndrome is caused by a mutation in the PTEN gene on chromosome 10 [84]. Affected patients have multiple hamartomas and an increased risk of developing breast or thyroid carcinoma at a young age.

It is especially important for women identified to be at potentially high risk to maintain breast awareness from a young age [85]. The recommendations for follow-up of individuals with an inherited predisposition to breast cancer, from the Cancer Genetics Studies Consortium, include monthly self-breast examination, beginning at age 18 to 21 years, annual, or semi-annual clinical breast examination commencing at age 25 to 35 years, and annual mammography from age 25 to 35 years [86]. The recommendations for optimal screening modality and frequency are currently not well described in planned prospective studies designed with mortality endpoints, and are largely based on expert opinion [87, 88]. Several studies have suggested that screening with MRI benefits women at high risk, as the sensitivity for detecting invasive breast cancer was higher for MRI compared to mammography or clinical breast examinations, although whether MRI provides a meaningful clinical benefit and improves survival requires further evaluation [89–92].

Currently, tamoxifen is the only drug to be approved for the risk reduction of breast cancer in high-risk individuals [93, 94]. The study that led to its approval was the phase III NSABP chemoprevention trial (BCPT-P1), which randomized 13,388 women at high risk for breast cancer to tamoxifen versus placebo for 5 years [95]. After a median follow-up of 54 months, a 49% reduction in the incidence of invasive breast cancer was observed for those receiving tamoxifen (p<0.00001). However, tamoxifen did not reduce the occurrence of ER-negative breast cancers and it remains questionable whether a reduction in the incidence of breast cancer will eventually lead to improvements in survival. Furthermore, identification of the ideal target population that would derive the most benefit from using tamoxifen for breast cancer prevention is urgently required, especially as the risks and benefits of tamoxifen are considerable. The side effects of tamoxifen in the NSABP trial included an increased risk of endometrial cancer, with a relative risk in the tamoxifen group of 2.5, increasing to 4.01 in women aged 50 years or older. Deep vein thrombosis and pulmonary emboli were also seen more often in the tamoxifen group, with women aged 50 years or older at highest risk (relative risk 1.7 for deep vein thrombosis, 3.0 for pulmonary emboli) [95].

The impact of tamoxifen on women with high genetic risk, such as BRCA1 or BRCA2 mutation carriers, is currently being evaluated. BRCA1 and BRCA2 gene sequencing was performed on all breast cancer cases (n=288) in women enrolled in the NSABP-P1 trial, and 19 cases were found to have the BRCA1 or BRCA2 mutation [95]. Five out of 8 patients with BRCA1 received tamoxifen, and 3 out of 11 patients with BRCA2 mutations received tamoxifen: 83% of BRCA1 breast tumors were ER-negative vs. 76% of BRCA2 breast tumors that were ER-positive, with results suggesting that tamoxifen reduces breast cancer incidence in BRCA2 carriers, but not in BRCA1 carriers, although the sample size was low. In contrast, another study showed that tamoxifen reduces the risk of contra-lateral breast cancer in women with BRCA1 or BRCA2 mutations [96]. Furthermore, studies have also shown that bilateral prophylactic oophorectomies also reduce the risk of breast cancer in BRCA1 or BRCA2 mutation carriers, indicating the efficacy of anti-hormonal intervention [97, 98].

It remains unknown whether tamoxifen can reduce the risk of breast cancer in BRCA1 mutation carriers. Preventive mastectomy and oophorectomy have also been shown to reduce subsequent breast cancer risk and should be considered potential options [99–107].

Girls and young women who have received mantle (mediastinal and/or axillary lymph node) radiotherapy for Hodgkin lymphoma are at significantly increased risk of developing breast cancer [108]. The risk of developing breast cancer is most pronounced in women treated during puberty (10 to 16 years). Among 1,380 children treated for Hodgkin lymphoma, the ratio of observed to expected breast cancer cases was 75-fold higher in women who received mantle radio-

therapy [108]. The actuarial cumulative probability of breast cancer was 35% at age 40 years. The increased risk of breast cancer is evident at 10 years following treatment, with further cases seen 15 years or more into follow-up. The long-term risk of developing breast cancer falls with increasing age at radiation exposure, demonstrating the predisposition to the development of breast cancer to be due to the exposure of mammary tissue to radiation during the pubertal growth phase. A reasonable recommendation for these patients is bi-annual mammographic screening beginning 8 years post-radiation until age 30 years and annually thereafter [109].

18.7.4 Psychosocial Issues

There are a variety of other psychosocial challenges for the young woman with breast cancer. Some of these are unique, as described below, and others are general to the age group, as described in other chapters in this book.

Younger women with breast cancer are likely to face unique concerns, and studies have shown them to be particularly vulnerable [110, 111]. In a retrospective study of 577 women aged 25 to 50 years when diagnosed to have breast cancer and disease-free for a mean of 6 years (range 2–10 years), their quality of life was, in general, inversely proportional to their age at diagnosis. The younger the patient, the worse the scores on emotional and social well being, vitality, and depression [111].

Young women frequently have concerns about the impact of the diagnosis on their partner and may have practical issues related to the care of young children during their treatment. Research suggests that peer support and self-help groups decrease feelings of social isolation, depression, and anxiety [112, 113]. Young age of onset of disease has been identified as a risk factor predicting adverse psychological outcomes, and very young women are especially vulnerable to psychological distress related to body image and sexuality. Loss of fertility may also be the source of psychological distress in young patients, with between 10 and 50% of women experiencing sexual problems following the diagnosis and treatment of breast cancer [114, 115]. Adjuvant chemotherapy and endocrine therapy may affect sexual response, and the induction of premature menopause may produce atrophic vaginitis. Physicians should be aware that these young patients have an increased risk of psychological problems and refer patients early for counseling.

18.8 Conclusions

Breast cancer is rare in adolescents and young women, with less than 1% of all breast cancer cases occurring before the age of 30 years. Invasive breast cancer in young women is more aggressive and associated with a worse prognosis than in older women. Breast cancers in young women are more often poorly differentiated, ER-negative, and have high proliferating fractions and lymphovascular invasion. Current evidence suggests that even when corrected for these risk factors, the prognosis is worse when the diagnosis occurs before age 40 years and especially before age 30 years.

Young women at high risk of developing breast cancer include those with germ-line mutations of BRCA1, BRCA2, Tp53, or PTEN, or patients who have previously received mantle irradiation for Hodgkin lymphoma. These women are candidates for screening and close follow-up from a young age.

Breast-conserving surgery in women <35 years old is associated with a higher risk of local recurrence than in older women. All young women should be considered at high risk by age alone and offered adjuvant therapy. The long-term toxicities of possible fertility impairment and premature menopause due to adjuvant therapies is a particular concern for these patients and require consideration when planning adjuvant chemo- and/or endocrine therapy. Adolescents and young women are particularly at risk from emotional and psychosocial problems and require appropriate support.

References

1. Bleyer WA, OLeary M, Barr R, Ries LAG (eds) (2006) Cancer Epidemiology in Older Adolescents and Young Adults 15 to 29 Years of Age, including SEER Incidence and Survival, 1975–2000. National Cancer Institute, NIH Pub. No. 06-5767, Bethesda MD; also available at www.seer.cancer.gov/publications

2. Surveillance Epidemiology, and End Results (SEER) Program Public–Use CD–ROM (1973–1997). National Cancer Institute, DCCPS, Cancer Surveillance Research Program, Cancer Statistics Branch, released April 2000, based on August 1999 submission

3. Bothroyd A, Carty H (1994) Breast masses in childhood and adolescence. Pediatr Radiol 24:81–85

4. Ferguson TB Jr, McCarty KS Jr, Filston HC (1987) Juvenile secretory carcinoma and juvenile papillomatosis: diagnosis and treatment. J Pediatr Surg 22:637–639

5. Rosen PP, Cranor ML (1991) Secretory carcinoma of the breast. Arch Pathol Lab Med 115:141–144

6. Serour F, Gilad A, Kopolovic J, Krispin M (1992) Secretory breast cancer in childhood and adolescence: report of a case and review of the literature. Med Pediatr Oncol 20:341–344

7. Adami HO, Malker B, Holmberg L, et al (1986) The relation between survival and age at diagnosis in breast cancer. N Engl J Med 315:559–563

8. Host H, Lund E (1986) Age as a prognostic factor in breast cancer. Cancer 57:2217–2221

9. De La Rochefordiere A, Asselain B, Campana F, et al (1993) Age as prognostic factor in premenopausal breast carcinoma. Lancet 341(8852):1039–1043

10. Walker RA, Lees E, Webb MB, Dearing SJ (1996) Breast carcinomas occurring in young women (< 35 years) are different. Br J Cancer 74:1796–800

11. Winchester DP, Osteen RT, Menck HR (1996) The National Cancer Data Base report on breast carcinoma characteristics and outcome in relation to age. Cancer 78:1838–1843

12. Kollias J, Elston CW, Ellis IO, et al (1997) Early-onset breast cancer: histopathological and prognostic consideration. Br J Cancer 75:1318–1323

13. Chung M, Chang HR, Bland KI, Wanebo HJ (1996) Younger women with breast carcinoma have a poorer prognosis than older women. Cancer 77:97–103

14. Swanson GM, Lin CS (1994) Survival patterns among younger women with breast cancer: the effects of age, race, stage, and treatment. J Natl Cancer Inst Monogr 16:69–77

15. Albain KS, Allred DC, Clark GM (1994) Breast cancer outcome and predictors of outcome: are there age differentials? J Natl Cancer Inst Monogr 16:35–42

16. Holli K, Isola J (1997) Effect of age on the survival of breast cancer patients. Eur J Cancer 33:425–428

17. Kroman N, Jensen MB, Wohlfahrt J, et al (2000) Factors influencing the effect of age on prognosis in breast cancer: population based study. BMJ 320(7233):474–478

18. Goldhirsch A, Glick JH, Gelber RD, et al (2001) Meeting highlights: International Consensus Panel on the Treatment of Primary Breast Cancer. Seventh International Conference on Adjuvant Therapy of Primary Breast Cancer. J Clin Oncol 19:3817–3827

19. Panel of the National Institutes of Health Consensus Development (2001) National Institutes of Health Consensus Development Conference Statement: Adjuvant Therapy for breast cancer, November 1–3, 2000. J Natl Cancer Inst 30:5–15

20. Schag CA, Ganz PA, Polinsky ML, et al (1993) Characteristics of women at risk for psychosocial distress in the year after breast cancer. J Clin Oncol 11:783–793

21. Bloom JR, Kessler L (1994) Risk and timing of counselling and support interventions for younger women with breast cancer. J Natl Cancer Inst Monogr 16:199–206

22. Roberts CS, Cox CE, Reintgen DS, et al (1994) Influence of physician communication on newly diagnosed breast patients' psychologic adjustment and decision-making. Cancer 74:336–341

23. Shavers VL, Harlan LC, Stevens JL (2003) Racial/Ethnic variations in clinical presentation, treatment and survival among breast cancer patients under 35. Cancer 97:134–147

24. Aebi S, De Ridder M, Vlastos G, et al (2006) Young age is a poor prognostic factor in women with stage I breast cancer Eur J Cancer Suppl 4:120

25. Ashley S, Royle GT, Corder A, et al (1989) Clinical, radiological and cytological diagnosis of breast cancer in young women. Br J Surg 76:835–837

26. Brand IR, Sapherson DA, Brown TS (1993) Breast imaging in women under 35 with symptomatic breast disease. Br J Radiol 66:394–397

27. Hochman MG, Orel SG, Powell CM, et al (1997) Fibroadenomas: MR imaging appearances with radiologic-histopathologic correlation. Radiology 204:123–129

28. Colleoni M, Rotmensz N, Robertson C, et al (2002) Very young women (<35 years) with operable breast cancer: features of disease at presentation. Ann Oncol 13:273–279

29. Nixon AJ, Neuberg D, Hayes DF, et al (1994) Relationship of patient age to pathologic features of the tumor and prognosis for patients with stage I or II breast cancer. J Clin Oncol 12:888–894

30. Dubsky PC, Gnant MF, Taucher S, et al (2002) Young age as an independent adverse prognostic factor in premenopausal patients with breast cancer. Clin Breast Cancer 3:65–72

31. Kothari AS, Beechey-Newman N, D'Arrigo C, et al (2002) Breast carcinoma in women age 25 years or less. Cancer 94:606–614

32. Xiong Q, Valero V, Kau V, et al (2001) Female patients with breast carcinoma age 30 years and younger have a poor prognosis: the M.D. Anderson Cancer Center experience. Cancer 92:2523–2528

33. Goldhirsch A, Gelber RD, Yothers G, et al (2001) Adjuvant therapy for very young women with breast cancer: need for tailored treatments. J Natl Cancer Inst Monogr 30:44–51

34. Aebi S, Gelber S, Castiglione-Gertsch M, et al (2000) Is chemotherapy alone adequate for young women with oestrogen-receptor-positive breast cancer? Lancet 355(9218):1869–1874

35. Shannon C, Smith IE (2003) Breast cancer in adolescents and young women. Eur J Cancer 39:2632–2642

36. Gonzalez-Angulo AM, Broglio K, Kau SW, et al (2005) Women age 35 years or younger with primary breast carcinoma: disease features at presentation. Cancer 103:2466–2472

37. Kurtz JM, Jacquemier J, Amalric R, et al (1990) Why are local recurrences after breast-conserving therapy more frequent in younger patients? J Clin Oncol 8:591–598

38. Arriagada R, Le MG, Contesso G, et al (2002) Predictive factors for local recurrence in 2006 patients with surgically resected small breast cancer. Ann Oncol 13:1404–1413

39. Voogd AC, Nielsen M, Peterse JL, et al (2001) Differences in risk factors for local and distant recurrence after breast-conserving therapy or mastectomy for stage I and II breast cancer: pooled results of two large European randomized trials. J Clin Oncol 19:1688–1697

40. Calle R, Vilcoq JR, Zafrani B, et al (1986) Local control and survival of breast cancer treated by limited surgery followed by irradiation. Int J Radiat Oncol Biol Phys 12:873–878

41. van Limbergen E, van den Bogaert W, van der Schueren E, Rijnders A (1987) Tumor excision and radiotherapy as primary treatment of breast cancer. Analysis of patient and treatment parameters and local control. Radiother Oncol 8:1–9

42. Kini VR, White JR, Horwitz EM, et al (1998) Long term results with breast-conserving therapy for patients with early stage breast carcinoma in a community hospital setting. Cancer 82:127–133

43. Voogd AC, Peterse JL, Crommelin MA, et al (1999) Histological determinants for different types of local recurrence after breast-conserving therapy of invasive breast cancer. Dutch Study Group on local Recurrence after Breast Conservation (BORST). Eur J Cancer 35:1828–1837

44. 43. Schnitt SJ, Connolly JL, Harris JR, et al (1984) Pathologic predictors of early local recurrence in Stage I and II breast cancer treated by primary radiation therapy. Cancer 53:1049–1057

45. Osteen RT, Connolly JL, Recht A, et al (1987) Identification of patients at high risk for local recurrence after conservative surgery and radiation therapy for stage I or II breast cancer. Arch Surg 122:1248–1252

46. Veronesi U, Marubini E, Del Vecchio M, et al (1995) Local recurrences and distant metastases after conservative breast cancer treatments: partly independent events. J Natl Cancer Inst 87:19–27

47. Fourquet A, Campana F, Zafrani B, et al (1989) Prognostic factors of breast recurrence in the conservative management of early breast cancer: a 25-year follow-up. Int J Radiat Oncol Biol Phys 17:719–725

48. Dewar JA, Arriagada R, Benhamou S, et al (1995) Local relapse and contralateral tumor rates in patients with breast cancer treated with conservative surgery and radiotherapy (Institut Gustave Roussy 1970–1982). IGR Breast Cancer Group. Cancer 76:2260–2265

49. Schnitt SJ, Abner A, Gelman R, et al (1994) The relationship between microscopic margins of resection and the risk of local recurrence in patients with breast cancer treated with breast-conserving surgery and radiation therapy. Cancer 74:1746–1751

50. Macmillan RD, Purushotham AD, Mallon E, et al (1997) Tumour bed positivity predicts outcome after breast-conserving surgery. Br J Surg 84:1559–1562

51. Early Breast Cancer Trialists' Collaborative Group (1998) Polychemotherapy for early breast cancer: an overview of the randomised trials. Early Breast Cancer Trialists' Collaborative Group. Lancet 352(9132):930–942

52. Early Breast Cancer Trialists' Collaborative Group (1998) Tamoxifen for early breast cancer: an overview of the randomised trials. Early Breast Cancer Trialists' Collaborative Group. Lancet 351(9114):1451–1467

53. Levine MN, Bramwell VH, Pritchard KI, et al (1998) Randomized trial of intensive cyclophosphamide, epirubicin, and fluorouracil chemotherapy compared with cyclophosphamide, methotrexate, and fluorouracil in premenopausal women with node-positive breast cancer. National Cancer Institute of Canada Clinical Trials Group. J Clin Oncol 16:2651–2658

54. Henderson IC, Berry DA, Demetri GD, et al (2003) Improved outcomes from adding sequential paclitaxel but not from escalating doxorubicin dose in an adjuvant chemotherapy regimen for patients with node-positive primary breast cancer. J Clin Oncol 21:976–983

55. Mamounas EP, Bryant J, Lembersky BC, et al (2005) Paclitaxel following doxorubicin/cyclophosphamide as adjuvant chemotherapy for node-positive breast cancer: Results from NSABP B-28. Proc Am Soc Clin Oncol 22:4 (abstract 12)

56. Nabholtz JM, Pienkowski T, Mackey J, et al (2002) Phase III trial comparing TAC (docetaxel, doxorubicin, cyclophosphamide) with FAC (5-fluorouracil, doxorubicin, cyclophosphamide) in the adjuvant treatment of node positive breast cancer patients: interim analysis of the BCIRG 001 study. Am Soc Clin Oncol 20:22a (abstract 141)

57. Citron M, Berry DA, Cirroncione C, et al (2003) Randomized trial of dose-dense versus conventionally scheduled and sequential versus concurrent combination chemotherapy as postoperative adjuvant treatment of node-positive primary breast cancer: First report of Intergroup trial C9741/Cancer and Leukemia Group B trial 9741. J Clin Oncol 21:1431–1439

58. Goldhirsch A, Gelber RD, Castiglione M (1990) The magnitude of endocrine effects of adjuvant chemotherapy for premenopausal breast cancer patients. The International Breast Cancer Study Group. Ann Oncol 1:183–188

59. Bianco AR, Del Mastro L, Gallo C, et al (1991) Prognostic role of amenorrhea induced by adjuvant chemotherapy in premenopausal patients with early breast cancer. Br J Cancer 63:799–803

60. Jonat W (2000) Zoladex versus CMF adjuvant therapy in pre/peri-menopausal breast cancer: tolerability and amenorrhea comparisons. Proc Am Soc Clin Oncol 19:87a (abstract 333)

61. Richards MA, O'Reilly SM, Howell A, et al (1990) Adjuvant cyclophosphamide, methotrexate, and fluorouracil in patients with axillary node-positive breast cancer: an update of the Guy's/Manchester trial. J Clin Oncol 8:2032–2039

62. Goodwin PJ, Ennis M, Pritchard KI, et al (1999) Risk of menopause during the first year after breast cancer diagnosis. J Clin Oncol 17:2365–2370

63. Boccardo F, Rubagotti A, Amoroso D, et al (2000) Cyclophosphamide, methotrexate, and fluorouracil versus tamoxifen plus ovarian suppression as adjuvant treatment of estrogen receptor-positive pre-/perimenopausal breast cancer patients: results of the Italian Breast Cancer Adjuvant Study Group 02 randomized trial. J Clin Oncol 18:2718–2727

64. Jakesz R, Hausmaninger H, Kubista E, et al (2002) Randomized adjuvant trial of tamoxifen and goserelin versus cyclophosphamide, methotrexate, and fluorouracil: evidence for the superiority of treatment with endocrine blockade in premenopausal patients with hormone-responsive breast cancer – Austrian Breast and Colorectal Cancer Study Group Trial 5. J Clin Oncol 20:4621–4627

65. Jonat W, Kaufmann M, Sauerbrei W, et al (2002) Goserelin versus cyclophosphamide, methotrexate, and fluorouracil as adjuvant therapy in premenopausal patients with node-positive breast cancer: The Zoladex Early Breast Cancer Research Association Study. J Clin Oncol 20:4628–4635

66. Davidson NE, O'Neill A, Vukov A, et al (1999) Effect of chemohormonal therapy in premenopausal, node + , receptor + breast cancer: an Eastern Cooperative Oncology Group phase III intergroup trial (E5188, INT-0101). Proc Am Soc Clin Oncol 18:249a (abstract 67)

67. Bines J, Oleske D, Cobleigh M (1996) Ovarian function in premenopausal women treated with adjuvant chemotherapy for breast cancer. J Clin Oncol 14:1718–1729

68. Meirow D (1999) Ovarian injury and modern options to preserve fertility in female cancer patients treated with high dose radio-chemotherapy for hemato-oncological neoplasias and other cancers. Leuk Lymph 33:65–76

69. Lower E, Blau R, Gazder P, Tummala R (1999) The risk of premature menopause induced by chemotherapy for

early breast cancer. J Womens Health Gen Based Med 8:949–954

70. Del Mastro L, Venturini M, Sertoli MR, Rosso R (1997) Amenorrhea induced by adjuvant chemotherapy in early breast cancer patients: prognostic role and clinical implications. Breast Cancer Res Treat 43:183–190

71. Fox K, Ball JE, Mick R, Moor HCF (2001) Prevention of chemotherapy-associated amenorrhoea with Leupro-lide in young women with early-stage breast cancer. Proc Am Soc Clin Oncol 20:25a (abstract 98)

72. Recchia F, Sica G, De Filippis S, et al (2002) Goserelin as ovarian protection in the adjuvant treatment of pre-menopausal breast cancer: a phase II pilot study. Anti-cancer Drugs 13:417–424

73. Lishner M (2003) Cancer in pregnancy. Ann Oncol 14:31–36

74. Anderson BO, Petrek JA, Byrd DR, et al (1996) Preg-nancy influences breast cancer stage at diagnosis in women 30 years of age and younger. Ann Surg Oncol 3:204–211

75. Zemlickis D, Lishner M, Degendorfer P, et al (1992) Maternal and fetal outcome after breast cancer in preg-nancy. Am J Obstet Gynecol 166:781–787

76. Clark RM, Reid, J (1978) Carcinoma of the breast in pregnancy and lactation. Int J Radiat Oncol Biol Phys 4:693–698

77. Bonnier P, Romain S, Dilhuydy JM (1997) Influence of pregnancy on the outcome of breast cancer: a case-con-trol study. Int J Cancer 72:751–755

78. Petrek J (1994) Breast cancer during pregnancy. Cancer 74:518–527

79. Doll D (1989) Antineoplastic agents and pregnancy. Semin Oncol 16:337–346

80. Tretli S, Kvalheim G, Thoreson S, Host H (1988) Sur-vival of breast cancer patients diagnosed during preg-nancy and lactation. Br J Cancer 58:382–384

81. Difronzo LA, O'Connell TX (1996) Breast cancer in pregnancy and lactation. Surg Clin North Am 76:267–278

82. Kroman N, Mouridsen HT (2003) Prognostic influence of pregnancy before, around and after diagnosis of breast cancer. Breast 12:516–521

83. Li FP, Fraumeni JF Jr (1969) Soft-tissue sarcomas, breast cancer, and other neoplasms. A familial syndrome? Ann Intern Med 71:747–752

84. Nelen MR, Padberg GW, Peeters EA, et al (1996) Local-ization of the gene for Cowden disease to chromosome 10q22-23. Nat Genet 13:114–116

85. Miller A (1997) Screening by breast self examination. In: Jatoi I (ed) Breast Cancer Screening. Springer, Ber-lin

86. Burke W, Daly M, Garber J, et al (1997) Recommenda-tions for follow-up care of individuals with an inherited predisposition to cancer. II. BRCA1 and BRCA2. Can-cer Genetics Studies Consortium. JAMA 277:997–1003

87. Brekelmans CT, Seynaeve C, Bartels CC, et al (2001) Effectiveness of breast cancer surveillance in BRCA1/2 gene mutation carriers and women with high familial risk. J Clin Oncol 19:924–930

88. Scheuer L, Kauff N, Robson M, et al (2002) Outcome of preventive surgery and screening for breast and ovarian cancer in BRCA mutation carriers. J Clin Oncol 20:1260–1268

89. Stoutjesdijk MJ, Boetes C, Jager GJ, et al (2001) Mag-netic resonance imaging and mammography in women with a hereditary risk of breast cancer. J Natl Cancer Inst 93:1095–1102

90. Warner E, Plewes DB, Shumak RS, et al (2001) Com-parison of breast magnetic resonance imaging, mam-mography, and ultrasound for surveillance of women at high risk for hereditary breast cancer. J Clin Oncol 19:3524–3531

91. Warner E, Plewes DB, Hill KA, et al (2004) Surveillance of BRCA1 and BRCA2 mutation carriers with magnetic resonance imaging, ultrasound, mammography, and clinical breast examination. JAMA 292:1317–1325

92. Kriege M, Brekelmans CT, Boetes C, et al (2004) Effi-cacy of MRI and mammography for breast-cancer screening in women with a familial or genetic predis-position. N Engl J Med 351:427–437

93. Fisher B, Costantino JP, Wickerham DL, et al (1998) Tamoxifen for prevention of breast cancer: report of the National Surgical Adjuvant Breast and Bowel Project P-1 Study. J Natl Cancer Inst 90:1371–1388

94. Chlebowski RT, Col N, Winer EP, et al (2002) American society of clinical oncology technology assessment of pharmacologic interventions for breast cancer risk reduction including tamoxifen, raloxifene, and aroma-tase inhibition. J Clin Oncol 20:3328–3343

95. King MC, Wieand S, Hale K, et al (2001) Tamoxifen and breast cancer incidence among women with inherited mutations in BRCA1 and BRCA2: National Surgical Adjuvant Breast and Bowel Project (NSABP-P1) Breast Cancer Prevention Trial. JAMA 286:2251–2256

96. Narod SA, Brunet JS, Ghadirian P, et al (2000) Tamoxi-fen and risk of contralateral breast cancer in BRCA1 and BRCA2 mutation carriers: a case-control study. Hereditary Breast Cancer Clinical Study Group. Lancet 356:1876–1881

97. Kauff ND, Satagopan JM, Robson ME, et al (2002) Risk-reducing salpingo-oophorectomy in women with a BRCA1 or BRCA2 mutation. N Engl J Med 346:1609–1615

98. Rebbeck TR, Lynch HT, Neuhausen SL, et al (2002) Prophylactic oophorectomy in carriers of BRCA1 or BRCA2 mutations. N Engl J Med 346:1616–1622

99. Hartmann LC, Schaid DJ, Woods JE, et al (1999) Effi-cacy of bilateral prophylactic mastectomy in women with a family history of breast cancer. N Engl J Med 340:77–84

100. Hartmann LC, Sellers TA, Schaid DJ, et al (2001) Efficacy of bilateral prophylactic mastectomy in BRCA1 and BRCA2 gene mutation carriers. JNCI Cancer Spectrum 93:1633–1637

101. Meijers-Heijboer H, van Geel B, van Putten WL, et al (2001) Breast cancer after prophylactic bilateral mastectomy in women with a BRCA1 or BRCA2 mutation. N Engl J Med 345:159–164

102. Rebbeck TR, Friebel T, Lynch HT, et al (2004) Bilateral prophylactic mastectomy reduces breast cancer risk in BRCA1 and BRCA2 mutation carriers: the PROSE Study Group. J Clin Oncol 22:1055–1062

103. Parazzini F, Braga C, La Vecchia C, et al (1997) Hysterectomy, oophorectomy in premenopause, and risk of breast cancer. Obstet Gynecol 90:453–456

104. Schairer C, Persson I, Falkeborn M, et al (1997) Breast cancer risk associated with gynecologic surgery and indications for such surgery. Int J Cancer 70:150–154

105. Meijer WJ, van Lindert AC (1992) Prophylactic oophorectomy. Eur J Obstet Gynecol Reprod Biol 47:59–65

106. Struewing JP, Watson P, Easton DF, et al (1995) Prophylactic oophorectomy in inherited breast/ovarian cancer families. J Natl Cancer Inst Monogr 17:33–35

107. Rebbeck TR, Levin AM, Eisen A, et al (1999) Breast cancer risk after bilateral prophylactic oophorectomy in BRCA1 mutation carriers. J Natl Cancer Inst 91:1475–1479

108. Bhatia S, Robison LL, Oberlin O, et al (1996) Breast cancer and other second neoplasms after childhood Hodgkin disease. N Engl J Med 334:745–751

109. Diller L, Medeiros Nancarrow C, Shaffer K, et al (2002) Breast cancer screening in women previously treated for Hodgkin disease: a prospective cohort study. J Clin Oncol 20:2085–2091

110. Northouse LL (1994) Breast cancer in younger women: effects on interpersonal and family relations. J Natl Cancer Inst Monogr 16:183–190

111. Ganz PA, Greendale GA, Peterson L, et al (2003) Breast cancer in younger women: reproductive and late health effects of treatment. J Clin Oncol 21:4184–4193

112. Farash J (1979) Effect of counselling on resolution of loss and body image following a mastectomy. Dissertation Abstracts International 39:4027B

113. Van den Borne H, Pruyn J, Van den Heuvel WJ (1987) Effects of contracts between cancer patients on their psychosocial problems. Patient Educ Couns 1:33–51

114. Partridge AH, Gelber S, Peppercorn J, et al (2004) Web-based survey of fertility issues in young women with breast cancer. J Clin Oncol 22:4174–4183

115. Schain WS, d'Angelo TM, Dunn ME, et al (1994) Mastectomy versus conservative surgery and radiation therapy. Psychosocial consequences. Cancer 73:1221–1228

Liver Tumors

Marcio H. Malogolowkin •
Arthur Zimmermann • Jack Plaschkes

Contents

19.1 Introduction

Primary neoplasms of the liver are rare in adolescents and young adults aged 15–29 years, accounting for only 1% of all neoplasms [1]. This is similar to the 1.1% incidence seen in individuals 0–14 years of age. Hepatoblastomas (HBLs) comprise over two-thirds of the malignant liver tumors in children, while hepatocellular carcinomas (HCCs) are the most common liver tumor seen in adolescents and young adults as well as in older adults.

In attempting to focus on cancer of adolescents and young adults aged 15–29 years, one finds oneself in as yet largely uncharted waters. On the more firm land on one side of the waters are the classical embryonal tumors occurring almost exclusively in children, and on the other, the carcinomas found invariably in adults.

Specifically for liver tumors, the two sides are represented by HBL in children and HCC in adults. Only rarely do both these tumors occur in adolescents or young adults. However, very little evidence-based information about the biology, epidemiology, treatment, and outcome of these rare events is available. Does HBL occurring outside the usual age peak of 3 years respond to the same treatment, and is the outcome as good? Is HCC in children, adolescents, and young adults similar in all respects to those seen in older adults, or are there relevant differences?

This chapter will review briefly the incidence, outcomes, etiology, and pathology of the liver tumors in adolescents and young adults. In an attempt to address the aforementioned questions, we will focus on HCC, and highlight the similarities and differences between this tumor in adolescents, young adults, and older adults. It is also the aim of this chapter to give directions for future research in this gray area.

19.2 Epidemiology

19.2.1 Incidence

The estimated incidence of liver and intrahepatic bile duct tumors increases with age from 2.0 per million in individuals 15–19 years of age to 14.6 per million for those 25–29 years of age (Table 19.1). According to the Surveillance, Epidemiology, and End Results (SEER) data, 404 adolescents and young adults in the United States were diagnosed with these tumors in the year 2000.

According to the SEER data collected between 1975 and 1998, a total of 9,300 individuals 15–29 years of age were diagnosed with liver tumors in the United States. Although these data include both liver and intrahepatic bile duct tumors, the occurrence of the latter tumors in individuals less than 29 years of age is extremely rare. The incidence of liver tumors is relatively constant between 5 and 35 years of age, but then it increases steadily with age (Fig. 19.1). The incidences of liver and intrahepatic bile duct tumors have increased progressively between 1975 and 2000; however, this increase is more pronounced in patients older than 45 years of age (Fig. 19.2). The male to female incidence ratio for liver tumors is close to 1.1 for individuals 15–29 years of age. However, this ratio steadily increases after 30 years of age, with a predominance of males being diagnosed with these tumors (Fig. 19.3).

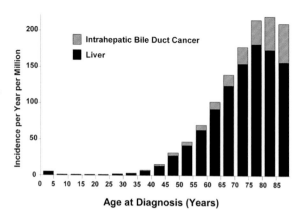

Figure 19.1

Relative incidence of liver (*solid bars*) and intrahepatic bile duct cancer (*hatched bars*) by age at diagnosis. United States SEER [1]

Liver tumors are more prevalent among Asians/Pacific Islanders, followed by African Americans when compared with whites and Hispanics in the USA.

Bosch et al., utilizing population-based cancer registries and the World Health Organization (WHO) mortality data bank, reported the incidence and mortality of liver cancers worldwide [2]. With an estimated 437,000 new cases in 1990, liver cancers rank fifth in frequency in the world, accounting for 5.4% of all human cancer cases. Liver cancer corresponds to 7.4% of all cancer cases among men and 3.2% of all cancers among women. The largest estimated concentrations of liver cancer cases are located in Eastern Asia (China, Hong Kong, Korea, Mongolia, and Japan), Middle

Table 19.1 Incidence, incidence trends, and number of new diagnoses of liver cancer; United States Surveillance, Epidemiology, and End Results (SEER)

Age at diagnosis (years)	15–19	20–24	25–29
United States population (in millions), year 2000 census	19.90	18.70	17.63
Average incidence, 1975–2000, per million	2.0	5.6	14.6
Average annual increase, 1975–2000, SEER	0	1.8	2.6
No. persons diagnosed with liver and intrahepatic bile duct cancer, year 2000, United States	41	105	258

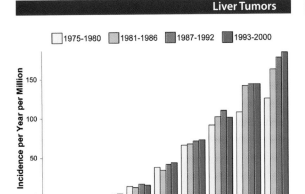

Figure 19.2

Incidence of liver and intrahepatic bile duct cancer by era and age in patients diagnosed before age 40 years. United States SEER [1]

Figure 19.3

Incidence of liver and intrahepatic bile duct cancer by gender, in patients diagnosed before age 40 years. United States SEER 1975–2000 [1]

Africa (Cameroon, Chad, Congo, and Equatorial Guinea), and in some Western African countries (Gambia, Guinea, Mali, and Senegal) [3]. The lowest concentration of liver cancer is seen in Northern Europe, Australia, New Zealand, and among the Caucasian populations in North and Latin America [3].

The data given above, although comprehensive, detailed, and useful for health-care planning, have one serious weakness as far as scientific value is concerned: these do not discriminate between wide ranges of clinically and histologically disparate tumors, including biliary carcinoma, which rarely occurs in adolescents and young adults. Even when only the strictly epithelial tumors (HBL and HCC) are considered together, the conclusions of such studies can hardly be considered relevant for HCC. For instance, in the past, since HCC is so rare in children and adolescents, these patients have consistently been treated according to the same prospective trials developed for children with HBL or according to adult guidelines.

The European Automated Childhood Cancer Information System data, based in France, which collects data from National Cancer Registries in Europe, has similar and other weaknesses, particularly since there is no standard method of collecting data from tumor registries in the various European countries.

The International Society of Pediatric Oncology (SIOPEL) studies have registered more than 685 cases of HBL and 119 of cases of HCC on the last 2 trials conducted during their 14 years of existence. Despite the fact that the incidence data in these international trials are not population based, they have provided important information on prognosis and survival of children and adolescents with these tumors.

19.3 Risk Factors and Etiology

HCCs appear to result from complications of previous hepatic damage due to metabolic or inflammatory disorders. Chronic infection with hepatitis B virus is the leading cause of HCC in children, adolescents, and young adults in Asia and Africa. However, in the Western countries, less than one-third of the adolescent or young adult patients diagnosed with HCC have an identifying cause such as hepatitis or other inflammatory liver disease [4, 5]. This is in marked contrast to older adults, in whom almost 90% of the cases are cirrhosis related, secondary to viral infection or alcohol consumption [6]. The prevention of a carrier state in children by a universal program of hepatitis B immunization has shown a dramatic decrease in the prevalence of chronic hepatitis B virus, and a decline in the rates of HCC in Taiwan among children less then 15 years of age [7].

Less frequently, HCC is associated with congenital diseases such as hereditary tryosinemia, biliary cirrhosis, glycogen storage disease, and alpha 1-antitrypsin deficiency [8–11]. Prolonged exposure to anabolic steroids, toxin-contaminated foods (aflatoxin), and potential hepatic carcinogens (pesticides, vinyl chloride, Thorotrast) have also been associated with the development of HCC [12–14].

19.4 Pathology and Biology

The four most common liver lesions in adolescents and young adults are reviewed below.

19.4.1 Hepatocellular Carcinoma, Adult Type

The pathologic features of HCCs are well established. HCCs are often multinodular and extensively invasive, and usually show hemorrhage, necrosis, and vascular invasion (Fig. 19.4). The main biological and patho-

logical features have been reviewed recently [15, 16], and to date, no differences have been recognized among children, adolescents, and adults in the biology and pathology of typical HCC and its variants. A systematic analysis of the significance of histopathologic risk factors identified in adult HCC patients [17] has yet to be performed in adolescents and young adults.

19.4.2 Fibrolamellar HCC

Fibrolamellar HCC (FL-HCC) occurs most often in young individuals. It is characterized by a single expanding mass with typical histological features consisting of large eosinophilic cells embedded in a copious collagen-rich stroma (Fig. 19.5) [18–20]. A clear-cell variant of FL-HCC exists [21]. The neoplasm has distinct immunohistochemical features [22], including reactivity for cytokeratin 7 [23]. FL-HCC accounts for about 30% of HCC in patients younger than 20 years of age. Typically, FL-HCC develops without underlying cirrhosis, viral infection, or metabolic disorders. The relationship between HCC and FL-HCC is not clear, although both lesions may occur in close association [24]. Alpha-fetoprotein (AFP) is frequently

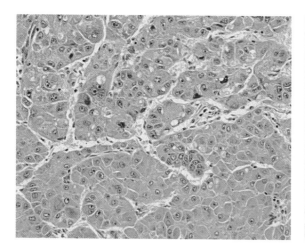

Figure 19.4

Hepatocellular carcinoma, trabecular type: thick plates without typical intervening sinusoids

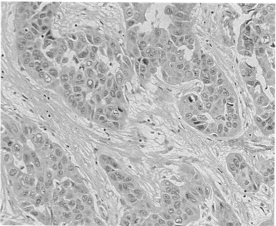

Figure 19.5

Fibrolamellar carcinoma: solid nests of large and eosinophilic cells are embedded in a collagen-rich stroma forming fibrolamellar structures

within normal levels, however these may be associated high serum vitamin B12 and transcobalamin I [25–28], elevated serum neurotensin [29], and expression of aromatase causing gynecomastia [30]. Whereas DNA fingerprinting has revealed genomic homogeneity of FL-HCC [31], there are striking differences in cytogenetic aberrations in primary FL-HCC and recurrent FL-HCC, probably caused by increasing genetic instability [32].

19.4.3 Transitional Liver Cell Tumor

Recently, a novel subset of liver cell tumors developing in older children and young adolescents has been recognized [33]. Among the first seven tumors described, six had initially been diagnosed as HBL. However, these hepatocellular lesions exhibit, for the age group involved, an unusual phenotype with respect to clinical presentation, pathology, and treatment response. Specifically, these tumors show a highly aggressive behavior, and reveal histology intermediate between HBL and HCC (Fig. 19.6). Immunohistochemically, all tumors analyzed so far were AFP-positive, and more than half disclosed nuclear reactivity for beta-

catenin, indicating mutations of the respective gene [33]. Based on the hypothesis that these tumors may reflect growth of a cell type situated between hepatoblasts and hepatocytes, the term "transitional liver cell tumor" was coined as a working formulation.

19.4.4 Hepatoblastoma

HBL is rare in adolescence and adulthood [34]. The pathology of HBL is the same in young and older subjects, and the criteria for histologic diagnosis have been reviewed recently (Fig. 19.7) [35]. HBL is associated with distinct cytogenetic aberrations and, in about 50%, genetic anomalies of the Wnt/beta-catenin signaling pathway have been detected [36]. Histogenetic aspects of HBL have been discussed [37]. There are intriguing situations whereby HCC occurs in combination with HBL [38], or HCC recurring as HBL [39], suggesting a possible at filiation. However, the carcinogenic pathways of HCC and HBL are different. HCCs show multiple chromosomal aberrations (mainly losses), whereas HBLs exhibit a low number of chromosomal changes [34, 36]. In contrast to HCC, p53 gene (and related genes) mutations are almost lacking

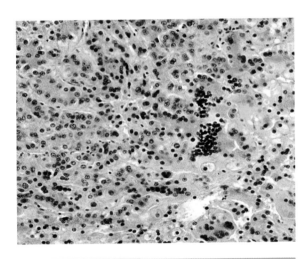

Figure 19.6

Transitional cell liver tumor: cells forming this neoplasm are morphologically situated between hepatoblasts and hepatocytes. Few multinuclear giant cells are seen

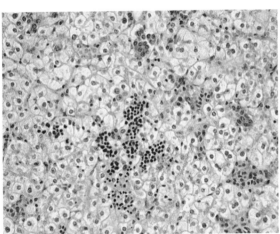

Figure 19.7

Hepatoblastoma, fetal morphology type: most of the tumor cells exhibit a clear cytoplasm. Extramedullary hemopoiesis is present

in HBL, and p53 protein overexpression is seen infrequently [15, 40–43]. Anecdotal survival information about 12 patients older then 12 years of age treated in the SIOPEL studies appears to be worse than for those in the younger age group.

19.5 Genetic and Molecular Mechanisms of Hepatocarcinogenesis

Recent publications have summarized the vast data now available on the genetic and molecular pathogenesis of human HCCs [36, 44, 45]. Briefly, the development of HCC is a slow, multistep process that is associated with changes in genomic expression that lead to alterations of the hepatocellular phenotype and the appearance and progression of a tumor. The development of HCC may take many years, and starts in the setting of chronic hepatitis or cirrhosis, with destruction of hepatocytes and inflammatory changes that alter the matrix and the microenvironment of the liver.

During the long pre-neoplastic stage (10–30 years), phenotypically altered hepatocytes appear. These abnormal hepatocytes frequently present quantitative changes in gene expression, such as elevation of expression of transforming growth factor-α and insulin-like growth factor-2, and functional inactivation of tumor-suppressor genes, like p53 and Rb, leading to the accelerated proliferation of hepatocytes. This leads to the production of monoclonal populations of aberrant and dysplastic hepatocytes that have telomerase erosion, microsatellite instabilities, and occasional structural aberrations in genes and chromosomes. The accumulation of these irreversible structural alterations continues through the development of dysplastic foci and nodules, and the emergence of HCC. The genetic changes observed in different HCC nodules are frequently distinct, suggesting heterogeneity in that the malignant hepatocyte phenotype is produced by the disruption of genes that function in different regulatory pathways, producing several molecular variants of HCCs.

Understanding the molecular pathogenesis of HCCs may provide us with clues about the critical regulatory pathways involved in tumor development, and create new opportunities for therapeutic intervention by either delaying the development of the mono-clonal dysplastic hepatocyte population or by interfering in the progression and metastatic spread of established HCCs.

19.6 Clinical Presentation and Diagnosis

The symptoms associated with HCC are usually of short duration, and most often patients present with an enlargement of the abdomen and an associated palpable right upper quadrant mass. Anorexia, weight loss, and abdominal pain are frequently seen in association with advanced disease. Rarely, it may present as an acute abdominal crisis secondary to tumor rupture. Jaundice, vomiting, fever, and pallor are rare. On physical examination, hepatomegaly is common, and a palpable hard mass is frequently found. If the tumor is associated with pre-existing inflammatory or metabolic diseases of the liver, signs associated with cirrhosis of the liver can be found, including splenomegaly and spider angiomata. Most frequently there is extensive involvement of the liver by the tumor, and often the tumor is multifocal in origin. The presence of ascites may suggest intra-abdominal extension, and at least one-third of patients present with metastatic involvement, with the lungs being the most common site of disease.

Mild normochromic-normocytic anemia can be seen, as well as thrombocytosis and occasionally polycythemia secondary to extrarenal secretion of erythropoietin. Hepatic enzymes can be elevated, however elevation of bilirubin is infrequent unless it is associated with cirrhosis of the liver.

AFP is the most valuable laboratory test for diagnosis and monitoring of hepatic tumors. AFP is a normal globulin that is present during fetal life, and is synthesized in the liver and fetal yolk sac. Elevated levels of AFP are seen during the newborn period, and adult levels are reached by about 1 year of age. The biologic half-life of AFP is 5–7 days. The level of AFP at diagnosis has been shown to be of prognostic value, and it can be utilized to monitor response to therapy and disease recurrence in HBLs [46]. AFP levels, however, can be normal in at least 30–50% of the patients with HCC. Lectin-affinity immunoelectrophoresis can differentiate AFP derived from malignant liver tumors from that derived from benign inflammatory or regenerative hepatic disease [47]. Levels of carcinoembryonic antigen and ferritin can also been increased in HCC [48]. The fibrolamellar variant of HCC can be associated with an abnormality of the vitamin B12 binding protein, which can occasionally be used to monitor disease status and response to therapy [25, 48]. Screening for viral hepatitis (B and C) should be performed in all patients.

Plain radiographs of the abdomen frequently demonstrate the presence of a right upper quadrant mass, and calcifications may be noted in approximately 6% of the malignant tumors [49]. Ultrasonography is a reliable and non-invasive imaging technique for establishing the presence of an intrahepatic mass. It aids in differentiating solid from cystic masses, and in determining the presence and extent of vascular invasion [50, 51]. Computed tomography (CT) scanning (including the chest) is the most commonly used imaging study to determine both local and distant extent of tumor involvement. Features like the presence of multiple lesions and portal hypertension may suggest the diagnosis of HCC [52, 53]. Due to the multiplanar nature of magnetic resonance imaging (MRI), this technique is rapidly replacing CT scan as a predictor of tumor resectability [54].

Arteriography has been used to help surgeons map the liver vasculature in planning for surgery; however, MRI/magnetic resonance angiography is being used increasingly for this purpose. Although gallium scan is used infrequently in the diagnosis of liver tumors, it may add in distinguishing between regenerating nodules of cirrhosis and tumors, since the regenerating nodules are usally gallium negative.

19.6.1 Differential Diagnosis

Some other liver tumors (non HBL and non HCC) that can occur in this age group should be considered in the differential diagnosis, and are discussed below:

19.6.1.1 Embryonal (Undifferentiated) Sarcoma of the Liver

This is a specific, well-described [55] but rare tumor which, although not to be confused with rhabdomyosarcoma, generally responds to the types of chemotherapy used in the treatment of that disease. It occurs mostly in older children and adolescents; 25% occur between the age of 11 and 20 years and 6% between 16 and 20 years. The tumor presents mainly as a large solitary mass often preceded by rather non-specific abdominal symptoms. Liver function is usually not compromised.

The imaging can be confusing in that, on ultrasound it appears solid, but on CT and MRI may show cystic elements even so far as to be misinterpreted as a solitary cyst [56]. Therefore histological diagnosis is essential and can show some specific (i.e., "polygonal") cells).

There is no standard treatment protocol and initially this tumor was considered to be highly malignant with a poor prognosis. This opinion has of late been revised, especially since the advent of pre-operative chemotherapy [57]. Most tumors respond very well to rhabdomyosarcoma-like therapy (i.e., VAC regimen with vincristine, actinomycin and cyclophosphamide) and to agents like doxorubicin, and cisplatin. When these tumors are resected completely the prognosis is relatively good [56]. With this approach in some personal experience, even some ruptured tumors are curable [58].

19.6.1.2 Angiosarcoma and Cholangiocarcinoma

These tumors rarely occur in this age group, except when associated with a predisposing disease such as biliary atresia. However, they should be considered as part of the differential diagnosis.

19.6.1.3 Benign Tumors

Focal Nodular Hyperplasia and Liver Cell Adenoma

These are essentially tumors of adults that are found most commonly in women taking oval contraceptives, but occasionally also occur in the age group under consideration here, although with no known hormonal etiology. In the Armed Forces Institute of Pathology Monograph (1977–1999), 20% of the total of the benign liver tumors seen in patients aged between 11 and 15 years were focal nodular hyperplasia (FNH).

Focal Nodular Hyperplasia

FNH often presents as an asymptomatic mass in the liver, which can mimic a well-differentiated carcinoma. However, there is usually a very specific scar-like lesion in the center, which differentiates it on imaging from this and from liver cell adenoma and other benign lesions [59]. In children it has been associated with other disorders such a sickle cell disease, vascular malformations, and limb hyperplasia [60]. It has also been described in children who have undergone treatment for solid tumors [61].

Liver Cell Adenoma

Liver adenomas have a bimodal distribution, occurring within the 1st year of life and then again over the age of 5 years. Liver adenomas can be quite large and present with abdominal symptoms, like distension and pain, and their growth is unpredictable.

Obviously, for benign lesions, the only possible treatment apart from the "watch, wait, and see" approach, is surgical excision. There are no hard and fast rules about which is best; the various guidelines are very flexible and the results of both approaches acceptable [62]. Basically, symptomatic lesions should be excised if feasible without too great a risk. None of these lesions poses a realistic risk of malignancy so that the "watch, wait, and see" approach with regular imaging and follow-up is quite appropriate.

19.6.2 Tumor Staging

Tumor staging is used to determine prognosis and in planning therapy. Since children and adolescents with HCC have been treated according to therapeutic trials for HBL, the staging classifications used by the pediatric groups are very different than those used by the adult oncology groups. In North America the most widely used staging system is based on the extent of tumor and surgical resectability [62–65]. The International Society of Pediatric Oncology (SIOP), however, has developed a pre-operative staging system (Pretreatment Extent of Disease System – PRETEXT; Fig. 19.8. PRETEXT relies on radiological staging using the main veins and bile ducts to identify the number of liver sec-

tors involved by the tumor [66, 67]. Since more than 70% of HCC in adults develop in cirrhotic livers, the conventional pre-treatment TNM staging system is clinically inadequate because it does not take in to consideration parameters of hepatic function. Instead, current staging systems used in adult liver cancer trials, such as the CLIP (Cancer of the Liver Italian Program) [68], the BCLC (Barcelona Cancer of the Liver Committee) [69], the CUPI (Chinese University Prognostic Index score) [70] and the Japanese Okemah system [71], incorporate the extent of disease and liver function, as determined by the Child's-Pugh system [72], to determine risk groups and for treatment planning.

In contrast, since adolescents and young adults frequently develop HCC without pre-existing cirrhosis, it would seem appropriate to use a system least depen-

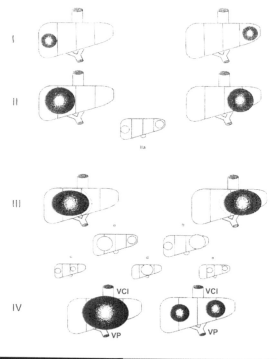

Figure 19.8

Pretreatment Extent of Disease System (PRETEXT) of the International Society of Pediatric Oncology (SIOP). *VCI* Inferior vena cava, *VP* portal vein

dent on the functional state of the liver, such as the TNM or PRETEXT system.

19.7 Treatment and Outcomes

Children and adolescents with HCC have up to now usually been treated according to clinical trials designed for the treatment of childhood HBL, and less commonly according to adult guidelines. Since these strategies are so different, they will be discussed separately in this chapter.

Complete tumor resection is the cornerstone of therapy for liver tumors and offers the only realistic chance of long-term disease-free survival [4, 5, 67, 73]. New surgical techniques and careful patient management during and after surgery have minimized the risks associated with liver resection and improved resection rates.

HCCs most often present as multi-focal tumors with vascular invasion and frequent metastases at diagnosis, making complete surgical excision almost impossible [5, 74]. Total hepatectomy followed by liver transplantation has been used successfully as an alternate surgical approach for un-resectable liver tumors. The use of liver transplant for the treatment of childhood HBL has been associated with satisfactory results [75–77]; however, the experience is still limited for the treatment of patients with HCC.

19.7.1 Adults with HCC

Worldwide HCC represents the third largest cause of cancer-related death. Since the main risk factor for HCC is liver cirrhosis caused by alcohol consumption and/or chronic infection by hepatitis B or C, primary prevention through vaccination (hepatitis B), implementation of adequate health standards, and antiviral treatment to prevent progression to cirrhosis (hepatitis C) may be the only effective ways to change this outcome. As discussed previously, a universal program of hepatitis B immunization has resulted in a decrease in hepatitis-B-virus-related HCC [7, 78]; however, no therapy has been demonstrated to be efficacious once cirrhosis develops. Therefore, surveillance aimed at early detection of the tumor and implementation of

effective therapy is the only option to diminish tumor-related mortality. The European Association for the Study of the Liver recommends that patients with cirrhosis who could undergo potentially curative treatment for HCC should have surveillance ultrasonography and serum AFP measurements made every 6 months [79].

The choice of treatment for adults with HCC has been based on the extent of disease and liver function. Treatment strategies can be divided in three groups: (1) patients with localized disease (early stage); (2) patients with advanced disease as determined by extensive hepatic involvement, vascular invasion, or presence of extrahepatic disease; and (3) patients with significant liver dysfunction (Child's-Pugh class C).

Treatment for patients with localized disease (i.e., with a single nodule <5 cm or with ≤3 nodules that are less then 3 cm in size) should be with curative intent since their 5-year survival rate may exceed 70% [80, 81]. Curative treatments, such as resection, liver transplantation, and percutaneous ablation have been associated with a high rate of tumor response and survival.

Resection is the treatment of choice for non-cirrhotic patients, but should be used with caution for cirrhotic patients to prevent post-operative liver failure. Optimal candidates are those without relevant portal hypertension and normal bilirubin levels [82]. Liver transplant is regarded as the ideal therapy because it theoretically cures both the tumor as well as the underlying liver disease [82–85]. However, this treatment is not readily available worldwide. In Western countries the shortage of cadaveric donors impacts negatively on the usefulness of transplantation [82, 86]. While adjuvant therapies have been used to prevent tumor progression while patients are on the waiting list, the benefit of these therapies have yet to be confirmed by randomized studies. The lack of sufficient cadaveric donors has prompted the use of living donor liver transplantation as a feasible alternative [87–89].

Percutaneous tumor ablation refers to the destruction of tumor cells by the intra-tumoral injection of chemical substances (ethanol, acetic acid, hot saline) or by modifying the temperature of tumor cells (radio-frequency, microwave, laser, and cryo-ablation) [90–96]. Percutaneous ethanol injection (PEI) is the most widely used method, and is well tolerated and of low cost. Patients in Child's-Pugh A treated with PEI have a 5-year survival rate of 50%. Radio-frequency ablation is now the second option. Some studies suggest that radio-frequency ablation is as efficacious as PEI, and requires fewer treatment sessions. However, it is associated with a higher number of severe side effects. Other techniques are either associated with increased complications or are still experimental.

Treatment for patients with advanced disease (multinodular tumors, vascular invasion, or presence of extra-hepatic disease) is generally considered palliative, since they are not aimed to cure but to control disease progression and prolong survival. Multiple approaches to palliation have been used for these patients, including arterial embolization with or without chemotherapy (chemo-embolization), systemic chemotherapy, hormonal therapy, internal radiation with ^{131}I lipiodol, immunotherapy, and others.

Arterial embolization with or without chemotherapy has been the most widely used treatment for these patients. Objective responses have been achieved in 15–55% of patients as have substantial delays in tumor progression and improvements in survival [97–102].

Systemic chemotherapy is the only therapeutic option for those patients with extrahepatic disease or portal venous system involvement. However, one needs to be careful in evaluating the reported results of this approach since the patients for whom systemic chemotherapy has been offered routinely are those with advanced disease and with compromised liver function. Poor liver function may lead to increased morbidity and mortality. The discouraging results obtained with past studies may in part reflect the need for adjusting the doses of the therapeutic agents to the degree of liver dysfunction. HCCs are considered widely chemotherapy resistant. Response rates from 15 to 35% have been reported with single agents, but durable remission is uncommon. The high incidence of overexpression of the multidrug resistance gene (MDR-1) and the gene product P-glycoprotein may in part explain some of this chemotherapeutic resistance of HCC [103–105]. Anthracyclines, like doxorubicin, epirubicin, and mitoxantrone, are among the most commonly used single agents for the treatment of HCC [106–110]. Other chemotherapeutic agents of the older generation that have been studied as single agents for the treatment of HCC include 5-fluorouracil [111–113], cisplatin [114, 115], and etoposide [116, 117]. The newer generation chemotherapeutic agents, like capecitabine [118], gemcitabine [119, 120], paclitaxel [121], and irinotecan [122] as single agents have not shown any better response and at times even shown lesser activity. Combination chemotherapy has helped improved responses rates, although the duration of remission has remained short, with no evidence of improvement in survival [123–130].

Using a four-drug systemic chemotherapy combination with cisplatin, recombinant interferon-α2b, doxorubicin, and 5-fluorouracil (PIAF regimen) Patt et al. achieved a complete pathologic remission in a case of disseminated HCC [131]. Leung et al. reported on 149 patients with HCC treated with a modified regimen using the same drug combination [132]. The objective response rate was 16.8%, with a complete response seen in 3 patients and a partial response in 22 patients. Although the response rate was not high, 16 patients had their disease rendered operable after chemotherapy. In eight patients a complete pathologic response was seen, and the remainder had greater than 95% necrosis. The median overall survival time for all patients was 30.9 weeks. Prognostic factors associated with increased response and survival were absence of cirrhosis and low bilirubin levels. The objective response rate was 50% for those patients with good risk factors.

The favorable results obtained with the PIAF regimen, especially when compared with previous trials of single or multiagent systemic chemotherapy, may be a result of the antiangiogenic activity of interferon-α [133, 134]. The expression of various angiogenic factors (e.g., vascular endothelial growth factor, platelet-derived endothelial growth factor, interleukin-8 (IL-8), cyclo-oxygenase-2, tumor necrosis factor-alpha) that lead to endothelial cell proliferation, migration, invasion, differentiation and capillary tube formation have been associated with the development and progression of HCCs. Recent evidence suggests that the addition of anti-angiogenic agents to conventional chemotherapy improves the efficacy against experimental drug-resistant cancer [135]. Thalidomide and bevacizumab, a monoclonal antibody to vascular endothelial growth factor, have anti-angiogenic activity and have been evaluated in phase II trials for HCC patients [136, 137].

The presence of estrogen and androgen receptors in HCC cells led to the rationale of using anti-hormonal therapy [138, 139]. Two large randomized phase III trials using the anti-estrogen tamoxifen showed no survival benefit for patients treated with this agent when compared with best available supportive care measures [140, 141].

Finally, there is no proven effective therapeutic option for patients with significant liver dysfunction (Child's-Pugh class C). These patients usually die within 6 months; therapy should thus focus on symptomatic relief to avoid unnecessary suffering.

Chemotherapy has become an important part of the therapy for children with HBL. It has been used as adjuvant therapy for patients who undergo complete tumor resection at the time of diagnosis, to induce tumor shrinkage pre-operatively in those tumors considered unresectable, or when primary resection is considered hazardous. Since HCCs are rare in children and adolescents in the Western world, they have consistently been treated according to therapeutic trials for HBL, despite the fact that the two malignancies are biologically different.

Katzenstein et al. [74] and Czauderna et al. [142] reported on the results of children and adolescents with HCC treated on the recently completed North American Intergroup Hepatoma study (INT-0098) and the first International Society of Pediatric Oncology liver tumor study (SIOPEL-1). Both studies utilized pre-operative chemotherapy in an attempt to increase surgical resectability, since this is the foundation for curative therapy for liver tumors.

Forty-six patients were entered onto the North American Intergroup Hepatoma study [74]. After initial surgery or biopsy all patients, 8 with stage I (completely resected tumors), 25 with stage III (unresectable tumor), and 13 with stage IV (metastatic disease) were randomized to receive cisplatin with either doxorubicin or 5-fluorouracil and vincristine. There was no difference in response or survival rates between the two treatment regimens.

Seven of the eight patients (88%) with complete tumor excision at time of diagnosis (stage I) followed by adjuvant cisplatin-based chemotherapy survived.

This was a significant improvement when compared with only 12 of 33 historical control patients (36%) treated before the routine use of adjuvant chemotherapy [74, 143]. This result suggests that adjuvant chemotherapy is of benefit for patients with completely resected HCC. In contrast, outcome was uniformly poor for patients with advanced-stage disease. Five-year event-free survival for stage III and IV patients was 23±9% and 10±9%, respectively. Tumor resection after neo-adjuvant chemotherapy was only feasible in two patients, and although they did have a prolonged survival they eventually died of recurrent disease.

Thirty-nine patients were entered onto the SIOPEL-1 study [142]. Of these, 2 had complete resection of the tumor at diagnosis followed by adjuvant chemotherapy, and 37 had pre-operative chemotherapy using cisplatin and doxorubicin. Tumor extent was determined by radiologic findings, and was classified according to the PRETEXT system. Disease was often advanced at the time of diagnosis, with 24 of 39 patients (62%) classified as PRETEXT III and IV. Metastases were identified in 31% of the patients, and extra-hepatic tumor extension, vascular invasion, or both in 39%. The tumor was multifocal in 56% of the patients. Although partial tumor response to therapy was observed in 49% (18/37) of the patients, complete tumor resection was achieved in only 36% (14/39). The results of this study were also unsatisfactory, with a 5-year event-free survival of 17% (6–30%). All long-term survivors had complete surgical excision of their tumor.

Twenty-one patients diagnosed with HCC were registered in the SIOPEL 2 study from March 1994 to May 1998, and data are available for 17 of those (personal communication, J. Plaschkes, 2004). Disease was advanced in most patients at diagnosis. Metastases occurred in 18% of the patients, extra-hepatic tumor extension and/or vascular invasion were found in 35% of patients, and the tumor was multi-focal in 53% of the patients. One patient died 17 days after diagnosis from massive gastrointestinal bleeding, having never received treatment. Thirteen of the 16 treated patients received pre-operative chemotherapy (SuperPLADO – cisplatin/carboplatin and doxorubicin). A partial response to pre-operative chemotherapy was observed in 6/13 cases (46%). Tumor resection was achieved in eight patients (47%; three at the time of diagnosis), and one had a liver transplant. Nine tumors (53%) never became operable. One patient was lost to follow-up just before planned surgery. Four of the resected patients were alive at a median follow-up time of 53 months (35–73 months). Twelve patients died due to progressive disease and one from surgical complications. The 3-year overall survival for this study was 22%.

In the SIOPEL-2 trial, treatment intensity was increased, compared with SIOPEL-1, by rapidly alternating the administration of cisplatin (every 14 days) with carboplatin and doxorubicin (personal communication, J. Plaschkes 2004). Despite this intensification of standard systemic chemotherapy, no improvement in event-free or overall survival has been achieved.

When we compare the results of these three studies with three North American studies conducted between 1973 and 1984 [144], the outcome for patients with HCC has shown no significant improvement, despite the improvements observed in surgical techniques, chemotherapy delivery, and patient support. It seems obvious that a completely new treatment approach is needed to increase HCC cure rate.

First described in 1956 by Edmonson [18] as a distinct pathologic variant, FL-HCC has been associated with a higher resection rate and better survival when compared with the typical pathologic variant of HCC both in adolescents and young adults [145–151].

The higher resection rate was not supported by the studies reported by Katzenstein et al. [152] and Czauderna et al. [142]. Ten of 46 patients (22%) entered onto the Intergroup Hepatoma study had a FL-HCC. Resectability at diagnosis and response to therapy was not different than for those patients with typical HCC. Patients with FL-HCC did not have a better outcome when compared with those with typical HCC; the 5-year event-free survival was 30±15% and 14±6%, respectively (p=0.18), although the median survival was longer for patients with FL-HCC. The same results were seen in the SIOPEL-1 study. Four out of 6 patients with FL-HCC died of the disease. However, their survival was much longer (25 months versus 11 months) than for the rest of the group.

Extent of disease (stage and PRETEXT) and presence of metastases at diagnosis were the two most important prognostic factors for patients diagnosed

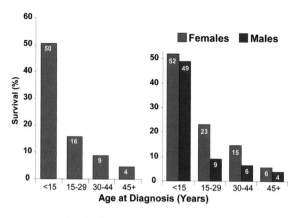

Figure 19.9

Five-year survival of patients with liver and intrahepatic bile duct cancer by age (*left panel*) and gender (*right panel*). United States SEER 1975–1998 [1]

with HCC and entered onto the Intergroup Hepatoma or SIOPEL-1 studies [142]. Advanced disease and/or presence of metastases at diagnosis were associated with a lower survival. Analysis of the Intergroup Hepatoma trial showed a trend toward improved event-free survival for those children with normal AFP level at diagnosis when compared with those with elevated levels, with 5-year event-free survival estimates of 29±12% and 10±6%, respectively (p=0.09) [152]. However, this finding was not confirmed by the SIOPEL-1 study [142]. AFP levels were low in eight of nine patients with FL-HCC in the Intergroup Hepatoma study and in all six patients in the SIOPEL-1 study [142].

Treatment of recurrent HCC in this age group has had dismal results. Due to the rarity of these tumors, very little experience has been gained from phase I and II trials. Hepatic arterial chemo-embolization refers to the intra-arterial administration of chemotherapeutic and vascular occlusive agents (generally gelatin) with anti-tumor agents. The most commonly used chemo-embolization agents are doxorubicin, mitomycin, and cisplatin [153–155]. Intra-arterial injection of anti-cancer agents results in a higher local concentration of drugs with reduced systemic side effects, while the

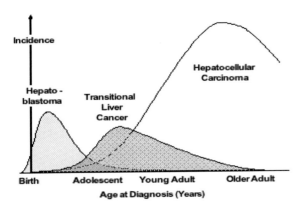

Figure 19.10

Conceptual depiction (not drawn to scale) of the overlap between pediatric and adult types of liver cancer, which may explain the type of liver cancer observed in older adolescents and young adults. *HB* Hepatoblastoma, *HCC* hepatocellular carcinoma, *AYA* adolescents and young adults

intra-arterial embolization causes ischemic necrosis of the tumor. This therapy has been used in a small number of children and adolescents with recurrent HCC while waiting for a donated liver to become available, or as adjuvant therapy in an attempt to allow tumor resection [156–159]. A major limiting factor for the success of this therapy is the status of the liver function; since in children and adolescents HCCs are rarely associated with liver cirrhosis and therefore they usually have normal liver function, chemo-embolization may be useful for these patients.

19.7.2 Mortality and Survival

The mortality rate of liver tumors has shown a significant decrease over time (1975–2000) for patients less than 45 years of age, but not for older patients (>45 years). Survival has improved significantly for individuals with liver tumors younger than 15 years of age since the introduction of a multi-disciplinary therapeutic approach after the 1980s. However, progress has been much slower for older individuals (>15 years of age). The survival of patients less than 15 years of age is close to 60%, while for those individuals between 15 and

29 years of age, survival is approximately 16% and steadily decreases with the advancement of age, as shown in Fig. 19.9. This is due to the fact that younger patients are predominantly diagnosed with HBLs, which are far more responsive to chemotherapy than HCC and bile duct tumors. Although survival is not different for males compared to females younger than 15 years of age, females have a much better survival in the group between 15 and 29 years of age (Fig. 19.5).

According to Bosch et al., mortality rate estimates worldwide present the same pattern to that observed with the incidence rates, with higher mortality rates seen in the developing countries when compared to those seen in developed countries [2].

19.8 Liver Cancer in Adolescents and Young Adults

One of the main striking differences between HCC in adults and a younger population is the absence of cirrhosis in the latter. Other differences are listed in the Table 19.2. The finding and description of a tumor in adolescents and young adults with characteristics in between HBL and HCC could be explained by a novel hypotheses postulating two different pathways of origin of the tumors with an overlap in the adolescent and the young adult age population (Fig. 19.10).

19.9 Future Perspectives

The overall survival for children and adults with HCC, with the exception of highly selected patients for whom complete tumor resection is feasible, continues to be dismal. In Western countries, where HCC in older adults is secondary to liver cirrhosis caused by alcohol consumption and/or chronic infection by hepatitis B or C, primary prevention through vaccination (hepatitis B), implementation of adequate health standards and antiviral treatment to prevent progression to cirrhosis (hepatitis C) may be the only effective ways to change this outcome. In Asia, and African countries HCC is related to chronic infection with hepatitis B virus acquired at birth or at an early age. Universal hepatitis B immunization programs will continue to dramatically

Table 19.2 Differences between adult and childhood hepatocellular carcinoma. *HBV* Hepatitis B virus

Clinical differences	Pediatric	Adult
Liver cirrhosis	<30%	70–90%
Incidence	0.5–1 per 10^6	3–150 per 10^5
Male:female ratio	2.5:1	3.8:1
Response to chemotherapy	40–49%	10–20%
Histology	High incidence of fibrolamellar hepato-cellular carcinoma	Lower incidence of fibrolamellar hepatocellular carcinoma
Associations (etiology)	Congenital metabolic diseases	HBV
	Congenital HBV vertical transmission	Toxins
	Biliary atresia	Hormonal factors
Endemic HBV regions	No	Yes

reduce the incidence of HCC in these countries. Since no therapy has been demonstrated to be efficacious once cirrhosis develops, surveillance aimed at early detection of tumors and implementation of effective therapy is the only option to diminish tumor-related mortality.

In contrast to the older adults in whom almost 90% of the cases of HCC are associated with cirrhosis, less than one-third of adolescent or young adult HCC patients have hepatitis or other inflammatory liver diseases. Furthermore, most of these young patients are in a good state of health and have normal liver function. Therefore, treatment choices for these patients should have a curative goal even at the expense of increased toxicity.

Tumor resection should be the therapy of choice for adolescents and young adults with localized disease. For those patients for whom up-front surgical resection is not feasible, the use of percutaneous tumor ablation or intra-arterial chemo-embolization has been associated with a high response rate and increased survival; however, failures are usually associated with local tumor recurrence. Therefore, future studies are needed to determine whether surgical resection of these lesions following local control measures, like chemoembolization or percutaneous ablation, can improve these results.

Unlike that for those with localized disease, treatment for patients with advanced unresectable or metastatic disease has not been associated with an improvement in the response rate or overall survival. Despite the aggressive use of systemic chemotherapy followed by an attempt at surgical resection, the pediatric clinical trials have failed to demonstrate an increase in tumor resectability and survival. Trials for adults with advanced and metastatic HCC, on the other hand, have been frequently designed with palliative intent due to the potential risks associated with the use of systemic chemotherapy in patients with hepatic dysfunction.

Recently, the use of systemic chemotherapy for the treatment of adults with advanced HCC with the PIAF regimen has resulted in an increased tumor response rate and resectability [132]. This favorable result may be due to the combination of chemotherapeutic agents with the anti-angiogenic activity of interferon-α.

Angiogenesis is important for the growth of both the primary and metastatic tumors. Therefore, drugs that inhibit angiogenesis may be useful in the treatment of malignant tumors. Angiogenesis is dependent on the interaction of various factors, such as vascular endothelial growth factor, platelet-derived endothelial growth factor, IL-8, cyclo-oxygenase-2, and tumor necrosis factor-alpha, which lead to endothelial cell proliferation, migration, invasion, and differentiation, and capillary tube formation. Various factors have already been associated with the development and progression of HCCs. Their expression have also been associated with histology grade, proliferative activity, invasion, and patient survival. Multiple studies have demonstrated that agents with antiangiogenic activity (e.g., TNP-470, thalidomide, angiotensin-converting enzyme inhibitors, aspirin) may reduce the size and frequency of development of experimentally induced

HCC in rats and inhibit tumor growth, invasion, and metastasis of human HCC in nude mouse models.

Based on these data and the encouraging results obtained for good-risk patients (non-cirrhotic and with low bilirubin levels) treated with the PIAF regimen, the development of studies using the combination of systemic chemotherapy and anti-angiogenic agents should be explored for the treatment of adolescents and young adults with HCC. The treatment should have as its main goal tumor shrinkage, allowing for complete excision of the tumor by conventional surgical resection or by liver transplant. These patients are ideal candidates for exploring the role of this therapeutic approach as well as other new chemotherapeutic regimens, and novel therapeutic approaches such as gene therapy as they become available.

In order to achieve this aim, however, broad collaboration and compromise between adult and pediatric oncologists on an international level will be necessary to successfully design and conduct a therapeutic trial for adolescents and young adults with HCC.

References

1. Bleyer A, O'Leary M, Barr R, Ries LAG (eds) (2006) Cancer Epidemiology in Older Adolescents and Young Adults 15 to 29 Years of Age, Including SEER Incidence and Survival: 1975–2000. National Cancer Institute, NIH Pub. No. 06-5767. Bethesda, MD, p 220
2. Bosch FX, Ribes J, Borras J (1999) Epidemiology of primary liver cancer. Semin Liver Dis 19:271–285
3. Feraly J, Parkin DM, Pisani P (1998) GLOBOCAN Graphical Package 1: Cancer Incidence and Mortality Worldwide. IARC Press, Lyons
4. Chen JC, et al (1998) Hepatocellular carcinoma in children: clinical review and comparison with adult cases. J Pediatr Surg 33:1350–1354
5. Czauderna P (2002) Adult type vs. childhood hepatocellular carcinoma – are they the same or different lesions? Biology, natural history, prognosis, and treatment. Med Pediatr Oncol 39:19–23
6. Di Bisceglie AM, et al (1998) NIH conference. Hepatocellular carcinoma. Ann Intern Med 108:390–401
7. Chang M, et al (1997) Universal hepatitis B vaccination in Taiwan and the incidence of hepatocellular carcinoma in children. Taiwan Childhood Hepatoma Study Group. N Engl J Med 336:1855–1859
8. Ishak KG (1991) Hepatocellular carcinoma associated with inherited metabolic diseases. In: Tabor E, Di Bisceglie AM, Purcell RH (eds) Etiology, Pathogenesis and Treatment of Hepatocellular Carcinoma in North America. Portfolio Publishing Company, The Woodlands, Texas, pp 91–103
9. Ugarte N, Gonzalez-Crussi F (1981) Hepatoma in siblings with progressive familial cholestatic cirrhosis of childhood. Am J Clin Pathol 76:172–177
10. Kharsa D, et al (1990) Adenome hepatique et carcinome hepatocellulaire chez deux freres ateints de glycogenose de type I. Gastroenterol Clin Biol 14:84–89
11. Eriksson S, Carlson J, Velez R (1986) Risk of cirrhosis and primary liver cancer in alpha 1-antitrypsin deficiency. N Engl J Med 296:1411–1412
12. Ishak KG (1979) Hepatic neoplasms associated with contraceptives and anabolic steroids. Recent Results Cancer Res 66:73–128
13. Sun Z, Lu P, Gail MH (1999) Increased risk of hepatocellular carcinoma in male hepatitis B surface antigen carriers with chronic hepatitis who have detectable aflatoxin metabolite M1. Hepatology 30:379–383
14. Christopherson WM, Mays ET (1987) Risk factors, pathology, and pathogenesis of selected benign and malignant liver neoplasm. In: Wanebo HH (ed) Hepatic and Biliary Cancer. Marcel Decker, New York, pp 17–43
15. Okuda K (2000) Hepatocellular carcinoma. Hepatology 32:225–237
16. Okuda K (2002) Natural history of hepatocellular carcinoma including fibrolamellar and hepato-cholangiocarcinoma variants. J Gastroenterol Hepatol 17:401–405
17. Lauwers GY, et al (2002) Prognostic histologic indicators of curatively resected hepatocellular carcinomas: a multi-institutional analysis of 425 patients with definition of a histologic prognostic index. Am J Surg Pathol 26:25–34
18. Edmonson H (1956) Differential diagnosis of tumors and tumor-like lesions of liver in infancy and childhood. Arch Dis Child 1:168–186
19. Craig JR, et al (1980) Fibrolamellar carcinoma of the liver: a tumor of adolescents and young adults with distinctive clinico-pathologic features. Cancer 46:372–379
20. McLarney JK, et al (1999) Fibrolamellar carcinoma of the liver: radiologic-pathologic correlation. Radiographics 19:453–471
21. Cheuk W, Chan JK (2001) Clear cell variant of fibrolamellar carcinoma of the liver. Arch Pathol Lab Med 125:1235–1238
22. Berman MA, Burham JA, Sheahan DG (1988) Fibrolamellar carcinoma of the liver: an immunohistochemical study of nineteen cases and review of the literature. Hum Pathol 19:784–794
23. Van Eyken P, et al (1990) Abundant expression of cytokeratin 7 in fibrolamellar carcinoma of the liver. Histopathology 17:101–107
24. Seitz G, et al (2002) Adult-type hepatocellular carcinoma in the center of a fibrolamellar hepatocellular carcinoma. Hum Pathol 33:765–769

25. Paradinas FJ, et al (1982) High serum vitamin B12 binding capacity as a marker of fibrolamellar variant of hepatocellular carcinoma. Br Med J 25:840–842

26. Sheppard KJ, et al (1983) High serum vitamin B12 binding capacity as a marker of the fibrolamellar variant of hepatocellular carcinoma. Br Med J 286:57

27. Wheeler K, et al (1986) Transcobalamin I as a "marker" for fibrolamellar hepatoma. Med Pediatr Oncol 14:227–229

28. Kane SP, et al (1978) Vitamin B12 binding protein as a tumour marker for hepatocellular carcinoma. Gut 19:1105–1109

29. Collier NR, et al (1984) Neurotensin secretion by fibrolamellar carcinoma of the liver. Lancet 1:538–540

30. Hany MA, et al (1997) A childhood fibrolamellar hepatocellular carcinoma with increased aromatase activity and a near triploid karyotype. Med Pediatr Oncol 28:136–138

31. Sirivatanauksorn Y, et al (2001) Genomic homogeneity in fibrolamellar carcinomas. Gut 49:82–86

32. Wilkens L, et al (2000) Cytogenetic aberrations in primary and recurrent fibrolamellar hepatocellular carcinoma detected by comparative genomic hybridization. J Clin Pathol 114:867–874

33. Prokurat A, et al (2002) Transitional liver cell tumors (TLCT) in older children and adolescents: a novel group of aggressive hepatic tumors expressing beta-catenin. Med Pediatr Oncol 39:510–518

34. Perilongo G, Plaschkes J, Zimmermann A (2002) Hepatic tumours. In: Souhami RL, Tannock I, Hohenberger P, Horiot JC (eds) Oxford Textbook of Oncology, Vol. 2. Oxford University Press, Oxford, pp 2657–2668

35. Rowland JM (2002) Hepatoblastoma: assessment of criteria for histologic classification. Med Pediatr Oncol 39:478–483

36. Buendia MA (2002) Genetic alterations in hepatoblastoma and hepatocellular carcinoma: common and distinctive aspects. Med Pediatr Oncol 39:530–535

37. Zimmermann A (2002) Pediatric liver tumors and hepatic ontogenesis: common and distinctive pathways. Med Pediatr Oncol 39:492–503

38. Postovsky S, et al (2001) Late recurrence of combined hepatocellular carcinoma and hepatoblastoma in a child: case report and review of the literature. Eur J Pediatr Surg 11:61–65

39. Dumortier J, et al (1999) Recurrence of hepatocellular carcinoma as a mixed hepatoblastoma after liver transplantation. Gut 45:622–625

40. Chen TC, Hsieh LL, Kuo TT (1995) Absence of p53 gene mutation and infrequent overexpression of p53 protein in hepatoblastoma. J Pathol 176:243–247

41. Kusafuka T, et al (1997) Mutation analysis of p53 gene in childhood malignant solid tumors. J Pediatr Surg 32:1175–1180

42. Pang A, et al (2003) Clinicopathologic significance of genetic alterations in hepatocellular carcinoma. Cancer Genet Cytogenet 146:8–15

43. Aoki T, et al (2004) Clinical value of alterations in p73 gene, related to p53 at 1p36, in human hepatocellular carcinoma. Int J Oncol 24:441–446

44. Feitelson MA, et al (2002) Genetic mechanisms of hepatocarcinogenesis. Oncogene 21:2593–2604

45. Thorgeirsson SS, Grisham JW (2002) Molecular pathogenesis of human hepatocellular carcinoma. Nature Genet 31:339–346

46. Van Tornout JM, Buckley JD, Ortega JA (1997) Timing and magnitude of decline in alpha-fetoprotein levels in treated children with unresectable or metastatic hepatoblastoma are predictors of outcome: a report from the Children's Cancer Group. J Clin Oncol 15:1190–1197

47. Tsuchida Y, et al (1989) Three different types of alpha-fetoprotein in the diagnosis of malignant solid tumors: use of a sensitive lectin-affinity immunoelectrophoresis. J Pediatr Surg 24:350–355

48. Ortega JA, Siegel SE (1993) Biological markers in pediatric solid tumors. In: Pizzo AP, Poplack DG (eds) Principles and Practice of Pediatric Oncology. Lippincott, Philadelphia pp 179–194

49. Miller JH, Gates GH, Stanley P (1977) The radiologic investigation of hepatic tumors in childhood. Radiology 124:451–464

50. Liu P, Daneman A, Stringer DA (1985) Diagnostic imaging of liver masses in children. J Can Assoc Radiol 36:296–300

51. de Campo M. de Campo JF (1988) Ultrasound of primary hepatic tumours in childhood. Pediatr Radiol 19:19–24

52. King S, et al (1993) Value of CT in determining the resectability of hepatoblastoma before and after chemotherapy. AJR Am J Roentgenol 160:793–799

53. Korobkin M, et al (1981) Computed tomography of primary liver tumors in children. Radiology 139:431–438

54. Boechat MI, et al (1988) Primary liver tumors in children: comparison of CT and MR imaging. Radiology 169:727–732

55. Stocker JT, Ishak KG (1978) Undifferentiated embryonal sarcoma of the liver. Report of 31 cases. Cancer 42:336–348

56. Chowdhary SK, et al (2004) Undifferentiated embryonal sarcoma in children: beware of the solitary liver cyst. J Pediatr Surg 39:E9–12

57. Bisogno G, et al (2002) Undifferentiated embryonal sarcoma of the liver in childhood : a curable disease. Cancer 94:252–257

58. Uchiyama M, et al. (2001) Treatment of ruptured undifferentiated sarcoma of the liver in children. J Hepatobil Pancreat Surg 8:87–91

59. Herman P et al. (2000) Hepatic Adenoma and focal nodular hyperplasia: differential diagnosis and treatment. World J Surg 24:372–376

60. Heaton ND, et al (1991) Focal nodular hyperplasia of the liver: a link with sickle cell disease. Arch Dis Child 66:1073–1074

61. Bouyn CL, et al (2003) Hepatic focal nodular hyperplasia in children previously treated for a solid tumour. Incidence risk factors and outcome. Cancer 97: 3103–3107

62. Reymond D, et al (1995) Focal nodular hyperplasia of the liver in children. Review of follow up and outcome. J Pediatr Surg 30:1590–1593

63. Reynolds M (1999) Pediatric liver tumors. Semin Surg Oncol 16:159–172

64. Evans AE, Land VJ, Newton WA Jr (1982) Combination chemotherapy in the treatment of children with malignant hepatoma. Cancer 50:821–826

65. Ortega JA, et al (1991) Effective treatment of unresectable or metastatic hepatoblastoma with cisplatin and continuous infusion doxorubicin chemotherapy: a report from the Children's Cancer Study Group. J Clin Oncol 9:2167–2176

66. MacKinlay G, Pritchard J (1992) A common language for childhood liver tumours. Pediatr Surg Int 7:325–326

67. Brown J, et al (2000) Pretreatment prognostic factors for children with hepatoblastoma – results from the International Society of Paediatric Oncology (SIOP) study SIOPEL 1. Eur J Cancer 36:1418–1425

68. The Cancer of the Liver Italian Program (CLIP) Investigators (2000) CLIP, Prospective validation of the CLIP score: a new prognostic system for patients with cirrhosis and hepatocellular carcinoma. Hepatology 31:840–845

69. Llovet JM, Bru C, Bruix J (1999) Prognosis of hepatocellular carcinoma: the Bclc staging classification. Semin Liver Dis 19:329–338

70. Leung TW, et al (2002) Construction of the Chinese University prognostic index for hepatocellular carcinoma and comparison with the TNM staging system, the Okuda staging system, and the cancer of the liver Italian program staging system: a study based on 926 patients. Cancer 94:1760–1769

71. The Liver Cancer Study Group of Japan (1994) Predictive factors for long term prognosis after partial hepatectomy for patients with hepatocellular carcinoma in Japan. Cancer 74: 2272–2280

72. Pugh RNH, et al (1973) Transection of the oesophagus for bleeding of oesophageal varices. Br J Surg 60:646–664

73. Tagge EP, et al (1992) Resection including transplantation for hepatoblastoma and hepatocellular carcinoma. J Pediatr Surg 21:292–297

74. Katzenstein HM, et al (2002) Hepatocellular carcinoma in children and adolescents: results from the Pediatric Oncology Group and the Children's Cancer Group intergroup study. J Clin Oncol 20:2789–2797

75. Reyes JD, et al (2000) Liver transplantation and chemotherapy for hepatoblastoma and hepatocellular cancer in childhood and adolescence. J Pediatr 136:795–804

76. Koneru B, et al (1991) Liver transplantation for hepatoblastoma. The American experience. Ann Surg 213:118–121

77. Otte JB, et al (2004) Liver transplantation for hepatoblastoma: results from the International Society of Pediatric Oncology (SIOP) study SIOPEL-1 and review of the world experience. Pediatr Blood Cancer 42:74–83

78. Chang MH (2003) Decreasing incidence of hepatocellular carcinoma among children following universal hepatitis B immunization. Liver Int 23:309–314

79. Bruix J, et al (2001) Clinical management of hepatocellular carcinoma: conclusions of the Barcelona-2000 EASL Conference. J Hepatol 35:421–430

80. Sakamoto M, Hirohashi S (1998) Natural history and prognosis of adenomatous hyperplasia and early hepatocellular carcinoma: multi-institutional analysis of 53 nodules followed for more than 6 months and 141 patients with single early hepatocellular carcinoma treated by surgical resection o percutaneous ethanol injection. Jpn J Clin Oncol 28:604–608

81. Takayama K, et al (1998) Early hepatocellular carcinomas an entity with high rate of surgical cure. Hepatology 28:1241–1246

82. Llovet JM, Fuster J, Bruix J (1999) Intention-to-treat analysis of surgical treatment for early hepatocellular carcinoma: resection versus transplantation. Hepatology 39:1434–1440

83. Mazzaferro V, et al (1996) Liver transplantation for the treatment of small hepatocellular carcinomas in patients with cirrhosis. N Engl J Med 334:693–699

84. Jonas S, et al (2001) Vascular invasion and histopathologic grading determine outcome after liver transplantation for hepatocellular carcinoma in cirrhosis. Hepatology 33:1080–1086

85. Yao FY, et al (2001) Liver transplantation for hepatocellular carcinoma: expansion of tumor size limits does not adversely impact survival. Hepatology 33:1394–1403

86. Yao FY, et al (2002) Liver transplantation for hepatocellular carcinoma: analysis of survival according to the intention-to-treat principle and dropout from the waiting list. Liver Transpl 8:873–883

87. Cronin D, Millis M, Siegler M (2001) Transplantation of liver grafts from living donors into adults: too much, too soon? N Engl J Med 344:1633–1637

88. Sarasin F, et al (2001) Liver donor liver transplantation for early hepatocellular carcinoma: a cost-effective perspective. Hepatology 33:1073–1079

89. Trotter J, et al (2002) Adult-to-Adult transplantation of the right hepatic lobe from living donor. N Engl J Med 14:1074–1082

90. Lau WY, et al (2003) Percutaneous local ablative therapy for hepatocellular carcinoma: a review and look into the future. Ann Surg 237:171–179

91. Lencioni R, et al (2004) Percutaneous ablation of hepatocellular carcinoma: state-of-the-art. Liver Transpl 10: S91–97

92. Livraghi T, et al (2004) Multimodal image-guided tailored therapy of early and intermediate hepatocellular carcinoma: long-term survival in the experience of a

single radiologic referral center. Liver Transpl 10:S98–106

93. Livraghi T (2003) Radiofrequency ablation, PEIT, and TACE for hepatocellular carcinoma. J Hepatobil Pancreat Surg 10:67–76

94. Okada S (1999) Local ablation therapy for hepatocellular carcinoma. Semin Liver Dis 19:323–328

95. Buscarini L, Buscarini E, Di Stasi M (2001) Percutaneous radiofrequency ablation of small hepatocellular carcinoma: long-term results. Eur Radiol 11:914–921

96. Lencioni RA, et al (2003) Small hepatocellular carcinoma in cirrhosis: randomized comparison of radiofrequency thermal ablation versus percutaneous ethanol injection. Radiology 228:235–240

97. Llovet JM, Bruix J (2003) Systematic review of randomized trials for unresectable hepatocellular carcinoma: chemoembolization improves survival. Hepatology 37:429–442

98. Groupe d'Etude et de Traitement du Carcinome Hepatocellulaire (1995) A comparison of lipiodol chemoembolization and conservative treatment for unresectable hepatocellular carcinoma. N Engl J Med 332:1256–1261

99. Zhang Z, et al (2000) The effect of preoperative transcatheter hepatic arterial chemoembolization on disease-free survival after hepatectomy for hepatocellular carcinoma. Cancer 89:2606–2612

100. Bruix J, et al (1998) Transarterial embolization versus symptomatic treatment in patients with advanced hepatocellular carcinoma: results of a randomized, controlled trial in a single institution. Hepatology 27:1578–1583

101. Lo CM, et al (2002) Randomized controlled trial of transarterial lipiodol chemoembolization for unresectable hepatocellular carcinoma. Hepatology 35:1164–1171

102. Raoul JL, et al (1997) Prospective randomized trial of chemoembolization versus intra-arterial injection of 131-I labeled-iodized oil in the treatment of hepatocellular carcinoma. Hepatology 26:1156–1161

103. Soini Y, et al (1996) Expression of P-glycoprotein in hepatocellular carcinoma: a potential marker of prognosis. J Clin Pathol 49:470–473

104. Huang CC, et al (1992) Overexpression of the MDR1 gene and P-glycoprotein in human hepatocellular carcinoma. J Natl Cancer Inst 84:262–264

105. Chou YY, et al (1997) Expression of P-glycoprotein and p53 in advanced hepatocellular carcinoma treated by single agent chemotherapy: clinical correlation. J Gastroenterol Hepatol 12:569–575

106. Johnson PJ, et al (1978) Induction of remission in hepatocellular carcinoma with doxorubicin. Lancet 1:1006–1009

107. Chlebowski RT, et al (1984) Doxorubicin (75 mg/m^2) for hepatocellular carcinoma: clinical and pharmacokinetic results. Cancer Treat Reports 68:487–491

108. Hochster HS, et al (1985) 4'Epidoxorubicin (epirubicin): activity in hepatocellular carcinoma. J Clin Oncol 3:1535–1540

109. Dunk AA, et al (1985) Mitozantrone as single agent therapy in hepatocellular carcinoma. A phase II study. J Hepatol 1:395–404

110. Vogel CL, et al (1977) A phase II study of adriamycin (NSC 123127) in patients with hepatocellular carcinoma from Zambia and the United States. Cancer 39:1923–1929

111. Falkson G, et al (1978) Chemotherapy studies in primary liver cancer: a prospective randomized clinical trial. Cancer 42:2149–2156

112. Tetef M, et al (1995) 5-Fluorouracil and high-dose calcium leucovorin for hepatocellular carcinoma: a phase II trial. Cancer Invest 13:460–463

113. Porta C, et al (1995) 5-Fluorouracil and D,L-leucovorin calcium are active to treat unresectable hepatocellular carcinoma patients: a preliminary results of a phase II study. Oncology 52:487–491

114. Melia WM, Westaby D, Williams R (1981) Diamminodichloride platinum (cis-platinum) in the treatment of hepatocellular carcinoma. Clin Oncol 7:275–280

115. Okada S, et al (1993) A phase 2 study of cisplatin in patients with hepatocellular carcinoma. Oncology 50:22–26

116. Melia WM, Johnson PJ, Williams R (1983) Induction of remission in hepatocellular carcinoma. A comparison of VP 16 with adriamycin. Cancer 51:206–210

117. Wierzbicki R, et al (1994) Phase II trial of chronic daily VP-16 administration in unresectable hepatocellular carcinoma. Ann Oncol 5:466–467

118. Lozano RD, et al (2000) Oral capecitabine (Xeloda) for the treatment of hepatobiliary cancers (hepatocellular carcinoma, cholangiocarcinoma, and gallbladder cancer). Proc Am Soc Clin Oncol 19:264a (abstract 1025)

119. Yang TS, et al (2000) Phase II study of gemcitabine in patients with advanced hepatocellular carcinoma. Cancer 89:750–756

120. Kubicka S, et al (2001) Phase II study of sytemic gemcitabine chemotherapy for advanced unresectable hepatobiliary carcinomas. Hepatogastroenterology 48:783–789

121. Chao Y, et al (1998) Phase II and pharmacokinetic study of paclitaxel therapy for unresectable hepatocellular carcinoma patients. Br J Cancer 78:34–39

122. O'Reilly EM, et al (2001) A phase II study of irinotecan in patients with advance hepatocellular carcinoma. Cancer 91:101–105

123. Patt YZ, et al (2003) Phase II trial of systemic continuous fluorouracil and subcutaneous recombinant interferon Alfa-2b for treatment of hepatocellular carcinoma. J Clin Oncol 21:421–427

124. Ji SK, et al (1996) Combined cis-platinum and alpha interferon therapy of advanced hepatocellular carcinoma. Korean J Int Med 11:58–68

125. Falkson G, et al (1987) A random phase II study of mito-xantrone and cisplatin in patients with hepatocellular carcinoma. An ECOG study. Cancer 60:2141–2145

126. Falkson G, et al (1984) Primary liver cancer. An Eastern Cooperative Oncology Group Trial. Cancer 54:970–977

127. Al-Idrissi HY, et al (1985) Primary hepatocellular carcinoma in the eastern province of Saudi Arabia: treatment with combination chemotherapy using 5-fluorouracil, adriamycin and mitomycin-C Hepato-gastroenterology 32:8–10

128. Bobbio-Pallavicini E, et al (1997) Epirubicin and etopo-side combination chemotherapy to treat hepatocellular carcinoma patients: a phase II study. Eur J Cancer 33:1784–1788

129. Baker LH, et al (1977) Adriamycin and 5-fluorouracil in the treatment of advanced hepatoma: a Southwest Oncology Group study. Cancer Treat Reports 61:1595–1597

130. Taieb J, et al (2003) Gemcitabine plus oxaliplatin for patients with advanced hepatocellular carcinoma using two different schedules. Cancer 98:2664–2670

131. Patt YZ, et al (1998) Systemic therapy with platinol, inter-feron alpha 2b, doxorubicin and 5-fluorouracil (PIAF) for treatment of non-resectable hepatocellular carcinoma. Proc Am Soc Clin Oncol 17:301a (abstract 1158)

132. Leung TW, et al (1999) Complete pathological remis-sion is possible with systemic combination chemother-apy for inoperable hepatocellular carcinoma. Clin Can-cer Res 5:1676–1681

133. Minischetti M, et al (2000) TNP-470 and recombinant human interferon-alpha2a inhibit angiogenesis syner-gistically. Br J Cancer 109:829–837

134. Lai CL, et al (1989) Recombinant alpha 2 interferon is superior to doxorubicin for inoperable hepatocellular carcinoma: a prospective randomised trial. Br J Cancer 60:928–33

135. Browder T, et al (2000) Antiangiogenic scheduling of chemotherapy improves efficacy against experimental drug-resistant cancer. Cancer Res 60:1878–1886

136. Schwartz JD, et al (2002) Thalidomide in hepatocellular carcinoma (HCC) with optional interferon-alpha upon progression. Proc Am Soc Clin Oncol 21:10b

137. Schwartz JD, et al (2005) Bevacizumab in hepatocellu-lar carcinoma in patients without metastasis and with-out invasion of the portal vein. Program and abstracts of the American Society of Clinical Oncology 2005 Gastrointestinal Cancers Symposium; January 27–29, 2005; Hollywood, Florida. Abstract 134

138. Nagasue N, et al (1985) Androgen receptors in hepato-cellular carcinoma and surrounding parenchyma. Gas-troenterology 89:643–647

139. Nagasue N, et al (1986) Estrogen receptors in hepato-cellular carcinoma. Cancer 57:87–91

140. Chow PK, et al (2002) High-dose tamoxifen in the treatment of inoperable hepatocellular carcinoma: a multicenter randomized controlled trial. Hepatology 3:1221–1226

141. Perrone F, et al (2002) Tamoxifen in the treatment of hepatocellular carcinoma: 5-year results of the CLIP-1 multicenter randomised controlled trial. Curr Pharm Des 8:1013–1019

142. Czauderna P, et al (2002) Hepatocellular carcinoma in children: results of the first prospective study of the International Society of Pediatric Oncology group. J Clin Oncol 20:2798–2804

143. Exelby PR, et al (1975) Liver tumors in children in the particular reference to hepatoblastoma and hepatocel-lular carcinoma: American Academy of Pediatrics sur-gical section survey – 1974. J Pediatr Surg 10:329–337

144. Haas JE, et al (1989) Histopathology and prognosis in childhood hepatoblastoma and hepatocarcinoma. Can-cer 64:1082–1095

145. Lack EE, Neave C, Vawter GF (1983) Hepatocellular carcinoma: review of 32 cases in childhood and adoles-cents. Cancer 52:1510–1515

146. Farhi DC, et al (1983) Hepatocellular carcinoma in young adults. Cancer 52:1516–1525

147. Craig J, et al (1980) Fibrolamellar carcinoma of the liver: a tumor of adolescents and young adults with dis-tinctive clinico-pathologic features. Cancer 46:372–379

148. Epstein BE, et al (1999) Metastatic nonresectable fibrolamellar hepatocellular carcinoma: prognostic fea-tures and natural history. Am J Clin Pathol 22:22–28

149. Saab S, Yao F (1996) Fibrolamellar hepatocellular carci-noma: case reports and a review of the literature. Digest Dis Sic 41:1981–1985

150. Altmann HW (1990) Some histological remarks on the fibrolamellar carcinoma of the liver. Pathol Res Pract 186:63–69

151. Rolfes DB (1987) Fibrolamellar carcinoma of the liver. In: Okuda K, Ishak KG (eds) Neoplasms of the Liver. Springer, New York, NY, pp 137–142

152. Katzenstein HM, et al (2003) Fibrolamellar hepatocel-lular carcinoma in children and adolescents. Cancer 97:2006–2012

153. Holladay ES, et al (1985) Conversion to resectability by intra-arterial infusion chemotherapy after failure of systemic chemotherapy. J Pediatr Surg 20:715–717

154. Groupe d'Etude et de Traitement du Carcinome Hepa-tocellulaire (1995) A comparison of lipiodol chemoem-bolization and conservative treatment for unresectable hepatocellular carcinoma. N Engl J Med 332:1256–1261

155. Rose DM, et al (1999) Transcatheter arterial chemoem-bolization as primary treatment for hepatocellular car-cinoma. Am J Surg 177:405–410

156. Malogolowkin MH, et al (2000) Feasibility and toxicity of chemoembolization for children with liver tumors. J Clin Oncol 18:1279–1284

157. Goiter S, et al (1987) Intraarterial chemotherapy with lipid contrast medium for hepatic malignancies in infants. Cancer 60:2886–2890

158. Ogita S, et al (1987) Intraarterial injection of anti-tumor drugs dispersed in lipid contrast medium: a choice for initially unresectable hepatoblastoma in infants. J Pediatr Surg 22:412–414

159. Sue K, et al (1989) Intrahepatic arterial injections of cis-platin-phosphatidylcholine-Lipiodol suspension in two unresectable hepatoblastoma cases. Med Pediatr Oncol 17:496–500

Colorectal Cancer

Wayne L. Furman • D. Ashley Hill • Michael LaQuaglia

Contents

20.1 Introduction

Colorectal cancer (CRC) is the third most common malignant tumor in adults [1]. It was estimated that, in the United States in 2004, 147,000 new cases of CRC were diagnosed and 56,730 would die of CRC [2]. The risk of CRC begins to increase at the age of 40 years, and patients less-than 40 years of age account for only 2–6% of all patients [3]. However, CRC is very unusual in children and adolescents (Fig. 20.1).

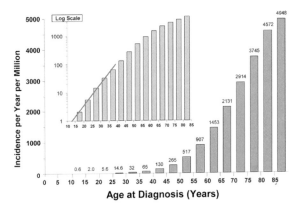

Figure 20.1

Incidence of colorectal carcinoma, United States SEER, 1975–2000. The diagonal line on the semilogarithmic inset chart indicates that the incidence is exponential below age 40 years and extrapolates to a lower age limit between 10 and 15 years for the youngest cases

20.2 Epidemiology

20.2.1 Incidence

The incidence of CRC increases exponentially as a function of age from 15 to 40 years (Fig. 20.1). Over 90% of CRC cases occur after the age of 50 years and are very unusual in children ≤20 years of age, with an estimated annual incidence of about one case in one million persons less than 20 years old in the United States. It is estimated that CRC accounts for 2.1% of all neoplasms in adolescents and young adults (AYA) between the ages of 15 and 29 years [1]. At St. Jude Children's Research Hospital, where over 20,000 children and adolescents with cancer have been seen since March 1962, 77 children ≤20 years of age have been diagnosed with CRC.

Relative to non-Hispanic whites and Hispanics/Latinos, African Americans/blacks have had a higher incidence of CRC and American Indians/Alaska Native have had a low incidence, differences in racial/ethnic incidence rates that are apparent by age 25 years (Fig. 20.2). Since the 1980s, the age-corrected incidence of CRC has been declining in the United States for adults over the age of 45 years (Fig. 20.3). Below this age, however, there has been no significant change in the incidence (Fig. 20.3).

The distribution by extent of disease at diagnosis did not differ as a function of age at diagnosis (Fig. 20.4). The proportion of patients with distant metastases, or with regional extension plus distant metastases was essentially the same in the age groups evaluated: 60% had regional extension and/or distant metastases.

20.2.2 Etiology

It is thought that, in adults, adenomatous polyps are precursors for the vast majority of CRCs. High fat intake and consumption of red meat and alcohol have been implicated as risk factors for the development of CRC. Use of cyclo-oxygenase-2 inhibitors and diets with increased fiber and calcium are believed to reduce the risk. How these factors contribute to CRC development in patients <20 years old is unknown.

Predisposing risk factors for CRC in AYA include inflammatory bowel disease, prior radiation exposure,

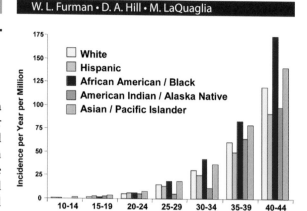

Figure 20.2

Incidence of colorectal carcinoma by race/ethnicity, United States SEER, 1992–2002 [1]

and certain hereditary conditions. Based on familial clustering studies, 20–30% of all CRC cases have a potentially definable inherited cause. However, for the majority of these cases the specific genes remain to be characterized [4]. Well-defined CRC pre-disposition syndromes account for only about 3–5% of all colon cancer and include Peutz-Jeghers syndrome, familial juvenile polyposis, hereditary mixed polyposis syndrome, hereditary non-polyposis colon cancer, and familial adenomatous polyposis [4]. The most common is familial adenomatous polyposis, which is inherited as a dominant trait with 90% penetrance and may be associated with the appearance of multiple cancers by the age of 37 years [5, 6]. Early diagnosis and total colectomy eliminates the risk of development of CRC for these patients. Other syndromes associated with CRC in young people include Turcot's syndrome [7], for which the frequent mutation of the adenomatous polyposis coli gene has been found [8], Oldfield's syndrome [9], and Gardner's syndrome [10]. There may be an association with neurofibromatosis and polyposis coli [11], and one individual with multiple adenomatous polyps and multiple colonic carcinomas had a constitutional deletion of the *p53* gene, also in association with neurofibromatosis [11].

For children and adolescents there is no evidence that a family history of bowel cancer confers a greater risk for the development of CRC before the age of

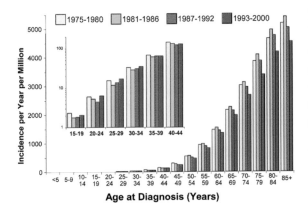

Figure 20.3

Incidence of colorectal carcinoma by era, United States SEER [1]

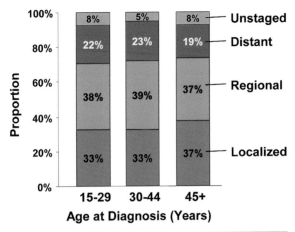

Figure 20.4

Proportion of colorectal carcinoma cases that are localized, have regional extension, or distant metastases at diagnosis, United States SEER, 1975–2000

20 years [12]. The risk for persons younger than 20 years belonging to families with hereditary CRC, cancer family syndromes, or familial juvenile polyposis is unclear. Most do not develop CRC until after the third decade of life. For example, the mean age for CRC development in patients with familial adenomatous polyposis is 39 years [13]. However, colon cancer in children as young as 5 years of age has been reported [14].

20.3 Biology/Pathology

There is extensive literature on the biology of adult CRC. In contrast, little has been published regarding the biology of this tumor in patients less than 21 years of age. As in adults, the histologic types of CRC include gland-forming non-mucinous adenocarcinomas (Fig. 20.5), mucinous adenocarcinomas (tumors in which >50% of the lesion is composed of mucin; Fig. 20.6), and signet-ring-cell carcinomas (tumors in which >50% of cells in the lesion contain intra-cellular mucin; Fig. 20.7). Signet-ring cells can occur within the mucin pools of mucinous adenocarcinoma or as a diffusely infiltrative process with minimal extra-cellular mucin. Well-differentiated neuro-endocrine carcinomas (carcinoid tumors) also occur in this age group, with the majority of colorectal carcinoid tumors occurring in the appendix [15]. Perhaps the most striking difference from adults with CRC is the finding reported by multiple authors of a high prevalence of mucinous tumors in AYA. In adults, mucinous CRC occurs in 2–4% of patients. In AYA, however, the prevalence approaches 50% [16–28]. La Quaglia et al. noted that the incidence of signet-ring carcinoma was 45% in a cohort of 29 patients with CRC who were less than or equal to 21 years of age at diagnosis [29]. Karnak et al. noted a prevalence of mucinous adenocarcinoma in 80% (13 patients of 20 patients reported) [17]. They also described one patient with Bloom's syndrome and another with a family history of colon cancer in this cohort. Rao et al. reported 30 patients seen at St. Jude Children's Research Hospital who were under the age of 30 years at the time of diagnosis and 25 of these had mucinous adenocarcinoma [26].

Mucinous adenocarcinoma has been shown in larger series of adults to be associated with a higher incidence of peritoneal, but not hepatic metastases, and a worse prognosis. Consorti et al., in a case-control study matched for age, sex, location, and Dukes stage, reported that patients with mucinous adenocarcinoma had a worse prognosis compared to those with non-mucinous adenocarcinoma [30]. Secco et al. noted that disease recurrence was more frequent with mucinous or signet-ring carcinomas [31]. They also reported that the 5-year survival rate was 45% for non-mucinous adenocarcinoma of the colorectum compared to 28% for mucinous tumors and 0% for signet-ring tumors. Primary signet-ring carcinomas of the colo-rectum have been associated with a higher percentage of stage III or IV tumors, and an increased frequency of peritoneal seeding, lower rate of hepatic metastases, and lower rate of curative resection when compared to non-signet-ring matched controls in adults [32]. Finally, Sugerbaker et al., in reporting patients with peritoneal carcinomatosis, noted that mucinous histology was an adverse prognostic factor [33].

Datta et al. reported micro-satellite instability (MSI) in 6 out of 13 patients who were under 21 years of age at diagnosis and who had available slides and paraffin blocks for analysis [34]. MSI-positive cancers were not associated with distinct clinical, histological, or familial features compared to MSI-negative cancers. However, MSI-positive cancers did have a significantly lower prevalence of *K-ras* mutation and of loss of heterozygosity (LOH) at 17p or 18q. Subsequent studies of early-onset CRC (unpublished data, Philip Paty laboratory, Memorial Sloane-Kettering Cancer Center) have shown *K-ras* mutation to be a strong prognostic marker associated with increased cancer mortality. In addition, cancers with *K-ras* mutation frequently develop aneuploidy of the *K-ras* locus at 12p21, with gain of the mutant *K-ras* allele and loss of the wild-type allele. The frequency and prognostic significance of these genetic changes in pediatric CRC is of considerable interest.

In summary, MSI status in adults correlates positively with early-age onset, positive family history of colon cancer, right-sided and poorly differentiated tumors, a distinct pattern of molecular genetic alterations (diploidy, low LOH, low prevalence of *K-ras* and *p53* mutations), favorable prognosis, and high risk of metachronous tumors. In a pilot study of 13 children and adolescents, the frequency of MSI was 46% and was associated with a low prevalence of LOH and *K-ras* mutations, but did not correlate with favorable prognosis or other clinicopathologic features. These data suggest that MSI positivity is associated with a unique pattern of molecular genetic development and has a different clinical course in childhood and adolescence.

20.4 Diagnosis: Symptoms and Clinical Signs

The presenting symptoms of AYA with CRC, similar to older adults, are usually non-specific. Rarely is the diagnosis made in an asymptomatic AYA patient. The

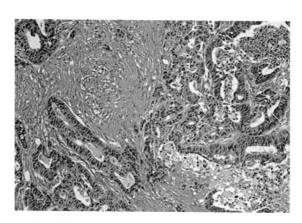

Figure 20.5

Moderately differentiated adenocarcinoma invading into pericolic fat in an adolescent/young adult patient

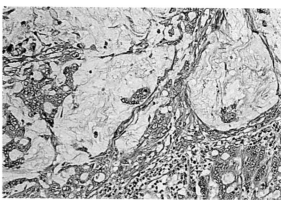

Figure 20.6

Mucinous adenocarcinoma characterized by large pools of blue mucin-containing malignant glands in an adolescent/young adult patient

most common symptom is vague, usually generalized abdominal pain [18, 26, 29, 35, 36]. Localizing abdominal pain is usually an indication of peritoneal involvement or perforation. This pain is occasionally suggestive of appendicitis [35, 37, 38]. Weight loss is relatively common according to our recent review of St. Jude patients in which approximately two-thirds noted weight loss [median loss 20 lbs (9.1 kg); range 5–81 lbs (2.3–36.8 kg)] [39]. Other less frequent associated symptoms include nausea, vomiting, constipation, diarrhea, pallor, anorexia, rectal bleeding, abdominal distension, dysuria, and intestinal obstruction [18, 26, 29]. In one review of 29 patients, 13 presented acutely whereas 16 had more chronic symptomatology [29]. In our experience, the duration of symptoms before diagnosis has ranged from 3 days to 12 months, with a median of 2 months [18]. A mass or fullness may or may not be palpable on physical exam [26, 35, 37]. Primary tumors of the right colon usually present with less symptomatology than do left-sided tumors, probably because the right colon has a larger diameter and a greater liquid content than the left side. Blood in stools or rectal bleeding is almost always associated with left-sided or rectal primaries.

Unfortunately, CRC is rarely thought of in the differential diagnosis of an adolescent with what would be considered "usual" symptoms for this diagnosis in an older patient, such as abdominal pain, change in bowel habits, and anemia. This has resulted in a delay in diagnosis and felt to be at least part of the reason why, according to several authors [36, 38] most AYA patients present with advanced-stage disease.

20.4.1 Staging

Staging is performed following the American Joint Commission on Cancer guidelines [40]. An attempt to assign a pre-operative, post-operative, and pathological stage should be made. This system is depicted in Table 20.1.

20.5 Treatment/Management

Since CRC is so rare in children and young adults, treatment guidelines for these young patients are usually extrapolated from adult trials. A multi-disciplinary approach is essential for managing these complex patients, and early referral to centers that are expert in the care of young patients with cancer will ensure the best possible outcome. Whenever possible, managing these patients on a clinical trial is preferable.

The diagnosis may be suspected when there is a history of cramping abdominal pain, change in bowel habits, unexplained weight loss, or hematochezia. If the diagnosis is suspected, the patient should undergo a flexible colonoscopy to the cecum unless the lesion is completely obstructing. Any intraluminal mass should be sampled via biopsy and notation made of concomitant polyps. If there are only a few polyps these should be removed for histological analysis. Computerized axial tomography of the chest, abdomen, and pelvis with both liver and lung windows should be done to identify peritoneal, or much less frequently hepatic and pulmonary metastases. ^{18}F-fluorodeoxyglucose-positron emission tomography imaging has the potential to detect malignant cells by their increased glucose metabolism, and is felt by many to be the best method for staging CRC in all localities. However, this modality is less useful in patients with mucinous histology, which is the histology seen in a majority of AYA patients. Both intrave-

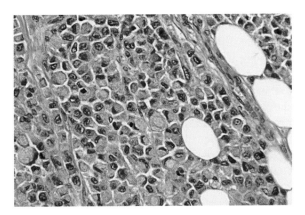

Figure 20.7

Signet-ring-cell carcinoma composed of individually dispersed tumor cells with a single large mucin droplet displacing the nucleus to the edge of the cell in an adolescent/young adult patient

Table 20.1 American Joint Committee on Cancer/International Union Against Cancer (AJCC/UICC) staging system for colorectal cancer [40]

Primary Tumor (T)		Regional Lymph Nodes (N)	
TX	Primary tumor cannot be assessed	NX	Nodes cannot be assessed (e.g., local excision only)
T0	No evidence of tumor in resected specimen (prior polypectomy or fulguration)	N0	No regional node metastases
		N1	1-3 positive nodes
Tis	Carcinoma in situ	N2	4 or more positive nodes
T1	Invades submucosa	N3	Central nodes positive
T2	Invades muscularis propria		
T3–T4	Depends on whether serosa is present	**Distant Metastases (M)**	
	If serosa present: T3 Invades through muscularis propria into subserosa, serosa (but not through), or pericolic fat within the leaves of the mesentery T4 Invades through serosa into free peritoneal cavity or through serosa into a contiguous organ	MX = Presence of distant metastases cannot be assessed M0 = No distant metastases M1 = Distant metastases present	
	If there is no serosa present (as in the distal two thirds rectum, posterior left or right colon): T3 Invades through muscularis propria T4 Invades other organs (vagina, prostate, ureter, kidney)		

nous and intraluminal contrast should be used both for tumor enhancement and identification of normal bowel. Hydronephrosis may be observed because of infiltration around the distal ureters from peritoneal metastases.

There is no specific tumor marker for colorectal adenocarcinoma in this age group, including carcinoembryonic antigen. Abnormalities of liver function tests, especially lactic dehydrogenase, may indicate hepatic involvement. There are no data evaluating use of the carcinoembryonic antigen in follow-up after therapy in AYA.

20.5.1 Surgery

Radical surgery with curative intent is the mainstay of treatment. In fact, if patients cannot be rendered surgically free of disease, they are rarely cured. Resection should follow guidelines established in adults. In particular, primary and secondary draining lymph node echelons should be removed. The basic surgical principles are removal of the major vascular pedicle supplying the tumor along with its lymphatics, and en bloc resection of any organs or structures attached to the tumor. At least a 5-cm margin of normal bowel should be obtained on either side of the tumor to minimize the possibility of an anastomatic recurrence [41]. Adequate lymph node resection is imperative because some patients with stage III tumors are cured by surgery alone. A minimum of 14 negative lymph nodes should be examined to define node-negative disease. The surgeon must also remember that the pattern of spread of mucinous CRC may be intra-peritoneal. Therefore an extensive exploration of the peritoneal surface including that overlying Gerota's fascia and the diaphragm should be undertaken at laparotomy. All peritoneal nodules should be removed if feasible.

If the diagnosis is not made pre-operatively or if the patient is urgently explored for an acute abdomen, and CRC is found, the surgeon should convert the procedure to a standard colon cancer resection with excision of draining lymphatics. This may necessitate closing the original wound (e.g., appendectomy incision) and using a midline approach.

Cases of localized recurrence may benefit from re-excision. Hyperthermic perfusion of the peritoneal cavity after colon resection and peritonectomy has been applied, but only in a few cases. There is not enough data to recommend this approach in all patients.

Unfortunately, in many AYA patients the initial surgery is not done as a cancer operation. In those instances, re-exploration of the abdomen, with the goals of resection of bowel with adequate margins and adequate lymph node sampling should be done at a center experienced with this type of surgery.

20.5.2 Radiation Therapy

The use of radiation therapy in children and young adults with CRC is dependent on the location of the primary disease. In general, radiation reduces the risk of local treatment failure in primary tumors in the rectal area, and occasionally it is useful in inoperable patients with localized disease. The indications for radiation therapy include extension of the tumor to surrounding organs or perforation of the visceral peritoneum (T_4). Radiation has been found to be more effective when given with concurrent continuous-infusion 5-fluorouracil (5-FU).

20.5.3 Adjuvant Chemotherapy

CRC that has been completely resected with adequate lymph node sampling (≥ 14 nodes) and does not invade through the muscularis propria (T_{1S-2}, N_0, M_0; Stage I–II) has an 80–90% overall survival rate when treated with surgery alone. Minimal follow-up recommendations according to the National Comprehensive Cancer Network include: history, physical exam, measurement of carcinoembryonic antigen levels every 3 months for 2 years and then every 6 months for a total of 5 years. Colonoscopy should be done yearly for 2 years and then every 2–3 years thereafter.

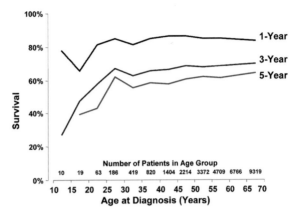

Figure 20.8

One-, 2-, and 5-year relative survival for patients with colorectal carcinoma by age; United States SEER, 1992–1998 [1]. The number of patients in each 5-year age group is listed above the abscissa

For patients whose tumor invades through the muscularis propria or into other organs or has either lymph node or distant metastases (T_{3-4}, N_{1-2}, M_{0-1}; Stage III–IV) adjuvant chemotherapy is necessary. For patients with stage III disease, 6 months of 5-FU and leucovorin (LV) has been standard treatment. Recently, combinations of 5-FU/LV with either irinotecan (FOLFIRI) or oxaliplatin (FOLFOX) have demonstrated improvements in response and survival. In addition, erbitux (cetuximab), a humanized monoclonal antibody against the epidermal growth factor receptor, and avastin (bevacizumab), a monoclonal antibody against the vascular endothelial growth factor have both recently been approved by the Food and Drug Administration for patients with advanced CRC.

20.6 Outcome

The outcome of AYA with CRC, similar to adults with this disease, is dependent on the extent of disease at diagnosis. As illustrated in Fig. 20.8, the overall survival for patients <30 years of age was lower than for older patients during the 1990s, whether the 1-, 2-, or 5-year

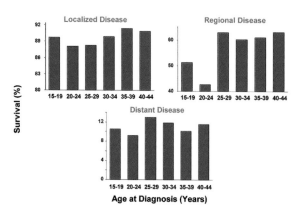

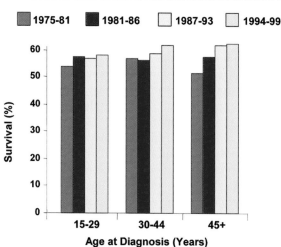

Figure 20.9

Five-year relative survival rate in patients with colorectal carcinoma who were less than 45 years of age at diagnosis, by stage of disease at diagnosis, United States SEER, 1975–2000 [1]

Figure 20.10

Five-year relative survival rate in patients with colorectal carcinoma by era, United States SEER [1]

survival rates are evaluated. For adolescents, the 5-year survival rate was about 40%, as opposed to the 60% rate achieved overall in patients over 30 years of age and regardless of the age group between 30 and 70 years.

The lower survival rate in patients diagnosed before age 30 years is not due to a more advanced stage at diagnosis in this age group as compared to older patients, as shown in Fig. 20.4. When survival rates are assessed within localized, regional, and distant disease presentations, a lower survival rates among 15- to 30-year-olds is apparent in each (Fig. 20.9).

When the 5-year survival rate is assessed by era of diagnosis (Fig. 20.10), the least amount of progress is apparent in patients less than 30 years of age.

The prognosis in younger patients has previously been reported to be dismal [16–19, 37, 42–47]. Explanations for the poor prognosis have included a delay in diagnosis because of its rarity, a greater percentage of patients having more advanced disease at presentation, and unfavorable histologic characteristics. The SEER data do not appear to substantiate the more advanced stage hypothesis. More likely, the different biology in the younger age group, lacking the sequential mutations induced in part by environmental carcinogens and driven more by MSI, are contributing to the worse prognosis.

20.7 Conclusions

CRC in AYA is rare, but of regular occurrence and repeated challenge. Past studies, mostly limited to collections of cases from single institutions, have suggested that AYA patients with CRC do worse in comparison to CRC in adults. This difference is partly explained by a higher frequency of mucinous histology and more advanced stage disease at diagnosis in these younger patients.

CRC in AYA is rare, accounting for about 2% of all neoplasms in patients between the ages of 15 and 29 years of age. Presenting symptoms, similar to adults, are often chronic, vague, and ill defined. Because of the young age, CRC is not considered early enough in the differential diagnosis. In contrast to adults, most of the reported cases in this young age group have mucinous or signet-ring-cell carcinomas. Although most large series suggest that AYA present with more advanced-stage disease, this is not borne out by the SEER data (Fig. 20.4). This discrepancy may be a result of selection bias in patients referred to academic centers and/or cases chosen for literature reports. AYA patients with localized CRC have an excellent prognosis and this diagnosis needs to be considered earlier in patients who present with vague abdominal complaints.

References

1. Bleyer WA, O'Leary M, Barr R, Ries LAG (eds) (2006) Cancer Epidemiology in Older Adolescents and Young Adults 15 to 29 Years of Age, including SEER Incidence and Survival, 1975–2000. National Cancer Institute, NIH Pub. No. 06-5767, Bethesda MD; also available at www.seer.cancer.gov/publications

2. Cancer Facts and Figures 2004. American Cancer Society, Atlanta, GA

3. Heys SD, O'Hanrahan TJ, Brittenden J, Eremin O (1994) Colorectal cancer in young patients: a review of the literature. Eur J Surg Oncol 20:225–231

4. Grady WM (2003) Genetic testing for high-risk colon cancer patients. Gastroenterology 124:1574–1594

5. Houlston RS, Murday V, Harocopos C, et al (1990) Screening and genetic counselling for relatives of patients with colorectal cancer in a family cancer clinic. BMJ 301:366–368

6. Dean PA (1996) Hereditary intestinal polyposis syndromes. Rev Gastroenterol Mex 61:100–111

7. Turcot J, Despres JP, St Pierre F (1959) Malignant tumors of the central nervous system associated with familial polyposis of the colon: report of two cases. Dis Colon Rectum 2:465–468

8. Hamilton SR, Liu B, Parsons RE, et al (1995) The molecular basis of Turcot's syndrome. N Engl J Med 332:839–847

9. Oldfield MC (1954) The association of familial polyposis of the colon with multiple sebaceous cysts. Br J Surg 41:534–541

10. Gardner EJ (1962) Follow-up study of a family group exhibiting dominant inheritance for a syndrome including intestinal polyps, osteomas, fibromas and epidermal cysts. Am J Hum Genet 14:376–390

11. Pratt CB, Jane JA (1991) Multiple colorectal carcinomas, polyposis coli, and neurofibromatosis, followed by multiple glioblastoma multiforme. J Natl Cancer Inst 83:880–881

12. Pratt CB, George SL (1982) Epidemic colon cancer in children and adolescents? In: Correa P, Haenszel W (eds) Epidemiology of Cancer of the Digestive Tract. Martinus Nijhoff, The Hague/Boston/London, pp 127–146

13. Burt RW (2000) Colon cancer screening. Gastroenterology 119:837–853

14. Distante S, Nasioulas S, Somers GR, et al (1996) Familial adenomatous polyposis in a 5 year old child: a clinical, pathological, and molecular genetic study. J Med Genet 33:157–160

15. Spunt SL, Pratt CB, Rao BN, et al (2000) Childhood carcinoid tumors: the St Jude Children's Research Hospital experience. J Pediatr Surg 35:1282–1286

16. Minardi AJ Jr, Sittig KM, Zibari GB, McDonald JC (1998) Colorectal cancer in the young patient. Am Surg 64:849–853

17. Karnak I, Ciftci AO, Senocak ME, Buyukpamukcu N (1999) Colorectal carcinoma in children. J Pediatr Surg 34:1499–1504

18. Odone V, Chang L, Caces J, et al (1982) The natural history of colorectal carcinoma in adolescents. Cancer 49:1716–1720

19. Lamego CM, Torloni H (1989) Colorectal adenocarcinoma in childhood and adolescent. Report of 11 cases and review of the literature. Pediatr Radiol 19:504–508

20. Donaldson MH, Taylor P, Rawitscher R, Sewell JB Jr (1971) Colon carcinoma in childhood. Pediatrics 48:307–312

21. Baughman BB (1969) Carcinoma of the colon in childhood. J Ky Med Assoc 67:895–898

22. Harvey DR, Paradinas FJ (1975) Multiple carcinomas of the large and small bowel in childhood. Postgrad Med J 51:672–676

23. Smith MA, Golding RL, Katz A (1976) Carcinoma of the colon in a child. S Afr Med J 50:879–880

24. Pratt CB, Rivera G, Shanks E, et al (1977) Colorectal carcinoma in adolescents implications regarding etiology. Cancer 40:2464–2472

25. Todani T, Watanabe Y (1982) Rectal carcinoma with a large amount of mucin production in childhood – report of a case. Z Kinderchir 36:73–75

26. Rao BN, Pratt CB, Fleming ID, et al (1985) Colon carcinoma in children and adolescents. A review of 30 cases. Cancer 55:1322–1326

27. Salas E, Urdaneta MT (1985) Cancer of the colon in childhood. Report of 2 cases. G E N 39:248–258

28. Rose RH, Axelrod DM, Aldea PA, Beck AR (1988) Colorectal carcinoma in the young. A case report and review of the literature. Clin Pediatr (Phila) 27:105–108

29. LaQuaglia MP, Heller G, Filippa DA, et al (1992) Prognostic factors and outcome in patients 21 years and under with colorectal carcinoma. J Pediatr Surg 27:1085–1089

30. Consorti F, Lorenzotti A, Midiri G, Di Paola M (2000) Prognostic significance of mucinous carcinoma of colon and rectum: a prospective case-control study. J Surg Oncol 73:70–74

31. Secco GB, Fardelli R, Campora E, et al (1994) Primary mucinous adenocarcinomas and signet-ring cell carcinomas of colon and rectum. Oncology 51:30–34

32. Tung SY, Wu CS, Chen PC (1996) Primary signet ring cell carcinoma of colorectum: an age- and sex-matched controlled study. Am J Gastroenterol 91:2195–2199

33. Sugarbaker PH, Schellinx ME, Chang D, et al (1996) Peritoneal carcinomatosis from adenocarcinoma of the colon. World J Surg 20:585–591

34. Datta RV, Laquaglia MP, Paty PB (2000) Genetic and phenotypic correlates of colorectal cancer in young patients. N Engl J Med 342:137–138

35. Hoerner M (1958) Carcinoma of the colon and rectum in persons under twenty years of age. Am J Surg 96:47–53

36. Karnak I, Ciftci AO, Senocak ME, Buyukpamukcu N (1999) Colorectal carcinoma in children. J Pediatr Surg 34:1499–1504

37. Radhakrishnan CN, Bruce J (2003) Colorectal cancers in children without any predisposing factors. A report of eight cases and review of the literature. Eur J Pediatr Surg 13:66–68

38. Brown RA, Rode H, Millar AJ, Sinclair-Smith C, Cywes S (1992) Colorectal carcinoma in children. J Pediatr Surg 27:919–921

39. Hill D, Rao B, Cain A, et al (2000) Colorectal carcinoma: a clinicopathologic review of 71 cases from St. Jude Children's Research Hospital. Proc Am Soc Clin Oncol 19:2000 (abstract 983)

40. Greene FL, Page DL, Fleming ID, et al (eds) (2002) AJCC Cancer Staging Manual, 6th edn. Springer Verlag New York, NY

41. Rodriguez-Bigas M, Lin EH, Crane CH (2003) Adenocarcinoma of the colon and rectum. In: Kufe D, Pollock R, Weichselbaum R, et al (eds). Cancer Medicine. 2. BC Deck, Hamilton, Ontario, pp 1635–1665

42. Sharma AK, Gupta CR (2001) Colorectal cancer in children: case report and review of literature. Trop Gastroenterol 22:36–39

43. Sebbag G, Lantsberg L, Arish A, et al (1997) Colon carcinoma in the adolescent. Pediatr Surg Int 12:446–448

44. Ferguson E Jr, Obi LJ (1971) Carcinoma of the colon and rectum in patients up to 25 years of age. Am Surg 37:181–189

45. Andersson A, Bergdahl L (1976) Carcinoma of the colon in children: a report of six new cases and a review of the literature. J Pediatr Surg 11:967–971

46. Steinberg JB, Tuggle DW, Postier RG (1988) Adenocarcinoma of the colon in adolescents. Am J Surg 156:460–462

47. Cain AS, Longino LA (1970) Carcinoma of the colon in children. J Pediatr Surg 5:527–532

Models of Care and Specialized Units

Ian Lewis • Sue Morgan

21.1 Introduction

This chapter is based on the premise that services can, and should, be reorganized in such a way as to better meet the many and varied needs of teenagers and young adults with cancer. Cancer in adolescence is relatively rare and yet presents challenging management problems, both medical and psychosocial. The context for proposing change is the perception that traditional models of care are not meeting these needs adequately.

In the United Kingdom, a national charity, the Teenage Cancer Trust (TCT), was set up originally with the explicit aim of championing the needs of teenagers with cancer, principally by promoting the concept of, and providing capital for, specific inpatient facilities. Several such sponsored units have opened in major cancer centers during the past decade, yet there has been limited formal evaluation of these centers, and the concept of such units remains the subject of professional medical controversy [1]. To some extent, controversy exists because evidence has not been sought formally and because some clinicians doubt the need to consider teenagers and young adults as an identifiable and separate group, believing that cancers occurring in this group should be managed within a more traditional model of care.

In this chapter, we examine the case for considering the special needs of teenagers and young adults with cancer. We consider which elements of care should be within a teenage-and-young-adult-specific patient pathway; describe how models and paradigms of care are evolving to meet these needs; address some of the barriers or obstructions to change; and describe how these might be overcome.

21.2 Aims of Care and the Patient Pathway

The aims of care for all patients, irrespective of age at diagnosis or type of cancer, should be to maximize the chance of survival whilst minimizing the physical, psychological, and social cost of survivorship.

In order to achieve this objective, a patient pathway that provides the key elements of diagnosis and treatment must be developed, as exemplified in Fig. 21.1. The first step is the referral process, which, in the United Kingdom, is most commonly from general practitioner to general physician, surgeon, or pediatrician, followed usually by further referral to an oncologist. It is clear that this period should be as short as possible.

The next element is the formal medical evaluation of the patient for histological diagnosis, disease staging, and the assessment of underlying health status, including comorbidity. The following step incorporates the need to inform the patient and family about these findings, to advise and decide on an initial treatment plan, and to discuss entry into a clinical trial if appropriate. This presumes an informed consent process.

Treatment then commences, varying considerably depending on the diagnosis and staging, but for many patients will include one or more of chemotherapy, radiotherapy, or surgery. For some, it may continue for many months or even years. This all demands close collaboration and multidisciplinary teamwork. Patients require a wide range of supportive care that is both medical (to treat or prevent major treatment-related effects) and psychosocial (to help and sustain them and their families through immensely stressful and challenging experiences). At the conclusion of successful treatment, patients embark on appropriate follow up, having completed an end-of-treatment evaluation, proceeding thereafter to assessment and management of any long-term or late effects of treatment. Sadly, treatment might be unsuccessful initially, or disease may recur either during treatment or some time after its completion. Usually patients then require further evaluation of disease status and discussion about a new therapeutic strategy. For many, this will involve further therapy with curative intent but, for some, further treatment will not

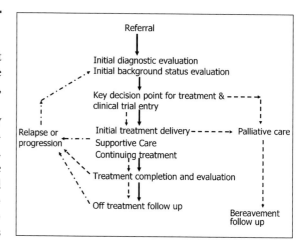

Figure 21.1

Patient pathway – the minimal model

be curative and they embark on a palliative course that may be brief or may last for months or even years.

This path, however, is rudimentary as it provides little detail of the specific requirements for any one patient and needs to be expanded to identify the services that may need to be provided at each of these steps. Pathways for children differ from those for adults, and there are differing pathways for different cancer diagnoses.

21.3 Teenagers and Young Adults Have Special Needs

Working with teenagers and young adults can be both stimulating and challenging. These young people are experiencing a period of life when they are initiating major tasks including establishing their personal identity, experiencing independence, making occupational choices, and developing philosophical and lifestyle options.

Periods of hospitalization and illness may contribute to increased dependence on parents, who quite naturally feel protective and may want to take over care. Reliance on family for financial support and on health-care professionals for treatment contributes to this loss of independence. The effects of chemotherapy, surgery, or radiotherapy will affect identity and self-esteem [2], which, combined with effects on fertility, may also influence the young person's sexual confidence. Peer contact will decrease at a time when peer group acceptance is crucial.

Illness and treatment changes the lifestyle of teenagers. Education can be disrupted and future occupational plans may be changed, either because of therapy or because of a real or perceived threat to life.

21.3.1 What do Young People Say They Need?

In designing and delivering services, it is essential to take the experiences and views of patients and their carers into account. It is imperative that the young people are given a "voice and a choice" in their care, as this helps to inform and underpin everything that is developed for them. Given the opportunity, young people will say what they want from services and those who provide them. They are an interesting, challenging and rewarding group and will "tell it as it is!"

There is an informative, although not extensive, literature that reveals some insights into the concerns of young people with cancer and how their management might be improved. Major elements of the direct cancer experience that concern young people include the possibility of disease recurrence, changes in body image, personal relationships with friends, family or partners, reintegration into education, and job prospects [3–6]. Whilst some issues are cancer specific, others are shared by many young people who do not have cancer. Teenagers and young adults with cancer need to be seen firstly as young people and only then with cancer.

One key element identified in several publications is the requirement for clear, appropriate, and comprehensive information at all stages as this allows for participation and a level of control in decision-making factors that relate positively to self-image and help with adjustment [7–9]. Patients need to be able to make choices for themselves.

The qualities of health professionals that young people favor to communication have been identified [7]. These included the ability to listen and to express concern, professional expertise, and honesty. In contrast, an impersonal manner, excessive jargon, haste, and a perceived generation gap impaired communication.

There are not many studies of young people's views of health services. One study assessed the views of young people about their care [10]. In addition, evidence has been gathered at three TCT-sponsored events held between 2001 and 2004 that have brought together several hundred young people with cancer who have experienced treatment in a range of settings. The views expressed by these young people seem consistent. In ranking those factors deemed to be essential, the most important was to "get better" and a desire to return to normal. A large majority indicated their willingness to travel long distances to get the necessary expertise and environment. Young people want to have treatment directed by professionals expert in their disease, preferably in a specialized center that caters specifically for their age group. To know that they are not the only young persons with cancer can have a very positive impact on their journey, and many strong bonds are formed in the process. Peer support can be vital to self-esteem in the pursuit of normality. This need was followed by the desire to keep up with their education in order to maintain parity with their peers who do not have cancer.

Wherever possible, young people want to be provided with their own space, so that they can mix with their own peer group in an age-appropriate environment and have experienced professionals who can guide them expertly in order to help them with their individual needs [8].

Whenever asked, young people want to be able to access family and friends and, if possible, to be at home or close to home. This desire is outweighed strongly by the willingness to travel to specialized centers if this means that outcome might be improved. Finally, an important factor, which has been identified often but for which evidence is sparse, is the widely expressed perception of significant and avoidable delay in the initial diagnosis and referral. Many young people, particularly those with solid tumors, provide stories of numerous attendances and assessments before referral for investigations leading to a correct diagnosis. This causes them enormous concern, often expressed as "I don't want other people to experience this."

21.4 Developing a Pathway to Meet the Needs of Teenagers and Young Adults

21.4.1 Centralization of Care and Access to Clinical Trials

There appears to be fairly strong evidence from pediatric oncology that centralization of care improves outcome for rare tumors or those requiring complex treatment [11–13]. Further evidence has been published to support the benefits of specialized cancer care in adults [14].

The specific evidence for teenagers and young adults is mixed. Patients with testicular tumors have better outcome with centralized care [15]. In a study of teenagers and young adults with leukemias in the United Kingdom presenting between 1984 and 1994, increased survival over this interval was demonstrated and it did not vary with category of hospital [16]. This study was undertaken before the development of specific Teenage and Young Adult units. In contrast, evidence from the United States of treatment of acute lymphoblastic leukemia [17], and from Germany, of the treatment of Ewing sarcoma [18], suggests that centralized care with an intensive pediatric regimen is better. A study of teenagers and young adults aged 15 to 24 years with cancer in Yorkshire between 1984 and 1994 demonstrated differences in outcome between geographical areas [19]. Whilst the exact reasons are unclear, it is possible that one factor may have been different patterns of care, as patients from the area with the poorest outcome were least likely to be referred to the specialized center. There is also evidence to suggest that centralized care reduces physical late effects. A study of children with Wilms tumor demonstrated that those not treated in specialized centers might be overtreated [20].

There is similar literature to support the contention that patients entered into clinical trials often have higher survival rates, especially for less common cancers. Trial entry has never been found to be associated with lower survival rates [21]. There is therefore some evidence supporting the recommendation that centralized treatment and access to clinical trials should be important elements of care for teenagers and young adults in order to maximize survival.

21.4.2 Improving Psychological, Social, and Educational Support

Psychological, social, and educational outcomes are important factors that must be taken into account when planning services for teenagers and young adults. It is intuitive that these particular outcomes are likely to be improved if teenagers and young adults receive care in an environment designed for young people, where they can meet others of similar age, and where staff are expert in and can focus on the needs of adolescents. However, there is little firm evidence to support this belief and psychosocial outcome studies are needed to compare results of teenagers and young adults treated in different settings. In the absence of clear evidence of better outcome, it would be reasonable to measure benefit by comparing process outcomes between traditional and new models. These should include comparison of rapidity of diagnosis, the clarity and quality of information received, choices about treatment, access to clinical trials, availability of psychological and peer support, facilitation of education, and existence of facilities designed for young people.

21.4.3 Cancer-Specific or Teenagers-and-Young-Adults-Specific Multidisciplinary Teams: is There a Conflict?

In expounding our view of the needs of teenagers and young adults, it is clear that a tension continues to exist between providing centralized care in a unit specializing in a particular malignant disease and in a unit specializing in the care and needs of young people. To some extent, we view this tension as spurious, perpetuated by different factions of health-care professionals. It might be thought that the best solution for young people would be to create an environment that combines these elements to ensure that teenagers and young adults benefit from both. This requires individual clinicians and groups to commit to working in new ways, thereby providing multidisciplinary teams expert in both the specific cancers and the needs of young people.

Whelan uses similar arguments to promote the case that, where possible, the optimal model is a unit designed specifically for young people and staffed by a

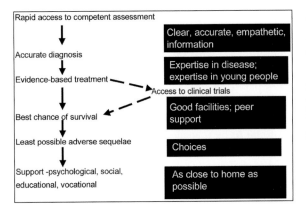

Figure 21.2

Patient pathway – the expanded model

skilled multiprofessional team expert in both the care of teenagers and young adults and their diseases [22].

This is a challenging agenda, given that teenagers and young adults develop a wide range of cancers that encompasses both pediatric and adult types of tumors and that pediatric and adult teams currently have very different ways of working. Adult oncology multidisciplinary teams are "site specific" and shaped by the disciplines required to treat the person with a specific form of cancer. The volume of patients is high and time for individual patients and families at a premium. The pediatric model is somewhat different, having a philosophy of care that is family centered rather than disease centered, and tends to be more holistic in its approach. There is usually a lower volume of patients, thus allowing more time for team meetings and reflective practice.

Nevertheless, bringing those from pediatric and adult backgrounds together to form a Teenage and Young Adult multidisciplinary team should be a core aim if teenagers and young adults are to have their needs for disease-related expertise and psychosocial support met appropriately. This should be a place for referrals, discussion and dissemination of knowledge, identifying patterns of care, and should become the focus for developing a local database concentrating on this age range. The Teenage and Young Adult multidisciplinary team needs to develop close relationships with several site-specific teams so that additional expertise can be harnessed for the benefit of patients.

This provides an opportunity to develop a forum for discussing the many ethical issues and treatment controversies that occur in these patients.

What should emerge eventually is a single, equitable model of delivery of care, tailor-made to these young patients and their family/carers, allowing equal access to expert diagnostic, treatment, and support services regardless of their disease or referring physician.

21.4.4 What Might a Single Pathway for Teenagers and Young Adults Look Like?

Currently there is little predictable in the experiences of teenagers and young adults with cancer and many elements of chance in any one patient's journey. A pathway should be evidenced-based if possible and take into account the expressed wishes and experience of those undertaking the journey. Figure 21.2 is an attempt to unify these factors into a single pathway based on the input of young people and incorporating competencies and requirements rather than particular places, people, or professional interest groups.

The first element of this pathway identifies the need for early diagnosis. This imposes responsibility on young people themselves to learn how to recognize symptoms or signs of concern and then seek appropriate professional help or advice. It demands also that health-care professionals listen to young people and make early referrals for specialized assessment. Examples of these circumstances include increasing public awareness amongst young men of the importance of testicular self-examination, and providing evidence that patients are being referred rapidly from primary or secondary care to specialized cancer services with a reduction in time from initial symptoms to commencing treatment.

Much of the rest of the pathway might appear self evident, yet the evidence from the literature, and reports of many young people's personal experiences, tell a very different story.

As outlined earlier in this chapter, young people find themselves managed by a wide range of medical teams, many of whom have little understanding of their needs. Both in the United States [23] and in the United Kingdom, only a minority appear to be given the opportunity to participate in clinical trials.

For many patients it is not known if late effects of therapy are taken into account appropriately when treatment is planned. It is recognized, however, that many young people report not having adequate information about fertility risks at the time of starting treatment and many "adult" treatment protocols pay little regard to cardiac, renal, and audiological toxicity monitoring.

Many young people report not being encouraged to continue with their education through treatment and are sometimes actively discouraged by well-meaning professionals. In addition, there are often less than adequate resources available to "adult" teams to provide the level of psychological and social support needs of teenagers and young adults.

It is perhaps for these reasons that there has been such strong pressure for and movement towards providing specialized facilities and health-care teams. Young people need to be offered the opportunities to choose, if they wish, to have their management coordinated by a professional team that is expert in young people and in the cancers from which they suffer. They should have access to a team that has developed age- and developmentally appropriate methods of communication, and which can provide necessary support. They should be able to undergo treatment in facilities that meet their very particular needs where they can meet other young people similarly affected, and where the needs of parents, partners, family, and friends can also be addressed. They should be given the opportunity to spend as much time as possible at home, or close to home, whilst still receiving the benefit of expert supervision and access to clinical trials.

21.5 An Action Plan For Teenagers and Young Adults With Cancer

In the United Kingdom there is formal recognition by government and professional organizations that adolescents have special health needs [24–26]. There have been similar formal recommendations specifically for young people with cancer with the Expert Advisory Group in Cancer to the Chief Medical Officers of England and Wales recognizing these needs and recommending the formation of specialized units for adolescents [27].

Despite this strong recommendation, there was, and remains, little understanding in the health-care community of what this might mean and how to proceed. The original focus, as proposed by the TCT, was for separate facilities and the provision of physical areas or units for young people within institutions, with the idea that teenagers and young adults would continue to be managed by their current health-care teams. There was no broad recognition that staff might need special training or development in order to meet the particular needs of teenagers and young adults with cancer, or that it might be necessary to develop specialized teams.

For those who set out on this path, the best hope of success appeared to lie in encouraging pediatric and adult disciplines to work together. There were threats to many entrenched beliefs and ways of working. Developing services for teenagers and young adults with cancer has been challenging and fraught with difficulties, most obviously inertia, or even obstruction, from professional colleagues, financial constraints within institutions, and a lack of understanding by commissioners of healthcare of the need for change. Despite these barriers, there has been a notable change in the climate such that this agenda is moving forward at a reasonable pace into a slightly less chilly, and at times even warm, atmosphere.

21.5.1 Past and Current Practice

In discussing how far we have moved down the road toward an ideal pathway for all teenagers and young adults with cancer, it will help to describe factors that influence current practice. These include patterns of how, where, and by whom teenagers and young adults are treated at present. This focuses largely on practice in the United Kingdom, where it is apparent that teenagers were, and are still, subject to a lottery in which decisions about referrals and patterns of care have developed in an apparently ad hoc manner.

21.5.2 Patterns of Care

These vary for different ages and diagnoses and are depicted pictorially for several diagnostic categories in Fig. 21.3.

21.5.2.1 Patients under 15 Years of Age

In the United Kingdom, nearly all children and young people below 15 years of age are now referred to one of the 22 major United Kingdom Children's Cancer Study Group (UKCCSG) pediatric oncology centers for management. This has been a progressive change. Prior to the mid-1970s, when pediatric oncology began to be recognized as a separate specialty, most children received their treatment locally, under the care of general pediatricians or surgeons. Following the establishment of children's cancer centers, there was a rapid change in referral patterns such that, by the early 1980s, the majority of children aged 0–9 years were treated centrally.

Interestingly, it took up to a decade longer before the majority of young adolescents aged 10–14 years achieved similarly high referral rates to children's cancer centers. As an example, in the period 1992–1994, only 58% of those aged 13 to 14 years and 73% of those aged 10 to 12 years were registered with UKCCSG centers, compared to 85% of those aged 0–9 years. Although never formally analyzed, it is now accepted that, during this time, adult specialists were treating many young teenagers in adult settings. There was only gradual and sometimes grudging acceptance by these specialists that young people would gain benefit from being treated in an environment more generally designed for them, where staff were more likely to understand their developmental, psychological, educational, and social needs. Perhaps more importantly, pediatric oncology centers and teams also became more expert in treating those cancers occurring most commonly in this age group and providing patients with access to appropriate clinical trials.

21.5.2.2 Patients Aged 15 to 19 Years

Pediatric Oncology Teams

Throughout the past 20 years, there has been a small but increasing number of young people over the age of 15 years managed by pediatric oncology teams. This group can be divided largely into three.

The first consists of patients diagnosed before the age of 15 years and treated in a children's cancer center,

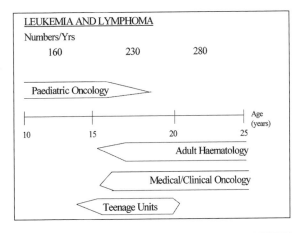

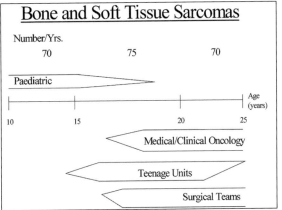

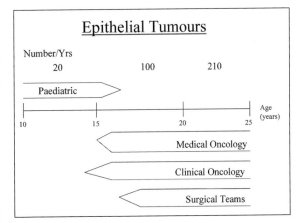

Figure 21.3

Current patterns of care. *Number/Yrs* refers to approximate number of expected cases in the United Kingdom by 5-year age band

who suffered a relapse as an older teenager or young adult. These young people and their families often request treatment in a familiar environment by the team known to, and trusted by, them.

The second group is made up of patients over 15 years newly diagnosed with cancers deemed to be "pediatric" in nature, most commonly bone sarcomas, acute lymphoblastic leukemia, or the rarer diagnoses in this age group of embryonal tumors.

The third group comprises patients aged over 15 years but deemed to have "pediatric" needs. In some geographical areas, formal service guidance has included the requirement that patients of 16 years, or in full-time secondary education, be treated in a children's setting. Elsewhere, the direction of referral has been determined by the referring clinician. The reasons given why older teenagers are referred to pediatric centers vary, but are often accompanied by a perception that the young person is relatively immature. This can be determined often by the size of the young person – a 6-foot-tall 15-year-old boy being thought capable of receiving treatment in an adult environment whilst a 5.5-foot-tall 17-year-old might be deemed to be treated more appropriately within a children's service. The direction of referral often takes place without any structured assessment of educational capability or social support mechanisms, although the numbers in this age group referred to pediatric teams have been small. In 1995, less than 100 young people of 15 years or over were registered as being treated at UKCCSG centers. Since then the number registered has increased but, as there has been also a growth in the number of units designed specifically for teenagers during this time period, it is not possible to disentangle those referred to children's teams from those referred to Teenage and Young Adult units that happen to be colocated with pediatric oncology units.

Adult Oncology Teams

The majority of young people over 15 years continue to be managed by teams whose work is mostly with older adults. This is often determined by the pathological diagnosis, but a range of factors, some of them more rational than others, have determined the team taking the lead in treating young people.

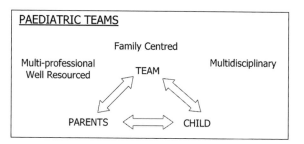

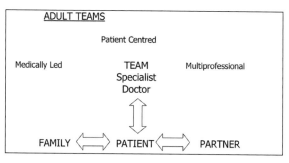

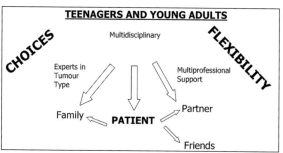

Figure 21.4
Paradigms of care

As an example, a young person with a lymphoma may be referred to and treated by a variety of teams. Most patients with lymphoma are managed by clinical hematology teams, but a substantial number are managed by medical oncology teams, depending on the setting or personal interest of the clinicians involved. The type of team can vary between, or even within, individual hospitals. Many young people are referred to major cancer centers, but a large number continue to be managed in more local settings where a teenager with cancer is a relative rarity.

Adult teams treat most young people with sarcomas or germ-cell tumors, although patterns of care vary. The adult oncology community has demonstrated clearly the value of centralized treatment for testicular tumors in young men [15] and nowadays, structured multidisciplinary teams within cancer centers manage the majority. In contrast, many young women with ovarian tumors are managed by predominantly surgical gynecological teams, often in district hospitals.

There is a similar pattern for sarcomas. In England and Wales, the majority of young people with bone sarcomas have their diagnostic and definitive surgery in one of two specialized surgical centers, with adjuvant chemotherapy delivered in pediatric, medical, or clinical oncology settings, usually in cancer centers. In contrast, soft-tissue sarcomas are often investigated initially and treated in district hospital settings by surgical teams. They may be seen in cancer centers or by specialized teams only if deemed to be more complex or if disease recurs.

Epithelial tumors appear to be managed mainly in local units. In a study of patterns of referral for young people aged 15–23 years in Yorkshire (United Kingdom), only a small proportion were treated in a hospital not in their own district [28]. This implied that only the minority of carcinomas were referred to specialized centers. Nasopharyngeal cancer and breast cancers were referred more frequently than other epithelial cancers, reflecting the importance of radiotherapy in accepted management. There is little evidence in the literature to suggest that patterns of care have changed significantly in more recent years.

21.5.2.3 Patients Aged 20 Years and Over

Treatment for young people over 20 years is generally very similar to that observed in those aged 15–19 years, with the majority being managed in adult units and with very few, if any, being managed in children's services. There is a perception that a small but increasing number of young people under 30 years old are being managed in Teenage and Young Adult Units.

21.5.3 Paradigms of Care, Communication, and Interaction

There are quite marked differences in how teams from differing disciplines interact with patients, and these can have a notable effect on how relationships and trust develop between young people, their families or partners, and the professional teams. These differences are illustrated in Fig. 21.4.

21.5.3.1 Children's Teams

Pediatric professionals work within the classic triad of professionals, parents, and patient. Clearly, very young children are not able to express complicated ideas verbally and, whilst they can be enormously expressive in several ways, most of the complex discussion and decision-making tends to take place between professionals and parents or carers. Pediatricians and children's nurses are trained to observe and listen to children so that some assessment of their views can be made. As children get older, their contribution to decision-making becomes more apparent, although decisions and discussions remain an intricate process in which parents' views tend to predominate.

Pediatric oncology teams have been relatively well resourced, with a high staff:patient ratio. A culture of multidisciplinary and multiprofessional working has become embedded into practice, which should be family-centered in approach. It is axiomatic that this approach combined with extensive multicenter, national, and international collaboration in the development of clinical trials and other studies, has been the reason why advances have been incorporated rapidly into pediatric oncology practice, thereby improving patient outcomes.

21.5.3.2 Adult Teams

Professionals working with adults who have cancer tend to work within a more classical medical model of a lead doctor interacting directly with the patient. This doctor–patient relationship is at the core of practice and is based on confidentiality and consent. The patient rather than the family is at the center of this particular care paradigm and other family members or partners interact with the professional team largely through the consent of the patient. Medical, clinical, and hematological oncology practice tends to be strongly medically led with other professionals providing a supporting role. Historically much of the focus of adult teams has been on older patients and there is much logic in this as the number of older patients who develop cancer is large. The emphasis has been often on treating with largely palliative intent whilst paying particular attention to unwanted acute side effects.

In contrast to pediatric oncology, resources have been more stretched and staff/patient ratios smaller. This implies less time for complex interaction and less reliance on professional support. The proportion of patients entered into multi-center clinical trials is much lower, although increasing this number in adults with malignant disease is a key objective of the National Cancer Research Institute and Network.

21.5.3.3 Teenage and Young Adult Teams

Patterns for teenagers and young adults with cancer are really only just emerging but the evidence base is starting to increase. It is clear that teenagers and young adults do not fit easily into either of the classic pediatric or adult paradigms of interaction.

Cancer nearly always interferes with normal physical and psychosocial developmental processes of young people. It is paramount, therefore, that professionals dealing with teenagers and young adults develop knowledge of and sensitivity to such issues, whilst recognizing that considerable flexibility is required to meet the needs of each individual.

This requires an approach that utilizes elements of both classic pediatric and adult models. Professionals should interact predominantly with the patient. They should, however, be sensitive to the needs and wishes of each individual and actively encourage patients to be accompanied and supported. For younger teenagers this is virtually always by parents, legal carers, or other family members, but for older teenagers or young adults it could be partners, friends or any combination of these. It is not uncommon to have a number of people accompanying teenagers and young adults with cancer. Individual choices can also change. The 14 year old who comes accompanied by her parents and who defers largely to their wishes may well develop into the 18 year old who brings her boyfriend and who may wish to override the advice of all around her. At 20, however, she may wish her parents to come as well, and also take and listen to advice from those around her. This demands an approach

that is both flexible and offers choices. It is almost impossible for this to be feasible without an extensive multi-professional and multi-disciplinary team.

Typically, patients in the teenage and young adult group have a much lower rate of entry into clinical trials than children. This reality is likely to be multi-factorial, but one important factor has been the perceived 'difficulty' of engaging young people in complex discussion. There is no fundamental reason for thinking that teenagers and young adults are less likely to consent to clinical trials than patients in any other age group.

21.5.3.4 Teenage and Young Adult Units and Teams

The first unit identified specifically as being for adolescents with cancer is sited at the Middlesex Hospital in London. This 10-bedded facility was opened in 1990 and focused predominantly on the care of young people with bone sarcomas [29]. Since then other units have opened, each reflecting local influences that have determined which cancers are managed within or outside of them and which clinicians are involved primarily in the care of patients.

Some of these Teenage and Young Adult units opened as an adjunct to the local adult oncology facility, whilst others have developed predominantly as an adjunct to pediatric oncology services. It has been less common for units to be developed by joint collaboration between adult and pediatric oncology teams but examples of this do exist.

Most of these units started with a combination of professional goodwill and charitable support. Funding from formal National Health Service sources has been sporadic, dependent upon local champions harnessing evidence and sympathetic commissioners of healthcare being prepared to listen. As a result there has been no standard package of funding nor pattern of development. Some units continue to exist because staff expanded their roles voluntarily from their original remit whilst others have had varying degrees of specific funding which may have included nursing staff, medical staff and other support staff.

The impetus for formation of these units has come from a combination of professional awareness, patient pressure, and lobbying by the voluntary sector. Despite notable successes to date, it is worth pointing out that it is still only the minority of cancer centers in the UK that have any specific facilities for young people. Even where these do exist, there is often disagreement between different groups of professionals about the value of such units. It seems that clinical hematologists are the medical professional group that has the most difficulty with the concept of managing young people within age-specific facilities.

When Teenage and Young Adult units were first created, the emphasis was on external appearances, albeit as a means of improving care and providing peer support. The need for bright and cheerful surroundings was paramount, with elements of "home" such as a sitting room with sofas to lie down on, a kitchen area to make drinks and snacks, and teenage-friendly facilities including TVs, pool table, DVD player, and computers with Internet access. These were to be places where their friends and family could visit without embarrassment, to provide an environment that enabled them to maintain a sense of normality and continuation of their lives. As these units have taken shape over the last 10 years, it has become apparent to those caring for this group of patients that the work is challenging and demands special skills. This has led to increasing numbers of staff either being appointed specifically to Teenage and Young Adult units or changing their roles to provide a greater proportion of time to this service. Expertise has been developing in both the management of the particular cancers experienced by teenagers and young adults and in their specific supportive care and psychosocial needs.

21.5.3.5 Virtual Units and Peripatetic Teams

In the absence of specific facilities it has been possible, nevertheless, to develop some services for young people by offering a "service without walls." Examples exist where specialized psychosocial support and expertise can be offered to the teenagers and young adults as a peripatetic service. In our own service in Leeds (United Kingdom), a team of professionals (i.e., nurse, social worker, learning mentor, and youth worker) can help provide some elements of care to those young people who cannot, for whatever reason, be cared for within the confines of our inpatient facility. The team works alongside, not instead of, the specialized hospital-based teams. Patients and their families can be visited at home, in their local hospital, or at work/school, and can have access to a system that offers advice, support, disease and treatment expertise, and a base for them to contact at any time, for any reason. The inclusion of a youth worker in this team facilitates patients' access to a network of other young people with cancer and overcomes some of the isolation they experience. Virtual units can become the foundation of definitive units, as the former have the capability of defining and, to a certain extent, quantifying the need for future developments.

There is a national review taking place currently of services for children and young people with cancer by the National Institute of Clinical Excellence, which is aimed at producing firm guidance to commissioners of healthcare by July 2005. This guidance encompasses those aged up to their mid-20s (www.nice.org.uk child and adolescent cancer).

Interestingly, whilst the United Kingdom may have taken the lead in developing adolescent cancer units, units are now being developed in several other countries including Australia and France.

21.6 Conclusions

In this chapter we have demonstrated ways in which services could be reorganized to meet the needs of the teenager or young adult with cancer. The path that will lead to the implementation of such developments is not a particularly easy one to take, and many obstacles may be placed in the way of establishing such best practice for this specific, separate group. However, we recommend that this does not deter those professionals who both understand the need and are in a position to influence change.

All-too-often, services have evolved in an unplanned way, with the result that these appear to serve the needs and predilections of professionals rather than consumers who then have to try to fit in. We believe it is feasible to outline a single generic pathway for teenagers and young adults with cancer that will require tailoring for each individual's specific disease and personal circumstances. We believe that this will provide optimal care for young people and is worth striving for, but we know that it will happen only when the grip of professional ownership is loosened and the needs of young people are addressed as the primary concern.

References

1. Lewis IJ (1996) Cancer in adolescence. Br Med Bull 52:887–897
2. Thompson J (1988) Adolescents with cancer. In: Tiffany R, Webb H (eds) Oncology for Nurses and Health Care Professionals, vol 2. Harper and Row, London, pp 254–261
3. Eiser C (1996) The impact of treatment: adolescents' views. In: Selby P, Bailey C (eds) Cancer and the Adolescent. BMJ Publishing, London, pp 264–275
4. Lynam MJ (1990) Examining support in context: a redefinition from the cancer patient's perspective. Sociol Health Ill 12:169–194
5. Pendley JS, Dahlquist LM, Dreyer ZA (1997) Body image and psychosocial adjustment in adolescent cancer survivors. J Pediatr Psychol 22:29–43
6. Roberts CS, Severinsen C, Carraway C, et al (1997) Life changes and problems experienced by young adults with cancer. J Psychol Oncol 15:15–25
7. Dunsmore J, Quine S (1995) Information, support and decision making needs and preferences of adolescents with cancer: implications for health professionals. J Psychosocial Oncol 13:39–56
8. Evans M (1996) Interacting with teenagers with cancer. In: Selby P, Bailey C (eds) Cancer and the Adolescent. BMJ Publishing, London, pp 251–263
9. Jamison RN, Lewis S, Burish TG (1986) Psychological impact of cancer on adolescents: self-image, locus of control, perception of illness and knowledge of cancer. J Chron Dis 39:609–617
10. Wilkinson J (2003) Young people with cancer – how should their care be organised? Eur J Cancer Care 12:65–70
11. Peppercorn JM, Weeks JC, Cook EF, Joffe S (2004) Comparison of outcomes in cancer patients treated within and outside clinical trials: conceptual framework and structured review. Lancet 363:263–270
12. Stiller CA (1988) Centralisation of treatment and survival rates for cancer. Arch Dis Child 63:23–30
13. Stiller CA (1994) Centralised treatment, entry to trials and survival. Br J Cancer 70:352–362
14. Selby P, Gillis C, Haward R (1996) Benefits from specialised cancer care. Lancet 348:313–318
15. Harding PJ, Paul J, Gillis CR, Kaye SB (1993) Management of malignant teratoma: does referral to specialist units matter? Lancet 341:999–1002
16. Stiller CA, Benjamin S, Cartwright RA, et al. (1999) Pattern of care and survival for adolescents and young adults with acute leukaemia – a population based study. Br J Cancer 79:658–665
17. Nachman J, Sather HN, Buckley JD, et al. (1993) Young adults 16–21 years of age at diagnosis entered on Childrens Cancer Group acute lymphoblastic leukemia and acute myeloblastic leukemia protocols. Results of treatment. Cancer 7:3377–3385
18. Paulussen M, Ahrens S, Juergens HF (2003) Cure rates in Ewing tumor patients aged over 15 years are better in pediatric oncology units. Results of GPOH CESS/EICESS studies. Proc Am Soc Clin Oncol 22:816 (abstract 3279)
19. Wilkinson JR, Feltbower RG, Lewis IJ, et al (2001) Survival from adolescent cancer in Yorkshire, UK. Eur J Cancer 37:903–911
20. Pritchard J, Stiller CA, Lennox EL (1989) Overtreatment of children with Wilms' tumour outside paediatric oncology centres. BMJ 299:835–836
21. Stiller C (2002) Epidemiology of cancer in adolescents. Med Pediatr Oncol 39:149–155
22. Whelan J (2003) Where should teenagers with cancer be treated? Eur J Cancer 39:2573–2578
23. Bleyer WA (2002) Cancer in older adolescents and young adults: epidemiology, diagnosis, treatment, survival, and importance of clinical trials. Med Pediatr Oncol 38:1–10
24. Department of Health (1991) Welfare of Children and Young People in Hospital. Department of Health, London
25. Department of Health (2003) The National Service Framework for Children, Young People and Maternity Services. First Module – Standard for Hospital Services. Department of Health, London
27. Department of Health (1995) A Policy Framework for Commissioning Cancer Services. A report by the Expert Advisory Group on Cancer to the Chief Medical Officer of England and Wales. Department of Health, London
26. Royal College of Paediatrics and Child Health (2003) Bridging the Gap: Health Care for Adolescents. The Intercollegiate Working Party on Adolescent Health, London
28. Selby P, Rider L, Joslin C, Bailey C (1996) Epithelial cancer. In: Selby P, Bailey C (eds) Cancer and the Adolescent. BMJ Publishing, London, pp 39–53
29. Souhami RL, Whelan J, McCarthy JF, Kilby A (1996) Benefits and problems of an adolescent cancer unit. In: Selby P, Bailey C (eds) Cancer and the Adolescent. BMJ Publishing, London, pp 276–283

Drug Compliance by Adolescent and Young Adult Cancer Patients: Challenges for the Physician

Benjamin Gesundheit • Mark L. Greenberg •
Reuven Or • Gideon Koren

Contents

22.1 Introduction

The terms *compliance* and *adherence* describe the behavior of following advice or instructions, and these terms are used interchangeably. In the medical context, compliance refers mostly to drug intake, but may also include adherence to diet, lifestyle, and other therapeutic modalities including medical follow-up. Noncompliance can be manifested as failure to fill the prescription, failure to take the prescribed drug, and incorrect frequency, timing, or dosage of drug administration. Correctly defined, misunderstanding the instructions of the health-care provider does not constitute noncompliance, but since this reason is raised frequently by the patient, a striking lack of understanding may reflect an underlying problem of noncompliance. Likewise, refusal of treatment might be considered as noncompliance at its extreme, as the case of the 13-year-old boy Tyrell Dueck, who refused treatment for osteosarcoma [1], even though the total lack of agreement to accept any treatment is a different issue.

Compliance may imply acceptance and accommodation to a dominant force (i.e., the physician dictates and the patient accepts). In the current climate of practice, however, the treatment process is ideally a partnership between the patient and the health-care providers, and therefore, compliance has to be redefined as an agreement between the patient and his health-care providers to restore or maintain the patient's health [2]. The best definition for compliance is the extent to which the patient's behavior coincides with medical or health advice [3–4].

Lack of compliance transcends the boundaries of disease categories and age groups. The number of research articles on patient compliance increased from 15 per year in the mid-1970s to more than 100 per year in recent years [5]. Although an abundance of literature is available on compliance issues in the adult cancer patient, little research exists on compliance of children [6, 7], and particularly of adolescents with cancer [8, 9].

The clinical implications of poor drug compliance are enormous. Noncompliance with oral chemotherapy may play a role in the long-term prognosis of childhood leukemia [10, 11], in the relapse rate [12–14], and in the graft survival after transplantation [15]. The prednisone nonadherence rate in adolescents and young adults with acute lymphoblastic leukemia (ALL) or Hodgkin disease was 52% according to the measured drug levels [12, 16]. The noncompliance in adolescent outpatients with cancer was 59% [11]. In a study of compliance using blood levels of 6-mercaptopurine in children with ALL, one-third of patients had undetectable levels of drug [14, 17]. The rate of compliance in pediatric and adolescent patients with cancer ranges from 40 to 60% [9]. With the advent of more successful treatment for childhood and adolescent cancer, the compliance factor is gaining greater importance because therapy is given currently with curative, rather than only palliative intent.

Thus, the implications of poor drug compliance by teenagers with cancer are enormous, and preventing this major factor of therapeutic failure is a paramount challenge for clinicians. Furthermore, the compliance of physicians and their prescription pattern of maintenance chemotherapy in ALL may contribute substantially to the success or failure of treatment, and improved physicians' compliance may improve the prognosis of the disease [18]. In order to understand the behavior of drug compliance, it is important to realize that for the adolescent with cancer, very often it is not survival of the disease in the future, but rather survival of the treatment in the present that is crucial [19].

Strict adherence to chemotherapeutic protocols is essential to secure optimal outcome. In clinical trials, noncompliance may lead to an overestimation of required dosage and may lead to significant toxicity

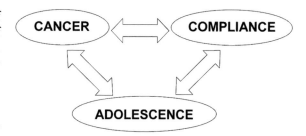

Figure 22.1
Cancer, adolescence, and compliance

and morbidity if drug dosage is increased because of perceived lack of response, or if the compliance of a patient suddenly improves. Drug noncompliance may obscure the actual rate of adverse reactions and may lead to a waste of resources. The availability of venous access ports and easy-to-operate pumps make the administration of parenteral chemotherapy at home ("home care") possible, but this introduces a new dimension to the issue of noncompliance.

22.1.1 Compliance: Definition and History, Cultural Changes During the Last 50 Years

Historically, Hippocrates (470–410 BCE, Greece) expressed in his famous oath his concerns about patients' noncompliance: "Keep watch also on the fault of patients which often make them lie about the taking of things prescribed" [20, 21]. Compliance with drug therapy for acute diseases and symptoms is often better than for chronic diseases [22]. Along with these therapeutic goals, social and legal changes of rights and the autonomy of the patient have caused major changes in the patient–physician relationship (PPR). The involvement of the patient and his consent for treatment is crucial, and nowadays no therapeutic modality is conceivable without the full cooperation of the patient.

Research on compliance focused initially on noncompliers and on the reasons for failure to adhere to instructions about medication given by patients: inadequate supply of medication, forgetfulness, misunderstanding of instructions, errors, discontinuation of treatment because symptoms have cleared, resistance

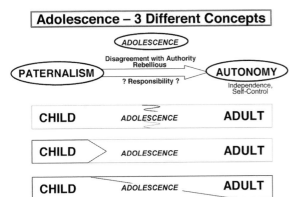

Figure 22.2

Childhood, adolescence and adulthood – three different approaches

22.2.1.1 Cancer and Adolescence

Cancer is very often the first personal encounter of the adolescent with death. The diagnosis of cancer and its treatment cause loss of control and increased dependency, when parents and physicians tend to protect the patient from facing the risks of morbidity and mortality. This situation may interfere with normal psychological development during adolescence.

The unclear line of responsibilities regarding the administration of drugs in the adolescent age group affects drug compliance [8, 26]. Parents of adolescents tend to be too optimistic regarding the compliance of their adolescent children with oral chemotherapy [27]. Adolescents have been described both as "abusers of nonprescribed drugs" and as "nonusers of prescribed drugs." Scare techniques also have been found to be rarely effective [28].

of the child, apparent ineffectiveness of the medication, or side effects [23]. More recently, research has aimed to identify the risk factors and predictors of noncompliance by more objective measures.

22.2 Conclusions

22.2.1 Cancer, Compliance, and Adolescence: Definitions and Interactions

The diagnosis of cancer has major effects on the patient's life. The fear of death and the severe adverse effects of treatment cause major stress for the patient and his family. The patient is often discouraged and copes suboptimally with his diagnosis and the aggressive treatment (Fig. 22.1).

Adolescence is commonly defined as the age range between 11 and 20 years, 12 and 19 years, or 13 and 25 years. Others define adolescence as a stage between childhood and adulthood, or as an overlap of both childhood and adulthood (Fig. 22.2). Adolescence has been described as a period of life characterized by "sturm and strife", rebellious behavior, and disagreement with parents and other authority figures [24]. Adolescence entails a process of growth and development when the healthy individual gains more control and independence [25].

22.3 Assessment of Compliance

Identification of noncompliance is important in explaining the absence of a therapeutic response, targeting individuals for intensive intervention, and the selection of appropriate compliance-improving strategies. Unfortunately, poor compliance is difficult to anticipate because of the lack of clear factors that predict which children will be compliant. Moreover, this assessment must include parents and other family members, which may complicate the process. Once lack of drug compliance is suspected, factors associated with noncompliance or patients at risk for noncompliance should be identified and targeted for intervention.

Both indirect and direct methods have been used to identify and monitor patients' compliance (Table 22.1), with advantages and shortcomings for each technique. Measurement of compliance over a short period of time may not reflect long-term patterns [29] and methods used for research purposes may not be practical for routine clinical use. An individualized approach should be chosen for each patient according to the conditions, personality of the patient, and the healthcare providers. A combination of different techniques, particularly direct and indirect methods, might be particularly useful. Compliance studies using patients' and parents' questionnaires have demonstrated a rather high correlation with objectively measured compliance [30]. In adolescents with cancer, a strong correlation was found between subjectively reported compliance and the blood levels of medication [9].

22.3.1 Indirect Methods

Reports from patients and parents as to whether drugs are being administered are a valuable and practical way to get a first impression in clinical practice. Questioning patients per se tends to increase adherence by serving as a reminder to take the medication [31]. Therefore, interviews on drug compliance may serve as an effective intervention [9]. Self-reports of noncompliance are often more accurate than self-reports of compliance [32]. The questions used in such investigations should be nonthreatening and nonjudgmental.

Written reports, diaries, and questionnaires, in which patients or family members record drug intake, may be helpful in obtaining more accurate data from the patient in order to monitor drug compliance.

Pill counts may document a discrepancy between the number prescribed and/or reported to be taken and the number of remaining pills. The value of this method may be limited in clinical practice, because patients may not always bring their medications to the clinic visit and drugs could have been vomited, spilled, or spit out [31]. In addition, patients may intentionally discard unused medications; this is known as the "parking-lot effect," or "pill dumping effect" [33].

Physicians tend to overestimate drug compliance [34]. Noncompliance is often suspected with treatment failure, but clinical outcome or absence of side effects cannot be used as reliable indications of noncompliance, since the disease does not always respond to the treatment [6] and side effects do not always correlate with drug intake.

22.3.2 Direct Methods

When noncompliance is suspected on clinical grounds, direct methods to assess compliance may be useful. These include measurement of drug levels in the blood or urine [11] and specific tracers added to the drug for better monitoring [31]. However, this information typically reflects only recent ingestion of the drug and patients may alter their compliance just prior to the test [35].

The leukocyte count may serve as a surrogate marker for the oral intake of 6-mercaptopurine, as may the clinical and hematological side effects of steroids. Yet there is not necessarily a linear correlation between the clinical or laboratory effects and the amount of drug ingested.

Recently, various microelectronic automated devices such as the Medication Event Monitoring System (MEMS, Aprex Corporation, Fremont, California) offer a major advantage to monitor compliance [36, 37], particularly in noncooperative patients [38]. Microprocessors in the cap of these standard drug containers record every bottle opening as a presumptive dose. MEMS can monitor compliance over a period of time. For the individual patient, MEMS may help to determine the pattern of noncompliance and differentiate between poor compliance and pharmacodynamic or pharmacokinetic mechanisms leading to

Table 22.1 Indirect and direct methods to assess patient compliance (after Matsui [39]). *MEMS* Medication Event Monitoring System

Indirect methods	Direct methods
Patient and parental report	Measurement of drug levels in blood/urine
Interview, questionnaires	Measurements of tracers added to drugs
Pill count	Surrogate markers for drug intake (e.g., leukocyte count)
Physcian's estimate	Automated devices (MEMS)
Clinical outcome	

low drug levels [39]. The use of electronic compliance monitoring has resulted in the recognition of different patterns of drug noncompliance, which can then be addressed better by the physician. For instance, the compliance with the evening dose tends to be higher than with the morning dose, possibly due to more intensive parental supervision in the evening than in the busy hours of the morning. Dose omissions are the most common dosing errors [40], and include incorrect dosage, premature discontinuation of the drug, and failure to fill the prescription, which was found in 5 to 20% of cases [41]. Studies with MEMS showed the pattern of "drug holidays," defined as a period of 3 or more drug-free days, often during holidays or weekends [42]. An improvement in compliance several days prior to a scheduled medical visit has been observed and has been called the "toothbrush effect" or "white-coat compliance" [35, 43]. The data obtained from parents and patients can be studied systematically with MEMS and the results of drug dosing patterns of noncompliant children would be useful in designing a more appropriate medication regimen for those children. The expense and the incorrect use of electronic monitoring devices are major drawbacks for a broad clinical use of MEMS [6]. Less expensive electronic compliance monitors would be more practical for widespread use, particularly in noncompliant adolescents with cancer.

22.3.3 Risk Factors and Predictors of Noncompliance

A variety of factors may influence patient's compliance (Table 22.2): (A) the disease and its treatment, (B) demographic and social factors, and (C) the child's and the parents' knowledge and attitudes toward the disease and its treatment. Clinically, these factors might be important indices of suspicion, but they are

Table 22.2 Factors predicting drug compliance (modified from Tebbi 1993 [8])

A. Features of treatment and adverse effects of medication	Duration of treatment Physical characteristics of medication Number of medications Number of doses each administration Mode of administration Administered by healthcare provider vs. self-administered drugs Cost Number, severity, and expectations of side effects Appearance (color, taste, and size) of the tablets
B. Demographic and social factors	Age and sex of child Family socioeconomic status Marital status of mother Parent of child responsible for medication Parent accompanies child to provider Effect of child's illness on family life
C. Child's and parents' knowledge and attitudes	Purpose of medication Dosage Frequency To-do list No overflow of information regarding long-term ("U-shaped" correlation) Belief about the effectiveness of the medication Beliefs about cancer cure Satisfaction with medical care received Control over health outcomes Instructions about medication given and understood Satisfaction with information about the disease and treatment

not reliable as predictors of the patient's drug compliance [44].

22.3.3.1 Features of Treatment and Adverse Effects of Medication

The severity of the disease as assessed by physicians has not been found to correlate with compliance [22]. Compliance may be related to the duration of treatment, the physical characteristics of the drugs such as the number of these, the number of doses for each administration and the mode of administration. The cost, and the appearance, color, and size of tablets can all influence drug compliance. Palatability is a very critical factor in children [45, 46]. Compliance is higher with medications administered by a health-care provider when compared with self-administered drugs. Compliance decreases significantly over the duration of treatment when the treatment exceeds 5 days [2]. In a study of 46 children and adolescents with cancer and 40 of their parents, compliance, judged by response to questionnaires and by bioassays, was >80% at 2 weeks of therapy and decreased to 60% by 20 weeks [9]. Compliance is better with drugs having less or milder side effects and among patients whose expectations about side effects were worse or about the same as what actually occurred. However, others have found no correlation between side effects and compliance [9]. In some studies compliance may be decreased by complex regimens, prolonged therapies [47], oral self-administered medication and regimens causing severe side effects. Compliance tends to decrease sharply soon after the child's symptoms have improved and is generally lower in the treatment of asymptomatic conditions or with preventive medications [48].

22.3.3.2 Demographic and Social Factors

The studies analyzing the correlation of compliance with demographic and social factors have been controversial and did not demonstrate any evident relationship [22]. Patients aged about 10 years of age tend to be good compliers, as opposed to very poor compliance at the age of about 17 years. The child's illness has an effect on the life of the whole family; strong family cohesiveness, positive attitudes of others, and availability of help and support by the family enhance compliance [49–51], whereas family dysfunction may be a risk factor for noncompliance [22]. The socioeconomic status of the family per se does not necessarily correlate with compliance. The compliance of children of single parents or of children coming without company to the clinic visits tends to be reduced [52].

22.3.3.3 Parents' and Child's Knowledge and Attitudes

The child's understanding of the disease has a major impact on compliance. The interaction and communication with the health-care provider are crucial. Educational conversations shortly after diagnosis are often not very effective due to the emotional trauma at that time. Misunderstanding and forgetting are aggravated by stress, and during the visit to the physician up to 50% of advice and instructions are forgotten almost immediately [53]. Only 50% of instructions given by physicians are recalled immediately following the visit [32]. Therefore, repeated discussions with the health-care providers, a written contract, and a home-support person to clarify the responsibility of drug administration tend to enhance compliance. Positive effects on compliance were found if the health-care provider relates in a friendly and respectful way to the patient, shows interest in the child [54], and believes in the efficacy of the treatment [55]. Better compliance is correlated with more visits to the physician, with patients attending specialized and private clinics, probably due to individualized attention [56], and better understanding of instructions. Defining with the parents the responsibility for drug administration improves compliance [9, 57].

The nature of the knowledge of the disease is critical: Practical knowledge about the purpose of the treatment, and dosage and frequency of drug intakes enhances compliance, whereas an overload of information extending beyond the practical aspects of the regimen like lifelong consequences, side effects, and prognosis, may result in discouragement and futility, and therefore in a "U-shaped" correlation with compliance [58]. The attitude and the belief system [59] of the patient may correlate with good compliance and outcome [16].

22.4 Discussion

Noncompliance with therapy is widespread among adolescents with cancer, who are at particularly high risk, since their malignancies may have a poorer prognosis than those of younger children and the state of mind of the adolescent may interfere significantly with adherence to treatment. Therefore, the importance of compliance in adolescents with cancer cannot be overemphasized.

In order to develop with the family and the healthcare team an individualized approach for each patient, we suggest a checklist for the physician (Table 22.3). Continuous educational efforts and reinforcement should be tailored to meet the needs of the individual patient during various stages of the disease and intervening social and medical changes. It is through proper education and personalized needs assessment and intervention that progress toward better compliance can be made [8].

Communication skills are crucial to identify and to address noncompliance. Only few patients object when a compliance measurement is proposed and its rationale explained [60]. Treatment goals should be discussed in collaboration with the patient and his family. Explicit instructions should be provided. The prescribed regimen should be simple and tailored to the patient's daily routine. Written information including educational handouts, self-monitoring calendar, schedules ("road maps"), and brief telephone reminders might improve communication [61].

A positive, hopeful ,and encouraging attitude will improve compliance as part of the relationship between the physician and his patient. A careful review of the risk factors listed above may guide clinicians to identify problems. For noncompliant patients, different measures might be appropriate: More frequent visits for follow-up, social support, monitoring drug levels in blood or urine, replacing oral self-administered medication with parenteral medication, and finally, using sophisticated electronic pill containers. Favorable results using behavioral strategies, such as self-monitoring, contracting, and reinforcement programs, have been obtained with chronic disease treatment regimens [22].

Table 22.3 Suggestions to improve compliance. *PPR* Patient-physician relationship

1.	Think about the compliance of each of your patients.
2.	Address compliance with your patient and his family and listen to them very carefully.
3.	Regularly report issues of compliance in the patient's chart, including the attitude of the family and friends.
4.	Discuss compliance with your team of health providers.
5.	Reduce forgetfulness and misunderstanding of your explanation with detailed written information including schedules ("road maps"), calendars, and other reminders.
6.	Involve the patient and his family to share and define responsibility. Questionnaires and personal charts for the patient may be very helpful.
7.	Check Table 22.2 and consider individual improvements.
8.	A positive and hopeful attitude with encouragement will enhance compliance and well being of the patient and his family.
9.	For noncompliant patients consider [i] More frequent visits for follow-up [ii] Provide immediate and extended family and social support [iii] Monitor drug levels in blood and urine [iv] Replacing oral self-administered medication by parenteral medication [v] The use of sophisticated electronic pill boxes
10.	Assess your own skills to address issues of compliance. Try to improve your PPR. Feedback of your skills!

Patients' adherence to physicians' instructions depends very much on the interpersonal skills of the physician and her/his ability to understand the patient's personality and needs. The complexity of compliance leads to reflections on the mission of the physician, defined as the holistic management of the patient and on the PPR. As suggested by Emanuel and Emanuel [62], there are different models for the PPR in the adult population (Table 22.4). The relationship may differ significantly in various clinical situations for which different models may be appropriate. Historically, there has been a shift in the PPR from paternalism to increased autonomy of the patient. The principle of "autonomy" has a different role in these four models, increasing from left to right. Similar shifts have occurred in nonmedical professions such as politics, education, religion, and law. The ideal modern model of PPR is the deliberative model, in which the physician is a teacher and friend of the patient, and the dialogue deals with the worthiness of health-related values. The patient's autonomy is a moral self-development, supported by the physician's values, which are relevant to the patient. Particularly for a longstanding relationship during cancer treatment, the deliberative model of PPR seems to be most appropriate [63].

The four models of PPR for adults of Emanuel and Emanuel [62] have to be modified for pediatric patients and their families. The autonomy of the child is limited by definition, but is certainly not absent. In adolescent cancer patients, all of these models may apply simultaneously. Over the longstanding treatment of cancer, the adolescent patient may actually mature and undergo a development through all four models of the PPR. His individual psychological maturation parallels the historical development of the four models. From a very minimal role in the paternalistic model, the autonomy according to the informative model expects the patient to accept the technical facts and the professional expertise of the physician. According to the interpretative model, the autonomy of the patient

Table 22.4 Four models of the PPR (after Emanuel and Emanuel 1992) [62]

Conflict between autonomy (patient) <–> paternalism, health (physician)				
Model	Paternalistic	Informative (scientific, "engineering")	Interpretative	Deliberative
Role of Physician (Paternalism, Health)	Guardian of health, dictates to the patient	Provides facts, technical expert	Provides facts, technical expert –> Interpret and elicit patient's values "counselor"	Teacher/friend Dialogue on the worthiness of health-related values
Role of patient (autonomy)	Minimal function	Autonomy = values fixed	Autonomy = Self-understanding	Autonomy = moral self-development
Comments	"Patient control"; justified only in emergency situation	Lack of care and understanding the patient, no self-reflection and deliberation; based on trend of specialization and impersonalization of medicine, physician is a technologist. Justified in walk-in-clinic, consultations	Place for "second-order desires", particularly if conflicting values in patient present and ongoing relationship Physician's values unwittingly imposed upon the patient (shift to paternalism)	Ideal concept of autonomy; physician's role for patient; physician's values are relevant to the patient Patient's and physician's values are incommensurable

means self-understanding of his disease [64], whereas in the deliberative model the autonomy is a moral self-development during the dialogue with the physician.

It is evident that the PPR plays a crucial role in drug compliance for adolescent patients with cancer. During the longstanding treatment of the patient with cancer, a mutual trust is essential to ensure cooperation and compliance.

The quality of the PPR influences adherence with therapy, showing better results with patients who were treated consistently by the same physician than patients treated by different physicians on different occasions [47]. Adherence is usually better with patients treated by pediatricians in private practice than by pediatricians in a hospital setting [28]. Understanding the parents' major concerns and meeting their expectations from the medical visit during the prolonged time of active treatment and follow-up are extremely important for successful compliance [65]. Therefore, the physician should develop his/her skills toward a longstanding dialogue with cancer patients and their families. Continuous educational effort from both patients with their families and the health-care team are necessary [66].

The essential role of compliance needs more attention in order to prevent therapeutic failures. Most of the research on compliance has been conducted in the adult population, and these issues are not yet well studied in pediatrics. There is a need to improve education of the patient and his health-care providers with respect to compliance.

The training of all physicians, and particularly of oncologists, should address the importance of compliance. Input from clinical psychology and communication skills are crucial to improve the PPR, particularly in chronic diseases. Physicians caring for children should be educated to have a high index of suspicion for drug noncompliance. Identification of potential barriers to compliance may allow for early intervention to ensure compliance and minimize the negative consequences of inappropriate administration of medications.

Compliance remains a poorly understood subject and a source of frustration for today's practitioners. Clinical research to identify noncompliers and to treat them optimally is crucial. Research on compliance does not only address the patient and his psychology, but also has a major impact on drug development and treatment regimens [60]. Moreover, the attitudes to better understand and address noncompliance may improve the well being of the patient and the overall quality of the PPR.

References

1. Kondro W (1999) Boy refuses cancer treatment in favour of prayer. Lancet North Am Ed 353:1078
2. Fletcher RH (1989) Patient compliance with therapeutic advice: a modern view. Mt Sinai J Med 56:453–458
3. Haynes RB, McDonald H, Garg AX, Montague P (2002) Interventions for helping patients to follow prescriptions for medications. Cochrane Database Syst Rev 2: CD000011
4. Haynes RB, Sackett DL, Taylor DW (1979) Compliance in Health Care. Johns Hopkins University Press, Baltimore xvi, p 516
5. Vander Stichele R (1991) Measurement of patient compliance and the interpretation of randomised clinical trials. Eur J Clin Pharmacol 41:27–35
6. Matsui D, Hermann C, Klein J, et al (1994) Critical comparison of novel and existing methods of compliance assessment during a clinical trial of an oral iron chelator. J Clin Pharmacol 34:944–949
7. Shope JT (1988) Compliance in children and adults: review of studies. Epilepsy Res Suppl 1:23–47
8. Tebbi CK (1993) Treatment compliance in childhood and adolescence. Cancer 71:3441–3449
9. Tebbi CK, Cummings KM, Zevon MA, et al (1986) Compliance of pediatric and adolescent cancer patients. Cancer 58:1179–1184
10. Macdougall LG, McElligott SE, Ross E, et al (1992) Pattern of 6-mercaptopurine urinary excretion in children with acute lymphoblastic leukemia: urinary assays as a measure of drug compliance. Drug Monit 14:371–375
11. Smith SD, Rosen D, Trueworthy RC, Lowman JT (1979) A reliable method for evaluating drug compliance in children with cancer. Cancer 43:169–173
12. Festa RS, Tamaroff MH, Chasalow F, Lanzkowsky P (1992) Therapeutic adherence to oral medication regimens by adolescents with cancer. I. Laboratory assessment. J Pediatr 120:807–811
13. Smith SD, Cairns NU, Sturgeon JK, Lansky SB (1981) Poor drug compliance in an adolescent with leukemia. Am J Pediatr Hematol Oncol 3:297–300
14. Snodgrass W, Smith S, Trueworthy R (1984) Pediatric clinical pharmacology of 6-mercaptopurine: lack of compliance as a factor in leukemia relapse. Proc Am Soc Clin Oncol 3:204

15. Meyers KE, Weiland H, Thomson PD (1995) Paediatric renal transplantation non-compliance. Pediatr Nephrol 9:189–192

16. Tamaroff MH, Festa RS, Adesman AR, Walco GA (1992) Therapeutic adherence to oral medication regimens by adolescents with cancer. II. Clinical and psychologic correlates. J Pediatr 120:812–817

17. Lansky SB, Smith SD, Cairns NU, Cairns GF (1983) Psychological correlates of compliance. Am J Pediatr Hematol Oncol 5:87–92

18. Peeters M, Koren G, Jakubovicz D, Zipursky A (1988) Physician compliance and relapse rates of acute lymphoblastic leukemia in children. Clin Pharmacol Ther 43:228–232

19. Whyte F, Smith L (1997) A literature review of adolescence and cancer. Eur J Cancer Care 6:137–146

20. Edelstein L (1987) Ancient Medicine. Johns Hopkins University Press, Baltimore and London

21. Prioreschi P (1995) The Hippocratic Oath: a code for physicians, not a Pythagorean manifesto. Med Hypotheses 44:447–462

22. Rapoff MA, Barnard MU (1991) Compliance with pediatric medical regimens. In: Cramer JA, Spilker B (eds) Patient Compliance in Medical Practice and Clinical Trials. Raven, New York, p 73

23. Daschner F, Marget W (1975) Treatment of recurrent urinary tract infection in children. II. Compliance of parents and children with antibiotic therapy regimen. Acta Paediatr Scand 64:105–108

24. Tebbi CK (1983) Care for adolescent oncology patients. In: Higby DJ (ed) Supportive Care in Cancer Therapy. Martinum Nijhoff, Boston, pp 281–309

25. Adams GR (2000) Adolescent development: the essential readings. In: Essential Readings in Developmental Psychology. Blackwell, Oxford UK, Malden, Mass, ix, p 345

26. Tebbi CK, Richards ME, Cummings KM, et al (1988) The role of parent–adolescent concordance in compliance with cancer chemotherapy. Adolescence 23:599–611

27. Levenson PM, Copeland DR, Morrow JR, et al (1983) Disparities in disease-related perceptions of adolescent cancer patients and their parents. J Pediatr Psychol 8:33–45

28. Litt IF, Cuskey WR (1980) Compliance with medical regimens during adolescence. Pediatr Clin North Am 27:3–15

28. Matsui DM (1997) Drug compliance in pediatrics. Clinical and research issues. Pediatr Clin North Am 44:1–14

29. Friedman IM, Litt IF (1986) Promoting adolescents' compliance with therapeutic regimens. Pediatr Clin North Am 33:955

30. Shope JT (1980) Intervention to improve compliance with pediatric anticonvulsant therapy. Patient Couns Health Educ 2:135–141

31. Rodewald LE, Pichichero ME (1993) Compliance with antibiotic therapy: a comparison of deuterium oxide tracer, urine bioassay, bottle weights, and parental reports. J Pediatr 123:143–147

32. Liptak GS (1996) Enhancing patient compliance in pediatrics. Pediatr Rev 17:128–134

33. Rudd P, Byyny RL, Zachary V, et al (1989) The natural history of medication compliance in a drug trial: limitations of pill counts. Clin Pharmacol Ther 46:169–176

34. Sackett DL (1991) Helping patients follow the treatments you prescribe. In: Sackett DL, Haynes RB, Guyatt GH (eds) Helping patients follow the treatments you prescribe. Clinical epidemiology: a basic science for clinical medicine. Little Brown, Boston, p 249

35. Feinstein AR (1990) On white-coat effects and the electronic monitoring of compliance. Arch Intern Med 150:1377–1378

36. Claxton AJ, Cramer J, Pierce C (2001) A systematic review of the associations between dose regimens and medication compliance. Clin Ther 23:1296–1310

37. Cramer JA (1995) Microelectronic systems for monitoring and enhancing patient compliance with medication regimens. Drugs 49:321–327

38. Diaz E, Levine HB, Sullivan MC, et al (2001) Use of the Medication Event Monitoring System to estimate medication compliance in patients with schizophrenia. J Psychiatry Neurosci 26:325–329

39. Matsui D, Hermann C, Braudo M, et al (1992) Clinical use of the Medication Event Monitoring System: a new window into pediatric compliance. Clin Pharmacol Ther 52:102–103

40. Urquhart J (1994) Role of patient compliance in clinical pharmacokinetics. A review of recent research. Clin Pharmacokinet 27:202–215

41. Beardon PH, McGilchrist MM, McKendrick AD, et al (1993) Primary non-compliance with prescribed medication in primary care. BMJ 307:846–848

42. Kruse W, Koch-Gwinner P, Nikolaus T, et al (1992) Measurement of drug compliance by continuous electronic monitoring: a pilot study in elderly patients discharged from hospital. J Am Geriatr Soc 40:1151–1155

43. Blowey DL, Hebert D, Arbus GS, et al (1997) Compliance with cyclosporine in adolescent renal transplant recipients. Pediatr Nephrol 11:547–551

44. Roth HP, Caron HS (1978) Accuracy of doctors' estimates and patients' statements on adherence to a drug regimen. Clin Pharmacol Ther 23:361–370

45. Dajani AS (1996) Adherence to physicians' instructions as a factor in managing streptococcal pharyngitis. Pediatrics 97:976–980

46. Powers JL, Gooch WM III, Oddo LP (2000) Comparison of the palatability of the oral suspension of cefdinir vs. amoxicillin/clavulanate potassium, cefprozil and azithromycin in pediatric patients. Pediatr Infect Dis J 19:S174–180

47. Fotheringham MJ, Sawyer MG (1995) Adherence to recommended medical regimens in childhood and adolescence. J Paediatr Child Health 31:72–78

48. Jay S, Litt IF, Durant RH (1984) Compliance with therapeutic regimens. J Adolesc Health Care 5:124–136

49. Cummings KM, Becker MH, Kirscht JP, Levin NW (1982) Psychosocial factors affecting adherence to medical regiments in a group of hemodialysis patients. Med Care 20:567–580

50. Griffith S (1990) A review of the factors associated with patient compliance and the taking of prescribed medicines. Br J Gen Pract 40:114–116

51. Richardson JL, Marks G, Johnson CA, et al (1987) Path model of multidimensional compliance with cancer therapy. Health Psychol 6:183–207

52. Gordis L, Markowitz M, Lilienfeld AM (1969) Studies in the epidemiology and preventability of rheumatic fever. IV. A quantitative determination of compliance in children on oral penicillin prophylaxis. Pediatrics 43:173–182

53. Ley P (1979) Memory for medical information. Br J Soc Clin Psychol 18:245–255

54. Becker MH, Maiman LA (1975) Sociobehavioural determinants of compliance with health and medical care recommendations. Med Care 13:10–24

55. Rosenstock IM (1988) Enhancing patient compliance with health recommendations. J Pediatr Health Care 2:67–72

56. Evans L, Spelman M (1983) The problem of non-compliance with drug therapy. Drugs 25:63–76

Chapter 22

57. Tebbi CK, Zevon MA, Richards ME, Cummings KM (1989) Attributions of responsibility in adolescent cancer patients and their parents. J Cancer Educ 4:135–142

58. Hamburg BA, Inoff GE (1982) Relationships between behavioural factors and diabetic control in children and adolescents: a camp study. Psychosom Med 44:321–339

59. Tebbi CK, Mallon JC, Richards ME, Bigler LR (1987) Religiosity and locus of control of adolescent cancer patients. Psychol Rep 61:683–696

60. Urquhart J (1999) The impact of compliance on drug development. Transplant Proc 31:39S

61. Finney JW, Friman PC, Rapoff MA, Christophersen ER (1985) Improving compliance with antibiotic regimens for otitis media. Randomised clinical trial in a pediatric clinic. Am J Dis Child 139:89–95

62. Emanuel EJ, Emanuel LL (1992) Four models of the physician–patient relationship. JAMA 267:2221–2226

63. Balint J, Shelton W (1996) Regaining the initiative. Forging a new model of the patient–physician relationship. JAMA 275:887–891

64. Katz J (1986) The Silent World of Doctor and Patient. Free Press Collier Macmillan, New York London, xxi, p 263

65. Mattar ME, Yaffe SJ (1974) Compliance of pediatric patients with therapeutic regimens. Postgrad Med 56:181–185, 188

66. Maiman LA, Becker MH, Liptak GS, et al (1988) Improving pediatricians' compliance-enhancing practices. A randomised trial. Am J Dis Child 142:773–779

Psychological Support

Christine Eiser • Aura Kuperberg

Contents

23.1 Introduction

Diagnosis of cancer during adolescence is especially challenging. Typically, adolescence is a time of major freedom and increasing independence from parents and family. A diagnosis of cancer challenges adolescents' views about their invulnerability, threatens their self-esteem, and compromises all aspects of quality of life. Treatments are associated with major changes in physical appearance and physical energy. Long-term educational goals can be seriously compromised by hospitalization and health complications. These obstacles and roadblocks may derail normal adolescent development and interfere with transition into adulthood. These potential difficulties merit the establishment of innovative specialized programs to ensure treatment management and create a seamless transition from adolescence to young adulthood. This chapter will highlight the challenges of transitioning from diagnosis to long-term survivorship, pediatric to adult medical care, and psychological and economic dependence to independence. Due to limited space, we will be unable to cover issues relating to end-stage disease in adolescence, which is covered in Chap. 24. From empirically based studies and descriptive articles, those psychological approaches that have been, in our experience, the most useful will be discussed.

23.2 From Diagnosis to Aftercare

The cancer experience has been likened to a journey, or progression through the seasons of the year. The focus following diagnosis is on acquisition of information, acute care, and management. This is followed by an extended period from the end of intensive treatment through to a period of watchful waiting and fear of relapse, then a period of permanent survival with concern for adverse late effects, and finally an ultimate resolution. Obviously, the journey is long, if not a lifetime, and rarely is it fully completed.

23.2.1 Diagnosis

Any negative life event creates changes that can be stressful and that require adaptation on the part of the individual. The initial period after such an event is critical, and the inability to cope during that period can be a precipitating factor in the development of long-term problems. Behavior patterns exhibited during this period are likely to become fixed and may shape behavior during subsequent phases [1], suggesting the benefits of an early and ongoing rehabilitation program [2]. Kaplan et al. [3] have emphasized the importance of developing appropriate "psychosocial tools" during the initial period, which can be utilized throughout the treatment course and beyond. Ross [4] emphasizes the need to be aware of the critical phases through which the adolescent cancer patient and family pass, and to determine the nature of the intervention based on a clear understanding of those phases.

Efforts directed at mitigating developmental disruption and increasing quality of life must begin at the time of diagnosis [2]. Normalcy and belonging to a peer group is paramount, yet the onset of illness and treatment side effects make the adolescent patient feel and look different. The loss of normalcy in terms of appearance, body integrity, and daily activities is often of greater concern for the adolescent than the potential loss of life [5].

A sense of control plays a part in adolescent development, and has implications for treatment adherence [6–8]. Giving adolescents options and choices is one way to regain a sense of control for young patients and foster the adolescent's cooperation, and this can best be achieved through a concerted effort by staff and family. To enhance a patient's sense of mastery and sense of control, List et al. [2] suggest education regarding the illness, simple and understandable explanations about the cancer experience, written directions

on treatment procedures and medical schedules [6–8], and teaching coping strategies, such as guided imagery.

It is inevitable that adolescents will have much more difficulty accepting a diagnosis of cancer compared with children. Their greater cognitive competence, knowledge, and experience mean that they are likely to be much more aware of the potential seriousness of the disease. Adolescents typically see themselves as invulnerable [9], and knowledge of a life-threatening disease is therefore extremely challenging.

In addition to accepting the diagnosis, adolescents may be expected to make decisions about treatment or participation in clinical trials. These are very difficult decisions for anyone. Adolescents may take into account different considerations compared with those of adults. For example, in making decisions about amputations or limb salvage, adults may focus on long-term issues, body image, and potential impact on interpersonal relationships. Adolescents may put more weight on whether they can continue contact sports. In the longer term, they may come to regret this decision.

Social support has been linked to positive adjustment [10, 11], and reduced feelings of uncertainty [11, 12] found adolescents able to adapt to cancer in the context of strong family and social support. Yet adolescent patients can experience emotional isolation both within their families [5] and from their peers [13]. Adolescents report that parents expect to see them as strong, upbeat, and pleasant [14]. Social isolation is a major concern of adolescents, and peer reactions leave many adolescents feeling very lonely [14]. In an effort to counteract isolation, Haluska et al. [15] suggest that the medical staff allow the adolescent patient every opportunity to maintain social networks of friends and family by encouraging visits, providing social opportunities in the hospital, and emphasizing the importance of attending school. However, not all sources of support are perceived as positive. Manne and Miller [16] suggest that mother-adolescent conflict be an appropriate target for psychosocial interventions.

Other factors influence adjustment and a positive transition through the treatment course. A sense of hopefulness [17, 18] and maintenance of self-esteem

[10] have been identified as "protecting mechanisms" and relevant in the care for adolescents during treatment [10]. Developing care strategies to promote self-esteem and hope includes identifying the patient's positive abilities, giving genuine and honest feedback [10], and encouraging certain self-initiated behaviors [18]. Haase [19] found that resilient adolescents frequently use the defensive coping strategy of denial in dealing with their cancer experience. Although denial plays an important role in adjusting to a cancer diagnosis, if left unchecked it may have a long-term adverse effect.

23.3 Pediatric-, Adolescent- or Adult-Based Care?

Typically, adolescents are cared for in pediatric wards, although some may be admitted to adult care units. Neither is optimal. On pediatric units, adolescents may be disturbed by the noise and crying of younger children, and they usually find the toys and books unsuitable. On the other hand, adolescents on adult wards can be highly distressed, finding little to talk about with elderly and sometimes dying patients [20]. Teenagers typically want personal space to play music or use personal computers, for example, and an opportunity to be with others of the same age.

The solution is provision of adolescent units wherever possible. In the United Kingdom, the first Teenage Cancer Unit opened in 1990 and has been followed by similar units in major oncology centers. The advantages of such units include specialist medical care of cancers that typically affect this age group: acute leukemias, Hodgkin and non-Hodgkin lymphomas, brain tumors, sarcomas, and germ-cell tumors. In addition, the medical staff is specially trained to deal with the social and psychological consequences of cancer for this age group. The units seem to be well received by patients [21]. Advantages for patients include contact with specialist nurses who are not only experts in cancer care but also in touch with teenage issues, opportunities to share experiences with similar others, involvement of parents, and opportunities to take part in activities and education. More formally, there is little evidence that survival rates are improved. However,

given the excellent rates of survival in conditions such as Hodgkin lymphoma, it is "unnecessarily narrow to consider this as exclusive justification for Units" [22].

23.3.1 When Treatment Ends

Given the frequent report of anxiety, fear, and feelings of vulnerability, MacLean et al. [23] suggest psychological care target patients as they transition from on-treatment to off-treatment. The authors suggest implementing a formal conference to address unfinished business, accurately assess relapse, and administer a quality of life assessment to determine an intervention plan that will enhance long-term psychological adjustment. This transition is covered in Chap. 30.

23.3.2 Follow-up Care

As described in Chap. 30, many survivors experience physical or psychological late effects depending on treatment received. Follow-up care is therefore considered essential for many survivors, with the aim to identify problems early and provide appropriate intervention, as well as to inform them about risks to future health.

Although the nature of the problems survivors face is increasingly well described, there is as yet no consensus on how best to provide long-term care. Procedures are far from standard across centers [24, 25]. The results from a postal questionnaire in the United States concluded that few programs exist that focus on long-term care for survivors into adulthood [24]. Indeed, only 44% of responding institutions had mechanisms in place for continued care of adult survivors. The vast majority employed pediatric staff in the follow-up care, and only 13% of programs involved adult oncologists. According to the survey respondents, the major barriers to providing long-term follow-up care were: patient's uncertainty about the need for follow-up; unwillingness to be followed up; and difficulties locating adult survivors. In a similar study in the United Kingdom, Taylor et al. [25] also found large disparities in care between treatment centers.

Thus, the evidence suggests that follow-up is far from systematic and more needs to be done to assess how long-term care should be provided to this patient group, as described in Chaps. 31 and 32. Taylor et al. (2004) advise that a subset of survivors may benefit from permanent transfer to primary care, whereas a proportion of patients with complex needs should receive specialist-led hospital-based care in an adult environment. Likewise, strategies have been proposed for the development of follow-up programs [26]. For example, telephone or postal surveys may be adequate for those who receive low-risk chemotherapy or surgery alone. Rosen [27] argues that adult clinics for adolescents and young adults with cancer have several major benefits. First, the transition to adult care can provide a positive and optimistic sense of future that indicates life after a serious illness; a sense of graduation. Second, adult clinics can provide a more suitable environment in which to discuss age-relevant health information, such as contraception, sexuality, and fertility. Third, given the importance placed on follow-up care for cancer survivors, an adult environment can avoid having the young adult cancer survivors feeling that they have outgrown the service provided by pediatricians and consequently become lost to follow-up. Several authors have suggested multidisciplinary clinics that combine the skills of pediatricians, adult oncologists, and nursing staff to provide comprehensive care for the range of medical issues survivorship can entail [23, 28].

In terms of psychological support, follow-up clinics need to offer reassurance as well as advice and education [29]. Traditional health promotion advice is needed regarding the risks associated with smoking or sunbathing, for example. In addition, these young people face additional risks to their health depending on past treatment. Problems that require some psychological intervention include those related to weight-gain following treatment, infertility, or reduced cardiac function. As more is learned about possible late effects, questions need to be asked about how such risk information is best communicated to survivors. They have a right to know about such risks, but care must be taken not to create unnecessary anxiety. Where possible, information about risk needs to be associated with information about what the individuals can realistically do to ensure their own health. Some examples are given in the following section.

23.4 Long-Term Issues

23.4.1 Body Image

Many survivors are at risk of obesity, low bone density, and have poor body image. A healthy lifestyle involving exercise may be a first step toward minimizing these late effects of cancer. Participation in sports activities among survivors seems to be similar to the general population. Survivors who participate in sports were more likely to report having access to health insurance and medical care by a local physician, although there were no differences based on age, race, socioeconomic status, body mass index, time since diagnosis, length of treatment, and time since completed treatment [30]. Males were found to exercise more than females, a difference typically also found in the general population.

Survivors who are overweight need particularly sensitive counseling and motivation to take part in regular activity. As these problems are recognized in the general community, several community-based programs are being reported. It is likely that similar approaches will also be beneficial for survivors of cancer.

23.4.2 Fertility

Infertility is potentially a side effect, especially for those treated with radiotherapy below the diaphragm or chemotherapy with alkylating agents, as covered in Chap. 27 and considered in Chaps. 24, 25, and 30 . It is established in other settings that infertility can cause considerable distress, although individuals differ substantially in their psychological reactions [31]. Information about possible infertility and its impact on psychological function in cancer survivors was investigated by Green et al. [32]. Interviews conducted with 15 male survivors suggested that survivors varied greatly in how prepared they were for such information, with some being well prepared while others regarded it as "a bolt from the blue." The most common emotional response was anger. However, emotional responses varied greatly. Three coping styles were identified. A first group wanted no further counseling and chose to get on with their lives as best as possible. A second group included those who were prepared to think about infertility to a limited degree. This group reflected at length about the information but chose not to discuss the matter further with friends or medical staff. The third group wanted more information (about alternative routes to parenthood) and engaged important others in discussions about what to do.

Of significance is the finding of great and unpredictable variability in reactions that makes it difficult to recommend a single approach to information giving and counseling about infertility in the clinic. Undoubtedly there is a certain amount to be learned from the experience of those working in other infertility clinics, and it is likely that the importance of this issue will become greater as greater numbers of survivors reach adult life.

23.4.3 Employment

Survivors of childhood cancer report prejudice in the workplace and indeed may be less likely to be employed than peers or healthy siblings [33]. Particularly for those with physical or cognitive disability, realistic vocational guidance is essential. In addition, other research is needed to determine survivors' attitudes to work and employment.

23.5 Adolescence to Young Adulthood – The Developmental Transition

23.5.1 Unique Challenges of Adolescence

Adolescents with cancer are faced with several interrelated developmental challenges that impact transition to adulthood and must be considered in the provision of psychological care. These include: (1) developing a positive body image, (2) forming a sense of identity and achieving economic and emotional independence, (3) developing a firm sexual identity, and (4) attaining a clear goal orientation with regard to a future career [14].

23.5.1.1 Positive Body Image

Many adolescents report that the treatment is worse than the disease [1], and the bodily changes that accompany chemotherapy and radiation make it more difficult to develop a positive body image [34]. While on treatment, satisfaction with body image was found to be related to gender, age, education level, and the frequency of changes in appearance caused by chemotherapy [35]. The effect on physical appearance is especially disruptive for females [36]. Pendley et al. [37] examined body image in adolescents who completed treatment and found that adolescents who had been off treatment longer reported more negative body image perceptions. Findings suggest that body image concerns do not develop until several years after treatment termination. Persistent negative perceptions may result in a loss of sex appeal and virility [34]. A distorted body image, whether based on reality or not, produces feelings of inferiority, low self-esteem, and incompetence. These findings suggest that more attention should be paid to adolescents who perceive changes in their appearance and help them develop a positive body image [35].

23.5.1.2 Sense of Identity and Independence

During adolescence, individuals struggle to separate and formulate their own unique identity [38]. Identity formation among adolescent survivors of childhood cancer has been found to differ from that of healthy adolescents, with a greater frequency of survivors than healthy peers falling within foreclosed identity status and tendency to foreclose prematurely on a career choice [39, 40]. Factors associated with the foreclosed identity status include a cancer diagnosis, symptoms of posttraumatic stress disorder, and family functioning characterized by greater levels of conflict. The tendency to foreclose may be adaptive in adolescent cancer survivors by serving a protective function in assisting survivors to cope with the stressors of the cancer experience [39]. Counseling is recommended to mitigate the stressors of cancer and its treatment [40].

The onset of illness threatens attempts to establish independence [41] with imposed dependence on family and medical staff, compliance to treatment, and loss of control [2]. Emotional separation from parents is often complicated by parental overprotectiveness [14]. Furthermore, the new and unfamiliar role as "patient" increases dependence and can lead to a sense of helplessness at the very time when normal development involves breaking away and establishing independence [36].

Cancer necessarily restricts the freedom normally typical of adolescence [42]. Adolescent cancer patients can be resentful about the sudden restrictions imposed upon them, which are seen as symbolic of the perceived lack of control over their own lives and their dependent role [43].

23.5.1.3 Sexual Identity

The course of normal sexual development is also likely to be affected by a diagnosis of cancer during adolescence. The inherent lack of privacy that accompanies the illness is likely to inhibit or delay social exploration, while overprotective parents may limit the time spent away from the family. At the same time, there may be fewer peer contacts in the school environment and fewer opportunities for social exploration. Koocher et al. [41], for example, found that adolescent girls with physical impairments had more difficulty establishing intimate relationships than similar girls without impairments. Concerns about late effects from the disease and treatment are superimposed on age-related issues such as establishing intimate relationships, defining physical attractiveness, and preparing for marriage and family [14].

23.5.1.4 Future Career Goals

The development of future goals and clear objectives is influenced by the way the adolescent feels about him or herself, about the physical limitations brought about by the illness, and by ongoing socialization and peer group experiences. The constant need to "catch-up" in school and the general unpredictability of the future can frustrate and demoralize the adolescent cancer patient. The sense of uncertainty and ambiguity about the future and the threat of recurrence of the disease may taint the future outlook [14].

23.6 Treatment Approaches to Meet the Developmental Challenges of Adolescents and Young Adults

Various forms of psychosocial support have been suggested in working with adolescents and young adults as they attempt to cope with cancer, including individual therapy, camps, cognitive behavioral techniques, and support groups. Given the significance of peer relationships and the reality that a cancer diagnosis may lead to physical and emotional isolation, peer-based interventions can play an important role in psychological adjustment. Therapeutic group work appears to have several advantages over individual psychotherapy. Group interaction allows members to feel that they give, as well as receive, which can serve to enhance self-esteem and lessen feelings of powerlessness. The experience of sharing with others provides a sense of community and reduces the sense of isolation so common among cancer patients. However, most intervention studies have examined primarily group treatment for adult cancer patients, concluding in general that such group interventions can be effective [42]. Little empirically based knowledge is available regarding adolescent and young adult survivors and the benefits of group treatment models [43a] Moreover, encouraging adolescent cancer patients to participate in a group program is a major challenge [5].

There is limited evidence that individual counseling may be appropriate in some cases. Cain et al. [44] studied adult female cancer patients who attended psychoeducational counseling sessions over a 6-month period. After the 6-month period, the patients were significantly less depressed and anxious, had more knowledge about their illness, developed better relationships with their caregivers, experienced fewer sexual difficulties, and participated in more leisure activities.

The psychosocial needs of adolescents with cancer can be met through a variety of support programs focusing on school reintegration, learning coping methods such as relaxation and hypnosis techniques, and participating in peer-based programs. Such programs should be offered routinely rather than in a response to a crisis. While there is a need for crisis-initiated interventions, such programs are a last resort and tend to foster stigmatization, alter effective treatment, and discourage self-help [45].

Studies on the effectiveness of camping programs suggest that this type of program can enhance a cancer patient's self-esteem as well as improve family communications [46]. This line of research was extended in two studies of adolescents with cancer who partici-pated in a summer camp [47, 48]. These researchers found that camp participation improved adolescents' knowledge about cancer, even in the absence of formal educational programs. They also found that relation-ships formed at the camp were maintained after the camp itself. Their key finding was the shared experi-ence with other camp participants; it was valuable in bringing about better quality peer relationships and a higher degree of knowledge about the medical and psychological aspects of cancer.

Most studies on group treatment for adolescents with chronic illness are descriptive, but in general, show that group interventions can be effective. The opportunity to actively participate and to have recipro-cal relationships can be a welcome respite from the nonreciprocal and passive roles patients play in the typical medical environment [49]. This is a particularly significant issue for adolescents. Ross [4] observed that adolescents who associated with others having similar medical conditions were more successful in develop-ing positive self-images. Moreover, the use of groups for adolescents can give them an opportunity for peer reinforcement not otherwise available [50]. Given the fact that the adolescents' mode of coping is often asso-ciated with their support from a peer group, organized but informal groups can play an important role in this area.

23.6.1 Impact Cancer, a Transition Model

For over 16 years, the Teen Impact program – housed at Children's Hospital Los Angeles – has served thou-sands of adolescents and young adults on and off can-cer treatment throughout the Southern California area [50]. The program is appropriate both for those on treatment as well as survivors.

Capitalizing on the adolescent need for peer rela-tionships and groups, Teen Impact has developed a comprehensive multidimensional psychosocial treat-ment model that provides age-appropriate activities such as support groups, 3-day retreats, and special events to help the adolescent navigate the obstacles of illness and treatment.

To assist with the transition into young adulthood, the program has established a three-tiered transition

model of care for adolescents across the developmen-tal path. To incorporate the issue of transition very early, a support group was developed for patients in the latency age range, 9 to 11 years. Conducted con-currently, the adolescent group serves patients between 12 and 22 years of age. Trained mentors, 18 to 22 years of age, who are former Teen Impact participants, attend adolescent group meetings to help younger members, recruit new patients, and assist with pro-gram design and supportive activities on the 3-day retreats. Long-term young adult survivors serve as counselors and cocounselors on the retreats. The con-cept of reciprocity, giving rather than always receiving, plays a major role in helping adolescents with cancer begin to define who they are and where they are going – important developmental tasks. Through curricu-lum-based training and ongoing supervision, the maturing adolescent is given the opportunity to help younger members and the newly diagnosed patient to cope with the onset of illness. Thus, this model paral-lels the targeted developmental needs of the popula-tion, while fostering the transitional process from ado-lescence to adulthood.

Teen Impact incorporates a family-centered approach, based on research that, despite the increased need for peer support during adolescence, families, and partic-ularly mothers, play a major role in the lives of these patients. Cancer is a family disease and all members need help. Supporting all family members will not only help the family as a whole, but will also enhance com-munication between parents and the adolescent patient to prevent parent-adolescent conflict and encourage honest dialogue. Teen Impact provides a bilingual par-ent group and a sibling group to meet the unique needs of individual family members and enhance the func-tioning of the family system.

Clinical observations and patient testimonials sug-gest that group-related participation encourages dis-cussions associated with being an adolescent and young adult with a life-threatening illness, creates a sense of normalcy by belonging to a supportive net-work of peers, empowers through cancer-related edu-cation, enhances coping skills by sharing strategies on how to deal with the illness, builds self-esteem through positive interpersonal interactions, and encourages treatment adherence by providing hope. The finding that Teen Impact members used a broader variety of strategies for coping than the comparison group of nonparticipants implies that the intervention may have been successful in teaching a range of coping skills [51].

Several underlying mechanisms may contribute to the overall effectiveness of the group experience, with the most apparent being the fact that group members model coping behavior and provide mutual support for one another. Whatever the specific mechanisms, however, it seems clear that group approaches can be effective in working with adolescents with cancer.

23.7 Conclusions

The diagnosis of cancer during adolescence threatens normal physical and psychological development. While younger children may be somewhat protected by their limited ability to understand the implications of the illness, adolescents may be well-informed and fully aware about the seriousness of their condition. As a group, therefore, they may be more vulnerable psychologically than either children or adults. For this reason, comprehensive programs of care must involve provision for psychological support, both in the immediate period after diagnosis and in the long-term.

Acknowledgments

Christine Eiser is supported by Cancer Research-UK (CP 1019/0104). Aura Kuperberg is supported by Health Promotion and Outcomes, Children's Center for Cancer and Blood Diseases, Children's Hospital Los Angeles

References

1. Ross JW (1982) The role of the social worker with long term survivors of childhood cancer and their families. Soc Work Health Care 7:1–13
2. List MA, Ritter-Sterr C, Lansky SB (1991) Cancer during adolescence. Pediatrician 18:32–36
3. Kaplan SL, Busner J, Weinhold C, Lenon P (1986) Depressive symptoms in children and adolescents, and their families. J Am Acad Child Psychiatry 26:727–787
4. Ross JW (1978) Social work intervention with families of children with cancer: the changing critical phases. Soc Work Health Care 3:257–272
5. Stuber M, Gonzalez S, Benjamin H, Golant M (1995) Fighting for recovery: group interventions for adolescents with cancer and their parents. J Psychother Pract Res 4:286–296
6. Jamison, RN, Lewis S, Burish T (1986) Cooperation with treatment in adolescent cancer patients. Adolesc Health Care 7:162–167
7. Lansky SB, Smith SD, Cairns NU, Cairns GF (1983) Psychological correlates of compliance. Am J Pediatr Hematol Oncol 5:87–92
9. Erickson EH (1959) Identity and the life-cycle. Psychol Issues 1:164
8. Smith KE, Gotlieb S, Gurwitch RH, Blotcky AD (1987) Impact of a summer camp experience on daily activity and family interactions among children with cancer. J Pediatr Psychol 12:533–542
10. Ritchie MA (2001) Sources of emotional support for adolescents with cancer. J Pediatr Oncol Nurs 18:105–110
11. Trask PC, Paterson AG, Trask CL, et al (2003) Parent and adolescent adjustment to pediatric cancer: association with coping, social support, and family function. J Pediatr Oncol Nurs 20:36–47
12. Neville K (1998) The relationships among uncertainty, social support, and psychological distress in adolescents recently diagnosed with cancer. J Pediatr Oncol Nurs 15:37–46
13. Nichols ML (1995) Social support and coping in young adolescents with cancer. Pediatr Nurs 21:235–240
14. Ettinger RS, Heiney SP (1993) Cancer in adolescents and young adults. Cancer Suppl 71:3276–3280
15. Haluska HB, Jessee PO, Nagy MC (2002) Sources of social support: adolescents with cancer. Oncol Nurs Forum 29:1317–1324
16. Manne S, Miller D (1998) Social support, social conflict, and adjustment among adolescents with cancer. J Pediatr Psychol 23:121–130
17. Hendricks-Ferguson VL (1997) An analysis of the concept of hope in the adolescent with cancer. J Pediatr Oncol Nurs 14:73–80
18. Hinds PS (2000) Fostering coping by adolescents with newly diagnosed cancer. Semin Oncol Nurs 16:328–336
19. Haase J (1997) Hopeful teenagers with cancer: living courage. Reflections 32:20
20. Wilkinson J (2003) Young people with cancer – how should their care be organised? Eur J Cancer 12:65–70
21. Gehan S (2003) The benefits and drawbacks of treatment in a specialist Teenage Unit – a patient's perspective. Eur J Cancer 39:2681–2683
22. Whelan J (2003) Where should teenagers be treated? Eur J Cancer 39:2573–2578

23. MacLean WE, Foley GV, Ruccione K, Sklar CA (1996) Transitions in the care of adolescents and young adult survivors of childhood cancer. Cancer 78:1340–1344

24. Oeffinger KC, Eshelman DA, Tomlinson GE, Buchanan GR (1998) Programs for adult survivors of childhood cancer. J Clin Oncol 16:2864–2867

25. Taylor A, Hawkins M, Griffiths A, et al. (2004) Long-term follow-up of survivors of childhood cancer in the UK. Pediatr Blood Cancer 42:161–168

26. Wallace WH, Blacklay A, Eiser C, et al (2001) Developing strategies for long term follow up of survivors of childhood cancer. BMJ 323:271–274

27. Rosen DS (1993) Transition to adult health care for adolescents and young adults with cancer. Cancer 71:3411–3414

28. Boyle MP, Farukhi Z (2001) Strategies for improving transition to adult cystic fibrosis care, based on patient and parent views. Pediatr Pulmonol 32:428–436

29. Eiser C (2004) Children with Cancer: Their Quality of Life. Lawrence Erlbaum, USA

30. Elkin TD, Tyc VL, Hudson M, Crom D (1998) Participation in sports by long-term survivors of childhood cancer. J Psychosoc Oncol 16: 63–73

31. Morrow K, Thoreson R, Penney L (1997) Predictors of psychological distress among infertility clinic patients. J Consult Clin Psychol 63:163–167

32. Green D, Galvin H, Horne B (2003) The psychosocial impact of infertility on young male cancer survivors: a qualitative investigation. Psychooncology 12:141–152

33. Hudson MM, Mertens AC, Yasui Y, et al. (2003) Health status of adult long-term survivors of childhood cancer: a report from the Childhood Cancer Survivor Study. JAMA 290:1583–1592

34. Zeltzer LK, Zeltzer PM, LeBaron S (1983) Cancer in adolescents. In: Smith MS (ed) Chronic Disorders in Adolescence. John Wright, Littleton, MA, pp 253–275

35. Wu LM, Chin CC (2003) Factors related to satisfaction with body image in children undergoing chemotherapy. Kaohsiung J Med Sci 19:217–224

36. Zeltzer LK, Ellenberg L, Rigler D (1980) Psychologic effects of illness in adolescents: crucial issues and coping styles. J Pediatr 97:132–138

37. Pendley JS, Dahlquist LM, Dreyer Z (1997) Body image and psychosocial adjustment in adolescent cancer survivors. J Pediatr Psychol 22:29–43

38. Erickson EH. (1959). Identity and the life-cycle. Psychological Issues 1: 164.

39. Madan-Swain A, Brown RT, Foster MA, et al (2000) Identity formation in adolescent survivors of childhood cancer. J Pediatr Psychol 25:105–115

40. Stern M, Norman SL, Zevon MA (1991) Career development of adolescent cancer patients: a comparative analysis. J Couns Psychol 38:431–439

41. Koocher GP, O'Malley JE (1981) The Damocles Syndrome. Psychosocial Consequences of Surviving Childhood Cancer. McGraw-Hill, New York

42. Vugia H (1991) Support groups in oncology: building hope through the human bond. J Psychosoc Oncol 9:89–107

43. Farrell F, Hutter JJ (1980). Living until death: adolescence with cancer. Health Soc Work 5:35–38

43a. Plante WA, Lobato D, Engel R (2001) Review of group interventions for pediatric chronic conditions. J Pediatr Psychol 26:435–453

44. Cain EN, Kohorn EI, Quilan DM, et al (1986) Psychosocial benefits of a cancer support group. Cancer 57:183–189

45. Kellerman J, Zeltzer L, Ellenberg L, et al (1980) Psychological effects of illness in adolescence. I. Anxiety, self-esteem, and perception of control. J Pediatr 97:126–131

46. Benson PJ (1987) The relationship between self-concept and a summer camping program for children and adolescents who have cancer. J Assoc Pediatr Oncol Nurs 4:42–43

47. Bluebond-Langner M, Perkel D, Goertzel T, et al (1990). Children's knowledge of cancer and its treatment: impact of an oncology camp experience. J Pediatr 116:207–272

48. Bluebond M, Perkel D, Goetzel T (1991) Pediatric cancer patients' peer relationships: the impact of an oncology camp experience. J Psychosoc Oncol 9:67–80

49. Chesler MA, Yoak M (1984) Difficulties for providing help i a crisis: Relationship between parents of childen with cancer their families. In Kobalk, HB (ed), Helping patients and their families. San Francisco: Jossey-Bass.

50. Carr-Gregg M, Hampson R (1986) A new approach to the psychosocial care of adolescents with cancer. Med J Aust 145:580–583

51. Kuperberg AL (1996) The relationship between perceived social support, family behavior, self-esteem, and hope on adolescents' strategies for coping with cancer. Diss Abstr Int A Humanit Soc Sci 56:3744

Psychosocial Support

Brad J. Zebrack • Mark A. Chesler •
Anthony Penn

Contents

24.1 Introduction

This chapter focuses on the psychosocial impact of cancer on adolescents and young adults and provides a basis for therapeutic recommendations provided in the chapter on psychologic support by Eiser and Kuperberg (Chap. 23). It examines the unique developmental and psychosocial issues and subsequent needs of these young people as they occur throughout a continuum of survivorship, as well as approaches to address those needs. In contrast to the aforementioned chapter, which primarily addresses the patient undergoing active therapy, this chapter focuses on patients and survivors together because the experience of young adulthood stimulates responses to a personal history of childhood cancer that may differ from those evident in earlier developmental periods. Young adulthood is a time of increased vulnerability to stress and presents cancer survivors with major developmental challenges above and beyond those faced by other young people [1]. For example, gaining independence, establishing one's sense of identity, negotiating interpersonal relationships (including intimacy and forming families), as well as making important decisions about education and employment, all require a focus, in most individuals for the first time, on the medical, cognitive, or psychosocial effects of cancer treatment.

Chesler and Barbarin's [2] Stress-coping model is useful for organizing psychosocial issues across five dimensions: intellectual, practical, interpersonal, emotional, and existential. The utility of this model comes from its organization of the cancer experience into observable categories of stress, coping responses and strategies, and sources of social support. It helps identify patient and survivor needs from perspectives incorporating quality of life, positive adaptation, and family systems, thereby informing the development of interventions that address psychopathologic disease prevention as well as health promotion.

24.2 Intellectual Issues

24.2.1 Information About Cancer Diagnosis, Prognosis, and Treatment

Communicating information to adolescent and young adult cancer patients can be a sensitive issue. Some patients prefer to be shielded from direct communication about their cancer; others may desire to assume a more prominent position in the information flow and management of their care. For instance, Young and colleagues [3] report that parents most often manage what and how their children are told about cancer, and that young people vary in their preferences as to how much information should be disclosed to them. Last and van Veldhuizen [4] found that while the majority of young people with cancer prefer to be fully informed about their disease, approximately one-third of the young adult patients surveyed preferred not to know. Nonetheless, in general, the adolescent and young adult patients' desire for information is a chief concern. They typically express preferences for face-to-face communication with health professionals that is open, honest, nonjudgmental, respectful, and inclusive of them in the formulation of treatment plans [5, 6].

Researchers and clinicians alike have stressed the importance of adolescents and young adults receiving adequate and direct information about their cancer history and related risks (e.g., late effects, including in fertility, risks for second cancers, potential genetic effects on offspring [7–9]). Survivors themselves often express desires for services related to diet and nutrition, supportive counseling, health insurance, assistance with career planning, guidelines for appropriate long-term medical follow-up, and access to community physicians familiar with oncologic late-effects, and meeting other long-term survivors [10, 11].

24.2.2 Information Seeking

Adolescent and young adult survivors of childhood cancer often lack critical information regarding their cancer and its treatment, including information about the types and dosages of chemotherapy, and in some cases even the type of cancer they had, along with knowledge about potential long-term physical effects [12]. The active process of seeking and obtaining information about cancer appears to be related to improved self-confidence [8], and young survivors who preferred and received open communication about their diagnosis and prognosis at the initial stage of disease also showed significantly less anxiety and depression later [4]. Yet, adolescents' and young adults' attitudes about information-seeking may change over time, depending on cultural backgrounds or beliefs about cancer, health or illness. The extent to which survivors and their family members perceive risks of relapse or a "need to know" may also influence information-seeking.

As adolescent and young adult cancer patients complete treatment, grow older, become geographically mobile (e.g., move away from their families of origin and from their source of medical/oncologic care), and become more solely responsible for their own healthcare, the process of seeking and accessing healthcare is often perceived to be stressful [13]. Selecting employer-offered or other group health-insurance packages, or finding a doctor are all new experiences for cancer survivors to handle on their own. In these regards, survivors and health professionals alike have identified significant barriers or obstacles to obtaining appropriate follow-up care, including survivors' lack of knowledge about relevant and appropriate care, limitations with regard to health insurance and financial resources, as well as healthcare providers' lack of knowledge about relevant long-term survivorship issues [14, 15].

24.3 Practical Issues

24.3.1 The Hospitalization Experience, Including Pain and Painful Procedures

As adolescent and young adult patients undergo diagnostic procedures and subsequent treatment, they meet innumerable health-care professionals and ancillary hospital staff who will be involved in their care for an extended period of time. Diagnostic tests, curative and palliative therapies, and subsequent side effects often bring discomfort, pain, nausea, vomiting, fevers and infections, fatigue, changes in appetite, altered bodily appearance, and sleep disturbances. While subject to these painful procedures and treatments, adolescent cancer patients have reported a lost sense of control over their lives [16]. End-of-life care presents special difficulty as emotional stress increases, physical functioning deteriorates and pain management becomes an issue.

24.3.2 School and Work

Adolescent and young adult patients and survivors confront myriad disruptions in the worlds of school and work as a direct result of cancer diagnosis and treatment. Returning to school represents the continuation of "normal" life, as junior high and high school attendance for all and college for some are vital social and developmental activities for this population. Regular school attendance is vital to foster normal development and to prevent isolation from peers and social regression [17]. Research suggests the importance of encouraging adolescents to participate in school activities as fully as possible, since positive school experiences can reduce teenagers' maladaptive emotional responses to the disease and its treatments by helping them feel academically accomplished and socially accepted [18]. It also helps reestablish normal life patterns and a renewed sense of control and stability.

In the United States, state and local school districts are required by law to provide a free, appropriate elementary and secondary education in the least restrictive environment for all young people needing special attention/education, including students with cancer or a cancer history whose medical problems might adversely affect their educational performance [19]. For those whose physical conditions place them at risk of further health problems, homebound or hospital-based education may be necessary. When possible, however, preference should be given to the regular school environment, and if this is not possible, the hospital-based school [20].

With regard to educational achievement, employment, and living situations, studies indicate that most patients and survivors are functioning well and leading normal lives [21, 22]; yet many young adult cancer patients and survivors report having experienced restricted role function at work and in daily activities, including social discrimination and rejection in employment and military opportunities [23–27]. Some also experience difficulty maintaining or obtaining independent or family-based health insurance, encounter financial strain, and attain lower income levels when compared to other noncancer groups [9, 24, 25, 28].

Subsets of survivors also experience impaired achievement in education, employment, and social and family goals when compared to others [24, 29–31]. In particular, central nervous system (CNS) tumor patients/survivors and leukemia survivors treated with cranial radiation are much less likely to complete high school, attain an advanced graduate degree, or follow normal elementary or secondary school paths when compared to survivors of other cancer types and to healthy controls [29, 32]. CNS tumor survivors also are more likely to be unemployed, have a health condition that affects their ability to work, and enroll in learning disabled programs [33]. In a Childhood Cancer Survivor Study that monitors a multi-institutional epidemiologic cohort of over 16,000 survivors, use of special education services was reported by 23% of survivors in comparison to only 8% of siblings, with the greatest differences observed among female survivors who were diagnosed before age 6 years, and most notably among survivors of CNS tumors, leukemia, and Hodgkin lymphoma [34].

24.4 Interpersonal Issues

24.4.1 Relationship with Parents

The literature suggests that seriously ill young people tend to become more dependent upon their parents, at least temporarily. For adolescents and young adults, this may involve regression from recently achieved independence into a prior dependent relationship. As young people with cancer try to deal with or discuss the illness with their parents, they sometimes discover that they have quite different coping strategies. Just as symmetry in coping strategies is an important factor in spousal interaction, it affects child–parent interactions as well. Parents may want to discuss issues with their children that the children do not wish to discuss, or vice-versa, perhaps because doing so evokes issues or feelings that for so long have been buried in the past. Parents also may express or manifest emotional distress quite differently than their children. Some young people with cancer desire to protect their parents and not share their deepest worries with them, perhaps out of guilt for what their parents are going through, or perhaps just because they can see how upset their parents are [2, 35].

24.4.2 Relationships with Peers

Problems with establishing close interpersonal relationships have been reported among long-term survivors and appear to be associated with longer duration of treatment and more recent illness [36]. Gray [37] reports that cancer survivors describe improvements in social relationships (as compared to controls), but also feel greater disappointment in those relationships, suggesting that this disappointment is a result of having higher expectations of those relationships. Indeed, a common theme arising out of survivor meetings and present in the medical literature is the notion that prior social networks may fail to provide the type or kind of support that long-term survivors seek, and may even cause additional stress [38].

Although adolescents with cancer may be thought of as being more socially isolated than their healthy peers, empirical evidence does not support this assertion. In general, adolescents with cancer have been shown to be similar to peers on numerous dimensions of psychological and social functioning [39]. However, adolescents and young adults with cancer commonly experience changes in friendships and a sense of isolation from friends due to lengthy time away from home, school, or work for treatments, and many friendships may fall by the wayside over time [40, 41]. Specifically, adolescents and young adults report feeling that some friends are no longer able to relate to their life situation and get uncomfortable continuously talking with the

patient about cancer, resulting in feelings of being "different" and apprehensive about forming new friendships [40, 42]. Consequently, many of these young people form (or would like to form) new friendship circles, often with other cancer patients and survivors with whom they can relate to their current life situation and past experience with cancer.

According to Heiney [43], studies have found that there is a general lack of knowledge about the anatomy and physiology of reproduction among adolescents generally. This comes at a time when most adolescents display heightened curiosity about sexuality, and some begin to experiment with intimacy and sex. Reviewing the impact of cancer treatment on sexuality, intimacy and relationships, Thaler-DeMers [44] suggests that the issue of sharing one's cancer history with a new partner is particularly salient to a young adult survivor population, and Roberts et al. [45] report that relevant issues arising in a group intervention study among young adult survivors included concerns about fertility and raising children. With regard to family planning, Schover and colleagues [46] identify salient relationship-oriented concerns for young adults, including infertility, reproductive problems, desire for children in the future, sperm banking, concerns about the health of their offspring, and genetic risks, pregnancy concerns and complications, and attitudes about having children after cancer.

24.5 Emotional Issues

24.5.1 Psychological Distress

Current research suggests that 15–30% of childhood and young adult cancer survivors are seriously troubled psychologically, or significantly more likely than various comparison groups to report distress [1, 31, 47, 48]. These problems include a wide range of psychosocial adjustment difficulties, such as delayed social maturation, mood disturbances, academic difficulties, job and insurance discrimination, increased health concerns, and relationship problems. These findings suggest that a cancer diagnosis during childhood continues to interfere with the ability of many survivors to master the developmental tasks of young adulthood

[49]. Comparative studies of survivors have demonstrated significantly greater psychological distress in childhood cancer survivors as compared to various comparative groups when measured by standardized psychometric scaling techniques [28, 50, 51].

In contrast, several other investigators demonstrate that, on aggregate, adolescent and young adult cancer survivors score in the normal range on standardized psychometric measures and live normal social lives with no evidence of significant mental or emotional distress, thereby being quite similar to peers without a history of cancer in terms of their psychosocial adjustment and quality of life [22, 52–56].

In some instances, psychological and quality of life outcomes among young adult survivors are the same as, if not better than those among comparison populations [57–61]. In a study of young adult survivors of childhood leukemia and lymphoma, Gray and colleagues [55] indicate that, compared with their peers, survivors reported significantly more positive emotional health status, less negative mood or affect, a higher motivation for intimacy (i.e., thinking about others, concern for others), more perceived personal control, and greater satisfaction with control in life situations. Maggiolini and colleagues [62] showed that teenagers cured of leukemia showed a more positive and mature self-image when compared to student peers.

In general, the psychosocial literature on survivors of pediatric cancer suggests that cancer universally alters the way survivors view themselves and that these alterations can be positive or negative and both positive and negative [63]. In particular, adolescents have reported a sense of relief upon completion of therapy, but also ambivalence related to perceived loss of social ties (i.e., with other adolescents with cancer, with health-care providers who have come to know them, with the health-care system), and fears of life without the protective "crutch" of effective treatment [64]. The aforementioned series of studies vary substantially in their theoretical frames, inquiry methods, and samples of informants. By examining them on aggregate, a reasonable summary argues that some young adult and childhood cancer survivors have managed to grow in positive ways as a result of their cancer experience. Most probably are relatively normal in psychosocial terms and on most psychosocial measures, and an important minority experience ongoing psychological and/or social adjustment problems. Moreover, most survivors, even those apparently doing quite well, continue to be concerned about the physical, psychological, and social quality of their current and future lives.

24.5.2 Posttraumatic Effects

A recently emerging literature on stress, threat, and trauma provides a new and different paradigm for examining and understanding emotional responses to life-threatening situations like cancer. Recent conceptualization of cancer as a psychological "trauma" has furthered our understanding of the long-term psychological effects of cancer and its treatment, with studies assessing the symptoms of posttraumatic stress indicating that anywhere from 10 to 30% meet the criteria for posttraumatic stress disorder, and an additional proportion meet the criteria for at least one trauma symptom [65]. Reporting symptoms of posttraumatic stress appears to be associated with survivors' retrospective subjective appraisal of life threat at the time of treatment and the degree to which the survivor experienced that treatment as "hard" or "scary," as well as with general anxiety, history of other stressful life experiences, less time since end of treatment, female gender, and lack of family or social support.

A new trauma paradigm raises the possibility that some people may not just survive such stress and trauma, but that they may "thrive" or achieve "posttraumatic growth" as a result, and they may create or experience a higher quality of life than prior to the stress [66, 67]. As Folkman and Greer [68] argue, the focus on "psychiatric symptoms, such as anxiety and depression…obscure the struggle for psychological well-being and the coping processes that support it," and Paterson et al. [69] discuss how some people can transform their lives by responding to an illness in ways that enhance the quality and meaning of their lives. Some cancer survivors report positive growth as a function of how they and their families dealt with their illness and appear significantly better adjusted psychosocially in comparison with population norms or healthy controls groups [57, 70, 71]. Even so, these young people still worry about their physical health status, their self-esteem and identity, their immediate family's welfare, relating with the social world and being "different", reintegrating with the school system, possibilities for the future (including access to life and health insurance, jobs and career options, and understanding genetic compromises stemming from treatment), and continued care from a skilled and attentive medical system [72–74].

24.5.3 Coping

Research has addressed the factors and variables associated with coping and adjustment among adolescents and young adult cancer patients and survivors. For example, positive thinking or maintaining a positive outlook on the future is commonly reported as a coping strategy for adolescent and young adult cancer patients and survivors [13]. In a quality-of-life assessment of 176 adolescent and young adult survivors, Zebrack and Chesler [75] observed that having a sense of purpose in life and perceiving positive changes as a result of cancer were associated with positive quality of life.

Some investigators have suggested that the aforementioned aspects of positive adaptation or meaning-making may in fact suggest that denial is a common coping style among adolescent and young adult patients who maintain a positive outlook for the future [71, 76, 77]. However, adolescents and young adults with cancer can experience positive self-images and life outlooks without necessarily "denying" their true condition or fears [78]. Clearly, patients' and survivors' denial of their problems associated with cancer treatment (e.g., treatment refusal and noncompliance, ignoring signs of relapse or infections, engaging in health-risk-taking behavior) is unproductive and maladaptive, but denial of some of the discomforting emotions associated with cancer (anxiety about recurrence, worry about peer acceptance, obsession about a healthy long-term future, feeling like a victim) may be very adaptive and productive. In these instances, denial may even lead to the adoption of disease-preventing and health-promoting behaviors or the assumption of a positive life future and possibility of long-term personal growth. Yet, gaining knowledge of one's cancer treatment and effects also has been shown to be associated with positive adaptation and coping [8].

24.5.4 The Importance of Social, Peer, and Family Support

During a period of time in which individuals increasingly experiment with and seek relationships and social support, a diagnosis of cancer has the obvious potential to subvert normal adolescent and young adult development. At the same time, a perception of high levels of social support can help teens and young adults with cancer cope with their illness and overcome the feeling that they are alone. Kyngas et al. [8] found that social support was the major coping strategy used by adolescents to deal with cancer, with support coming from family, friends, and health-care providers, although the family was perceived to be the most important source of emotional support. Actively seeking support also has been demonstrated to be associated with positive adjustment [8, 79].

Several studies identify family support and cohesiveness as a most important contributor to positive adjustment [80] and family functioning as the single best predictor of distress, with poorer family functioning predictive of greater distress [81]. In addition, Trask and colleagues [82] report that adolescent and parental adjustment are related to one another, and suggest that the ability of teenage patients to cope with their illness is dependent upon their parents' ability to cope, and vice-versa. Lynam [83] found that the supportive role of the family is demonstrated through several actions and perceptions in the parent–child relationship. Notably, Lynam found that a reciprocal supportive relationship exists in which young adults share information about their condition with family members to allay their mutual concerns, but in some cases filter information that they felt would burden their family with excessive worry.

24.5.5 Support Groups

There exists a perception among some oncologists and parents that attending survivors meetings or support groups, spending time with other cancer survivors, and revisiting the cancer experience may be maladaptive and prevent survivors from integrating with other so-called "normal" peers. Yet, there exists no empirical evidence to suggest this is the case. In contrast, Roberts et al. [45] report the results of a support group intervention for young adults that led to improvements in psychological well-being. Topics covered included anxiety about health and physical well-being, worry about fertility and raising children, relationship problems, financial concerns, and body image. The authors noted that the group quickly developed a level of cohesion and suggested that the quickness and ease with which this happened was demonstrative of the need and desire for support among these participants.

An important issue for adolescent and young adults is the decision of if, when, and how to share information about cancer with their peers. An even more delicate issue is what and how much to say about their illness to new acquaintances, and particularly those for whom a long-term intimate relationship may be possible. Faced with the potential for varied reactions, young people with cancer may lose confidence because of their uncertainty about whether and how they will be accepted. When loss of opportunities for social interaction with peers is severe, it is experienced as a major deprivation that multiplies other stresses of the illness. When positive interaction with peers occurs, it helps ease the stress of coping with the illness and renews youngsters' adaptive capacities.

Thus, participation in teenage or young adult oncology camps, outdoor adventure programs, cancer survivor day picnics and family retreats offer opportunities for life experiences that promote successful achievement of age-appropriate developmental tasks. For instance, a dramatic wilderness adventure provides adolescents undergoing therapy with extraordinary experiences that boost self image and facilitate coping skills [84]. An 8-day adventure trip for 17 young adult survivors of childhood cancer provided participants with an opportunity for physical challenges and resulted in reports of improvements in self-confidence, independence, and social contacts [85]. In general, opportunities for peer involvement provide these young people a chance to address areas of concern such as coping with uncertainty, dependency versus autonomy, social exclusion, separation processes, body image, intimacy, sexuality and fertility, and occupations with others whom they can observe as sharing similar experiences.

24.6 Existential/Spiritual Issues

In the face of a life and death diagnosis, which is rare and totally unexpected for people their age, adolescent and young adult patients and survivors also experience a sense of existential crisis, a challenge to their sense of the normal order of things and the way they have assumed the world should work. Their faith in the continuity and predictability of life obviously is threatened. Especially because the precursors of adolescent and young adult cancers are largely unknown to the medical and scientific community, patients' often experience a high level of uncertainty about their current and future place in the world.

24.6.1 Uncertainty

Uncertainty has been defined by young people with cancer as more than living with the unknown, but also as not knowing what to expect [86]. Survivors in their teens and young adult years also suggest that, while uncertainty can be a source of distress, it also can be a catalyst for personal growth, a deepened appreciation for life, greater awareness of life purpose, development of confidence and resilience, and optimism [87].

Having a positive life attitude, belief in one's own resources, belief in God, earlier positive life experiences, and willingness to fight against the disease also have been identified as important resources for coping with cancer [8]. Nichols [88] reports the use of spiritual support as a coping behavior for teenage patients, but waning as the length of illness increased. Many young people report that their religious faith was tested by the cancer experience; most who experience such a test report that their faith has been strengthened by their experience, if not by the fact that they survived. Others, with or without a strong religious orientation or commitment, report a greater sense of existential clarity, a form of psychospiritual adaptation and growth that takes the form of knowledge about the meaning and purpose of their life, a sense that God would not give them more than they could handle, and a willingness to accept the uncertainty of life [88, 87].

Reflecting the notion that "a positive future exists for oneself," the concept of hope has been investigated in adolescent and young adult patients, with findings indicating a positive association between being hopeful and psychosocial adjustment [89]. In an investigation involving patients aged 8 to 18 years old, increased hopefulness and decreased feelings of helplessness were the most important factors associated with positive coping and decreased anxiety [90], with hopefulness reflected in patients' comments about attending school, future careers, and marriage.

24.7 Conclusion

Adolescents and young adults with cancer often report a desire for more information – about their diagnosis, prognosis, treatment, and potential short- and long-term effects. These desires are often not expressed to the medical staff or parents, and thus often go unmet. Moreover, young people with cancer often do not share with their parents the full extent of the pain and anxiety that they experience during the treatment process. They observe and understand their parents' distress and often hide their own concerns in order not to further worry or add to their parents' strain.

In addition to anxiety about the future course of medical treatment, young adult survivors of childhood cancer report worry about body image, sexual identity, and fertility. Such issues are part of a normal developmental process in this age group, but become more potent in the context of a serious and chronic illness. Moreover, these concerns may be further escalated in the case of unsettled peer relationships, as absence from school during treatment often changes the young person's relationships with former friends and neighbors. For some, school absence results in educational disadvantage and delayed preparation for higher education or career progress. The same holds true for young adults in their work and social worlds, where employment becomes disrupted, where they may be subject to prejudice and discrimination, and where young adults feel uncertain or burdened about how much to disclose about their cancer to employers, coworkers and friends.

In the end, the majority of young adult cancer survivors appear to be psychologically well-adjusted, even when acknowledging the visible and limiting physical effects of treatments. Overall, these young people

experience emotions and behave in ways that are normative for this age population. On the other hand, a substantial minority experience posttraumatic stress, a form of emotional and psychosocial disability that requires psychological counseling of some form. An important minority appear to experience posttraumatic growth and are able to transform their lives in ways that represent more positive outlooks and competencies than one would have expected prior to their diagnosis and treatment. Given the full range of these responses, including the possibility that some teenagers and young adults surviving cancer can exhibit signs of greater emotional stability and security, intervention programs that historically have focused on alleviating stress and preventing negative outcomes (such as posttraumatic stress symptoms) must be complemented by programs focusing on promoting successful achievement of age-appropriate developmental tasks and positive psychological and emotional growth.

References

1. Hobbie WL, Stuber M, Meeske K, et al (2000) Symptoms of posttraumatic stress in young adult survivors of childhood cancer. J Clin Oncol 18:4060–4066
2. Chesler M, Barbarin O (1987) Childhood Cancer and the Family. Brunner/Mazel, New York
3. Young M, Dixon-Woods M, Windridge KC, Heney D (2003) Managing communication with young people who have a potentially life threatening chronic illness: qualitative study of patients and parents. BMJ 326:305–309
4. Last B, Veldhuizen V (1996) Information about diagnosis and prognosis related to anxiety and depression in children with cancer aged 8–16 years. Eur J Cancer 32:290–294
5. Ljungman G, McGrath PJ, Cooper E, et al (2003) Psychosocial needs of families with a child with cancer. J Pediatr Hematol Oncol 25:223–231
6. Orr DP, Hoffmans MA, Bennetts G (1984) Adolescents with cancer report their psychosocial needs. J Psychosoc Oncol 2:47–59
7. Hudson MM, Tyc VL, Jayawardene DA, et al (1999) Feasibility of implementing health promotion interventions to improve health-related quality of life. Int J Cancer 12:138–142
8. Kyngas H, Mikkonen R, Nousiainen E, et al (2001) Coping with the onset of cancer: Coping strategies and resources of young people with cancer. Eur J Cancer

Care 10:6–11

9. Oeffinger KC, Mertens AC, Hudson MM, et al (2004) Health care of young adult survivors of childhood cancer: a report from the Childhood Cancer Survivor Study. Ann Fam Med 2:61–70

10. Lozowski SL (1993) Views of childhood cancer survivors. Cancer 15:3354–3357

11. Zebrack BJ, Chesler MA (2000) Managed care: the new context for social work in health care – implications for survivors of childhood cancer and their families. Soc Work Health Care, 31:89–104

12. Kadan-Lottick NS, Robison LL, Gurney JG, et al (2002) Childhood cancer survivors' knowledge about their past diagnosis and treatment: Childhood Cancer Survivor Study. JAMA 287:1832–1839

13. Enskar K, Carlsson M, Golsater M, Hamrin E (1997) Symptom distress and life situation in adolescents with cancer. Cancer Nurs 20:23–33

14. Mertens AC, Cotter KL, Foster BM, et al (2004) Improving health care for adult survivors of childhood cancer: recommendations from a Delphi panel of health policy experts. Health Policy 69:169–178

15. Zebrack BJ, Eshelman DA, Hudson M, et al (2004) Health care for childhood cancer survivors: insights and perspectives from a Delphi panel of young adult survivors of childhood cancer. Cancer 100:843–850

16. Kameny RR, Bearison DJ (2002) Cancer narratives of adolescents and young adults: a quantitative and qualitative analysis. Children Health Care 31:143–173

17. Deasy-Spinetta P (1993) School issues and the child with cancer. Cancer 71:3261–3264

18. Die-Trill M, Stuber ML (1998) Psychological problems of curative cancer treatment. In: Holland JC (ed) Psychooncology. Oxford University Press, New York, pp 897–906

19. Brophy P, Kazak AE (1994) Schooling. In: Johnson FL, O'Donnell EL (eds) The Candlelighters Guide to Bone Marrow Transplants in Children. Candlelighters Childhood Cancer Foundation, Bethesda pp 68–73

20. Searle NS, Askins M, Bleyer WA (2003) Homebound schooling is the least favorable option for continued education of adolescent cancer patients: a preliminary report. Med Pediatr Oncol 40:380–384

21. Green DM, Zevon MA, Hall B (1991) Achievement of life goals by adult survivors of modern treatment for childhood cancer. Cancer 67:206–213

22. Moe PJ, Holen A, Glomstein A, et al (1997) Long-term survival and quality of life in patients treated with a national ALL protocol 15–20 years earlier: IDM/HDM and late effects? Pediatr Hematol Oncol 14:513–524

23. Bloom JR, Hoppe RT, Fobair P, et al (1988) Effects of treatment on the work experiences of long-term survivors of Hodgkin disease. J Psychosoc Oncol 6:65–80

24. Dolgin MJ, Somer E, Buchvald E, Zaizov R (1999) Quality of life in adult survivors of childhood cancer. Soc Work Health Care 28:31–43

25. Jacobson Vann JC, Biddle AK, Daeschner CW, et al (1995) Health insurance access to young adult survivors of childhood cancer in North Carolina. Med Pediatr Oncol 25:389–395

26. Jankovic M, Van Dongen-Melman JE, Vasilatou-Kosmidis H, Jenney ME (1999) Improving the quality of life for children with cancer. European School of Oncology Advisory Group. Tumori 85:273–27957. new line

26. Apajasalo M, Sintonen H, Siimes M, et al (1996) Health-related quality of life of adults surviving malignancies in childhood. Eur J Cancer 32A:1354–1358

27. Somerfield MR, Curbow B, Wingard JR, et al (1996) Coping with the physical and psychosocial sequelae of bone marrow transplantation among long-term survivors. J Behav Med 9:163–184

28. Kornblith AB, Anderson J, Cella DF, et al (1992) Hodgkin disease survivors at increased risk for problems in psychosocial adaptation. Cancer 70:2214–2224

29. Langeveld NE, Ubbink MC, Last BF, et al (2003) Educational achievement, employment and living situation in long-term young adult survivors of childhood cancer in the Netherlands. Psychooncology 12:213–225

30. Novakovic B, Fears TR, Horowitz ME, et al (1997) Late effects of therapy in survivors of Ewing's sarcoma family tumors. J Pediatr Hematol Oncol 19:220–225

31. Zeltzer LK, Chen E, Weiss R, et al (1997) Comparison of psychologic outcome in adult survivors of childhood acute lymphoblastic leukemia versus sibling controls: a cooperative Children's Cancer Group and National Institutes of Health study. J Clin Oncol 15:547–556

32. Kingma A, Rammeloo LA, Der Doew-Van Den Berg A, et al (2000) Academic career after treatment for acute lymphoblastic leukemia. Arch Dis Child 82:353–357

32. Mostow EN, Byrne J, Connelly RR, Mulvihill JJ (1991) Quality of life in long-term survivors of CNS tumors of childhood and adolescence. J Clin Oncol 9:592–599

34. Mitby PA, Robison LL, Whitton JA, et al (2003) Utilization of special education services and educational attainment among long-term survivors of childhood cancer. Cancer 97:1115–1126

35. Zebrack B, Chesler M, Orbuch T, Parry C (2002) Mothers of survivors of childhood cancer: their worries and concerns. J Psychosoc Oncol 20:1–26

36. Mackie E, Hill J, Kondryn H, McNally R (2000) Adult psychosocial outcomes in long-term survivors of acute lymphoblastic leukaemia and Wilms' tumour: a controlled study. Lancet 355:1310–1314

37. Gray RE (1992) Persons with cancer speak out: reflections of an important trend in Canadian health care. J Palliat Care 8:30–37

38. Chesler M, Barbarin O (1984) Difficulties of providing help in a crisis: relationships between parents of children with cancer and their friends. J Soc Iss 40:113–134

39. Noll R, Bukowski W, Davies W, et al (1993) Adjustment in the peer system of adolescents with cancer. J Pediatr Psychol 18:351–364

40. Dunlop JG (1982) Critical problems facing young adults with cancer. Oncol Nurs Forum 9:33–38

41. Chesler MA, Weigers M, Lawther T (1992) How am I different? Perspectives for childhood cancer survivors on change and growth. In: Green DM, D'Angio G (eds) Late Effects of Treatment for Childhood Cancer. Wiley and Sons, New York, pp 151–158

42. Adams HS (2003) Young adults with cancer. Cure 2:36–41

43. Heiney SP (1989) Adolescents with cancer: Sexual and reproductive issues. Cancer Nurs 12:95–101

44. Thaler-Demers D (2001) Intimacy issues: Sexuality, fertility, and relationships. Semin Oncol Nurs 17:255–262

45. Roberts C, Piper L, Denny J, Cuddeback G (1997) A support group intervention to facilitate young adults' adjustment to cancer. Health Soc Work 22:133–141

46. Schover LR, Rybicki LA, Martin BA, Bringelsen KA (1999) Having children after cancer: a pilot survey of survivors' attitudes and experiences. Cancer 86:697–709

47. Glover DA, Byrne J, Mills JL, et al (2003) Impact of CNS treatment on mood in adult survivors of childhood leukemia: a report from the Children's Cancer Group. J Clin Oncol 21:4395–4401

48. Stuber M, Christakis DA, Houskamp B, Kazak AE (1996) Posttrauma symptoms in childhood leukemia survivors and their parents. Psychosomatics 37:254–261

49. Richardson R, Baron Nelson M, Meeske K (1999) Young adult survivors of childhood cancer: attending to emerging medical and psychosocial needs. J Pediatr Oncol Nurs 16:136–144

50. Zebrack B, Gurney JG, Oeffinger KC, et al (2004) Psychological outcomes in long-term survivors of childhood brain cancer: a report from the Childhood Cancer Survivor Study. J Clin Oncol 22:999–1006

51. Zebrack BJ, Zeltzer LK, Whitton J, et al (2002) Psychological outcomes in long-term survivors of childhood leukemia, Hodgkin disease and non-Hodgkin lymphoma: a report from the Childhood Cancer Survivor Study. Pediatrics 110:42–52

52. Calaminus G, Weinspach S, Teske C, Gobel U (2000) Quality of life in children and adolescents with cancer: first results of an evaluation of 49 patients with the PEDQOL questionnaire. Klin Pediatr 212:211–215

53. Crom DB, Chathaway DK, Tolley EA, Mulhern RK, Hudson MM (1999) Health status and health-related quality of life in long-term survivors of pediatric solid tumors. Int J Cancer 12:25–31

54. Eiser C, Hill JJ, Vance YH (2000) Examining the psychological consequences of surviving childhood cancer: systematic review as a research method in pediatric psychology. J Pediatr Psychol 25:449–460

55. Gray RE, Doan BD, Schermer P, FitzGerald AV, Berry MP, Jenkin D, Doherty MA (1992) Psychologic adaptation of survivors of childhood cancer. Cancer 70:2713–2721

56. Wasserman AL, Thompson EI, Wilimas JA, Fairclough DL (1987) The psychological status of survivors of childhood/adolescent Hodgkin disease. Am J Dis Child 141:626–631

57. Apajasalo M, Sintonen H, Siimes M, Hovi L, Holmberg C, Boyd H, et al (1996) Health-related quality of life of adults surviving malignancies in childhood Europ J Cancer, 32A:1354–1358

58. Evans SE, Radford M (1995) Current lifestyle of young adults treated for cancer in childhood. Arch Dis Child 72:423–426

59. Greenberg DB, Kornblith AB, Herndon JE, et al (1997) Quality of life for adult leukemia survivors treated on clinical trials of Cancer and Leukemia Group-B during the period 1971–1988– predictors for later psychologic distress. Cancer 80:1936–1944

60. Norum J, Wist E (1996) Psychological distress in survivors of Hodgkin disease. Support Care Cancer 4:191–195

61. Norum J, Wist E (1996) Quality of life in survivors of Hodgkin disease. Qual Life Res 5:367–374

62. Maggiolini A, Grassi R, Adamoli L, et al (2000) Self-image of adolescent survivors of long-term childhood leukemia. J Pediatr Hematol Oncol 22:417–421

63. Smith K, Ostroff J, Tan C, Lesko L (1991) Alterations in self-perceptions among adolescent cancer survivors. Cancer Invest 9:581–588

64. Weekes DP, Kagan S H (1994) Adolescent completing cancer therapy: meaning, perception, and coping. Oncol Nurs Forum 21:663–670

65. Erickson SJ, Steiner H (2001) Trauma and personality correlates in long term pediatric cancer survivors. Child Psychiatry Hum Dev 31:195–213

66. Carver CS (1998) Resilience and thriving: issues, models, and linkages. J Soc Iss 52:245–266

67. Harvey M (1996) An ecological view of psychological rauma and trauma recovery. J Trauma Stress 9:3–23

68. Folkman S, Greer S (2000) Promoting psychological well-being in the face of serious illness: When theory, research and practice inform one another. Psychooncology 9:11–19

69. Paterson B, Thorne S, Crawford J, Tarko M (1999) Living with diabetes as a transformational experience. Qual Health Res 9:786–802

70. Arnholt U, Fritz G, Keener M (1993) Self-concept in survivors of childhood and adolescent cancer. J Psychosoc Oncol 11:1–16

71. Elkin TD, Phipps S, Mulhern P, Fairclough D (1997) Psychological functioning of adolescent and young adult survivors of pediatric malignancy. Med Pediatr Oncol 29:582–588

72. Meadows A, Black B, Nesbit M, et al (1993) Long-term survival: clinical care, research and education. Cancer 71:3213–3215

73. Weigers ME, Chesler MA, Zebrack BJ, Goldman S (1998) Self-reported worries among long-term survivors of childhood cancer and their peers. J Psychosoc Oncol 16:1–24

74. Zeltzer L (1993) Cancer in adolescents and young adults. Cancer 71:3463–3468

75. Zebrack BJ, Chesler MA (2002) Quality of life in long-term survivors of childhood cancer. Psychooncology 11:132–141

76. Phipps S, Srivastava D (1997) Repressive adaptation in children with cancer. Health Psychol 16:521–528

77. Zeltzer LK, Kellerman J, Ellenberg L, et al (1980) Psychologic effects of illness in adolescence: II. Impact of illness in adolescents – crucial issues and coping styles. J Pediatr 97:132–138

78. Zebrack BJ, Chesler MA (2001) Health-related worries, self-image, and life outlooks of long-term survivors of childhood cancer. Health Soc Work 36:245–256

79. Meijer SA, Sinnema G, Bijstra JO, et al (2002) Coping styles and locus of control and predictors for psychological adjustment of adolescents with a chronic illness. Soc Sci Med 54:1453–1461

80. Newby WL, Brown RT, Pawletko TM, et al (2000) Social skills and psychological adjustment of child and adolescent cancer survivors. Psychooncology 9:113–126

81. Hill JM, Kornblith AB, Jones D, et al (1998) A comparative study of the long term psychosocial functioning of childhood acute lymphoblastic leukemia survivors treated by intrathecal methotrexate with or without cranial radiation. Cancer 82:208–218

82. Trask PC, Paterson AG, Trask CL, et al (2003) Parent and adolescent adjustment to pediatric cancer: associations with coping, social support, and family function. J Pediatr Oncol Nurs 20:36–47

83. Lynam MJ (1995) Supporting one another: the nature of family work when a young adult has cancer. J Adv Nurs 22:116–125

84. Stevens B, Kagan S, Yamada J, et al (2004) Adventure therapy for adolescents with cancer. Pediatr Blood Cancer 43:278–284

85. Elad P, Yagil Y, Cohen LH, Meller I (2003) A jeep trip with young adult cancer survivors: lessons to be learned. Support Care Cancer 11:201–206

86. Woodgate RL, Degner LF (2002) "Nothing is carved in stone!": uncertainty in children with cancer and their families. Eur J Oncol Nurs 6:191–202

87. Parry C (2003) Embracing uncertainty: an exploration of the experiences of childhood cancer survivors. Qual Health Res 13:227–246

88. Nichols ML (1995) Social support and coping in young adolescents with cancer. Pediatr Nurs 21:235–240

89. Hinds PS (2000) Fostering coping by adolescents with newly diagnosed cancer. Semin Oncol Nurs 16:317–327

90. Ritchie MA (2001) Self-esteem and hopefulness in adolescents with cancer. J Pediatr Oncol Nurs 16:35–42

Health-Related Quality of Life

Ernest R. Katz • Tasha Burwinkle •
James W. Varni • Ronald D. Barr

Contents

25.1 Introduction

With continuing advances in medical diagnosis and treatment, the focus on the individual cancer patient's perceptions of his or her health and well-being has assumed increasing importance [1]. The term "health-related quality of life" (HRQL) has been used at times in an imprecise manner along with other terms such as health status, functional status, and quality of life [2–4]. Quality of life is a global concept encompassing many different components according to the choice of the user [5]. HRQL, however, focuses more specifically on the wide-ranging implications that disease and treatment may have on an individual's appraisal of important aspects of life [5–7]. HRQL has been defined as a multidimensional construct [8, 9], consisting at a minimum of the physical, psychological, and social domains recommended by the World Health Organization [10], as well as the impact of disease-specific and treatment-related symptoms on a patient's self-perceptions of functioning [11–14]. More recent characterizations of this construct have also included spiritual and existential aspects of experience [15].

Although most medical research continues to focus on the overall survival rates of disease and the development of new treatments, HRQL research has proven to be valuable in monitoring and evaluating patient progress. By focusing on the patient's perspective of his or her experience, the hidden benefits and costs of illness and therapy are elucidated beyond that which is learned by measuring objective parameters of health alone [16]. In this way, monitoring HRQL in cancer patients is expected to enhance overall clinical outcomes [17]. It has been suggested that HRQL is critical to effective cancer care, second in importance only to survival itself [18, 19].

Within the field of oncology, Aaronson [20] has identified five purposes of researching HRQL: (1) to describe the nature and extent of functional and psychological problems that patients encounter during the course of their disease; (2) to determine norms for psychosocial problems for specific patient groups; (3) to screen patients for involvement in appropriate behavioral or psychopharmacological intervention programs; (4) to monitor patient care in order to improve the way that treatment is provided; and (5) to evaluate competing behavioral, psychosocial or medical treatment protocols. Ganz [21] has suggested that HRQL assessment will facilitate improvements in the quality of medical care provided to cancer patients (e.g., by informing healthcare providers of their patient's subjective experiences, they will be better able to tailor supportive interventions and improve quality).

HRQL research has become a salient factor in randomized, controlled clinical trials for new medical treatments [22, 23]. For example, HRQL questionnaires are used increasingly in cost effectiveness/utility analyses, and play an important role in the clinical documentation of the efficacy of new drugs and the quality of care for purchasers [14, 24, 25]. In adult oncology, HRQL measures have been well-incorporated into clinical trials, clinical practice improvement strategies, and healthcare services and research evaluation [4, 26]. In pediatric practice, these measures have only more recently begun to generate widespread interest and investigation [1, 22, 27, 28]. Particular sensitivity to developmental issues is needed when considering adolescents and young adults with cancer, for whom the diagnosis and treatment impact virtually every aspect of their lives [6, 29–33].

The adolescent with cancer moving into adulthood faces many unique psychological and emotional challenges [29, 34–37]. Adolescence is a period when peers play an increasingly significant role in how a young person views the world; a time for establishing autonomy and independence from parents and family [38, 39]. Other major changes associated with this period include beginning significant relationships, establishing future educational and career goals, and making a start toward financial security [40]. Cancer and its treatment creates unique and difficult additional challenges for young people, including frequent hospitalizations, separation from family and friends, coping with changes in appearance and physical abilities, disruption of schooling, traumatic medical procedures, and the uncertainty of survival [37, 41, 42]. Cancer in adolescents and young adults often requires a return to dependence on parents and caregivers, leading to real and perceived disruptions in the forward momentum of life and a decrease in quality of life [32, 33, 36, 37].

Adolescent and young adult survivors of cancer in childhood face many barriers in their transition from pediatric to adult care, including the lack of familiarity with long-term side-effects of pediatric cancers and therapy by adult physicians and other healthcare providers [34]. Appropriate follow-up care may be delayed or postponed indefinitely because of difficulties in insurance coverage for health screening and surveillance [43]. Young adult survivors may be reluctant to switch their care from pediatric practitioners and clinical settings they have come to know and trust over many years to new, adult practitioners with whom they may not easily establish a rapport [34]. They may avoid appropriate follow-up medical care altogether, or they may choose not to inform their adult providers about their cancer experience due to anxiety about the past, fear of losing insurance coverage due to a preexisting condition, or the desire to be "like everyone else" who does not have a cancer history [34, 37].

The purpose of the current chapter is to review critical issues and methods for the meaningful assessment and evaluation of HRQL in adolescent and young adult childhood cancer patients and survivors. We will also offer recommendations for the inclusion of HRQL into clinical trials and health surveillance programs to promote optimal HRQL and health outcomes in this population.

25.2 Dimensions Used in Measuring HRQL

According to Berzon et al. (1993), the measurement of HRQL should include an assessment of "physical, mental, psychological, and social health, as well as global perceptions of function and well being." Other components (sometimes referred to as dimensions, domains, categories, or attributes) that may be assessed also include pain, energy and fatigue, sleep, appetite, cognitive functioning, role functioning, and specific symptoms related directly to the disease or treatments [1, 20, 44–45]. According to Fayers and Machin [26], there is a causal relationship between disease-specific symptoms and HRQL; therefore, it is important to include the domain of "symptoms related to illness and treatment" when assessing HRQL. In cancer populations, pain, fatigue, nausea, and cognitive impairments are symptoms likely to be assessed.

25.3 Generic and Cancer-Specific Measures of HRQL

Three main purposes for HRQL assessments have been delineated by Guyatt et al. [11]: discrimination, evaluation, and prediction. The purpose of discrimination is to distinguish the burden of morbidity among groups or individuals at a point in time; this is especially useful in cross-sectional studies, in which the reliability of the measure is essential. Evaluation involves assessment of change in HRQL over time, which is particularly helpful in longitudinal studies in which the responsiveness of the measure is crucial. HRQL measures are used less often for prediction, such as determining how well these measures relate to prognosis.

HRQL measures may be either generic in scope, assessing broad and global issues, or more specific and targeted to unique subpopulations of patients. Generic measures are useful in the measurement of HRQL across diverse patient populations or disease groups, allowing for group comparisons. Generic HRQL measures may, however, be unresponsive to changes in specific conditions [11] and may fail to provide adequate data about specific disease symptoms and treatment-related side effects of relevance to particular disease groups [46]. In these cases, use of a disease-specific measure may provide a more accurate assessment of HRQL.

Disease-specific measures provide substantial and comprehensive analysis of the HRQL of patients suffering from specific conditions [47, 48]. Such measures generally contain a symptom checklist, in addition to disease and treatment-related issues that characterize a specific disease. In this way, disease-specific measures

are more sensitive to clinical change in patients with a particular illness, which may result from including only important aspects of HRQL that are relevant to the patients being studied [11, 46, 49].

25.4 Measuring HRQL in Adolescents vs Adults

Most published HRQL research in cancer focuses on adults. However, as child-mortality rates for cancer decline and the number of adolescent and young adult survivors continues to increase, conducting HRQL research with this age range is of critical importance [2, 50]. In addition, with a significant proportion of young people diagnosed with cancer presenting during their adolescent years, focusing specifically on this age range is an increasingly important issue [51]. Because of differences in developmental issues faced at different ages, however, adjustment to illness and treatment presents unique challenges across the adolescent age span [37].

Health in adolescents and young adults is defined as the ability to participate fully in developmentally appropriate activities [12, 43]. As in older adults, this ability requires physical, psychological, emotional, and social energy [12]. However, assessing HRQL in youths is different than assessing HRQL in adults for several reasons. First, measuring HRQL in the general population of adolescents and young adults can be more difficult due to the relative lack of illness in this age group when compared to older adults ([12]. Therefore, any HRQL measure to be used in this group must be extremely sensitive to small differences in health and changes over time [4, 12, 52]. Second, young people who have significant problems with HRQL may present with impaired or delayed physical, emotional, or intellectual development rather than a sudden, specific occurrence of a symptom or abnormality [12, 53]. This failure to develop appropriately may happen slowly over time, and may be difficult to capture in one measurement. Therefore, the timing of the assessment of HRQL in young people is crucial.

The dimensions typically assessed in HRQL research (i.e., physical function, role function, social/peer function, emotional well-being, effects of disease and treatments) are often utilized in both adult and youth HRQL studies [14, 52, 54]. However, the context in which the components of HRQL are measured may differ between adults and adolescents. For example, in some adult HRQL instruments that measure physical functioning, more value is placed upon independence and autonomy within that domain [54, 55]. Although it is also important to assess physical functioning in young patients, it would be inappropriate to place heightened value on independence, since it is expected that adolescents and young adults living at home would require more assistance than autonomous adults [54].

Another contextual difference arises when examining the way young people are required to function at school and with friends versus the way adults must function in the workplace and with social groups [54]. Although both of these functions are addressed in the domains of role and social functioning, the different context requires that different questions be raised for adults and younger subjects. These differences in context should be considered by researchers as they develop appropriate HRQL instruments for adolescents and young adults.

Although by definition the measurement of HRQL requires input from the individual, the accuracy or validity of self-report HRQL measures is sometimes questionable [6, 56]. A person may have a cognitive or motor impairment, or be too sick to respond appropriately to HRQL questionnaires[5, 6, 8]. This point becomes even more salient when assessing adolescents and young adults with brain tumors who may have cognitive impairments due to their disease and treatment [6, 56, 57].

25.5 Self Report vs. Proxy Reports (i.e., Parent, Provider, or Caregiver)

Reliance on parental proxy assessments of an adolescent's internal and external functioning is somewhat questionable [4, 54], as the parents' own anxieties and uncertainties about the future may influence their HRQL reports for their offspring [58]. Studies have consistently shown imperfect concordance rates between self-report and parental proxy ratings for children and adolescents with asthma, cystic fibrosis, chronic headache, limb deficiencies, and cancer [1, 14, 59]. This lack of agreement between proxy and self-

report is known as "cross-informant variance" and is even present with well-standardized measures [22, 60]. One reason for this discrepancy may be that, despite the fact that parents know their progeny better than anyone else, it is difficult for most parents to assess and interpret the internal emotional states of their children.

Researchers have discovered that, in general, agreement among parental proxy informants and their offspring tends to be higher for externalizing problems (e.g., aggression, hyperactivity, behavior problems) and lower for internalizing problems (e.g., depression, anxiety, pain, nausea) [52, 61, 62]. Because parents' perceptions of HRQL in their adolescent or young adult offspring are likely to influence healthcare utilization [63], and because there may be instances in which patients may not be able to provide self-report of their HRQL (either due to cognitive difficulties, unwillingness to participate, or because they do not feel well), parental proxy reports continue to be very important to clinical care [14, 64]. Parental proxy reports are especially useful when adolescent or young adult patients are living with their parents. It is expeditious and prudent to utilize HRQL measures that include both self-report and parental proxy report in order to consider both perspectives [1].

In adult HRQL research, proxies who have been used to provide HRQL ratings of an ill person include significant others/caregivers and healthcare providers [57, 65] von Essen [66] conducted a recent review of all proxy ratings of adult patient HRQL, and supported the use of proxy reports together with self reports whenever possible. This review emphasizes that self report is the preferred rating to consider when the patient is cognitively intact and a reasonable reporter. Differences in patient-proxy ratings for adults tend to be most pronounced for ratings of emotional functioning, similar to pediatric studies that demonstrate weaker concordance between parent and child ratings for internalizing behaviors [65].

25.6 HRQL Measurement and Clinical Cancer Care

During the past decade, clinicians and researchers have explored the value, appropriateness, and feasibility of integrating HRQL assessments into the daily routines of oncology clinics [19, 66, 67]. Researchers have found that physicians vary greatly in their ability to encourage patients to provide specific information about their quality of life, and patients vary in their ability to clearly express their problems and concerns [68]. This may be a particular problem with adolescents and physicians of the opposite gender [69].

Without appropriate and consistent provider–patient communication, physicians and healthcare providers may not fully appreciate their patients' symptoms, they may misjudge a patient's physical functioning, and they may be unable to gauge the patient's level of psychological distress [68]. Although patients frequently express a desire to feel understood by their physicians, many patients believe that it is only appropriate to raise issues about the effects of treatment on their daily lives and emotional states if their physicians indicate that it is acceptable to do so [68, 70]. Although oncologists generally feel it is essential that they discuss physical symptoms with their patients during medical appointments, they usually defer to their patients to raise psychosocial issues [68]. This situation may lead to a "conspiracy of silence," whereby psychosocial topics are not discussed because both physicians and patients are reluctant to raise such issues without a clear signal from the other that this is appropriate and desired. In these cases, formal HRQL assessments can be instrumental in helping patients communicate to their physicians and other healthcare providers areas of concern that may not be discussed otherwise. Furthermore, by monitoring HRQL, clinicians can evaluate symptom management, medical adherence, daily functioning, and the coping abilities of patients and their families.

In adult patients' communication with their physicians during outpatient palliative care visits, it has been demonstrated that patients' self-reported HRQL is the most powerful predictor of discussing HRQL issues with their physicians [71]. Even in patients experiencing serious HRQL problems, however, emotional functioning and fatigue were not addressed approximately 50% of the time in the absence of HRQL assessments. In pediatric research, investigations of psychosocial health as the "new hidden morbidity" has demon-

strated the continuing underidentification of psychosocial problems in routine practice and in tertiary care for children with chronic health conditions [63, 72]. These findings suggest that the value of systematic assessment of HRQL concerns utilizing screening methods similar to diagnostic laboratory tests. Similar to laboratory tests for biological disease, screening for HRQL morbidity in a patient population requires a standardized test with established reliability and validity [63].

HRQL measures may serve as standardized screening instruments for identifying physical and psychosocial health concerns from the perspectives of both the patient and the parent at the point of service [Table 25.1] [73]. For example, the American Academy of Pediatrics [74] has suggested that an integrated model of palliative care should include pain and symptom management at diagnosis and throughout the course of the condition, regardless of the ultimate outcome. From this perspective, all young subjects diagnosed with a potentially life-threatening condition should be screened on a regular basis for HRQL concerns and provided with appropriate palliative therapies based on these serial screenings. In this way, regardless of the potential for cure, they would be managed with optimal HRQL as an essential health outcome goal. This integrated measurement and targeted intervention approach would work well for evaluating and managing the HRQL of adolescents and young adults with cancer.

In addition to the assessment of patient groups, HRQL instruments can also be used to evaluate the physical and psychological functioning of individual patients. An individual patient can be compared to other patients with the same diagnosis and phase of treatment, to gain an understanding of his or her functioning relative to a group of similar patients (e.g., symptoms of nausea, pain, and emotional distress in an individual with newly diagnosed cancer in comparison to published data on a group of similar patients). This approach can be especially relevant in situations where patients with the same clinical criteria respond on HRQL instruments in different ways [11]. For example, two patients may indicate difficulties in different areas; one may report more problems with physical functioning while the other reports more problems in emotional or social functioning dimensions. A careful assessment of those areas of dysfunction for individual patients can aid a physician or mental health professional in designing specific treatment interventions.

A second use for HRQL assessment in individual patients is to monitor HRQL over time, to evaluate the efficacy of a particular treatment or to monitor health outcomes over the course of survivorship. If a patient's HRQL scores decrease from one visit to the next, a clinician can examine alternative treatments that may be more successful, or consider initiating if a survivor's status has deteriorated [Meeske K, personal communication]. Likewise, if a patient's scores increase after beginning a new treatment, the physician or nurse can conclude that the treatment is working [11].

25.7 Selected HRQL Measures for Adolescents and Young Adults

The current HRQL assessment strategy across pediatric and adult disorders has focused on the development and utilization of generic scales that evaluate the same basic domains and questions for all disorders, and can be benchmarked with healthy individuals for comparison purposes [14, 26, 75]. In addition to these generic measures, modules have been developed that focus on specific disease or cancer groups (e.g., breast cancer, prostate cancer, pediatric patients on active treatment), and finally symptom-specific modules such as pain, fatigue, and palliative care [1, 19]. In selecting measures for a specific application, such as a psychosocial outcome for a clinical chemotherapy

Table 25.1 Generic health-related quality of life (HRQL), disease-specific HRQL, and symptom-specific scales for adolescents and young adults with cancer*

Type	Instrument	Age (years)	Number of Items	Domains	Respondents
Generic HRQL Instruments					
Pediatric Quality of Life Inventory™ (PedsQL™) [4]		2–18	23	Physical, emotional, social, school	Parents of children 2–18 years Children 5–18 years
Child Health and Illness Profile [77]		11–17	153	Risks, discomfort, satisfaction, disorders, achievement, resilience	Adolescent
SF-36 [78]		14+	36	Physical, role-physical, bodily pain general health, vitality, social, role-emotional, mental health	Adolescent Young Adult
Cancer-Specific HRQL Instruments					
Pediatric Quality of Life Inventory™ (PedsQL™) Cancer Module [1]		2–18	27	Pain and hurt, nausea, procedural anxiety, treatment anxiety, worry, cognitive problems, perceived physical appearance, communication	Parents of children 2–18 years Children 5–18 years
FACT-G [79]		18+	27	Physical well-being, social/family well-being, emotional well-being, functional well-being	Young adult
EORTC QLQ-C30 [80])		18+	30	Physical, cognitive, emotional, social, role, fatigue, pain, nausea/vomiting	Young adult

Table 25.1 (continued)

Type	Instrument	Age (years)	Number of Items	Domains	Respondents
Pain Instruments					
Varni-Thompson Pediatric Pain Questionnaire (PPQ) [81]		5–19	35	Pain intensity, sensory, affective, evaluative, pain location, interference	Parents of children 5–18 years Children 5–18 years
Waldron-Varni Pediatric Pain Coping Questionnaire [82]		5–16	41	cognitive self-instruction, problem-solving, distraction, seeks social support, catastroph-izing/helplessness	Parents of children 5–16 years Children 5–16
McGill Pain Questionnaire [83]		18+	20	Total score	Young adult
West Haven-Yale Multidimensional Pain Inventory (MPI) [84]		18+	61	Pain severity, interference, life control affective distress, support from others, self-perception of disability	Young adult
Fatigue Instruments					
Pediatric Quality of Life Inventory™ (PedsQL™) Multidimensional Fatigue Scale [1]		2–18	18	General fatigue, sleep/rest fatigue, cognitive fatigue	Parents of children 2–18 years Children 5–18 years
Schwartz Cancer Fatigue Scale [85]		18+	28	Physical, emotional, cognitive, temporal	Young adult
Fatigue Symptom Inventory [86]		18+	13	Fatigue interference, fatigue duration, fatigue intensity	Young adult
Multidimensional Fatigue Inventory [87]		18+	20	General fatigue, physical fatigue, mental fatigue, reduced motivation, reduced activity	Young adult

*This list does not include preference-based instruments that provide utility scores for HRQL, such as the Quality of Well-Being scale [88], the EuroQOL 5D [89], and the Health Utilities Index [90]

trial, great care must be devoted to the selection of scales that focus on the exact behaviors and components that are likely to be sensitive to treatments under evaluation [76]. Table 25.1 lists several selected generic, disease-specific, and symptom-specific HRQL scales for use with adolescents and young adults, along with the recommended age range for administration, number of items, domains assessed, and respondents for each measure. Scales included in this table were selected to illustrate approaches that follow similar assessment models in adolescents and adults with cancer.

25.8 Barriers to the Use of HRQL Measures and Proposed Solutions

While HRQL assessments appear to have potential usefulness in the clinical setting, their use has been limited due to a number of barriers, as noted in Table 25.2. The attitudes of physicians and healthcare providers regarding HRQL assessment with their patients are critical to the adoption of these assessment tools. Unfortunately, the concerns expressed by providers are rarely based on empirical considerations, with many physicians believing that it is only practical to assess HRQL within randomized clinical trials or in palliative care situations [67].

In clinical settings, a bias may exist toward the use of qualitative approaches to assess HRQL, with the belief that such methods are less burdensome and intrusive than standardized quantitative methods. As mentioned previously, the use of a standardized assessment tool can enhance patient–provider communication and ensure that the patient's concerns and needs are adequately understood. Legitimate concerns about burdening patients and staff with time-consuming questionnaires of limited value can be addressed by designing brief instruments (to reduce respondent burden), developed with focus groups and cognitive interviews to hear the views of patients and family members, and by careful attention to the methodological details, involved in establishing the reliability and validity of instruments to be used [8, 23].

The perception by some physicians and other healthcare providers that HRQL measures are neither sufficiently associated with nor predictive of subtle changes in physiological parameters is not accurate. In fact, small-to-medium correlation effect sizes have been found between perceived HRQL and physiological parameters across a broad range of diseases [91]. The fact that HRQL measures correlate modestly with clinical outcomes suggests that physiological parameters and perceptual ratings are relatively independent. No one laboratory or subjective measure of patient functioning is inherently better for determining the general outcome of a treatment or clinical intervention by itself. Measures across modalities measure different things, and the clinical incorporation of data from multiple sources, including HRQL, will generally lead to better clinical decisions [91]. HRQL measures are not proxies for physiological parameters, but rather provide a more comprehensive evaluation of patient functioning across multiple life domains. The "gold standard" of comprehensive cancer care is only possible when multidimensional assessment leads to targeted interventions based on the clinical data and the patient's perceived needs [4, 27, 92].

25.9 Facilitating Clinical Decision-Making with HRQL Data

The impact of an HRQL measurement instrument on clinical decision-making can be tested under the working hypothesis that HRQL measurement must occur at the point of service for each individual patient in order to improve healthcare outcomes [93]. In adult primary care, computer-generated feedback of HRQL findings, accompanied by problem-specific resource and management suggestions, has resulted in subsequent improvements in patient mental health functioning [104].

Table 25.2 Barriers to utilization of HRQL measures in clinical practice

(1)	Physicians and health-care providers may not be convinced that standardized HRQL measures are sensitive to individual differences in response to illness and treatment.
(2)	The use of HRQL measures may require additional resources such as personnel, time, money, and computer scoring systems.
(3)	Measurement of HRQL might interfere with clinic operation.
(4)	The information provided might already be available through conventional evaluation methods (e.g., interviews or other assessments of mood).

Health status survey research methods have relied traditionally on paper-and-pencil procedures, administered by interviewers, or self-administered by respondents [95]. Recent technological advances, however, have enabled the use of laptop and palmtop lightweight computers in the assessment of HRQL. Computer-assisted assessment as a screening methodology may facilitate shared clinical decision-making, including the identification of areas of need at the point of service, and interventions to enhance HRQL [96, 97]. For instance, a one-page report might be generated electronically to provide a brief summary of symptoms and problem areas for the individual patient on a real-time basis, and may influence clinical decision-making of the healthcare team [65].

Investigators of HRQL have found that the use of electronic questionnaires versus conventional paper questionnaires increases the completeness of data and the speed of data flow, and decreases the workload of handling data [24]. As personal computers are now ubiquitous in clinical oncology settings, computerized HRQL questionnaires might become very useful to the integration of HRQL assessment in oncology clinics. The results of a small study by Detmar and Aaronson [65] indicate that, when done correctly, computer-based HRQL assessment is feasible in the daily routine of an outpatient clinic. These findings are supported by the work of Berry and colleagues [98]. Providing physicians and patients with printouts of computerized graphical summaries of patients' current and previous scores enables providers and patients to take more responsibility for bringing up HRQL issues and use their time efficiently to focus on issues that warrant further discussion [65, 99].

The application of computer-assisted assessment technology to the measurement of patient self-report and parent/other proxy-report in clinical care may reduce some of the burden associated with the administration and completion of standardized HRQL instruments. Data suggest that individuals are more truthful providing personal data in this manner, with electronic communications perceived as more private than completing written forms [100]. Computer and web-based assessment strategies also represent a developing method that young people, generally well experienced with the technology, may find appealing in its application to HRQL [101]. New applications of touch-screen and talking methods of administration may hold great promise for increasing access and evaluation of low-literacy populations who might otherwise be excluded, including survivors who may be cognitively impaired as a result of their illness or treatment [102].

When HRQL scores are available at the point of service, patient and parent/other perceptions of the patient's physical and psychosocial health can inform clinical decisions by the healthcare provider [1]. Varni et al. [103] demonstrated the benefits of routine clinic HRQL assessments, whereby the clinic physician reviewed the measure during patient examinations and addressed problems indicated by the measure. This is similar to the findings of Detmar and Aronson [65] in a group of patients with cancer.

Previous research with adult patients, however, has demonstrated that simply providing primary care physicians with HRQL screening information without specific resource and management suggestions was not sufficient in either changing healthcare provider behavior or changing patient HRQL outcomes [104]. Linking HRQL findings directly to referral resources may reduce the barrier to implementation further by facilitating the process of problem identification and appropriate intervention.

25.10 Risk Prediction

Risk prediction is of increasing importance for caregivers of adolescent and young adult cancer survivors who need to be provided with ongoing health surveillance to monitor the possible late effects of illness and treatment [34]. In addition, health insurance purchasers, payers, and policy makers also need this information to allocate resources appropriately [105]. Predicting resource utilization is key to managing defined populations in a prospective payment system and for proactively case-managing those at greatest risk of poor health. When practitioners know in advance which survivors are most likely to experience debilitating late effects of illness and treatment, they are able to target those individuals in order to minimize or prevent morbidity and associated costs.

Progress in predicting health outcomes in adolescent and young adult survivors has been made, but is hampered by lack of good transition services for adolescents and incomplete access to ongoing surveillance for adult patients [51]. Being able to demonstrate the usefulness of HRQL measurement in identifying adolescents and young adult patients with the greatest needs, while simultaneously demonstrating the cost advantages of providing timely targeted interventions to address those needs, may ultimately provide the driving force for incorporating HRQL measurement in clinical practice [105]. A recent report by Danmark-Wahnefried and colleagues [106] identified a positive correlation between HRQL and exercise behavior in childhood cancer survivors. These data suggest that screening specific quality of life domains can help target individuals in need of targeted health-promoting interventional strategies.

25.11 Conclusions

Efforts to understand and improve the HRQL of patients are now recognized as necessary components of clinical trials and comprehensive cancer care, throughout the entire temporal trajectory of cancer: at diagnosis, during active treatment, at the end of treatment, and across long-term survival. If the patient relapses, needs palliative care, and approaches death, the ongoing monitoring of HRQL can help maximize psychosocial and health outcomes to the best degree possible [107, 108].

The continuity of active healthcare and health surveillance across the lifespan makes it imperative that HRQL evaluation be an ongoing process that may begin during childhood or adolescence, and is maintained into adulthood. Adolescents and young adults face unique developmental challenges associated with their age and life experience that make HRQL assessment especially challenging. The need to use appropriate and sometimes different measurement instruments as a teenager transitions to young adulthood requires care and further study to ensure seamless attention to HRQL variables.

Much has been accomplished over the last decade in the development of clinically reliable and valid assessment instruments, but the process of implementing current knowledge into clinical trials and decision-making is not yet standard practice. HRQL assessment needs to become a regular part of medical care and health surveillance like other basic laboratory measures, and HRQL data need to be made available to clinical providers in real-time to facilitate care and maximize health outcomes. Computerized and web-based technologies need to be developed and evaluated to increase the usage and utility of HRQL assessment and monitoring strategies to aid clinicians and researchers, and increase their acceptability to adolescent and young adult patients.

Further research on HRQL methodology in adolescents and young adults is required to help attain the promise of more effective therapy and supportive care that can be delivered when the patient is in greatest need and most receptive to intervention. Future investigations should attempt to determine which measures work best for specific adolescent and young adult populations, and whether participation in clinical trials is associated with improved HRQL. Research needs to evaluate how improved HRQL may be associated with better adherence to follow-up care, and whether prospective HRQL assessment is associated with better health outcomes. We need to determine whether electronic assessment and scoring strategies provide empirical advantages over traditional paper-and-pencil versions. Finally, given the increasing multiculturalism of numerous populations, the interaction between HRQL and culture, acculturation, language, socioeconomic status, and educational level must be examined. These efforts will greatly improve our understanding of HRQL, and pave the way to more effective medical and psychosocial interventions to improve health outcomes in adolescents and young adults with cancer.

References

1. Varni JW, Burwinkle T, Katz ER, et al (2002) The PedsQL™ in pediatric cancer: reliability and validity of the Pediatric Quality of Life Inventory™ Generic Core Scales, Multidimensional Fatigue Scale, and Cancer Module. Cancer 94:2090–2106
2. Eiser C (2004) Children with Cancer: The Quality of Life. Lawrence Erlbaum Associates, Mahwah, New Jersey

3. Greenfield S, Nelson, EC (1992) Recent developments and future issues in the use of health status assessment measures in clinical settings. Med Care 30:MS23–41
4. Varni JW, Seid M, Kurtin PS (1999) Pediatric health-related quality of life measurement technology: a guide for health care decision makers. J Clin Outcomes Manag 6:33–40
5. Eiser C (1995) Choices in measuring quality of life in children with cancer: a comment. Psychooncology 4:121–131
6. Eiser C, Vance YH, Horne B, et al (2003) The value of the PedsQL™ in assessing quality of life in survivors of childhood cancer. Child Care Health Dev 29:95–102
7. Reaman GH, Haase GM (1996) Quality of life research in childhood cancer: the time is now. Cancer 78:330–1332
8. Cella D (1998) Quality of life. In: Holland JC (ed) Psychooncology. Oxford University Press, New York, pp 1135–1146
9. Testa MA, Simonson DC (1996) Assessment of quality-of-life outcomes. N Engl J Med 334:835–840
10. World Health Organization (1948) Constitution of the World Health Organization basic document. World Health Organization, Geneva, Switzerland
11. Guyatt GH, Feeny DH, Patrick DL (1993) Measuring health-related quality of life. Ann Intern Med 118:622–629
12. Jenney EM, Kane RL, Lurie N (1995) Developing a measure of health outcomes in survivors of childhood cancer: a review of the issues. Med Pediatr Oncol 24:145–153
13. Pal DK (1996) Quality of life assessment in children: a review of conceptual and methodological issues in multidimensional health status measures. J Epidemiol Commun Health 50:391–396
14. Varni JW, Seid M, Rode CA (1999) The PedsQL™: measurement model for the pediatric quality of life inventory. Med Care 37:126–139
15. Zebrack BJ, Zeltzer LK (2003) Quality of life issues in cancer survivorship. Curr Probl Cancer 27:198–211
16. Schwartz CE, Sprangers MAG (2002) An introduction to quality of life assessment in oncology: the value of measuring patient reported outcomes. Am J Manag Care 8:s550–s559
17. American Society of Clinical Oncology (ASCO) (1996) Outcomes of cancer treatment for technology assessment and cancer guidelines. J Clin Oncol 14: 671–679
18. Frost MH, Sloan JA (2002) Quality of life measurements: a soft outcome – or is it? Am J Manage Care 8:S574–S579
19. Roila F, Cortesi E (2001) Quality of life as a primary end point in oncology. Ann Oncol 12:S3–S6
20. Aaronson NK (1991) Methodologic issues in assessing the quality of life of cancer patients. Cancer 67:844–850
21. Ganz PA (1995). Impact of quality of life outcomes on clinical practice. Oncology 9:S61–65
22. Varni JW, Katz ER, Seid M, et al (1998) The Pediatric Cancer Quality of Life Inventory (PCQL). I. Instrument development, descriptive statistics, and cross-informant variance. J Behav Med 21:179–204
23. Varni JW, Katz ER, Seid M, et al (1998) The Pediatric Cancer Quality of Life Inventory-32 (PCQL-32). I. Reliability and validity. Cancer 82:1184–1196
24. Drummond HE, Ghosh S, Ferguson A, et al (1995) Electronic quality of life questionnaires: a comparison of pen-based electronic questionnaires with conventional paper in a gastrointestinal study. Qual Life Res 4:21–26
25. Feeny D, Furlong W, Barr RD, et al (1992) A comprehensive multi-attribute system for classifying health status survivors of childhood cancer. J Clin Oncol 10:923–928
26. Fayers PM, Machin D (2000) Quality of life: assessment, analysis, and interpretation. Wiley, New York
27. Drotar D (1998) Measuring Health-Related Quality of Life in Children and Adolescents. Lawrence Erlbaum, Mahwah, New Jersey
28. Mulhern RK, Ochs J, Armstrong FD, et al (1989) Assessment of quality of life among pediatric patients with cancer. J Consult Clin Psychol 2:130–138
29. Barr RD (2001) Paediatric update: the adolescent with cancer. Eur J Cancer 37:1523–1530
30. Holland J, Gooden-Piels J (2000) Principles of psychooncology. In: Holland JF, Frei E (eds) Cancer Medicine, 5th edn. BC Decker, Hamilton, Ontario, pp 943–958
31. Katz ER, Dolgin MJ, Varni JW (1990) Cancer in children and adolescents. In: Gross AM, Drabman RS (eds) Handbook of Clinical Behavioral Pediatrics. Plenum Press, New York, pp 129–146
32. Whyte F, Smith L (1997) A literature review of adolescence and cancer. Eur J Cancer Care 6:137–146
33. Zeltzer LK (1993) Cancer in adolescents and young adults: psychosocial aspects. Cancer Suppl 71:3463–3468
34. Keene N, Hobie W, Ruccione K (2000). Childhood Cancer Survivors: a Practical Guide to Your Future. O'Reilly and Associates, Sebastapol, Ca
35. McLean WE, Foley GB, Ruccione K, Sklar C (1996) Transitions in the care of adolescent and young adult survivors of childhood cancer. Cancer 78:1340–1344
36. Nessim C, Ellis J (1991) Cancervive: the challenge of life after cancer. Boston, Houghton Mifflin
37. Zebrack BJ, Chesler MA (2004) The impact of cancer on pediatric and young adult patients and their families: psychosocial issues. National Cancer Institute White Paper
38. Brown RT, Madan-Swain A, Lambert R (2003) Posttraumatic stress symptoms in adolescent survivors of childhood cancer and their mothers. J Trauma Stress 16:309–318
39. Feldman SS, Elliot GR (1990) At the Threshold: The Developing Adolescent. Harvard University Press, Cambridge, MA

40. Miller B, Keane C (1992) Encyclopedia and Dictionary of Nursing and Allied Health, 3rd edn. WB Saunders, Toronto

41. Barbarin OA (1990) Adjustment to serious childhood illness. In: Lahey BB, Kazdin E (eds) Advances in Clinical Child Psychology 13. Plenum, New York, pp 377–403

42. Varni JW, Blount RL, Quiggins DJ (1998). Oncologic disorders. In: Ammerman RT, Campo JV (eds) Handbook of Pediatric Psychology and Psychiatry, Vol. 11. Disease, Injury, and Illness. Allyn and Bacon, Boston, pp 190–221

43. Zebrack BJ, Eshelman DA, Hudson MA, et al (2004) Insights and perspectives from a Delphi panel of young adult survivors of childhood cancer. Cancer 100:843–850

44. Berzon R, Hays RD, Shumaker SA (1993) International use, application and performance of health-related quality of life instruments. Qual Life Res 2:367–368

45. Wilson I, Cleary PD (1995) Linking clinical variables with health-related quality of life. JAMA 273:59–65

46. Sprangers MG, Cull A, Bjordal K, et al (1993) The European Organization for Research and Treatment of Cancer approach to quality of life assessment: guidelines for developing questionnaire modules. Qual Life Res 2:287–299

47. Bullinger M, Ravens-Sieberer U (1995) Health-related quality of life assessment in children: a review of the literature. Rev Eur Psychol Appl 45:245–254

48. Graham P, Stevenson J, Flynn D (1997) A new measure of health-related quality of life for children: preliminary findings. Psychol Health 12:655–665

49. Deyo RA, Patrick, DL (1989) Barriers to the use of health status measures in clinical investigation, patient care, and policy research. Med Care 27:S254–268

50. Pantell RH, Lewis CC (1987) Measuring the impact of medical care on children. J Chronic Dis 40:99–115

51. Bleyer WA, Tejeda H, Murphy SM, et al (1997) National cancer clinical trials: children have equal access, adolescents do not. J Adolesc Health 21:366–373

52. Varni JW, Rode CA, Seid M, et al (1999) The Pediatric Cancer Quality of Life Inventory-32 (PCQL-32). II. Feasibility and range of measurement. J Behav Med 22:397–406

53. Katz ER, Madan-Swain A (2006) Maximizing school and social outcomes in children and adolescents with cancer. In: Brown RT (ed) Comprehensive Handbook of Childhood Cancer and Sickle Cell Disease. A Biopsychosocial Approach. Plenum, New York, pp 313–338

54. Parsons SK, Brown AP (1998) Evaluation of quality of life of childhood cancer survivors: a methodological conundrum. Med Pediatr Oncol Suppl 1:46–53

55. Karnofsky JA, Burchenal JH (1949) The clinical evaluation of chemotherapeutic agents in cancer. In: McLeod CM (ed) Evaluation of Chemotherapeutic Agents. Columbia University Press, New York, 1191–1205

56. Meeske K, Katz ER, Palmer SN, et al (2005) Parent and proxy-reported health related quality of life and fatigue in pediatric cancer patients diagnosed with brain tumors and acute lymphoblastic leukemia. Cancer 101:2116–2125

57. Sneeuw KCA, Aaronson NK, Osoba D, et al (1997). The use of significant others as proxy raters of the quality of life of patients with brain cancer. Med Care 35:490–506

58. Dahlquist L, Czyzewski D, Jones C (1996) Parents of children with cancer: a longitudinal study of emotional distress, coping style, and marital adjustment 2 and 20 months after diagnosis. J Pediatr Psychol 21:541–554

59. Feeny D, Juniper EF, Ferrie PJ, et al (1998) Why not just ask the kids? Health-related quality of life in children with asthma. In: Drotar D (ed) Measuring Health-Related Quality of Life in Children and Adolescents. Lawrence Erlbaum Associates, Mahwah, NJ, pp 171–186

60. Varni JW, Katz ER, Colegrove R, Dolgin M (1995). Adjustment of children with newly diagnosed cancer: cross-informant variance. J Psychosoc Oncol 13:23–38

61. Achenbach TM, McConaughy SH, Howell CT (1987) Child/adolescent behavioral and emotional problems: implications of cross-informant correlations for situational specificity. Psychol Bull 101:213–232

62. Varni JW, Seid M, Kurtin PS (2001) The PedsQL™ 4.0: reliability and validity of the Pediatric Quality of Life Inventory™ Version 4.0 Generic Core Scales in healthy patient populations. Med Care 39:800–812

63. Varni JW, Setoguchi Y (1992) Screening for behavioral and emotional problems in children and adolescents with congenital or acquired limb deficiencies. Am J Dis Child 146:103–107

64. Meeske K, Katz ER, Palmer SN, et al (2004) Parent proxy-reported health related quality of life and fatigue in pediatric patients diagnosed with brain tumors and acute lymphoblastic leukemia. Cancer 101:2116–2125.

65. Von Essen L (2004) Proxy ratings of patient quality of life: factors related to patient-proxy agreement. Acta Oncol 43:229–234

66. Detmar SB, Aaronson NK (1998) Quality of life assessment in daily clinical oncology practice: a feasibility study. Eur J Cancer 34:1181–1186

67. Taylor KM, MacDonald KG, Bezjak P, DePetrillo AD (1996) Physicians' perspectives on quality of life: an exploratory study of oncologists. Qual Life Res 5:5–14

68. Detmar SB, Aaronson NK, Muller WM, Schornagel JH (2000) How are you feeling? Who wants to know? Patients' and oncologists' preferences for discussing health-related quality of life issues. J Clin Oncol 18:3295–3301

69. Fritz G, Williams J (1988) Issues of adolescent development for survivors of childhood cancer. J Am Acad Child Adolesc Psychiatry 27:712–715

70. Detmar SB, Muller MJ, Schornagel IH, et al (2002) Health-related quality of life assessments and patient–physician communication. JAMA 288:3027–3034

71. Detmar SB, Muller MJ, Wever DD, et al (2001) Patient–physician communication during outpatient palliative

treatment visits: an observational study. JAMA 285:1351–1357

72. Costello EJ, Edelbrock C, Costello AJ, et al (1988) Psychopathology in pediatric primary care: the new hidden morbidity. Pediatrics 82:415–424

73. Varni JW, Burwinkle T, Seid M, Zellner J (2002) The PedsQL™ as a population health measure: implications for states and nations. Qual Life Newsl 28:4–6

74. American Academy of Pediatrics (2000) Palliative care for children. Pediatrics 106:351–357

75. Varni JW, Burwinkle T, Seid M, Skarr D (2003). The PedsQL™ 4.0 as a Pediatric population health measure: feasibility, reliability, and validity. Ambul Pediatr 3:329–341

76. Fairclough DL (2002) Design and Analysis of Quality of Life Studies in Clinical Trials: Interdisciplinary Statistics. Chapman and Hall/CRC, New York

77. Starfield B, Riley AW, Green BF, et al (1995) The adolescent child health and illness profile. A population-based measure of health. Med Care 33:553–566

78. Ware JE, Sherbourne CD (1992) The MOS 36-item short form health survey (SF-36): I. Conceptual framework and item selection. Med Care 30:473–481

79. Cella DF, Tulsky DS, Gray G, et al (1993) The Functional assessment of cancer therapy scale: development and validation of the general measure. J Clin Oncol 11:570–579

80. Aaronson NK, Ahmedzai S, Bergman B, et al (1993) The European Organization For Research and Treatment of Cancer QLQ-C30: a quality of life instrument for use in international clinical trials in oncology. J Natl Cancer Inst 85:365–376

81. Varni JW, Thompson KL, Hanson V (1987) The Varni/Thompson Pediatric Pain Questionnaire: I. Chronic musculoskeletal pain in juvenile rheumatoid arthritis. Pain 28:27–38

82. Varni JW, Waldron SA, Gragg RA, et al (1996) Development of the Waldron/Varni Pediatric Pain Coping Inventory. Pain 67:141–150

83. Melzack R (1975) The McGill Pain Questionnaire: major properties and scoring methods. Pain 1:277–299

84. Kerns RD, Turk DC, Rudy TE (1985) The West Haven-Yale Multidimensional Pain Inventory (WHYMPI). Pain 23:345–356

85. Schwartz AL (1998) The Schwartz Cancer Fatigue Scale: testing reliability and validity. Oncol Nurs Forum 25:711–717

86. Hann DM, Jacobsen PB, Azzarello LM, et al (1998) Measurement of fatigue in cancer patients: development and validation of the Fatigue Symptom Inventory. Qual Life Res 7:301–310

87. Smets EMA, Garssen B, Bonke B, DeHaes JCJM (1995). The Multidimensional Fatigue Inventory (MFI) psychometric qualities of an instrument to measure fatigue. J Psychosom Res 39:315–325

88. Kaplan RM, Anderson JP (1996) The general health policy model: an integrated approach. In: Spilker B (ed) Quality of Life and Pharmacoeconomics in Clinical Trials, 2nd edn. Lippincott-Raven, Philadelphia, pp 309–332

89. Rabin R, de Charro F (2001) EQ 5D: a measure of health status from the EuroQol Group. Ann Med 33:337–343

90. Furlong WJ, Feeny DH, Torrance GW, Barr RD (2001) The Health Utilities Index (HUI) system for assessing health-related quality of life in clinical studies. Ann Med 33:375–384

91. McHorney CA (2002) The potential clinical value of quality of life information. Med Care 40:III56–III62

92. Feeny D, Furlong W, Mulhern RK, et al (1999) A framework for assessing health-related quality of life among children with cancer. Int J Cancer Suppl 12:2–9

93. Wetzler HP (2000) The future of health status assessment. Am J Manag Care 6:121–123

94. Rubenstein LV, McCoy JM, Cope DW, et al (1995) Improving patient quality of life with feedback to physicians about functional status. J Gen Intern Med 10:607–614

95. Fowler FJ Jr (1993) Survey Research Methods (2nd edn). Sage, Newbury Park

96. Higginson I, Carr A (2001) Using quality of life measures in the clinical setting. BMJ 322:1297–1300

97. Tamburini M (2001) Health-related quality of life measures in cancer. Ann Oncol 12:S7–S10

98. Berry DL, Trigg LJ, Lober WB, et al (2004) Computerized symptom and quality of life assessment for patients with cancer Part I: development and pilot testing. Oncol Nurs Forum 31:895–904

99. Mullen KH, Berry DL, Zierler BK (2004) Computerized symptom and quality of life assessment for patients with cancer, Part II: acceptability and usability. Oncol Nurs Forum 31:896–903

100. Webster K, Cella D, Yost K (2003) The Functional Assessment of Chronic Illness Therapy (FACIT) Measurement System: properties, applications, and interpretation. Health Qual Life Outcomes 16:79

101. Eysenbach G (2003) The impact of the Internet on cancer outcomes. CA Cancer J Clin 53:356–371

102. Hahn EA, Cella D, Dobrez D, et al. (2004) The talking touchscreen: a new approach to outcomes assessment in low literacy. Psychooncology 13:86–95

103. Varni JW, Seid M, Knight TS, et al (2002) The PedsQL™ 4.0 Generic Core Scales: sensitivity, responsiveness, and impact on clinical decision-making. J Behav Med 25:175–193

104. Rubenstein LV, Calkins DR, Young RT, et al (1989) Improving patient function: a randomized trial of functional disability screening. Ann Intern Med 111:836–842

105. Seid M, Varni JW, Kurtin PS (2000) Measuring quality of care for vulnerable children: challenges, conceptualization of a pediatric outcome measure of quality. Am J Med Qual 15:182–188

106. Danmark-Wahnefried W, Werner C, Clipp EC, et al (2005) Survivors of childhood cancer and their guardians: current health behaviors and receptivity to health promotion programs. Cancer 103:2171–2180

107. Apolones G (2003) Clinical and outcome research in oncology: the need for integration. Health Qual Life Outcomes 1:3

108. Bradlyn RS, Ritchey AK, Harris CV, et al (1996) Quality of life research in pediatric oncology: research methods and barriers. Cancer 78:1333–1339

Rehabilitation and Exercise

Marilyn J. Wright

26.1 Introduction

Rehabilitation and exercise are essential components of comprehensive cancer care, as the disease and its treatments present many challenges to functional independence and health. For adolescents and young adults (AYA) these challenges are compounded by the complex developmental transitions that take place during this time of life. Rehabilitation programs focus on the prevention or alleviation of physiological and psychosocial impairments, the promotion of participation in age-appropriate activities, and the enhancement of quality of life. The overall goal is the achievement of an independently functioning and self-sufficient individual who has a satisfying social and emotional life and is a contributing member of society within the limits of their disease and environment. An adolescent's goal may be simply to get life back to normal.

There is a paucity of studies specific to rehabilitation and exercise for AYA with cancer. Strategies for clinical practice are based therefore on general principles of rehabilitation, evidence- and theory-based knowledge regarding motor learning, physiology, and psychology, and information extrapolated from studies of cancer patients of all ages. These are linked with an understanding of the physical and psychosocial events and tasks inherent to adolescence and young adulthood.

26.2 General Principles of Rehabilitation

General principles of rehabilitation regarding goals, decision-making, and therapeutic approaches should be incorporated into all stages of cancer care: at diagnosis, throughout treatment, following treatment, and in some cases at the end of life. Goals should be realistic, promote participation in meaningful life activities, and have measurable outcomes. These should be individualized depending on the unique needs and strengths of each patient and family, support systems, and environment. Goals may need to be readjusted, based on ongoing assessment of a constantly changing array of impairments and associated problems. The patient and family should be involved in decision-making regarding goals, wishes, preferences, and ways to achieve these, as a sense of control regarding interventions will result in more effective programs [1]. It is important to educate the AYA and relevant family members about the implications of cancer-related impairment, the importance of rehabilitation and exercise, and optimal activities and strategies to achieve their goals. This enables them to make informed decisions and may promote motivation and compliance. They need to be encouraged also to accept some responsibility for their outcomes. Healthcare professionals and others in the community can support them in their efforts and provide specific programs and interventions, but for the best results, the day-to-day and long-term follow-through have to be adopted by the recipient.

In some cases, compromises among the goals of the adolescent, the parent and the health care team will have to be made. The latter must be sensitive to individual differences in short-term and long-term needs, values, culture and the day-to-day variation in how the adolescent and family are coping physically and emotionally. Services are interdisciplinary, involving potentially many different health care professionals. These may include physiotherapists, occupational therapists, child life specialists, psychologists, speech and language pathologists, nurses, physicians, recreation therapists, dieticians, and social workers. Ongoing communication and collaboration are imperative.

26.3 Rehabilitation and Exercise Needs

The International Classification of Functioning, Disability, and Health [2] provides a standard language

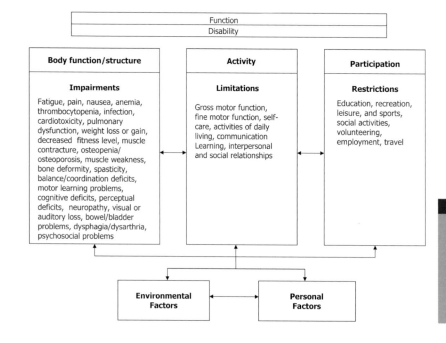

Figure 26.1

Potential impairments, activity limitations, and participation restrictions encountered by adolescents and young adults receiving treatment for cancer and framework for the description of health and health-related states to classify and address rehabilitation assessment, options, treatments, methods of service delivery and outcomes. The tool recognizes the interactions among the dimensions of body -anatomic structure and physiological function; activity – the execution of a task or action by an individual (capacity); and participation – an individual's involvement in life situations (performance). Problems within these dimensions are termed respectively impairments, activity limitations, and participation restrictions. The model also considers the impact of contextual environmental and personal factors on function.

The potential issues within these dimensions encountered by those receiving treatment for cancer that could impact on rehabilitation are outlined in Fig. 26.1. Although all of these may impact on intervention and must be considered when planning goals and intervention strategies, only those most pertinent to physical rehabilitation are discussed.

26.3.1 Body Structure and Function

Cancer and its treatment can result in numerous impairments in body structure and function. Problems vary within the course of treatment and vary greatly among patients. There is a wide range in the burdens of morbidity, even in patients receiving the same treatment.

Fatigue (a feeling of weariness, tiredness, or lack of energy) is a very common and pervasive complication of cancer treatment that may persist after therapy is completed. Fatigue can be physical, mental, or emotional. It contributes to the overall morbidity of the disease and has a significant impact on quality of life if it causes patients to reduce their level of activity and participation. The etiology is most likely multifactorial but includes a reduction in oxygen delivery to the cells [3]. Davies et al. [4] categorized fatigue in children and adolescents receiving treatment for cancer as typical tiredness (normal tiredness from regular activities or circumstances), treatment fatigue (energy lost greater than energy replenished resulting from hospitalization, disrupted sleep, pain, chemotherapy, radiation therapy, anemia, and psychological or emotional stress), or shutdown fatigue (sustained or profound loss of energy resulting in disengagement with surroundings).

Procedural, treatment-associated, and cancer-related pain, are common and concerning problems during cancer treatment [5]. Pain can limit activity to the extent that bed rest is necessary and can affect the quality and quantity of sleep. Specific examples include neuropathic, steroid-induced, and osteoporotic bone pain.

Reduced cardiovascular and pulmonary function [6] as well as poor exercise tolerance, fitness, and endurance [7] can occur. Anthracycline-induced cardiomyopathy can cause reduced exercise capacity [8].

Weight loss or weight gain can be problematic. The prevalence of obesity in the general population is increasing in many countries; a disturbing trend associated with undesirable body image, poor self-esteem, and the risk of subsequent higher morbidity and mortality rates [9]. These issues concerning obesity are amplified in AYA receiving and following treatment for cancer. Mechanisms may include cranial irradiation, chemotherapy, inactivity, and improper diet [10].

Musculoskeletal impairments are also prevalent. Osteopenia is a common complication of cancer therapy. Contributing factors include high-dose corticosteroids and possibly reduced activity during times of illness [11]. Treatment with corticosteroids can result also in myopathy of the proximal musculature [3, 12]. Lack of activity due to bed rest, malaise, fatigue, or nausea also contribute to muscle weakness. Loss of range of motion, leading potentially to contracture, is a secondary impairment resulting from weakness and immobility. Vincristine-induced neuropathy can contribute to this problem. Skeletal impairments such as amputation, deformity resulting from limb-sparing procedures, and scoliosis can occur due to tumors and their treatment.

Central nervous system (CNS) damage can result in cognitive and perceptual deficits and abnormal muscle tone. Spasticity can cause pain and interfere with hygiene and functional independence [12] These problems, compounded by other impairments such as weakness, decreased range-of-motion, and obesity, can contribute to multisystem impairments such as difficulties with balance, coordination, and motor learning [13].

26.3.2 Activity and Participation

Physical and psychosocial impairments can impact potentially on all areas of activity and participation, and activity limitations and participation restrictions can impact reciprocally on impairments. Limitations in motor function are obvious in many AYA treated for bone and CNS tumors. More subtle limitations in gross motor proficiency have been documented during and following treatment in adolescents with leukemia and lymphoma [14, 15]. Problems with fine motor skills including poor handwriting, manual dexterity, and drawing performance have also been identified [16].

Self-care skills such as bathing, toileting, dressing, personal care, and grooming can be affected. This can be devastating for adolescents who are striving to be independent and maintain their privacy. Other activities of daily living such as household tasks or yard work may be limited. These may not be priorities for adolescents, but they are important skills to learn to enable independent living as an adult.

Learning, cognitive, and language skills may be affected due to neurosurgery, radiation therapy, or other CNS treatments, and may affect participation in educational, social, and other activities. Oral motor dysfunction of neurogenic or mechanical origin, which may disrupt communication and eating, can be a significant impairment.

Participation in normal activities may also be affected by isolation restrictions, hospitalization, or preconceived ideas of people encountered by AYA in their schools and community. Teachers, coaches, employers, or even family members may overprotect or overrestrict the AYA with cancer.

Research in this area includes a study of leisure-time physical activity in adolescents receiving treatment for cancer that documented decreased participation and feelings of less competence while on treatment, with improvement following treatment. Those who remained active throughout their cancer experience reported better self-concept, perception of physical abilities, interactions with parents, and same and opposite sex relationships; many of the psychosocial areas that are compromised in AYA with cancer [17].

Long-term follow-up of AYA treated for acute lymphoblastic leukemia (ALL) has identified similar findings; the subjects felt less competent in physical activities, were less likely to participate in physical versus sedentary activities, enjoyed physical education less, and were more prone to sports injury. These findings were associated with decreases in health-related quality of life [18]. These AYA would have been less likely to reap the potential physical and psychological benefits of physical activity.

Activities in which AYA receiving treatment for cancer do participate when not feeling well or hospitalized include sedentary pastimes such as watching television, using the Internet, or playing video games. These pursuits have been linked to obesity [9]. A tendency to partake in these activities may continue following completion of treatment, resulting in further inactivity and long-term problems.

26.4 Intervention

26.4.1 Physical Activity

The most researched, efficacious, and efficient intervention to address physical impairments, activity limitations, participation restrictions, and reduced quality of life in people receiving treatment for cancer is physical exercise. Studies of various exercise interventions on adult populations have contributed most of the data that support the current understanding of the effects of exercise in AYA with cancer. Reviews of these studies have shown consistently that physical exercise following diagnosis has a clinically and statistically positive effect on many of the negative consequences of cancer and its treatment [19]. Exercise benefited physiological functions including aerobic capacity, muscle strength, flexibility, body composition and weight, hematological indexes, nausea, fatigue, pain, and diarrhea, and also had positive effects on many facets of psychological and emotional well-being including personality functioning, anxiety, depression, feeling of control, perceived physical competence, self-esteem, self-confidence, and satisfaction with life [3, 19, 20]. There is some evidence that physical activity can have an effect on the immune system, to reduce the risk of cancer recurrence and/or secondary malignancies and increase survival time. However, these data must be considered in the context of several methodological limitations inherent in the studies with respect to sampling, design, and outcome measures [3, 21].

Some studies of fatigue have included AYA. In a qualitative investigation of adolescents with cancer, clinical interventions identified as alleviating fatigue included maintenance of optimal fitness levels through an appropriate balance of rest and exercise, in addition to distraction and entertainment and relief from disease or treatment-related symptoms [4, 22]. A survey of cancer survivors who considered themselves athletes prior to diagnosis included young adults. Those who continued to exercise with modifications during treatment believed exercise made them less likely to develop health problems, and physical activity balanced with rest was an effective intervention for fatigue [23]. These studies have been complemented by the more rigorous research investigating the role of exercise in preventing and/or alleviating cancer-related fatigue in adults. This has demonstrated that increased physical exercise is associated with less fatigue during and after treatment [3, 19]. These findings are particularly important as the past recommendations of resting and avoiding physical effort can have a paradoxical effect. Inactivity induces further muscular wasting and loss of cardiorespiratory fitness and endurance, creating a self-perpetuating condition of further diminished activity, leading to easy fatigue and vice versa, which can be long lasting [3].

Sharkey et al. [7] found that an exercise program in AYA who had received anthracyclines resulted in increased exercise ability and a trend toward improved peak oxygen uptake and ventilatory anaerobic threshold. Children and adolescents who were encouraged to be physically active during treatment for ALL had less loss of passive range of motion compared to a group who did not receive activity intervention. Surgical procedures had been necessary in some of the patients in the nonintervention group [25].

To promote exercise in AYA receiving treatment for cancer, it is necessary to be aware of the determinants of physical activity. In addition to the many potential impairments, prediagnostic levels of activity influence participation during and following treatment [17]. Other predictors include individual factors such as physical and cognitive status, communication and

psychosocial abilities, gender, body mass index, feelings of competence, and perceived benefits. Environmental and personal factors such as available facilities, season, economics, alternative sedentary activities, social influences, cultural perspectives, preferences, and activity levels of family and peers; the educational influences of health professionals and educators, and the media are also influential [1]. These factors must be taken into consideration when working with AYA. Therapists must provide ongoing encouragement and reinforce the importance of regular activity. Ideally, participation in physical activity should take place throughout and following treatment. Efforts should be focused particularly on those individuals identified with low incentive, as they are most at risk for inactivity and its associated problems.

In addition to physical activity promoting health and well-being during treatment, there may be implications for long-term health, as adolescence is an important time for adopting healthy practices including preferences for activity or inactivity [25], which may impact on future fitness, obesity, bone density, and cardiovascular disease. This is particularly important for adult survivors of cancer who are at risk for multiple health problems.

The intensity, frequency, type, location, and progression of programs are based on medical condition, assessment, preferences, and goals. Exercise prescription in adult cancer studies is typically moderate-intensity exercise, 3–5 days per week, 20–30 min per session. However, low exercise intensities may achieve similar health benefits [19, 20]. Daily exercise with shorter, lighter-intensity bouts with rest intervals and slower progressions may be preferable for deconditioned patients [19]. These recommendations can be used for adolescents, but a consensus process developed recommendations for children and adolescents in the general population of participation in at least 1 h of moderately intensive physical activity daily, either continuous or spread throughout the day. Moderate intensity is activity equivalent to a brisk walk, such as that when the participant might feel warm or slightly out of breath. Those who do very little activity per day should start with 30 min per day. Activities that enhance muscle strength, flexibility, and bone health should be done twice weekly [26]. Exercise prescription should include warm-up and cool-down activities.

Types of exercise used most frequently in adult cancer patients were aerobic or cardiovascular endurance and occasionally strength training programs [19]. Activities included regular walking, treadmill walking, bicycle ergometry, or bed ergometry for hospitalized patients. Walking is the most common exercise for cancer patients [19, 27]. It is a natural, safe, and tolerable choice that relates directly to daily living and is conducive to AYA lifestyle, particularly if complemented with music or participation with peers. It is important for AYA to participate in activities in which they will experience personal accomplishment. Recreational pursuits are often the most preferred form of activity. Popular options include martial arts, dance, aerobics, swimming, walking, biking, and activities at fitness clubs. Some AYA are able to resume competitive sports, although adaptations may be necessary.

Individual lifestyle may influence the preference for type of program, varying from self-directed home programs to group exercise classes [27]. Alternatives should be offered, particularly for those who have a busy school or work life. The concept of "lifestyle physical activity interventions" has been an efficacious approach for youth treated for cancer. This approach focuses on increasing moderate-intensity activity through individualized programs that take into account individual, cultural, and environmental differences [28].

26.4.1.1 Precautions and Contraindications (Table 26.1)

It is important to be aware of the implications of cardiotoxicity, susceptibility to fractures, and other effects of cancer treatment on motor skills and balance when counseling AYA regarding exercise. Clinical concerns regarding the prescription of exercise for cancer patients have included the potentially immunosuppressive effect of vigorous exercise, fracture due to compromised bone integrity, and exacerbation of cardiotoxicity, pain, nausea, and fatigue. However, research is beginning to dispel many of the myths and fears about safety and feasibility [19]. Guidelines on

contraindications to participation in exercise programs for adults with cancer have been published but are not necessarily based on sound research [19, 27]. Precautions have included uncontrolled and unstable cardiac disease, certain metastatic lesions, and recent intracranial hemorrhage or deep-vein thrombosis with pulmonary embolism. Other recommendations include the avoidance of the following: high-intensity activities if the hemoglobin level is less than 80 g/l, activities that present a risk of bacterial infection if the absolute neutrophil count is less than 0.5×10^9/l, contact sports or high-impact activities that pose a risk of bleeding if the platelet count is less than 50×10^9/l [19], and power weight lifting if cardiomyopathy is a risk factor [29].

Patient symptomatology is the foremost guide for the intensity, duration, and mode of exercise employed during treatment for cancer [30]. It may be necessary to vary the intensity and frequency of exercise depending on treatment schedule and variations in response to therapy. Ideally, patients should receive individualized consultation.

Recommendations regarding a physically activity lifestyle should be part of a comprehensive program to effect an overall healthy lifestyle. Other healthy behaviors that should be addressed include proper diet, not smoking, sun protection, and regular checkups.

26.4.2 Other Specific Interventions

Adolescents with certain impairments, diagnoses, or treatments may require particular interventions. If a patient has or is at high risk for loss of range of motion, implementing the principles of treatment for contracture management may be indicated [12]. These may include prolonged stretch through positioning, serial casting, and the use of splints or orthoses. Orthoses may provide stability for protection from injury or enhancement of function. For example, ankle-foot orthoses may be used for significant vincristine neuropathy. These are sometimes unacceptable to adolescents due to cosmetic considerations and inconvenience. When neurological impairments are impacting on function or quality of life, a variety of therapeutic interventions, such as spasticity management techniques and motor learning prin-

Table 26.1 Potential issues impacting on rehabilitation programs for adolescents and young adults with cancer

Impairments of body function/structure Fatigue, pain, nausea		Activity Limitations Limitations in		Participation Restrictions Restricted partici-pation in
Thrombocytopenia, anemia		Gross motor function		Education
Cardiotoxicity, pulmonary dysfunction		Fine motor function		Recreation/leisure
Weight loss/weight gain, ↓fitness		Self-care		Sports
↓Range of motion/contracture		Activities of daily living		Social activities
Osteopenia/osteoporosis		Communication		Volunteering
Muscle weakness, bone deformity	↔	Learning	↔	Employment
Spasticity, balance/coordination deficits		Interpersonal relationships		Travel
Motor learning problems				
Cognitive deficits, perceptual deficits				
Sensory/motor neuropathy				
Visual and hearing deficits				
Bowel/bladder problems				
Dysphagia/dysarthria				
Psychosocial problems				
	↑		↑	
Contextual factors	Personal factors		Environmental factors	
	Gender		Accessibility	
	Age		Health care facilities	
	Family support		Community facilities	
	Peer support		Educational facilities	
	Culture		Climate, season, location	
	Spirituality		Societal attitude	
	Economic resources		Transportation	

ciples, may be incorporated into treatment [12, 13]. The etiology and nature of persisting fine motor and hand-writing problems are diverse, so individualized rehabilitation programs are warranted [16].

AYA undergoing amputations for bone tumors need to follow rehabilitation programs addressing strengthening, contracture management, prosthetic use, and adaptations for driving a car [30]. Therapy using orthopedic and gait-training principles is important for those having limb-sparing surgery. Guidelines for therapy vary depending on surgical protocols, specific procedures, and the amount of bone replaced.

Treatment principles involving cognitive strategies, generalization of learning, and behavioral approaches may need to be incorporated into rehabilitation programs. In some cases, a compensatory approach is necessary, requiring the use of adaptive equipment, or modification of environments or activities.

Pain management can be an important role for rehabilitation professionals. To augment the pharmacological management of pain, interventions such as massage, heat, cold, acupuncture, positioning, transcutaneous electrical stimulation, or behavioral techniques may be used. Appropriate precautions must be followed.

Interventions may involve the facilitation of safe and efficient swallowing for patients with pharyngeal dysfunction. Input for patients with dysarthria resulting from oral motor dysfunction of neurogenic or mechanical origin may involve the provision of communication devices or exercise.

26.4.3 Facilitating Participation

Various strategies are used to promote participation in an active life with respect to socialization, sports, leisure, recreation, education, volunteering, employment, and community. School reentry after a diagnosis of cancer can be very challenging, but is generally encouraged as it maintains some normalcy in life and allows for continued social and academic participation while providing hope for the future. Rehabilitation professionals may be involved in liaising with and educating school staff and peers about the diagnosis and its implications. Recommendations regarding positioning, lifting, and transferring, learning needs,

and physical education may facilitate the return to the educational setting. In school-based programs, therapists may prescribe equipment for accessibility and computer-based systems [31]. Going to college can present challenges of independence in learning, mobility, and self-care. Some postsecondary institutions may have programs to facilitate students with special needs. Vocational counseling is helpful for some AYA.

Families should be encouraged to access community recreational facilities, as these may be motivating, well equipped, and socially inviting. Alternatively or additionally, specialized groups or camps and adapted recreational programs provide opportunities for those who desire involvement with peers who are experiencing similar health issues.

26.4.4 Intervention for the Acutely Ill, Isolated, or Hospitalized Patient

Rehabilitation and exercise are very important for hospitalized patients. Goals for acutely ill patients will be focused on comfort and prevention of unnecessary secondary complications. Bed rest and immobility combined with cancer treatments can result in rapid loss of muscle strength, contracture, pulmonary complications, skin damage, and osteoporosis. Interventions to prevent these problems may include positioning, frequent change of position, active bed exercises, and breathing exercises and airway clearance techniques if respiratory function is compromised [32]. Patients should get out of bed for weight-bearing activities as soon as possible. Patients in isolation, such as recipients of bone marrow transplants, require encouragement and activity opportunities to remain mobile, maintain the ability to perform activities of daily living, and avoid boredom [32]. Stationary bicycles, ergometers, treadmills, or light weights can be used if appropriate disinfection protocols are employed. Performance of activities such as getting dressed, and if the isolation protocol allows, walking to the washroom or climbing stairs should be incorporated into the day. The temporary use of mobility or walking aids may facilitate early mobilization. A leave of absence from the hospital can be very beneficial physically and psychologically.

26.4.5 Palliative Care

Providing palliative care for a young person is very difficult for all involved. Rehabilitation input has been found to make a significant difference to the lives of patients with terminal cancer and their families by giving them the ability to participate in meaningful activities and decreasing the burden of care [33]. Rehabilitation professionals may be involved with facilitating function and optimizing comfort to help the young person and their family achieve the best possible quality of life. This is accomplished through applying rehabilitation principles and practices in respect to pain management and facilitation of independence in mobility and activities of daily living as tolerated and desired. Discharge from the hospital may be facilitated with appropriate environmental or mobility aids and assistive devices.

26.5 Conclusion

Adolescence and young adulthood can be a particularly difficult time to experience cancer and its treatment as there may be missed opportunities for participation in the normal daily activities and special events of these years. Rehabilitation professionals work collaboratively toward limiting impairment and facilitating optimal participation in the activities of importance to this group. There is a need for further research in all levels of functioning in this area.

References

1. Pender NJ (1998) Motivation for physical activity among children and adolescents. Ann Rev Nurs Res 16:139–172
2. World Health Organization (2001) International Classification of Functioning, Disability and Health. Geneva: http://www.who.int/classificaton/ict
3. Dimeo FC (2001) Effects of exercise on cancer-related fatigue. Cancer 92:1689–1693
4. Davies B, Whitsett, SF, Bruce A, McCarthy P (2002) A typology of fatigue in children with cancer. J Pediatr Oncol Nurs 19:12–21
5. Ljungman G, Gordh T, Sorensen S, Kreuger A (1999) Pain in paediatric oncology: interviews with children, adolescents and their parents. Acta Paediatr 88:623–630
6. Jenney MEM, Faragher EB, Morris Jones PH, Woodcock A (1995) Lung function and exercise capacity in survivors of childhood leukemia. Med Pediatr Oncol 24:222–230
7. Sharkey AM, Carey AB, Heise CT, Barber G (1993) Cardiac rehabilitation after cancer therapy in children and young adults. Am J Cardiol 71:1488–1490
8. Johnson D, Perrault H, Fournier J, et al (1997) Cardiovascular responses to dynamic submaximal exercise in children previously treated with anthracycline. Am Heart J 133:169–173
9. Anderson RE (2000) The spread of the childhood obesity epidemic. Can Med ASSOC J 163:1461–1462
10. Nysom K, Molgaard C, Holm K, et al (1998) Bone mass and body composition after cessation of therapy for childhood cancer. Int J Cancer Suppl 11:40–43
11. Haddy TB, Mosher RB, Reaman GH (2001) Osteoporosis in survivors of acute lymphoblastic leukemia. Oncologist 6:278–285
12. Kirshblum S, O'Dell MW, Ho C, Barr K (2001) Rehabilitation of persons with central nervous system tumors. Cancer 92:1029–1038
13. Olney SJ, Wright MJ (2000) Cerebral palsy. In: Campbell SK, Palisano RJ, Vander Linden DW (eds) Physical Therapy for Children. WB Saunders, Philadelphia, pp 533–570
14. Reinders-Messelink HA, Schoemaker MM, Snijders TAB, et al (1999) Motor performance of children during treatment for acute lymphoblastic leukemia. Med Pediatr Oncol 37:393–399
15. Wright MJ, Halton JM, Martin RF, Barr RD (1998) Long-term gross motor performance following treatment for acute lymphoblastic leukemia. Med Pediatr Oncol 31:86–90
16. Reinders-Messelink HA, Schoemaker MM, Snijders TA, et al (2001) Analysis of handwriting problems of children during treatment of acute lymphoblastic leukemia. Med Pediatr Oncol 33:572–576
17. Keats MR, Courneya KS, Danielsen S, Whitsett SF (1999) Leisure-time physical activity and psychosocial well-being in adolescents after cancer diagnosis. J Pediatr Oncol Nurs 16:180–188
18. Wright MJ, Galea RD, Barr RD (2003a) Self-perceptions of physical activity in survivors of acute lymphoblastic leukemia in childhood. Pediatr Exerc Sci 15:191–201
19. Courneya KS, Mackey JR, Jones LW (2000) Coping with cancer: can exercise help? Physician Sportsmed 28:49–51, 55–56, 66–68
20. Burnham TR, Wilcox A (2002) Effects of exercise on physiological and psychological variables in cancer survivors. Med Sci Sports Exerc 34:1863–1867
21. Fairey AS, Courneya KS, Field CJ, Mackey JR (2002) Physical exercise and immune system function in cancer survivors. Cancer 94:539–551
22. Hockenbury-Eaton M, Hinds PS (2000) Fatigue in children and adolescents with cancer: evolution of a program of study. Semin Oncol Nurs 16:261–272

23. Schwartz A (1998) Patterns of exercise and fatigue in physically active cancer survivors. Oncol Nurs Forum 25:485–491

24. Wright MJ, Hanna SE, Halton JM, Barr RD (2003b) Maintenance of ankle range of motion in children treated for acute lymphoblastic leukemia. Pediatr Phys Ther 15:146–152

25. Thompson AM, Humbert ML, Mirwald RL (2003) A longitudinal study of the impact of childhood and adolescent physical activity experiences on adult physical activity perceptions and behaviours. Qual Health Res 13:358–377

26. Cavill NS, Biddle S, Sallis JF (2001) Health enhancing physical activity for young people: statement of the United Kingdon expert consensus conference. Pediatr Exerc Sci 13:12–25

27. Jones LW, Courneya KS (2002) Exercise counselling and programming preferences of cancer survivors. Cancer Pract 10:208–215

28. Dunn AL, Andersen RE, Jakicic JM (1998) Lifestyle physical activity interventions – history, short- and long-term effects, and recommendations. Am J Prev Med 15:398–412

29. Hicks JE (1990) Exercise for cancer patients. In: Basmaijan JV, Wolf SL (eds) Therapeutic Exercise. Williams and Wilkins, Baltimore, Maryland, pp 351–369

30. Gillis TA, Donovan ES (2001) Rehabilitation following bone marrow transplantation. Cancer 92:998–1007

31. Stanger M (2000) Limb deficiencies and amputations. In: SK Campbell, RJ Palisano, DW Vander Linden (eds) Physical Therapy for Children. WB Saunders Company, Philadelphia, pp 370–397

32. O'Connor L, Blesch KS (1992) Life cycle issues affecting cancer rehabilitation. Semin Oncol Nurs 8:174–185

33. Santiago-Palma J, Payne R (2001) Palliative care and rehabilitation. Cancer 92:1049–1052

Adolescent and Young Adult Cancer Survivors: Late Effects of Treatment

Smita Bhatia • Wendy Landier •

Andrew A. Toogood • Michael Hawkins

Contents

27.1 Introduction

The overall incidence rate of cancer in 15- to 19-year-olds is twice that in younger persons [1]. Specifically, among adolescents 15 to 19 years of age in the United States during the 1990s there were 203 new cases per year per million persons, a rate that is 100% higher than the incidence of cancer in children less than 15 years of age. With the use of risk-based therapies, the overall 5-year survival rate is exceeding 75% [1]. Recent figures from the population-based National Cancer Registration System for England [2], which relate to cancers diagnosed in the year 2000, have been used to calculate the cumulative risk of developing cancer between the ages of 15 and 29 years inclusive. The cumulative risks are about 0.46% (or 1 in 217) for both males and females. Recent survival statistics for the United Kingdom indicate that about 75% of individuals diagnosed with cancer between the ages of 15 and 24 years survive at least 5 years [3]. Consequently, it is reasonable to anticipate, ignoring competing causes of death, that approximately 0.35% (or 1 in 286) of the population of adults aged over 30 years will eventually be survivors of cancer diagnosed between 15 and 29 years of age.

Unlike older cancer patients, adolescents and young adults tolerate the acute side effects of therapy relatively well. However, the use of cancer therapy can produce complications that may not become apparent until years later, hence the term "late effect" for late-occurring or chronic outcomes – either physical or psychological – that persists or develops beyond 5 years from the diagnosis of cancer. Approximately two out of every three survivors will experience at least one late effect [4–7] and about one out of four will experience a late effect that is severe or life-threatening [4, 6, 7]. These complications involve all organ systems.

Topics that will be reviewed in detail in this chapter include issues related to the potential adverse events faced by the survivors (Table 27.1), the options for providing survivorship care, and the future research opportunities that need to be explored (Table 27.2). We will review the known late effects in survivors of cancer occurring during adolescence and young adult-

hood, and discuss the relationship between these effects and individual therapeutic modalities (surgery, radiation, or single- and multiple-agent chemotherapy) or combined-modality regimens, including those used for blood and marrow transplantation. The resulting complications include cardiopulmonary compromise, endocrine dysfunction, renal impairment, gastrointestinal dysfunction, musculoskeletal sequelae, and subsequent malignancies. These complications are related not only to the specific therapy employed, but may also be determined by individual host character-

Table 27.1 Late effects associated with common therapeutic exposures. *AML* Acute myeloblastic leukemia, *MDS* myelodysplastic syndrome, *HIV* human immunodeficiency virus

Therapeutic exposure	Potential late effects
Vincristine, vinblastine	Peripheral neuropathy, Raynaud's phenomenon
Corticosteroids	Cataracts, osteopenia, osteoporosis, avascular necrosis
Mercaptopurine	Hepatic dysfunction, venoocclusive disease
Methotrexate (systemic)	Osteopenia, osteoporosis, renal dysfunction, hepatic dysfunction
Methotrexate (intrathecal)	Neurocognitive deficits, clinical leukoencephalopathy
Cytarabine (high-dose)	Neurocognitive deficits, clinical leukoencephalopathy
Anthracyclines	Cardiomyopathy, arrhythmias, secondary AML
Alkalyting agents	Hypogonadism, infertility, secondary AML/MDS
Busulfan, carmustine, lomustine	Pulmonary dysfunction
Cyclophosphamide, ifosfamide	Hemorrhagic cystitis, dysfunctional voiding, bladder malignancy, renal dysfunction (ifosfamide only)
Heavy metals (platinum)	Ototoxicity, peripheral sensory neuropathy, renal dysfunction, dyslipidemia
Etoposide, teniposide	Secondary AML
Bleomycin	Pulmonary dysfunction
Mantle radiation	Hypothyroidism, premature cardiovascular disease, cardiac valvular disease, cardiomyopathy, arrhythmias, carotid artery disease, scoliosis/kyphosis, second malignant neoplasm in radiation field (e.g., thyroid, breast), pulmonary dysfunction
Inverted Y radiation	Hypogonadism, infertility, adverse pregnancy outcome, second malignant neoplasm in radiation field (e.g., gastrointestinal)
Cranial or craniospinal radiation	Neurocognitive deficits, clinical leukoencephalopathy, cataracts, hypothyroidism, second malignant neoplasm in radiation field (e.g., skin, thyroid, brain), short stature, scoliosis/kyphosis, obesity
Splenectomy	Acute life-threatening infections
Blood products	Chronic viral hepatitis, HIV

istics. The research leading to our current state of knowledge began almost 30 years ago in single institutions and multi-institution consortia. With the recognition that large cohorts of survivors would be needed to evaluate the effects of multiple therapies on individuals treated for a variety of neoplasms at different ages, and with funding from the National Cancer Institute, the Childhood Cancer Survivor Study (CCSS) was established [8]. The publications of the CCSS include analyses of some of the late effects reported below; the web site may be accessed for more details – www.cancer.umn.edu/ltfu#ccss.

27.2 Medical Issues

27.2.1 Late Mortality

Overall mortality among adolescent and young adult cancer survivors has been described to be tenfold that of the general population [9, 10]. The CCSS assessed overall and cause-specific mortality in a retrospective cohort of 20,227 5-year survivors and demonstrated a 10.8-fold excess in overall mortality [9]. Risk of death was statistically significantly higher in females, individuals diagnosed with cancer before the age of 5 years,

and those with an initial diagnosis of leukemia or brain tumor. The excess mortality was due to death from primary cancer, second cancer, cardiotoxicity and non-cancer death, and existed for up to 25 years after the initial cancer diagnosis.

27.2.2 Second Primary Neoplasms

Etiological factors for the development of second primary neoplasms after cancer in adolescence and young adulthood include elements of treatment for the first primary neoplasm – particularly radiotherapy and chemotherapy, as well as genetic predisposition, hormonal factors, immunosuppression, and the potential interactions between these risk factors. Among survivors of cancer diagnosed in adolescence and young adulthood, during the initial years of follow-up there is relatively little opportunity for environmental factors (for example smoking, drinking, diet, and lifestyle influences) to be important etiologically, when compared with survivors of initial primary neoplasms diagnosed in middle age or older adulthood. We concentrate on second primary neoplasms occurring after those specific types of first primary neoplasm that occur more commonly in adolescence and young adulthood, and for which there is reliable large-scale

Table 27.2 Challenges in survivorship research

Treatment for cancer in young people undergoes constant change, including introduction of new:	– Therapeutic agents/combinations of agents – Radiation techniques – Surgical procedures – Supportive care agents/techniques
Most current data relates to outcomes within the first decade following treatment; only minimal data addresses longer-term outcomes	
Research is needed to:	– Determine the potential long-term impact of cancer therapy in the young – More clearly define survivors at greatest risk for specific outcomes – Identify genetic predisposition to certain key outcomes, including the role of gene–environment interactions – Identify the role of lifestyle choices (e.g., alcohol, tobacco, diet, exercise) and their impact on risk of late outcomes – Develop intervention strategies to prevent or minimize the impact of adverse late effects

evidence available, for example from large-cohort or case-control studies.

27.2.2.1 Second Primary Neoplasms after Hodgkin Lymphoma

A meta-analysis of previous studies has reported the risk of second primary leukemia to be 37-fold that expected (standardized incidence ratio, SIR) with a 95% confidence interval of 23, to 61-fold that expected [11]. The SIR for acute myeloid leukemia is higher than for other types of leukemia and is strongly associated with chemotherapy, which includes alkylating agents, particularly the MOPP (mechlorethamine, oncovorin, procarbazine, prednisone) regimen. There is no conclusive evidence indicating an independent effect of radiotherapy on the risk of leukemia, although some studies have suggested a link with the extent of radiotherapy. The excess risk of leukemia seems to diminish beyond 15 years from Hodgkin lymphoma, although the number of survivors followed beyond this interval is still relatively small [11].

In contrast to radiotherapy for Hodgkin lymphoma being, at most, weakly leukemogenic, it is associated with an increased risk of several solid cancers including: breast, lung, thyroid, stomach, bone, soft tissue, skin, and possibly colon and pancreas [12]. These excess risks of solid tumors tend to emerge by about a decade after Hodgkin lymphoma, and again, in contrast to leukemia, the excess risk is still increasing after 15 years of follow-up.

The risk of breast cancer after Hodgkin lymphoma was reviewed recently [13]. The risk of breast cancer is particularly excessive among women irradiated when young. For women irradiated under age 21 years, risks 15 to 25 times expected have been reported. The absolute excess risks have mostly been about 20 to 40 extra breast cancer cases per 10,000 survivors per year. Estimates of cumulative risk range from 12% at 30 years after treatment in the Nordic countries [14] to 17% by 30 years from treatment reported by the Late Effects Study Group [15].

The risk of breast cancer is also in excess of that expected following Hodgkin lymphoma diagnosed in young adulthood (ages 20–29 years), but the SIRs are lower than for those treated in childhood and adoles-

cence. Unfortunately, the lower SIRs are not necessarily accompanied by lower absolute excess risk, as several investigators reported absolute excess risks of comparable magnitude for patients treated between the ages of 20 and 29 years and below 20 years of age [13].

Two recently published studies investigated the effects of radiotherapy doses delivered to the breast and the effects of exposure to specific types of cytotoxic agents on subsequent breast cancer risk [16, 17]. The largest was a matched case-control study of cancer within a cohort of 3,817 female 1-year survivors of Hodgkin lymphoma diagnosed before age 31 years, within 6 population-based cancer registries [16]. The investigators assessed the relative risk of breast cancer in relation to radiation doses delivered to the breast and the ovaries, and the cumulative dose of alkylating agents received. Breast cancer developed in 105 survivors of Hodgkin lymphoma who were matched to 266 survivors without breast cancer. A radiation dose of at least 400 cGy to the breast was associated with a threefold increased risk, compared with individuals receiving lower radiation doses and no alkylating agents. The relative risk was eightfold at exposures of at least 4000 cGy. Increased risks persisted for at least 25 years following radiotherapy. Breast cancer risk declined with increasing number of alkylating agent cycles. The relative risk of breast cancer was low (0.4) among women who received at least 500 cGy to the ovaries compared with those given lower doses. The authors concluded that hormonal stimulation appears to be important for the development of radiation-induced breast cancer. Such a mechanism could potentially explain why breast cancer risk declines with age at irradiation for Hodgkin lymphoma, as women irradiated at age 30 years or older experience much lower excess risk than those irradiated before this age [13].

As breast cancer is a common disease in the general population, even modest SIRs may yield substantial increases in the absolute excess number observed. A surveillance strategy for women receiving supradiaphragmatic radiotherapy for Hodgkin lymphoma at less than 35 years of age has recently been published by the Royal College of Radiologists [18].

Doses of radiation to the lungs are substantial as a result of several radiotherapy field configurations used to treat Hodgkin lymphoma. In a review published in

1999 it was reported that the risk of lung cancer has consistently been in excess of that expected among Hodgkin lymphoma survivors [12]. Recently a large international collaborative case-control study of the role of radiotherapy, chemotherapy, and smoking in the development of lung cancer after Hodgkin lymphoma has been reported [19, 20]. It was ultimately based on 227 patients who developed second primary lung cancer and 455 matched controls who did not. An excess risk of lung cancer increased with both increasing number of cycles of alkylating agents (p for trend <0.001) and increasing radiation dose (p for trend <0.001). Statistically significant elevated risks of lung cancer were apparent within one to 4 years of treatment with alkylating agents, whereas the excess risks after radiotherapy began 5 years after treatment and persisted for more than 20 years. Tobacco use increased lung cancer risk more than 20-fold; risks from smoking appeared to multiply risks from treatment [19].

Excesses of cancers of several other sites have been observed after Hodgkin lymphoma including thyroid, stomach, bone, non-Hodgkin lymphoma (NHL), and melanoma [12].

27.2.2.2 Second Primary Neoplasms after Non-Hodgkin Lymphoma

A meta-analysis of studies available in 1999 indicated that among survivors of NHL, the observed numbers of the following second primary neoplasms were found to be in excess of the numbers expected: acute myeloid leukemia, Hodgkin lymphoma, lung cancer, melanoma, renal cancer, and brain cancer [11]. The authors concluded that the excess risk of acute myeloid leukemia is probably due to alkylating agent exposure; whilst the increased risk of Hodgkin lymphoma might be due to shared risk factors and susceptibility, but might also be partially explained by diagnostic misclassification.

27.2.2.3 Second Primary Neoplasms after Testicular Cancer

Excess risks of cancer of the stomach, bladder, bone, and connective tissue appear to be attributable to radiotherapy [12]. It also appears likely that there is some

increased risk of second primary leukemia resulting from chemotherapy use and that this may be related to use of etoposide, particularly in higher doses [21].

27.2.2.4 Second Primary Neoplasms after Breast Cancer

As noted in a review [12], before the implementation of breast-conserving surgery and localized radiotherapy to treat node-negative breast cancer, the principal method of local control was radical mastectomy and extensive radiotherapy to the chest wall and lymph nodes. Consequently, such women have experienced an excess risk of leukemias and cancers of the contralateral breast and lung, and possibly of esophagus, bone, connective tissue, and thyroid gland [22–26]. The risk of second primary leukemia is associated with radiotherapy (relative risk=1.8), alkylating agents (relative risk=6.5), and both (relative risk=17.4) [23]. The radiation dose to the contralateral breast can amount to several Grays and a review [12] has inferred that women irradiated in young adulthood are probably at increased risk of contralateral breast cancer, based mainly on one study [22]. However, another review [27] suggests no convincing evidence of such an effect. As the dose and effect appear to be less than substantial, it is possibly a question of statistical power that accounts for this apparent conflict. Women given radiotherapy who survived at least 10 years appear to have about double the risk of lung cancer experienced by nonirradiated women [24, 25, 28]. This risk is likely to be less following modern radiotherapy techniques. A recently published study [29] indicates that smoking is associated with a sixfold increased risk of second primary lung cancer, while radiotherapy was not significantly associated with an increased risk. However, another recent report of lung cancer in 3,515 breast cancer survivors, which was particularly informative as radiotherapy was subject to randomization and there was over 20 years of follow-up, reported a small increased risk associated with radiation use [30].

27.2.3 Cardiovascular Function

The anthracyclines doxorubicin and daunomycin are well-known causes of cardiomyopathy [31, 32].

Anthracyclines have a wide range of clinical activity, and about 40 to 50% of adolescent and young adult cancer survivors were treated with anthracyclines, making it one of the more common exposures. Chronic cardiotoxicity usually manifests itself as cardiomyopathy, pericarditis, and congestive heart failure. The incidence of cardiomyopathy is dose-dependent, and may exceed 30% among patients who received cumulative doses of anthracyclines in excess of 600 mg/m^2. With a total dose of 500 to 600 mg/m^2, the incidence is 11%, falling to less than 1% for cumulative doses less than 500 mg/m^2 [33]. This has formed the basis for considering 500 mg/^{2} as the threshold cumulative dose for cardiotoxicity. However, a lower cumulative dose of anthracyclines may place individuals at increased risk for cardiac compromise [34]. Kremer et al. evaluated the cumulative incidence of anthracycline-induced clinical heart failure in a cohort of 607 patients who had been treated with a mean cumulative anthracyclines dose of 301 mg/m^2 and were followed for a median of 6.3 years. A cumulative dose of anthracyclines greater than 300 mg/m^2 was associated with an increased risk of clinical heart failure (relative risk 11.8) compared with a cumulative dose lower than 300 mg/m^2. The estimated risk of clinical heart failure increased with time, and approached 5% after 15 years. In addition, several investigators have described subclinical anthracycline-induced myocardial damage.

Steinherz et al. found 23% of 201 patients to have echocardiographic abnormalities, a median of 7 years after therapy [35]. The median cumulative dose of doxorubicin received by these patients was 450 mg/m^2 (range 200 to 1275 mg/m^2). Lipshultz and colleagues evaluated cancer survivors who had received a median doxorubicin dose of 334 mg/m^2 (range 12 to 550 mg/m^2). They concluded that doxorubicin causes progressive elevation of afterload or depression of left-ventricular contractility in about 75% of the patients. However, the clinical relevance of subclinical myocardial injury is not clearly established, in part due to widely varying methods used to define and assess such injury.

These studies and others emphasize that cardiomyopathy can occur many years after completion of therapy (15 to 20 years), and that the onset may be spontaneous or coincide with exertion or pregnancy. During the third trimester, the cardiac volume increases, increasing the cardiac workload, leading to overt symptomology in women with left-ventricular dysfunction [36, 37]. Risk factors known to be associated with anthracycline-related cardiac toxicity include: mediastinal radiation, uncontrolled hypertension, exposure to other chemotherapeutic agents, especially cyclophosphamide, dactinomycin, mitomycin, dacarbazine, vincristine, bleomycin, and methotrexate, younger age, dyselectrolytemia such as hypokalemia and hypomagnesemia, and female gender [38].

Chronic cardiac toxicity associated with radiation alone most commonly involves pericardial effusions or constrictive pericarditis, sometimes in association with pancarditis [39]. Although 40 Gy of total-heart radiation dose appears to be the usual threshold, pericarditis has been reported after as little as 15 Gy, even in the absence of radiomimetic chemotherapy. Symptomatic pericarditis, which usually develops 10 to 30 months after radiation, is found in 2 to 10% of patients [40]. Subclinical pericardial and myocardial damage as well as valvular thickening may be common in this population [41], and symptomatic pericarditis may first appear as late as 45 years after therapy [42, 43].

Coronary artery disease has been reported following radiation to the mediastinum, although the mortality rate was not significantly higher in patients with Hodgkin lymphoma who had received mediastinal radiation than in the general population [44]. A Dutch study of Hodgkin lymphoma survivors reported a cumulative risk for ischemic heart disease of 21% at 20 years after radiation [45]. In another study following 415 Hodgkin lymphoma survivors, 10% developed coronary heart disease [46].

Prevention of cardiotoxicity is a primary focus of investigation. Certain analogs of doxorubicin and daunomycin, and liposomal anthracyclines, which appear to have decreased cardiotoxicity, with equivalent antitumor activity, are being explored. The anthracyclines chelate iron, and the anthracycline–iron complex catalyzes the formation of hydroxyl radicals. Agents that are able to remove iron from the anthracyclines, such as dexrazoxane, have been investigated as cardioprotectants. Clinical trials of dexrazoxane have been conducted with encouraging evidence of short-term cardioprotection [47, 48], although the long-term avoidance of cardiotoxicity with the use of this agent needs to be determined. In a recent prospective, randomized study of pediatric ALL patients, Lipshultz et al. have demonstrated that patients treated with doxorubicin at 300 mg/m^2 alone were more likely than those treated with dexrazoxane and doxorubicin to have cardiac injury as reflected by elevated troponin T levels (50% vs. 21%, $p<0.001$) and extremely elevated troponin T levels (32% vs. 10%, $p<0.001$), without compromising the antileukemic efficacy of doxorubicin (event-free survival was 83% at 2.5 years for both arms) [49]. However, longer follow-up is necessary to determine the influence of dexrazoxane on echocardiographic findings, and hence, the clinical significance of these findings. Lower doses of anthracyclines and reduced port sizes of radiation therapy may also help in decreasing the incidence of carditis. Management of survivors with asymptomatic deterioration of left-ventricular function is controversial. Angiotensin converting enzyme (ACE) inhibitors have been known to improve morbidity and mortality in patients with cardiomyopathy. There appear to be theoretical risks with such therapy in adolescence, since the ACE inhibitors, while lowering the afterload in the short-term, may also limit the cardiac growth potential by inhibiting cardiac growth factors. Thus, the role of ACE inhibitors and beta-blockers in asymptomatic survivors with cardiac dysfunction remains in question [50, 51].

Patients who received anthracycline chemotherapy need ongoing monitoring for late-onset cardiomyopathy, with frequency of evaluation based on total cumulative dose and age at the time of initial therapy. In addition to monitoring for cardiomyopathy, survivors who received radiation potentially impacting the heart (i.e., chest, spine, upper abdomen, or total body irradiation, TBI) also need monitoring for potential early-onset atherosclerotic heart disease, valvular disease, and pericardial complications. Specific recommendations for monitoring, based on age and therapeutic exposure, are delineated within the Children's Oncology Group (COG) Long-term Follow-up guidelines (described below).

27.2.4 Pulmonary Function

Pulmonary fibrosis and pneumonitis can result from pulmonary radiation. Thus, these problems are seen most often in patients with thoracic malignancies, notably Hodgkin lymphoma. Asymptomatic radiographic findings or restrictive changes on pulmonary function testing have been reported in more than 30% of such individuals [52–54]. Of 25 HD survivors treated with standard mantle radiation before age 35 years, 60% had an abnormal chest radiograph at a mean follow-up of 9 years [55]. Of the 19 who had pulmonary function testing, 89% had an abnormality, with 72% having a reduced diffusion capacity. None of the patients were symptomatic. These changes have been detected months to years after radiation therapy, most often in patients who suffered radiation pneumonitis during or shortly after therapy [56]. Clinically apparent pneumonitis with cough, fever, or dyspnea occurs in only 5 to 15% of patients, and is generally limited to those who received more than 30 Gy in standard fractions to more than 50% of the lung [56]. Craniospinal radiation for patients with malignant brain tumors and scatter from abdominal ports contribute to the development of late restrictive lung disease [57]. Obstructive changes have also been reported after conventional radiation therapy. Following blood and marrow transplantation, both restrictive and obstructive lung disease including bronchiolitis obliterans are well described [58, 59]. In one series [58], after 10 Gy TBI in a single fraction, 8% of patients had a forced expiratory volume in 1 s (FEV1)/vital capacity (VC) (a measure of obstructive lung disease) below 50% of normal at 3 years, and 29% had an FEV1/VC below 70% by that time.

On a molecular level, radiation-related pulmonary injuries in adolescents and young adults are likely to be mediated by cytokine production, which stimulates septal fibroblasts, increasing collagen production and resulting in pulmonary fibrosis [60, 61].

The incidence of radiation-induced late pulmonary toxicity has dramatically decreased in the last decade secondary to refined techniques of radiation therapy [62–64]. In a recently published study of patients with stage I and IIA Hodgkin lymphoma treated with radiation alone (40 to 45 Gy to involved fields), the late pulmonary effects observed were minimal [64]. While VC, residual volume, FEV1, the normal diffusing capacity of the lung for carbon monoxide (DLCO), and total lung capacity were significantly decreased at completion of radiation therapy compared with pre-treatment studies, all except DLCO returned to near normal within 1 year. The decrease in DLCO remained stable but the forced expiratory flow rate between 25 and 75% of VC had a significant decline at 3 years posttreatment compared with baseline studies. Use of more modest radiation doses also has contributed to decreased pulmonary toxicity [65].

In addition to radiation therapy, chemotherapeutic agents appear to be responsible for pulmonary disease in long-term survivors. Bleomycin toxicity is the prototype for chemotherapy-related lung injury, presenting as interstitial pneumonitis and pulmonary fibrosis [66, 67]. The chronic lung toxicity usually follows persistence or progression of abnormalities developing within 3 months of therapy. Like the acute toxicity, it is dose-dependent above a threshold cumulative dose of 400 units/m^2 and is exacerbated by concurrent or previous radiation therapy [68]. Above 400 units/m^2 in the absence of other risk factors, 10% of patients experience fibrosis [68]. At lower doses, fibrosis occurs sporadically in less than 5% of patients, with a 1 to 2% mortality rate. In some reports, bleomycin toxicity was anticipated on the basis of DLCO abnormalities.

Alkylating agents also are believed to cause chronic lung injury. As with bleomycin, carmustine and lomustine pulmonary toxicity is dose-related. Cumulative carmustine doses greater than 600 mg/m^2 result in a 50% incidence of symptoms [69]. A marked increase in pulmonary fibrosis appears at doses exceeding 1500 mg/m^2 [69]. Pulmonary fibrosis has also been observed in 16 to 40% of transplant recipients treated with cytotoxic conditioning agents including carmustine at doses of 500–600 mg/m^2; the incidence of fibrosis declines considerably when doses are limited to less than 300 to 450 mg/m^2 [70, 71]. Female patients are at a higher risk for this complication than their male counterparts. Case reports and small series suggest that cyclophosphamide can cause delayed-onset pulmonary fibrosis with severe restrictive lung disease in association with a marked reduction in the anteroposterior diameter of the chest [67, 72]. Melphalan and busulfan are also known to cause pulmonary fibrosis in a dose-related manner. Busulfan toxicity is most predictable in transplantation doses exceeding 500 mg, and may be associated with a progressive, potentially fatal restrictive lung disease. Lung injury associated with busulfan is characterized by diffuse interstitial fibrosis and bronchopulmonary dysplasia.

Additional factors contributing to chronic pulmonary toxicity include superimposed infection, underlying pneumonopathy (e.g., asthma), cigarette or respirator toxicity, chronic graft versus host disease, and the effects of chronic pulmonary involvement by tumor or reaction to tumor. Increased oxygen concentrations associated with general anesthesia or scuba diving have also been found to exacerbate pulmonary fibrosis [73, 74].

Monitoring for pulmonary dysfunction in cancer survivors includes asking about symptoms such as chronic cough (with or without fever) or dyspnea on yearly follow-up. All patients must understand the risks of smoking. The best approach to chronic pulmonary toxicity of anticancer therapy is preventive, and includes respecting cumulative dosage restrictions of bleomycin and alkylators, limiting radiation dosage and port sizes, and avoiding primary or secondhand smoke. Pulmonary function tests (including DLCO and spirometry) have been recommended as a baseline upon entry into long-term follow up for patients at risk, in patients with symptoms, or in those who require general anesthesia for any reason. Patients with risk factors for lung disease are discouraged from scuba diving.

27.2.5 Endocrine Function

The endocrine system is particularly susceptible to the long-term effects of cancer therapy. In a survey of the patients attending one late-effects clinic, 41% of patients had an endocrinopathy directly attributable to their disease or treatment [6]. This is likely to be an underestimate as it does not take into account the risk of growth hormone (GH) deficiency, which is now recognized to have important implications in adult life. Within the same group, a further 14% were reported to have problems related to fertility [6]. The endocrine system is particularly affected by radiotherapy, which impacts upon the normal function of the hypothalamic–pituitary axis, the thyroid, and the gonads. Chemotherapy can have a significant effect upon gonadal function, affecting steroid hormone secretion and reproductive potential.

27.2.6 Pituitary Function

Hypopituitarism, deficiency of one or more anterior pituitary hormones [growth hormone (GH), follicle-stimulating hormone (FSH), luteinizing hormone (LH), adrenocorticotrophic hormone (ACTH), and thyroid-stimulating hormone (TSH)], may be present at the diagnosis of cancer as a result of pathology in the sellar or suprasellar region that destroys normal pituitary tissue or disrupts the pituitary stalk, or may be a result of the treatments used, either surgery or irradiation. Deficiencies of the posterior pituitary hormones, antidiuretic hormone, and oxytocin, may occur in the presence of large suprasellar lesions such as a craniopharyngioma or germinoma, but are rarely caused by irradiation.

Patients at risk of radiation-induced hypopituitarism may have been treated for an intracranial tumor, malignancy of the nasopharynx, acute lymphoblastic leukemia (ALL) or with prepared for blood or marrow transplantation [75]. Pituitary dysfunction may develop several years after treatment and can be progressive; GH secretion is the most vulnerable to irradiation, followed by the gonadotropins, ACTH, and finally TSH [76, 77]. The risk of hypopituitarism increases with time from radiation and as the radiation dose increases [78]. Patients treated for ALL, the most common childhood malignancy, have been found to have abnormalities of GH secretion up to 25 years after they received prophylactic cranial irradiation at doses of 18 to 24 Gy [79]. Patients exposed to higher doses, such as those used to treat nasopharyngeal tumors or malignant brain tumors, are at greater risk; 50% will have abnormal GH secretion within 5 years of treatment and many will go on to develop other abnormalities of anterior pituitary function [77].

The majority of patients diagnosed with malignant disease between the ages of 15 and 30 years will have completed growth and development. However, GH is now known to play an important role throughout the adult lifespan, but particularly up to the age of 25 years. Studies have shown that GH-deficient adults complain of fatigue, have abnormal body composition (fat mass is increased and lean mass decreased), are osteopenic [80], and exhibit an adverse cardiovascular risk profile, which may contribute to the twofold increased cardiovascular mortality [81] observed in patients with hypopituitarism. GH replacement therapy, administered to adults as a single nightly injection, improves quality of life, increases lean mass, decreases fat mass, increases bone mineral density, and improves the cardiovascular risk profile. Although the improvements in the cardiovascular risk profile would support an improvement in cardiovascular risk, it is not yet known whether GH replacement therapy reduces mortality in adults [82].

GH is important for skeletal health, particularly in the years immediately after achieving final height, when it is vital to optimize peak bone mass, which is achieved in the middle of the third decade. A recent study in adolescents treated for GH deficiency during childhood has shown that continuing GH replacement beyond achievement of final height doubles the rate of bone mass accrual [83]. Thus young adults that develop GH deficiency may not reach peak bone mass, which will increase their risk of osteoporosis in the future. In a patient cohort that may have been exposed to other agents that have a negative impact upon bone mass, such as high-dose glucocorticoids, it is important to ensure that peak bone mass is achieved in order to minimize the risk of fracture in later life.

27.2.7 Gonadal Function

The ovaries and testes are sensitive to the effects of chemotherapy and radiotherapy. The risk of premature ovarian failure increases as the age at treatment increases; treatment before the age of 13 years is not associated with an increased risk, but treatment between the ages of 13 and 19 years is associated with a twofold increase in the risk of developing premature ovarian failure [84, 85]. This risk increases further as the age at cancer diagnosis increases. The majority of adolescent women undergoing treatment with combination chemotherapy will retain ovarian function. However, women undergoing blood and marrow transplant are at particular risk for ovarian failure. Some series suggest that the frequency of ovarian failure in women pretreated with high-dose alkylating agents may be as high as 100% [86].

The ovaries are particularly sensitive to radiation. Abdominal irradiation for Hodgkin lymphoma or

Wilms' tumor is associated with a high risk of ovarian failure. TBI used in preparation for blood and marrow transplantation is associated with ovarian failure in 100% of women at the time of treatment, of whom a small number will experience subsequent recovery of function [75].

In the male there are two aspects of testicular function to consider in those undergoing treatment for malignant disease: the germinal epithelium responsible for production of spermatozoa under the control of FSH, and the Leydig cells responsible for testosterone production under the control of LH. Chemotherapy, particularly alkylating agents such as cyclophosphamide and procarbazine, can cause failure of the germinal epithelium, resulting in oligospermia or azoospermia. Although Leydig cell function may be impaired, with testosterone levels in the low–normal range associated with an elevated LH level, testosterone deficiency is rarely seen following chemotherapy. Radiation to the testes can cause germinal epithelium failure at doses as low as 2 Gy. Doses in excess of 20 Gy result in Leydig cell failure and testosterone deficiency [87]. Men undergoing treatment known to cause azoospermia should be counseled and offered sperm banking, for use later in life when considering fertility.

Estrogen deficiency in women causes menopausal symptoms and abnormalities of cholesterol, which may impact upon cardiovascular risk. There is also increased loss of bone mass, and in younger women peak bone mass may be affected, increasing the risk of osteoporotic fractures. Testosterone deficiency in men causes reduced libido, erectile dysfunction, reduction in muscle mass, increased bone loss, and lipid abnormalities. Replacement therapy should be undertaken to promote well-being and to protect against osteoporosis and the risk of fracture in later life. Men should receive testosterone replacement either as a monthly intramuscular injection, via the transdermal route using patches or gels, or via the buccal mucosa. Women should receive estrogen therapy, which can be given orally or via the transdermal route. Women who have an intact uterus should receive progesterone during the latter part of the month to promote a menstrual bleed, reducing the risk of endometrial hyperplasia and subsequent development of endometrial carcinoma. The optimal dose of estrogen replacement in young women is not known; the oral contraceptive may provide too much estrogen, while the traditional hormone replacement therapy used in menopausal women may not provide sufficient estrogen. Further work is required to clarify this.

27.2.8 Other Endocrinopathies

Radiation may affect the thyroid gland. Patients that received radiation to the neck or craniospinal irradiation are at risk of thyroid dysfunction. This may take the form of hypothyroidism, thyrotoxicosis, or thyroid nodules, which may be malignant. Patients at risk should have regular thyroid function tests performed and their thyroid should be examined by palpation on an annual basis. Endocrine dysfunction of the thyroid should be managed as for any patient with hypo- or hyperthyroidism. The presence of nodules should be treated seriously and referral for thyroidectomy made where appropriate [88].

The parathyroid glands may also be affected by irradiation. Retrospective studies suggest that patients who received neck irradiation may be at increased risk of hyperparathyroidism compared with the background population, which may develop up to 50 years after irradiation [89].

Increasing numbers of patients are surviving malignant disease in early adult life. Endocrine dysfunction is one of the most common long-term effects of cancer therapy, and in many cases the endocrinopathy evolves with time. Such patients should remain under long-term follow-up in a multidisciplinary service, which includes an endocrinologist with experience in the conditions that these patients are likely to face.

27.2.9 Genitourinary Function

27.2.9.1 Renal

Long-term renal damage in individuals treated for cancer is most often associated with drugs such as cisplatin or ifosfamide, and radiation therapy. Cisplatin can damage the glomerulus and distal renal tubules, potentially causing diminished glomerular filtration rate (GFR) and electrolyte wasting, most commonly involving magnesium, calcium, potassium, and sodium [90].

Ifosfamide damages the proximal renal tubule, potentially resulting in Fanconi's renal syndrome (hypokalemia, hypophosphatemia, glucosuria, proteinuria, renal tubular acidosis, and rickets) [91]. Individuals at particular risk include those who received treatment with more than one nephrotoxic agent and those with concomitant renal damage related to surgery or radiation. Although the GFR may improve over time, the electrolyte wasting associated with ifosfamide therapy and hypomagnesemia associated with cisplatin therapy appear to persist in some patients [92, 93]. Yearly surveillance should include monitoring of serum creatinine, blood urea nitrogen and serum chemistries, urinalysis, and measurement of blood pressure. Ongoing management includes electrolyte replacement, treatment of hypertension, and avoidance of further nephrotoxic agents. Patients with a history of nephrectomy should be counseled regarding the importance of protecting the remaining single kidney. These patients should be cautioned to avoid potentially nephrotoxic agents (e.g., ibuprofen, aminoglycosides), maintain normal weight, obtain early intervention for urinary tract infections, and consult with their healthcare provider prior to participating in contact sports.

27.2.9.2 Bladder

Cyclophosphamide and ifosfamide are both capable of inducing hemorrhagic cystitis as a result of accumulation of acrolein in the bladder [94]. Urgency, frequency, and dysuria are symptoms commonly associated with hemorrhagic cystitis, which can be a long-term complication of cancer therapy in some patients [95]. Radiation to the pelvis or bladder can result in fibrosis and scarring, with resultant decreased bladder capacity and predisposition to urinary tract infections [96]. Bladder cancer has developed in some patients who received bladder-toxic agents during treatment for cancer [94]. Yearly urinalysis should be done in these patients to evaluate for the presence of microscopic hematuria.

27.2.10 Gastrointestinal Function

Fibrosis and enteritis are the most common pathologic abnormalities of the gastrointestinal tract in long-term survivors of cancer. These can arise as late complications of radiation to any site from the esophagus to the rectum [97–102], and have been associated with adhesions or stricture formation, sometimes with obstruction, ulcers, fistulae, and chronic enterocolitis or incontinence. Their frequency depends on the radiation dosage delivered by external beam or by brachytherapy. The stomach and small intestine appear to be more radiation sensitive than the colon or rectum. Overall, the incidence of fibrosis after 40 to 50 Gy is 5% and as high as 36% after 60 Gy or more. Most complications of intestinal fibrosis arise within 5 years, but strictures have developed as late as 20 years after treatment [97, 100, 102, 103]. Once they occur, radiation-induced gastrointestinal strictures may be progressive or recurrent. The incidence of clinically significant problems is enhanced by radiomimetic chemotherapy [98] or abdominal surgery [98, 103]. Abdominal surgery even without radiation can result in late-onset obstruction [104, 105].

Chemotherapy even in the absence of radiation therapy may be a cause of chronic hepatopathy. In several early prospective studies of patients given methotrexate for ALL or psoriasis, the incidence of biopsy-proven hepatic fibrosis was as high as 80% after 3–5 years of low-dose daily oral methotrexate [106, 107]. With intermediate doses of intravenous methotrexate, the incidence of fibrosis has been below 5% [108]. In general, and apparently in contrast to what occurs after radiation therapy, methotrexate-related hepatic fibrosis stabilizes or resolves after discontinuation of the drug. Radiation-induced or chemotherapy-related (in conservative or myeloablative doses) veno-occlusive disease, often fatal but sometimes transient, has been reported in a few cases [109].

Viral hepatitis, most often related to transfusion of blood products prior to 1992, is another cause of chronic liver disease in long-term survivors [110–112]. In one retrospective series of 658 cancer survivors who had been treated before routine screening of blood products, 117 (17.8%) were seropositive for hepatitis C [111]; 35% of these also were positive for hepatitis B with or without delta virus. Eighty percent of the seropositive patients had been transfused, so that in 20% other risk factors appeared to have been responsible. In one series of 10-year survivors of bone marrow transplantation for hematologic malignancy, hepatitis

C was the major risk factor for late development of cirrhosis: of 16 patients with cirrhosis, 15 had disease attributable to hepatitis C [113]. Hepatitis B has largely been eliminated in populations treated after 1972 [114].

The true incidence of hepatic pathology is undoubtedly higher than current numbers suggest because the presence of cirrhosis is seldom reflected by abnormal liver function tests or hepatomegaly, because hypertransaminasemia may be asymptomatic, and because liver biopsy procedures or liver scans are not routinely recommended after therapy. Thus, it is difficult to suggest foolproof guidelines for long-term follow-up. Patients at risk for gastrointestinal complications should be monitored by history or physical examination for hepatomegaly, icterus, and malabsorption. Especially for those patients with acute hepatotoxicity during therapy and for patients treated with hepatectomy, methotrexate, or hepatic radiation, the potential consequences of excessive alcohol and other high-risk behaviors should be emphasized. In such patients, we consider a posttreatment baseline screen including transaminase and bilirubin levels to be cost effective. Prothrombin time and serum albumin for evaluation of liver synthetic function may be indicated. If persistent, abnormalities should be evaluated further in collaboration with a gastroenterologist. The Center for Disease Control recommendations for hepatitis C screening include patients transfused or transplanted before 1992, even when transaminases are normal [115]. Hepatitis A and B testing should be considered in unimmunized patients with abnormal liver function tests.

Newer approaches to the treatment of gastrointestinal malignancy, including both administration of radiolabeled monoclonal antibodies for the therapy of hepatomas and intrahepatic arterial chemotherapy, have not yet been examined with respect to possible delayed effects.

27.2.11 Musculoskeletal and Related Tissues

Functional and cosmetic disabilities involving bone, teeth, muscle, and other soft tissues are common and are reported in up to one-third of survivors of various cancers affecting adolescents and young adults, notably solid tumors. Most clinically significant problems involve avascular necrosis (AVN), and osteoporosis (bone density ≥2.5 SD below mean)/osteopenia (bone density 1–2.5 SD below mean). Probably because most patients have already achieved their maximum growth at the time of diagnosis, leg length discrepancy does not appear to be a significant problem in Ewing sarcoma, in which the entire bone may receive as much as 70 Gy [116].

Young adult cancer survivors may also have reduced bone density, as measured by dual energy x-ray absorptiometry (DEXA) scans [117–119]. Although several studies have demonstrated decreased bone density at diagnosis in patients with ALL [120], osteopenia and osteoporosis are well-recognized to progress following exposure to corticosteroids or radiation therapy in doses used in patients with soft-tissue sarcomas or Ewing sarcoma [116]. Osteopenia in ALL survivors, as documented by quantitative computed tomographic scans, has also been related to cranial irradiation [121]. Exposure to radiation at a dose less than 25 Gy may result in osteopenia significant enough to cause spontaneous fractures, but which may go undetected by plain radiographs. Antimetabolites have been linked to decreased bone density in a manner that appears to be dose dependent. Following methotrexate, this problem appears primarily during therapy and resolves once the drug has been discontinued [122]. Both genders are at risk for reduced bone mineral density. Caucasians may be at greater risk than blacks [119]. Contributing factors include treatment-related gonadal and growth hormone failure, hyperthyroidism, poor calcium intake, and increased body weight [123, 124]. Some data suggest that bone density may increase 1 year off treatment of ALL, but that the risk of fracture remains high, suggesting that changes in bone architecture not assessable by DEXA scans may be relevant [120].

Avascular necrosis similarly is a radiographic diagnosis, which may be asymptomatic until the involved bone is subject to fracture or infection. Although AVN usually develops during therapy, the latency period has been as long at 13 years after treatment. Major risk factors are radiation therapy and systemic corticosteroids. Clinically significant AVN presenting as pain is well described in Hodgkin lymphoma and non-Hodgkin lymphoma, and in patients with ALL in whom the overall incidence has been about 5%, but in a more significant percent of adolescents [125–127; cf. also Chapter 6]. Dexamethasone appears to have more bone toxicity than equivalent doses of prednisone, and increased cumulative exposure conveys increased risk [126]. In one retrospective review, almost 15% of adolescents treated with dexamethasone experienced symptomatic AVN [128]. AVN most commonly involves the femoral heads, where it may be accompanied by slipped capital femoral epiphysis, but it has been described in virtually all locations and commonly is multifocal.

Detection and diagnosis of musculoskeletal and connective tissue toxicities depend largely upon anticipating these issues in vulnerable hosts, of taking a careful history, and performing a thorough physical examination. The need for diagnostic radiographs and appropriate referral in the case of clinically apparent disease is obvious. The relative benefit of surveillance radiographs of bones encompassed by radiation ports, and of bone densitometry is less clear. However, because of progress with various interventions (including the use of calcium supplementation, calcitonin, bisphosphonates, and sex hormone replacement in postmenopausal patients), a baseline DEXA scan has been recommended when survivors reach 18 years of age, with repeat studies as clinically indicated.

27.3 Delivering Survivorship Care

Chapters 29 (Access to Care after Therapy) and 30 (Information and Resources for Young Adults and Adolescents with Cancer) provide appropriate healthcare for survivors of cancer who are transitioning from pediatric to adult healthcare. As described in these chapters, this topic is emerging as one of the major challenges in medicine. Young cancer survivors, an especially high-risk population currently exceeding 270,000 in the United States, seek and receive care from a wide variety of healthcare professionals, including oncologists, medical and pediatric specialists, surgeons, primary care physicians, gynecologists, nurses, psychologists, and social workers [129]. The challenge arises from the heterogeneity of

this patient population treated with numerous therapeutic modalities in an era of rapidly advancing understanding of late effects. The Institute of Medicine has recognized the need for a systematic plan for lifelong surveillance that incorporates risks based on therapeutic exposures, genetic predisposition, lifestyle behaviors, and comorbid health conditions [129]. As described by Oeffinger [130], several key components are required for optimal survivorship care. These include: (1) longitudinal care utilizing a comprehensive multidisciplinary team approach, (2) continuity, with a single healthcare provider coordinating needed services, and (3) an emphasis on the whole person, with sensitivity to the cancer experience and its impact on the entire family.

Providing comprehensive risk-based care that is readily accessible to survivors presents a significant challenge. Although the number of young cancer survivors is ever increasing, healthcare professionals outside academic centers are unlikely to see more than a handful of survivors in their practice, and unless those patients share a similar diagnosis and receive similar treatment, there will likely be little similarity in their required follow-up care. Academic settings may allow for the establishment of a specialized multidisciplinary follow-up team to care for large numbers of survivors; however, the paucity of such centers and their limited geographic access often make them an option only for survivors who live nearby or who can afford time and expenses in order to travel to a distant center. Therefore, finding ways to educate local healthcare providers regarding needed follow-up is a priority. Efforts focusing on educating survivors regarding the indicated follow-up may be efficacious, with survivors in turn providing the necessary link in order to direct healthcare providers to specialized information regarding appropriate long-term follow-up care.

Regardless of the setting for follow-up, the first step in any evaluation is to have at hand an outline of the patient's medical history and comprehensive treatment summary (Table 27.3). Following completion of therapy, the treatment record and possible long-term problems should be reviewed with the patient and family. Correspondence between the treating oncologist and subsequent caretakers should address these potential long-term issues.

27.4 Recommendations for Screening

The development of standardized guidelines to screen young cancer survivors for potential complications has also presented substantial challenges. In contrast to the considerable literature describing treatment-related sequelae in young cancer survivors, specific recommendations for monitoring have generally been lacking. The development of screening recommendations in this population has been especially difficult due to continuing changes in cancer therapy, long latency periods required to evaluate many late treatment-related effects, multiple factors known to influence cancer-related health risks, and the unknown effects of aging on potential treatment-related complications. However, despite these challenges, two sets of clinical follow-up guidelines designed to guide care for young cancer survivors have recently been published and are described below.

The COG recently released risk-based, exposure-related guidelines (Long-Term Follow-Up Guidelines for Survivors of Childhood, Adolescent, and Young Adult Cancers) [131] that were designed specifically to direct follow-up care for patients who were diagnosed and treated for pediatric malignancies. These guidelines represent a set of comprehensive screening recommendations that are clinically relevant and can be used to standardize and direct the follow-up care for this group of cancer survivors with specialized healthcare needs. Implementation of these guidelines is intended to provide ongoing monitoring that facilitates early identification of and intervention for treat-

Table 27.3 Elements of a comprehensive therapeutic summary. *GVHD* Graft-versus-host disease

Topic	Data elements
Demographics	Name Date of birth Sex Race/ethnicity Record number/patient identification number
Diagnosis	Date/age at diagnosis Treating physician/institution Sites involved, stage, laterality, diagnostic details Pertinent past medical history Hereditary/congenital history Family history Relapse(s) dates/age at relapse(s), site(s) (if applicable)

Treatment	Treatment dates (initiated/completed)
	Protocols used
	Chemotherapy agents received, including:
	    Route of administration
	    Age at treatment
	    Cumulative doses for alkylators, anthracyclines, bleomycin, cytarabine, and methotrexate
	    Bioimmunotherapy
	Radiation fields, doses, dose fractions
	Surgical history
	Transfusion history
	Stem cell transplant(s), including donor source, preparative regimen, GVHD prophylaxis/treatment

Complications/late effects	Significant therapy-related complications (e.g., tumor lysis, septic shock, typhlitis, acute GVHD) Significant complications following completion of therapy (e.g., acute life-threatening infection following splenectomy, cardiomyopathy, second malignancies)

ment-related complications in order to increase quality of life for these patients. Specially tailored patient education materials, known as "Health Links," accompany the guidelines, offering detailed information on guideline-specific topics in order to enhance health maintenance and promotion among this population of cancer survivors. The entire set of guidelines, with associated Health Links, can be downloaded from www.survivorshipguidelines.org.

The Scottish Intercollegiate Guidelines Network (SIGN) has also released an evidence-based guideline (Long-Term Follow-up of Survivors of Childhood Cancer: A National Clinical Guideline). The SIGN guideline is targeted to provide a framework for the follow-up of young people who have survived cancer and covers five key areas, including growth, puberty and fertility, cardiac function, thyroid function, and neurodevelopment and psychological health. At this time, the guideline does not address long-term follow-up of the renal, pulmonary, gastrointestinal, ocular, auditory, or musculoskeletal systems and does not provide guidance regarding surveillance for second malignancies. The guideline can be downloaded in its entirety from www.sign.ac.uk.

27.5 Cancer Survivorship – Future Research Opportunities

Because of its heterogeneity, the growing population of young cancer survivors provides remarkable opportunities for research relating to the etiopathogenesis of cancer and early detection and prevention of adverse outcomes. Therapeutic exposures occurring at known time points, with close follow-up after the exposure, enables researchers to study testable hypotheses and to determine the effects of host and therapy-related factors in the development of adverse outcomes ranging from carcinogenesis and organ dysfunction to psychosocial consequences. Opportunities also exist to explore gene–environment interactions that may modify individual responses to treatment, as well as the susceptibility to develop adverse outcomes, thus providing insights into the identification of high-risk populations.

Notwithstanding the unique opportunities, several challenges exist to the conduct of survivorship research.

Cancer survivorship research is an evolving issue. With more than 20% of young cancer patients in need of better treatment options, new agents and combinations of agents are being developed [132]. Targeted therapies such as imatinab mesylate and other growth-factor inhibitors will probably contribute to increased survivorship. Evaluation of their late effects will need to keep in step with their increased usage. Recent refinements in radiation therapies such as conformal irradiation, and popularization of surgical techniques such as laparoscopy have been intended to minimize late effects. Evidence-based medicine will need to determine whether they will live up to this expectation. Advances in supportive care, including transfusions and hematopoietic growth factors, also require ongoing surveillance for identification of late effects. Furthermore, the influence of genetic profiles on susceptibility to late effects, as well as their interaction with lifestyle exposures such as tobacco, alcohol, and diet, is of growing interest, and has not been fully explored. However, the multifactorial etiology of the adverse effects, coupled with the heterogeneous nature of the patient population, necessitates large sample sizes within the context of well-characterized cohorts with complete long-term follow-up, and this remains the biggest challenge in conducting sound survivorship research.

In 1996, the National Cancer Institute established the Office of Cancer Survivorship (http://survivorship.cancer.gov), which promotes research into the effects of cancer and its treatment. To investigate adverse health outcomes among survivors, large-scale epidemiological investigations are required, particularly because of the complex and multifactorial etiology and rarity of many adverse outcomes. Two large ongoing cohort studies are addressing a wide spectrum of adverse health outcomes that may be increased following cancer and its treatment in the young. The CCSS was established in 1994 and comprised 25 clinical centers in the United States and Canada. Eligible cancer patients were aged under 21 years at diagnosis between 1 January 1970 and 31 December 1986 and survived at least 5 years [133]. Ultimately 20,276 survivors were accrued and baseline questionnaires have been completed by 69% of survivors (for further information visitwww.cancer.umn.edu/ccss and www.cancer.umn.

edu/ltfu). In 1998, the population-based British Childhood Cancer Survivor Study (BCCSS) was established [134]. Using the National Registry of Childhood Tumors, 18,123 individuals diagnosed with cancer before the age of 15 years between 1940 and 1991 and who survived at least 5 years were identified as eligible. The overall cohort will be used to study long-term survival and causes of late deaths and the incidence and etiology of second primary cancers. A postal questionnaire has been sent via primary care physicians to 14,550 survivors aged 16 years or older. Thus far, 10,205 questionnaires (70%) have been returned completed. For further information visit www.bccss.bham.ac.uk. Both of these research initiatives provide examples of the practicality and usefulness of large-scale follow-up of survivors employing minimally intrusive methodologies using mostly postal questionnaire and telephone contact. The considerable uncertainties relating to the long-term health of survivors of cancer diagnosed in adolescence and young adulthood provide a strong justification for comparable surveillance. It is important to distinguish between follow-up motivated by research and follow-up to address clinical need. Ideally, clinical follow-up should either provide demonstrable (evidence-based) benefit to the survivor, or be part of a clinical research investigation with clear and achievable objectives aimed at extending the evidence base. In relation to survivors of cancer in adolescence and young adulthood, the evidence base is currently very limited; nevertheless, it is important that guidelines for standardized clinical follow-up be used and regularly updated as the evidence base grows.

References

1. Reis LAG, Eisner MP, Kosary CL, et al (2001) SEER Cancer Statistics Review, 1973–1998. National Cancer Institute, Bethesda, MD
2. Office for National Statistics (2003) Cancer Statistics – Registrations: Registrations of cancer diagnosed in 2000, England. HMSO, London
3. Gatta G, Capocaccia R, De Angelis R, et al (2003) Cancer survival in European adolescents and young adults. Eur J Cancer 39:2600–2610
4. Garre ML, Gandus S, Cesana B, et al (1994) Health status of long-term survivors after cancer in childhood. Results of a uniinstitutional study in Italy. Am J Pediatr Hematol Oncol 16:143–152
5. Oeffinger KC, Eshelman DA, Tomlinson GE, et al (2000) Grading of late effects in young adult survivors of childhood cancer followed in an ambulatory adult setting. Cancer 88:1687–1695
6. Stevens MC, Mahler H, Parkes S (1998) The health status of adult survivors of cancer in childhood. Eur J Cancer 34:694–698
7. Vonderweid N, Beck D, Caflisch U, et al (1996) Standardized assessment of late effects in long-term survivors of childhood cancer in Switzerland: results of a Swiss Pediatric Oncology Group (SPOG) pilot study. Int J Pediatr Hematol Oncol 3:483–490
8. Robison LL, Mertens AC, Boice JD Jr, et al (2002) Study design and cohort characteristics of the Childhood Cancer Survivor Study: a multi-institutional collaborative project. Med Pediatr Oncol 38:229–239
9. Mertens AC, Yasui Y, Neglia JP, et al (2001) Late mortality experience in five-year survivors of childhood and adolescent cancer: the Childhood Cancer Survivor Study. J Clin Oncol 19:3163–3172
10. Moller TR, Garwicz S, Barlow L, et al (2001) Decreasing late mortality among five-year survivors of cancer in childhood and adolescence: a population-based study in the Nordic countries. J Clin Oncol 19:3173–3181
11. Boffetta P, et al (1999) Lymphomas. In: Neugut AI, Meadows AT, Robinson E (eds) Multiple Primary Cancers. Lippincott Williams and Wilkins, Philadelphia, pp 277–301
12. Inskip PD (1999) Second cancers following radiotherapy. In: Neugut AI, Meadows AT, Robinson E (eds) Multiple Primary Cancers. Lippincott Williams and Wilkins, Philadelphia, pp 91–135
13. Horwich A, Swerdlow AJ (2004) Second primary breast cancer after Hodgkin disease. Br J Cancer 90:294–298
14. Sankila R, Garwicz S, Olsen IH, et al (1996) Risk of subsequent malignant neoplasms among 1641 Hodgkin disease patients diagnosed in childhood and adolescence: a population-based cohort study in the five Nordic Countries. J Clin Oncol 14:1442–1446
15. Bhatia S, Yasui Y, Robison LL, et al (2003) High risk of subsequent neoplasms continues with extended follow-up of childhood Hodgkin disease: report from the Late Effects Study Group. J Clin Oncol 21:4386–4394
16. Travis LB, Nill DA, Dores GM, et al (2003) Breast cancer following radiotherapy and chemotherapy among young women with Hodgkin disease. JAMA 290:465–475
17. Van Leeuwen FE, Klokman WJ, Srovall M, et al (2003) Roles of radiation dose, chemotherapy and hormonal factors in breast cancer following Hodgkin disease. J Natl Cancer Inst 95:971–980
18. Ralleigh G, Given-Wilson R (2004) Breast cancer risk and possible screening strategies for young women following supradiaphragmatic irradiation for Hodgkin disease. Clin Radiol 59:647–650
19. Travis LB, Gospodarowicz M, Curtis RE, et al (2002) Lung cancer following chemotherapy and radiotherapy for Hodgkin disease. J Natl Cancer Inst 94:182–192

20. Gilbert ES, et al (2003) Lung cancer after treatment for Hodgkin disease: focus on radiation effects. Radiat Res 159:161–173

21. Sharir S, Jewett MAS (1999) Genitourinary Cancers In: Neugut AI, Meadows AT, Robinson E (eds) Multiple Primary Cancers. Lippincott Williams and Wilkins, Philadelphia, pp 365–396

22. Boice JD, Harvey EB, Blettner M, et al (1992) Cancer in the contralateral breast after radiotherapy for breast cancer. N Engl J Med 326:781–785

23. Curtis RE, Boile ID, Srovall M, et al (1992) Risk of leukaemia after chemotherapy and radiation treatment for breast cancer. N Engl J Med 326:1745–1751

24. Neugut AI, Robinson E, Lee WC, et al (1993) Lung cancer after radiation therapy for breast cancer. Cancer 71:3054–3057

25. Inskip PD Srovall M, Flannery JT (1994) Lung cancer and radiation dose among women treated for breast cancer. J Natl Cancer Inst 86:983–988

26. Harvey EB, Brinton LA (1985) Second cancer following cancer of the breast in Connecticut, 1935–82. Natl Cancer Inst Monogr 68:99–112

27. Daly MB, Costalas J (!999) Breast Cancer. In: Neugut AI, Meadows AT, Robinson E (eds) Multiple Primary Cancers. Lippincott Williams and Wilkins, Philadelphia, pp 303–317

28. Travis LB, Curtis RE, Inskip PD, Hankey BF (1995) Lung cancer risk and radiation dose among women treated for breast cancer (Letter). J Natl Cancer Inst 87:60–61

29. Ford MB, Sigurdson AJ, Petrulis ES, et al (2003) Effects of smoking and radiotherapy on lung carcinoma in breast carcinoma survivors. Cancer 98:1457–1464

30. Deutsch M, Land SR, Bègovic M, et al (2003) The incidence of lung carcinoma after surgery for breast carcinoma with and without postoperative radiotherapy. Cancer 98:1362–1368

31. Shan K, Lincoff AM, Young JB (1996) Anthracycline induced cardiotoxicity. Ann Intern Med 125:47–58

32. Grenier MA, Lipshultz SE (1998) Epidemiology of anthracycline cardiotoxicity in children and adults. Semin Oncol 25:72–85

33. Bossi G, Lanzarini L, Laudisa ML, et al (2001) Echocardiographic evaluation of patients cured of childhood cancer: a single center study of 117 subjects who received anthracyclines. Med Pediatr Oncol 36:593–600

34. Kremer LCM, van Dalen EC, Offringa M, et al (2001) Anthracycline-induced clinical heart failure in a cohort of 607 children: long-term follow-up study. J Clin Oncol 19:191–196

35. Steinherz LJ, Steinherz PG, Tan CTC, et al (1991) Cardiac toxicity 4 to 20 years after completing anthracycline therapy. JAMA 266:1672–1677

36. Pan PH, Moore CH (2002) Doxorubicin-induced cardiomyopathy during pregnancy: three case reports of anesthetic management for cesarean and vaginal delivery in two kyphoscoliotic patients. Anesthesiology 97:513–515

37. Hinkle AS, Proukou CB, Deshpande SS, et al (2004) Cardiovascular complications: cardiotoxicity caused by chemotherapy. In: Wallace H, Green DM (eds) Late Effects of Childhood Cancer. Oxford University Press, New York, pp 85–100

38. Lipshultz SE, Lipshultz SR, Mone SM, et al (1995) Female sex and higher drug dose as risk factors for late cardiotoxic effects of doxorubicin therapy for childhood cancer. N Engl J Med 332:1738–1743

39. Adams MJ, Hardenbergh PH, Constine LS, et al (2003) Radiation-associated cardiovascular disease. Crit Rev Oncol Hematol 45:55–75

40. Mill WB, Baglan RJ, Kurichetz P, et al (1984) Symptomatic radiation induced pericarditis in Hodgkin disease. Int J Radiat Oncol Biol Phys 10:2061–2065

41. Perraut DJ, Levy M, Herman JD, et al (1985) Echocardiographic abnormalities following cardiac irradiation. J Clin Oncol 3:546–551

42. Scott DL, Thomas RD (1978) Late onset constrictive pericarditis after thoracic radiotherapy. Br Med J 1:341–342

43. Haas JM (1969) Symptomatic constrictive pericarditis developing 45 years after radiation therapy to the mediastinum: a review of radiation pericarditis. Am Heart J 77:89–95

44. Boivin JF, Hutchinson GB, Lubin JH, et al (1992) Coronary artery disease in patients treated for Hodgkin disease. 69:1241–1247

45. Reinders JG, Heijman BJ, Olofsen-van Acht MJ, et al (1999) Ischemic heart disease after mantle-field irradiation of Hodgkin disease in long-term follow-up. Radiother Oncol 51:35–42

46. Hull MC, Morris CG, Pepine CJ, et al (2003) Valvular dysfunction and carotid, subclavian, and coronary artery disease in survivors of Hodgkin lymphoma treated with radiation therapy. JAMA 290:2831–2837

47. Bu'Lock FA, Gabriel HM, Oakhill A, et al (1993) Cardioprotection by ICRF187 against high dose anthracycline toxicity in children with malignant disease. Br Heart J 70:185–188

48. Wexler L (1998) Ameliorating anthracycline cardiotoxicity in children with cancer: clinical trials with dexrazoxane. Semin Oncol 25:86–92

49. Lipshultz SE, Rifai N, Dalton VM, et al (2004) The effect of dexrazoxane on myocardial injury in doxorubicin-treated children with acute lymphoblastic leukemia. N Engl J Med 351:145–153

50. Lipshultz SE, Lipsitz SR, Sallan SE, et al (2002) Long-term enalapril therapy for left ventricular dysfunction in doxorubicin-treated survivors of childhood cancer. J Clin Oncol 20:4517–4522

51. Silber JH, Cnaan A, Clark BJ, et al (2001) Design and baseline characteristics for the ACE Inhibitor After

Anthracycline (AAA) study of cardiac dysfunction in long-term pediatric cancer survivors. Am Heart J 142:577–585

52. Horning SJ, Adhikari A, Rizk N (1994) Effect of treatment for Hodgkin disease on pulmonary function: results of a prospective study. J Clin Oncol 12:297–305

53. Mefferd JM, SS D, Link MP (1989) Hodgkin disease: pulmonary, cardiac, and thyroid function following combined modality therapy. Int J Radiat Oncol Biol Phys 16:679–685

54. Nysom K, Holm K, Hertz H, et al (1998) Risk factors for reduced pulmonary function after malignant lymphoma in childhood. Med Pediatr Oncol 30:240–248

55. Morgan GW, Freeman AP, McLean RG, et al (1985) Late cardiac, thyroid, and pulmonary sequelae of mantle radiotherapy for Hodgkin disease. Int J Radiat Oncol Biol Phys 11:1925–1931

56. Wara WM, Phillips TL, Margolis LW, et al (1973) Radiation pneumonitis: a new approach to the derivation of time–dose factors. Cancer 32:547–552

57. Jakacki RI, Schramm CM, Bernadine R, et al (1995) Restrictive lung disease following treatment for malignant brain tumors: a potential late effect of craniospinal irradiation. J Clin Oncol 13:1478–1485

58. Springmeyer SC, Flournay N, Sullivan KM, et al (1983) Pulmonary function changes in long-term survivors of allogeneic marrow transplantation. In: Gale RP (ed) Recent Advances in Bone Marrow Transplantation. Alan R. Liss, New York, pp 343–353

59. Griese M, Rampf U, Hofmann D, et al (2000) Pulmonary complications after bone marrow transplantation in children: twenty-four years of experience in a single pediatric center. Pediatr Pulmonol 30:393–401

60. Kikkawa Y, Smith F (1993) Cellular and biochemical aspects of pulmonary surfactant in health and disease. Lab Invest 49:122–139

61. Rubin P, Finkelstein J, Shapiro D (1992) Molecular biology mechanisms in the radiation induction of pulmonary injury syndromes: interrelationship between the alveolar macrophages and septal fibroblast. Int J Radiat Oncol Biol Phys 24:93–101

62. Wohl ME, Griscom NT, Traggis DG, et al (1975) Effects of therapeutic irradiation delivered in early childhood upon subsequent lung function. Pediatrics 55:507–516

63. Hassink EAM, Souren TS, Boersma LJ, et al (1993) Pulmonary morbidity 10–18 years after irradiation for Hodgkin disease. Eur J Cancer 29A:343–347

64. Villani F, Viviani S, Bonfante V, et al (2000) Late pulmonary effects in favorable stage I and IIA Hodgkin Disease treated with radiotherapy alone. Am J Clin Oncol 23:18–21

65. Salloum E, Tanoue LT, Wackers FJ, et al (1999) Assessment of cardiac and pulmonary function in adult patients with Hodgkin disease treated with ABVD or MOPP/ABVD plus adjuvant low-dose mediastinal irradiation. Cancer Invest 17:171–180

66. Eigen H, Wyszomierski D (1985) Bleomycin lung injury in children: pathophysiology and guidelines for management. Am J Pediatr Hematol Oncol 7:71–78

67. Comis RL (1978) Bleomycin pulmonary toxicity. In: Carter SK, Crooke ST, Umezawa H (ed) Bleomycin: Current Status and New Developments. Academic Press, New York, p 279

68. Samuels ML, Johnson DE, Holoye PY, et al (1976) Large-dose bleomycin therapy and pulmonary toxicity: a possible role of prior radiotherapy. JAMA 235:1117–1120

69. Aronin PA, Mahaley MSJ, Rudnick SA, et al (1980) Prediction of BCNU pulmonary toxicity in patients with malignant gliomas: an assessment of risk factors. N Engl J Med 303:183–188

70. Wheeler C, Antin JH, Churchill WH, et al (1990) Cyclophosphamide, carmustine, and etoposide with autologous bone marrow transplantation in refractory Hodgkin disease and non-Hodgkin lymphoma: a dose-finding study. J Clin Oncol 8:648–566

71. Rubio C, Hill ME, Milan S, et al (1997) Idiopathic pneumonia syndrome after high-dose chemotherapy for relapsed Hodgkin disease. Br J Cancer 75:1044–1048

72. Bauer KA, Skarin AT, Balikian JP, et al (1983) Pulmonary complications associated with combination chemotherapy programs containing bleomycin. Am J Med 74:557–563

73. Goldiner PL, Schweizer O (1979) The hazards of anaesthesia and surgery in bleomycin-treated patients. Semin Oncol 6:121–124

74. Schwerzmann M, Seiler C (2001) Recreational scuba diving, patent foramen ovale and their associated risks. Swiss Med Wkly 131:365–374

75. Gleeson HK, Darzy K, Shalet SM (2002) Late endocrine, metabolic and skeletal sequelae following treatment of childhood cancer. Best Pract Res Clin Endocrinol Metab 16:335–348

76. Littley MD, Shalet SM, Beardwell CG, et al (1989) Hypopituitarism following external radiotherapy for pituitary tumours in adults. Q J Med 70:145–160

77. Lam KSL, Tse VKC, Wang C, et al (1991) Effects of cranial irradiation on hypothalamic–pituitary function – a 5-year longitudinal study in patients with nasopharyngeal carcinoma. Q J Med 78:165–176

78. Toogood AA (2004) Endocrine consequences of brain irradiation. Growth Horm IGF Res 14:S118–124

79. Brennan BM, Rahim A, Mackie EM, et al (1998) Growth hormone status in adults treated for acute lymphoblastic leukaemia in childhood. Clin Endocrinol 48:777–783

80. Cuneo RC, Salomon F, McGauley GA, et al (1992) The growth hormone deficiency syndrome in adults. Clin Endocrinol 37:387–397

81. Tomlinson JW, Holden N, Hills RK, et al (2001) Association between premature mortality and hypopituitarism. West Midlands Prospective Hypopituitary Study Group. Lancet 357:425–431

82. Toogood AA (2004) Cardiovascular risk and mortality in patients with growth hormone deficiency. In: Abs R,

Feldt-Rasmussen U (eds) Growth Hormone Deficiency in Adults: 10 years of KIMS, 1st edn. Oxford Pharmagenesis, Oxford, pp 63–74

83. Shalet SM, Shavrikova E, Cromer M, et al (2003) Effect of growth hormone (GH) treatment on bone in postpubertal GH-deficient patients: a 2-year randomized, controlled, dose-ranging study. J Clin Endocrinol Metab 88:4124–4129

84. Byrne J (1999) Infertility and premature menopause in childhood cancer survivors. Med Pediatr Oncol 33:24–28

85. Byrne J, Fears TR, Gail MH, et al (1992) Early menopause in long-term survivors of cancer during adolescence. Am J Obstet Gynecol 166:788–793

86. Sanders JE, Buckner CD, Amos D, et al (1988) Ovarian function following marrow transplantation for aplastic anemia or leukemia. J Clin Oncol 6:813–818

87. Howell SJ, Shalet SM (2002) Effect of cancer therapy on pituitary–testicular axis. Int J Androl 25:269–276

88. Jereczek-Fossa BA, Alterio D, Jassem J, et al (2004) Radiotherapy-induced thyroid disorders. Cancer Treat Rev 30:369–384

89. Rao SD, Frame B, Miller MJ, et al (1980) Hyperparathyroidism following head and neck irradiation. Arch Intern Med 140:205–207

90. Raney B HR, Cassady R, et al (1994) Late effects of cancer therapy on the genitourinary tract in children. In: Schwartz CL, Hobbie WL, Constine LS, Ruccione KS (eds) Survivors of Childhood Cancer: Assessment and Management. Mosby, St. Louis, pp 245–262

91. Pratt CB, Meyer WH, Jenkins JJ, et al (1991) Ifosfamide, Fanconi's syndrome and rickets. J Clin Oncol 9:1495–1499

92. Neglia JP, Nesbit ME (1993) Care and treatment of long-term survivors of childhood cancer. Cancer 71:3386–3391

93. Grossi M (1998) Management of long-term complications of pediatric cancer. Pediatr Clin North Am 45:1637–1658

94. Raney B, Heyn R, Cassady R, et al (1994) Late effects of cancer therapy on the genitourinary tract in children. In: Schwartz CL, Hobbie WL, Constine LS, Ruccione KS (eds) Survivors of Childhood Cancer: Assessment and Management. Mosby, St. Louis, pp 245–262

95. Green DM (1993) Effects of treatment for childhood cancer on vital organ systems. Cancer 71:3299–3305

96. Marina N (1997) Long-term survivors of childhood cancer: the medical consequences of cure. Pediatr Clin North Am 44:1021–1042

97. Mahboubi S, Silber RJ (1997) Radiation-induced esophageal strictures in children with cancer. Eur Radiol 7:119–122

98. Donaldson SS, Jundi S, Ricour C, et al (1975) Radiation enteritis in children: a retrospective review, clincopathologic correlation, and dietary management. Cancer 35:1167

99. Ettinger DS, Slavin RE (1977) Chronic radiation enteritis complicating non-Hodgkin lymphoma. South Med J 70:637–639

100. Localio SA, Stone A, Friedman M (1969) Surgical aspects of radiation enteritis. Surg Gynecol Obstet 129:1163–1172

101. Heyn R, Raney RB, Hayes DM, et al (1992) Late effects of therapy in patients with paratesticular rhabdomyosarcoma. J Clin Oncol 10:614–623

102. Paulino A, Wen BC, Brown CK, et al (2000) Late effects in children treated with radiation therapy for Wilms tumor. Int J Radiat Oncol Biol Phys 46:1239–1246

103. Roswit B (1974) Complications of radiation therapy: the alimentary tract. Semin Roentgenol 9:51–63

104. Olver IN, Pearl P, Wiernik PH, et al (1990) Small bowel obstruction as a late complication of the treatment of Hodgkin disease. Aust N Z J Surg 60:58558–8

105. Ritchey ML, Kelalis P, Breslow N, et al (1993) Small bowel obstruction following nephrectomy for Wilms' tumor. Ann Surg 218:654–659

106. Sharp H, Nesbit M, White J, et al (1969) Methotrexate liver toxicity. J Pediatr 74:818–819

107. Dahl MGC, Gregory MM, Schever PJ (1971) Liver damage due to methotrexate in patients with psoriasis. Br Med J 1:625–630

108. McIntosh S, Davidson DL, O'Brien RT, et al (1977) Methotrexate hepatotoxicity in children with leukemia. J Pediatr 90:1019–1021

109. Johnson FL, Balis FM (1983) Hepatopathy following radiation and chemotherapy for Wilms' tumor. Am J Pediatr Hematol Oncol 4:217

110. Strickland DK RC, Patrick CC et al (2000) Hepatitis C infection among survivors of childhood cancer. Blood 95:3065–3070

111. Locasciulli A, Testa M, Pontisso P, et al (1997) Prevalence and natural history of hepatitis C infection in patients cured of childhood leukemia. Blood 90:4628–4633

112. Cesaro S, Petris MG, Rosetti R, et al (1997) Chronic hepatitis C virus infection after treatment for pediatric malignancy. Blood 90:1315–1320

113. Strasser SI, Sullivan KM, Myerson D, et al (1999) Cirrhosis of the liver in long-term marrow transplant survivors. Blood 93:3259–3266

114. Dodd RY (1992) The risk of transfusion-transmitted infection. N Engl J Med 327:419–421

115. Rose VL (1999) CDC issues new recommendations for the prevention and control of hepatitis C virus infection. Am Family Phys 59:1321–1323

116. Tefft M, Lattin PB, Jereb B, et al (1976) Acute and late effects on normal tissue following combined chemo- and radiotherapy for childhood rhabdomyosarcoma and Ewing's sarcoma. Cancer 37:1201–1217

117. Aisenberg J, Hsieh K, Kalaitzoglou G, et al (1998) Bone mineral density in young adult survivors of childhood cancer. J Pediatr Hematol Oncol 20:241–245

118. Arikoski P, Voutilainen R, Kroger H (2003) Bone mineral density in long-term survivors of childhood cancer. J Pediatr Endocrinol Metab 16:343–353

119. Kaste SC, Jones-Wallace D, Rose SR, et al (2001) Bone mineral decrements in survivors of childhood acute lymphoblastic leukemia: frequency of occurrence and risk factors for their development. Leukemia 15:728–734

120. van der Suis IM, Keizer-Schrama S, van den Heuvel-Eibrink MM (2004) Bone mineral density in childhood acute lymphoblastic leukemia during and after treatment. Pediatr Blood Cancer 43:182–183

121. Gilsanz V, Carlson ME, Roe TF, et al (1990) Osteoporosis after cranial irradiation for acute lymphoblastic leukemia. J Pediatr 117:238–244

122. Nesbit M, Krivit W, Heyn R, et al (1976) Acute and chronic effects of methotrexate on hepatic, biliary, and skeletal systems. Cancer 37:1048–1057

123. Aisenberg J, Hsieh K, Kalaitzoglou G, et al (1998) Bone mineral density in young adult survivors of childhood cancer. J Pediatr Hematol Oncol 20:241–245

124. Henderson RC, Madsen CD, Davis C, et al (1996) Bone density in survivors of childhood malignancies. J Pediatr Hematol Oncol 18:367–371

125. Felix C, Blatt J, Goodman MA, et al (1985) Avascular necrosis of bone following combination chemotherapy for acute lymphocytic leukemia. Med Pediatr Oncol 13:269–272

126. Halton JM, Wu B, Atkinson SA, et al (2000) Comparative skeletal toxicity of dexamethasone and prednisone in childhood acute lymphoblastic leukemia. J Pediatr Hematol Oncol 22:369

127. Mattano LA, Sather HN, Trigg ME, et al (2000) Osteonecrosis as a complication of treating acute lymphoblastic leukemia in children: a report from the Children's Cancer Group. J Clin Oncol 18:3262–3272

128. Hewitt M WS, Simone JV (eds) (2003) Childhood Cancer Survivorship: Improving Care and Quality of Life. National Academies Press, Washington, DC

129. Oeffinger KC (2003) Longitudinal risk-based health care for adult survivors of childhood cancer. Curr Probl Cancer 27:143–167

130. Landier W, Bhatia S, Eshelman DA, et al (2004) Development of risk-based guidelines for pediatric cancer survivors: the Children's Oncology Group Long-term Follow-Up Guidelines from the Children's Oncology Group Late Effects Committee and Nursing Discipline. J Clin Oncol 22:4979–4990

131. Albritton K, Bleyer WA (2003) The management of cancer in the older adolescent. Eur J Cancer 39:2584–2599

132. Robison LL, Mertens AC, Boice JD, et al (2002) Study design and cohort characteristics of the Childhood Cancer Survivor Study: a multi-institutional collaborative project. Med Pediatr Oncol 38:229–239

133. Taylor A, Hawkins M, Griffins A, et al (2004) Long-term follow-up of survivors of childhood cancer in the UK. Pediatr Blood Cancer 42:161–168

Ethical Issues for the Adolescent and Young Adult Cancer Patient: Assent and End-of-Life Care

Susan Shurin • Eric Kodish

Contents

28.1 Introduction

The issues surrounding clinical decision-making facing families with adolescents and those facing young adults differ from those facing families with younger children and older adults. The nature of the involvement of adolescents and young adults in decision-making around his or her own life are summarized in Table 28.1

The extent to which an adolescent is informed, and therefore able to really participate in and consent to therapeutic decisions and interventions, changes radically as the family and the youngster become more educated and sophisticated in the course of their dealings with the healthcare system. In this chapter, we would like to use a case approach to explore some of the issues facing the patient, the family, and the medical caregivers [1–3]. "The case itself and the transcripts are fictitious, and not based on a single individual, but are rather an illustrative rendering based an our experience with similar patients."

The subject of this case study, Mark, was diagnosed with Ewing sarcoma when he was 14 years old. He was to begin his freshman year of high school, expecting to be the forward on his school's basketball team. His story is told below by his physician, his mother Sue, his father George, and by Mark himself.

Table 28.1 The nature of the involvement of adolescents and young adults in decision-making around his or her own life

Principal	Adolescent	Young adulthood
Autonomy (self determination)	Patient has only partial autonomy, shared with parents/guardians. Most adolescents in Western society do not have independent responsibilities, but others have some responsible for them	Patient has full autonomy, with right/ability to make independent decisions. Young adult may have newly assumed responsibilities
Consent	Legal requirement is for assent, with proxy consent given by parents/guardians	Legally able to consent without limitation
Avoidance of harm	Ability of patient to judge long-term, as opposed to short-term harm, may not be fully developed	Patient has more mature capacity to see complexities and long-term implications of decisions
Paternalism	Paternalism may be appropriate, limiting the patient's liberty to promote well-being	Paternalism – limiting liberty to prevent self-harm – is generally not deemed appropriate, and patients may make unwise decisions

28.2 Mark's Story at Diagnosis

28.2.1 July 20, 1998

28.2.1.1 Case Report Presented by the Attending Physician

Mark was referred for evaluation of pain in his left thigh of 6 months duration. My orthopedic colleague reviewed the films taken at the time of referral, and another set from 5 months ago, and found an expansile lytic lesion, which had increased in size between February and June. Biopsy showed Ewing sarcoma, and metastatic work-up, including bone marrow, was negative. In a 3-hour family meeting, which included our social worker and nurse practitioner, I explained the diagnosis, the prognosis, and my therapeutic recommendations to Mark and his parents.

Mark was impressively stoic. He allowed his parents to ask medical questions, but had few himself, mostly clarifying how his treatment would affect his school attendance and sports activities. His parents agreed readily to his enrollment on the Intergroup Ewing's Sarcoma Study (IESS). Mark said he wanted his parents to decide about his treatment, and was reluctant to sign the assent form presented, but did so when I

told him we could not begin until he signed the form. The discussion went well, and therapy will begin as soon as the central venous access device is in place.

28.2.1.2 Mark's Mother Sue's Diary Entry, July 20, 1998

This is the worst day of my life. We spent 3 hour with the doctor and nurse today – I thought it would never end! My beautiful baby has cancer. I cannot believe it – he has always been so healthy! He could die from this disease, he could die from this treatment, and he could lose his leg. His hair will fall out. There is no way he will be playing basketball this fall, and it is all he has ever wanted to do. If only I hadn't kept working when I was pregnant with him – I'll bet it is all the chemicals in the hair color I use every day at the shop. Or maybe it is from the pesticides George uses in his landscaping business. He has always made fun of the organic farmers – how I wish he had paid more attention and tried to do some of that! And the drugs they are planning to give him – speaking of poisons! One can make him sterile, one will damage his heart, one will ruin his kidneys, one has major allergic reactions, and they all make his hair fall out. And on top of that, they can give him leukemia! I am just so terrified, I can't even figure

ness in an adolescent directly affects far more than the patient. Respect for the dynamics of family systems, and of relationships between persons whose egos and identities are not easily separable is essential for the effective management of complex and ambiguous situations. While peer relationships are overwhelmingly important to adolescents, it is usually difficult for friends and classmates to either understand or adequately support a seriously ill teenager, especially if the illness interferes with the patient's ability to engage fully in common activities.

No individual can meet all the complex needs of any person with a chronic illness. The importance of a team approach is hard to overemphasize, as both professional roles and the personal characteristics of the professionals themselves are important to cover the many areas involved. Key roles can be filled by physicians, nurses, social workers, psychologists, spiritual caregivers, and family members and friends. The most important functions are ongoing throughout an illness, and reflect both changing circumstances (relapse, toxicities) and the developmental stages of individuals and families. Key functions include: Accurate diagnosis; identification of the patient's and family members' concerns and therapeutic options; communication of choices to patient and family; establishment of realistic goals; attention to management of symptoms; maintenance of hope; preparation for events, which respects the need to prepare for transitions, including the need to say goodbye.

28.5.2 Involvement of Adolescents in Decisions About Their Own Care

An ethical approach to involvement of adolescents in key decision-making regarding their care can be envisioned in the same context as involvement of human subjects in research. The principles of ethical practice outlined in the Belmont report [7] include respect for persons, beneficence, and justice. Respect for persons requires both recognition of individual autonomy, and protection of those with diminished autonomy. Application of these principles is particularly challenging to put into practice when dealing with adolescents, who have diminished, but not absent, autonomy. The stages of cognitive development are fluid throughout life, but

at no time changing more rapidly in ways which impact autonomy than in late adolescence. Ability to learn information, to comprehend the information learned, and to assess risks and benefits change dramatically during adolescence. Frontal lobe development continues well into adulthood, impacting skills in risk assessment and comprehension. All of these factors have substantial impact upon the ability of an adolescent to assess the complex issues facing any person with a potentially lethal disease. Emotional development is less linear than cognitive development. Once mastered, cognitive skills tend to be retained and dependably present, while skills for coping with overwhelming emotions usually come and go.

28.5.3 Impact of Symptom Control on Therapeutic Decisions

"Palliative care" addresses issues specifically related to morbidity, rather than mortality. Morbidity encompasses existential concerns (fear, anxiety, concerns about body image, sexual attractiveness, competence, depression, isolation, and abandonment), symptoms that are caused by the disease itself (pain, weight loss, dyspnea, gastrointestinal symptoms, lack of mobility), and therapy-related symptoms (hair loss, weight gain, nausea, vomiting, and mutilating surgical procedures, including amputation, evisceration, and venous access devices). Adequate attention to relief of symptoms can transform a devastating experience into one that is manageable, and which may even enhance personal growth and intimacy [8, 9].

28.5.4 Palliative Care Issues at Diagnosis

At the time of Mark's diagnosis, the key palliative issues concern control of disease- and therapy-related symptoms, which impact both quality of life and the ability or willingness of the adolescent to endure potentially life-saving therapy. Mark's expressed concerns reflect his level of maturity. He clearly comprehends that he has a serious and potentially fatal illness, but his focus is not on death. His major concerns deal with his ability to participate in sports, and the impact of his treatment on the issues of immediate importance in his life (school, friendships), and on his parents. Both he and his parents perceive the key decisions as ones in which their individual interests are totally aligned; this is a crucial point in his willingness to defer critical decisions to his parents. He is given full access to necessary information; he is able to focus on his adolescent concerns and allow his parents, particularly his father, to focus on the fully adult issues, and to endorse their decisions. Adequate attention to palliation is essential if he is to receive potentially curative therapy. While he may be submitting to rather than embracing toxic therapy, it cannot be administered if he refuses to accept it. Adequate palliation allows him not to focus on the toxicity of therapy or the possibility of a bad outcome [10].

Mark's situation is particularly fortunate: the family is intact; parents and teenager communicate well; there is no major conflict between Mark and his parents; Mark is realistic enough to be able to accept the toxicities of therapy in search of a longer-term good outcome. This is often not the case, and significant conflicts challenge the most skillful clinicians to persuade without coercion, to communicate information that a parent or patient may not be developmentally ready to process, and to resolve conflicts that have no satisfactory outcome.

For the physician, the primary challenges at diagnosis are communicating complex information and assisting the family and patient to achieve cognitive mastery and become her partners in achieving a common goal. Respect for autonomy can be demonstrated by providing information, teaching mastery skills, and attending to concerns that are common to most patients in this situation. Offering hope is largely a matter of focusing on the positive aspects of a reality, and minimizing the focus on the seeds of disaster. Most of the key issues are encompassed in good medical care, and can be addressed by expert nurses and physicians.

28.5.5 Palliative Care Issues at the End of Life

After several relapses, Mark no longer has a potentially curable illness. His impending death separates him from his parents [11, 12]. Optimal symptom control extends far beyond offering hope and conveying information. To adequately demonstrate respect for his autonomy, the physician must assist Mark and his parents as they struggle to communicate with each other. The poignancy of Mark's and his parents' individual narratives highlights the key challenges to such communication. Mark now has a very adult perspective on death [13]. He perceives his death not only as it ends his own life, but as it will devastate his parents [14]. Mark and both his parents are clinging emotionally to hope for a miracle, while recognizing cognitively that death is inevitable [15, 16]. All are very fearful that they may be failing each other by accepting the reality of a situation they cannot change.

Acknowledging autonomy requires that the physician in this tragic situation assist the members of the family to understand their own and each others expectations. She cannot honestly offer hope for cure. Their real fears of physical suffering, isolation, and abandonment must be addressed to provide adequate palliation in this situation [19, 20]. The frequency with which palliation of physical and existential symptoms is inadequately achieved testifies to the difficulty and complexity of managing these complex issues [19–22]. The physician's work in this situation involves far more than communicating information and ensuring mastery. Optimal palliative care to an adolescent at the end of life requires that the patient and key supportive family members and close friends establish common goals [23–25]. This is not always possible, even with the best medical, nursing, and psychological support [26, 27]. The challenge of facilitating this communication, without which it is not possible for Mark or his parents to make decisions that encompass their individual but intensely interlinked lives and psyches, is one of the greatest challenges to the ethical practice of medicine [10, 30, 31] While failure to succeed in this is common and inevitable, it is important for physicians to make a valiant effort to help families achieve the most elusive goal: peace with themselves and each other [33–35].

28.6 Biological Basis for Ongoing Development of Competence in Adolescents and Young Adults

A robust literature is emerging documenting the extent to which higher executive functions are highly relevant to the ability of older children and young adults to assume responsibility for decision-making in young adulthood [36, 37]. Two key functions that continue to mature throughout the third decade are executive functions and processing of emotions [38, 39]. Gray matter maturation flows posteriorly to anteriorly, in contrast to the pattern of other measures of brain development, with frontal lobe functions maturing last, showing the largest differences between teens and young adults [40]. The degree of myelination in the adult frontal cortex appears to relate to the maturation of cognitive processing and other executive functions. In contrast, parietal and temporal areas mediating language, spatial, and sensory functions are largely mature in the teen brain. The corpus callosum increases in size as long as measures of mentation continue to develop, usually into the early part of the fourth decade [41].

Functional magnetic resonance imaging of brain activity of normal volunteers who are imaged while they are identifying the emotions represented on pictures of faces demonstrates that young teens activate the amygdala, which mediates fear and other visceral reactions. With maturity, brain activity shifts to the frontal lobe, which is associated functionally with more reasoned perceptions and more mature performance on tests. On language skill tasks, activation shifts from the temporal lobe to the frontal lobe as teens mature, while functional changes parallel structural changes in temporal lobe white matter[42, 43].

The implications of these findings are that while adolescents may be cognitively capable of processing the information presented with any serious diagnosis, analyzing data, and remembering facts, their ability to organize and use such information is not fully developed, and the extent to which visceral responses may override rational analysis is even greater than it is in fully mature adults. Serious or life-threatening diagnoses are overwhelming to adults whose competence and right to make decisions about their own lives are not questioned. Over the course of the third decade of life, the ability to assume such responsibility continues to mature significantly in normal persons.

In the light of these developmental processes, consider how some of the key issues in decision-making and priorities might be impacted if Mark were a young adult, instead of an adolescent, at the time of his diagnosis.

28.6.1 An Alternate Scenario

Imagine that Mark were diagnosed at age 24 years, instead of 14 years. He is now 2 years out of college, having married his college sweetheart right after graduation. He and his wife bought a house just before their first child, now 1 year old, was born, and expect to have their second child in another year or so. He is a junior associate in a hedge fund firm. Now, he is diagnosed with Ewing sarcoma, with the same medical data outlined in the history provided.

Mark plays a central role in the economy of his household. As a husband and father, his presence and his income are essential for the security of his wife and child. While he may rely heavily upon his parents in facing this crisis, their role is consultative, and he is unlikely to expect them to make decisions for him. His wife is now his primary partner in making these decisions. The young couple has assumed the serious obligations of adulthood.

In the United States, a key issue that arises is that his access to healthcare is tied to his employment status, or that of his wife. If he does not have insurance, his family must deplete its resources to make him eligible for Medicaid programs. Either Mark or his wife must be employed with insurance for him to obtain the care that will enable him to have a chance of survival, supportive care, and control of symptoms. In a few short years, he has gone from having both responsible adults and social safety nets to buttress him, to making his own decisions and needing to obtain the resources needed to get care. Issues of the couple's reproductive future, his responsibility for his young family, and his work identity and career development are not hypothetical future questions, but pressing and immediate.

References

1. Goldman A, Christie D (1993) Children with cancer talk about their own death with their families. Pediatr Hematol Oncol 10:223–231
2. Hilden JM, Watterson J, Chrastek J (2000) Tell the children. J Clin Oncol 18:3193–3195

3. Raimbault G (1981) Children talk about death. Acta Paediatr Scand 70:179–182

4. Kodish E (ed) (2005) Ethics and Research with Children: A Case-Based Approach. Oxford University Press, USA

5. Kon AA (2006) Assent in pediatric research. Pediatrics 117:1806–1810

6. Miller VA, Drotar D, Kodish E (2004) Children's competence for assent and consent: a review of empirical findings. Ethics Behav 14:255–295

7. National Commission for the Protection of Human Subjects of Biomedical and Behavioral Research (1979) The Belmont Report: Ethical Principles and Guidelines for the Protection of Human Subjects of Research. Department of Health, Education, and Welfare, Washington DC

8. Nitschke R, Meyer WH, Sexauer CL, et al (2000) Care of terminally ill children with cancer. Med Pediatr Oncol 34:268–270

9. Wolfe J, Klar N, Grier H, et al (2000) Understanding of prognosis among parents of children who died of cancer: impact on treatment goals and integration of palliative care. JAMA 284:2469–2475

10. Himelstein BP, Hilden JM, Boldt AM, Weissman D (2004) Pediatric palliative care. N Engl J Med 350:1752–1762

11. Wolfe J (2000) Suffering in children at the end of life: recognizing an ethical duty to palliate. J Clin Ethics 11:157–163

12. Wolfe J, Friebert S, Hilden J (2002) Caring for children with advanced cancer: integrating palliative care. Pediatr Clin North Am 49:1043–1062

13. Sourkes BM (1996) The broken heart: anticipatory grief in the child facing death. J Palliat Care 12:56–59

14. Christ GAM (1984) Therapeutic strategies at psychosocial crisis points in the treatment of childhood cancer. In: Flomenhaft KCA (ed) Childhood Cancer: Impact on the Family. Plenum Press, New York, NY, 109–128

15. Christ GH (2000) Impact of development on children's mourning. Cancer Pract 8:72–81

16. Christ GH, Siegel K, Christ AE (2002) Adolescent grief: "It never really hit me…..until it actually happened." JAMA 288:1269–1278

17. Blueblond-Langner M (1978) The Private Worlds of Dying Children. Princeton University Press, Princeton, NJ

18. Sourkes BM (1991) Truth to life: art therapy with pediatric oncology patients and their siblings. J Psychosoc Oncol 9:81

19. Adams-Greenly M (1986) Psychological staging of pediatric cancer patients and their families. Cancer 58:449–453

20. Adams-Greenly M (1991) Psychosocial assessment and intervention at initial diagnosis. Paediatrician 18:3–10

21. Back AL, Arnold RM, Quill TE (2003) Hope for the best, and prepare for the worst. Ann Intern Med 138:439–443

22. Nitschke R, Meyer WH, Huszti HC (2001) When the tumor is not the target, tell the children. J Clin Oncol 19:595–596

23. Wolfe J, Grier HE, Klar N, et al (2000) Symptoms and suffering at the end of life in children with cancer. N Engl J Med 342:326–333

24. Hinds PS, Oakes L, Furman W, et al (2001) End-of-life decision making by adolescents, parents, and healthcare providers in pediatric oncology: research to evidence-based practice guidelines. Cancer Nurs 24:122–134

25. Wanzer SH, Federman DD, Adelstein SJ, et al (1989) The physician's responsibility toward hopelessly ill patients: a second look. N Engl J Med 320:844–849

26. Kreicbergs U, Valdimarsdóttir U, Onelöv E, Henter J-I, Steineck G (2004) Talking about death with children who have severe malignant disease. N Engl J Med 351:1175–1186

27. Feudtner C, Christakis DA, Zimmerman FJ, Muldoon JH, Neff JM, Koepsell TD (2002) Characteristics of deaths occurring in children's hospitals: implications for supportive care services. Pediatrics 109:887–893

28. Contro N, Larson J, Scofield S, et al (2002) Family perspectives on the quality of pediatric palliative care. Arch Pediatr Adolesc Med 156:14–19

29. Field MJ, Behrman RE, eds (2003) When Children Die: Improving Palliative and End-of-Life Care for Children and Their Families. The National Academies Press, Washington, DC

30. Himelstein BP, Hilden JM, Boldt AM, Weissmann D. Pediatric palliative care. N Engl J Med. 2004; 350:1752–1762

31. Contro N, Larson J, Scofield S, Sourkes B, Cohen H. Family perspectives on the quality of pediatric care. Arch Pediatr Adolesc Med. 2002; 156:14–19.

32. American Academy of Pediatrics (2000) Committee on Bioethics and Committee on Hospital Care: palliative care for children. Pediatrics 106:351–357

33. Berger AM, Portnenoy RK, Weissman DE (eds) (2002) Principles and Practice of Palliative Care and Supportive Oncology, 2nd edn. Lippincott Williams and Wilkins, Philadelphia, Pa

34. Block SD (2001) Psychological considerations, growth, and transcendence at the end of life: the art of the possible. JAMA 285:2898–2905

35. Burns JP, Truog RD (1997) Ethical controversies in pediatric critical care. New Horiz 5:72–84

36. Spinetta JJ (1974) The dying child's awareness of death: a review. Psychol Bull 81:256–260

37. Spinetta JJ, Rigler D, Karon M (1973) Anxiety in the dying child. Pediatrics 52:841–845

38. Rosso IM, Young AD, Femia LA, Yurgelun-Todd DA (2004) Cognitive and emotional components of frontal lobe functioning in childhood and adolescence. Ann N Y Acad Sci 1021:355–362

39. Sowell ER, Thompson PM, Holmes CJ, et al (1999) In vivo evidence for post-adolescent brain maturation in frontal and striatal regions. Nature Neurosci 2:859–861

40. Giedd JN, Blumenthal J, Jeffries NO, et al (1999) Brain development during childhood and adolescence: a longitudinal MRI study. Nature Neurosci 2:861–863

41. Thompson PM, Giedd JN, Woods RP, et al (2000) Growth patterns in the developing brain detected by using continuum mechanical tensor maps. Nature 404:190–193

42. De Luca CR, Wood SJ, Anderson V, et al (2003) Normative Data From the Cantab. I: Development of Executive Function Over the Lifespan. J Clin Exp Neuropsychol 25:242–254

43. Killgore WD, Yurgelun-Todd DA (2005) Social anxiety predicts amygdala activation in adolescents viewing fearful faces. Neuroreport 16:1671–1675

Access to Care after Therapy

Karen E. Kinahan • David R. Freyer •

Beverly Ryan • Mary Baron Nelson

Contents

29.1 Introduction

Obtaining access to appropriate medical care by young adults and adolescents is important for both newly diagnosed patients needing treatment and survivors who have completed therapy. Survivors who were treated as young adults require continued follow-up with their medical oncology teams to monitor for recurrence and for treatment-related sequelae. Young adult survivors who were treated for cancer as children similarly require long-term monitoring, but in addition face other major challenges associated with "coming of age," including finding access to competent, age-appropriate follow-up, obtaining medical insurance, completing school and/or finding employment, and completing psychosocial maturation. While all of these are essential for the realization of independent adulthood, the emphasis of this chapter is the provision of medical care in a framework that is optimal for the emerging adult survivor of childhood cancer.

29.2 Survivors of Young Adult Cancer

In contrast to the situation in pediatric oncology, formal programs appear to be uncommon and no uniform guidelines appear to exist for the long-term follow-up (LTFU) of survivors of cancer with onset in young adulthood [1]. In the United States, one factor contributing to this may be the markedly lower rate of enrollment of patients onto open clinical trials sponsored by the National Cancer Institute (<2% for those aged 20 to 29 years; see Chaps. 1 and 33) [2]. Patients not treated in the context of clinical trials lack the protocol-driven uniformity of required observations at specified time points in follow-up, and instead are reevaluated according to the prevailing opinions of treating oncologists, which may vary substantially. In clinical practice, some medical oncologists instruct young adult survivors that they have treated to return for extended follow-up both for disease recurrence and for long-term side effects. Other oncologists follow patients for a year or two post-therapy and then expect the patients to continue with their primary care physicians. In either setting, other factors may further impede compliance with follow-up by this patient population, although these have not been well studied. These include the generally lower level of concern for serious treatment-related morbidity (as patients were developmentally mature when treated), their geographical mobility, and insurance and employment issues in patients who are not yet vocationally stable. While important research has been done to study health-related quality of life in survivors of many young-adult malignancies, there is a need for studies of approaches to follow-up care in these patients.

29.3 Young Adult Survivors of Childhood Cancer

Like their counterparts treated for cancer as young adults, young adult survivors of childhood cancer also need to be monitored for disease recurrence, although this is less frequent in the latter group because of the longer time interval from diagnosis. In addition, childhood cancer survivors are at particular risk for late-onset complications of treatment. Studies indicate that over half of young adult survivors have at least one late effect, and about one-third have severe or moderately severe late complications [3–7]. However, a recent retrospective cohort analysis from the Childhood Cancer Survivor Study found that only 45% of survivors aged 20 to 24 years and 39% of those aged 25 to 29 years had a cancer-related medical visit in the 2 years prior to being queried [8]. Therefore, a critical task is to identify optimal approaches to ensure longitudinal care for these survivors, who began their encounter with cancer as children under the protection of their parents and pediatric providers, but must continue their follow-up as responsible adults. This course of events, characteristic of chronic illness in children generally, has been termed "transition of care." Because of their risk for late complications of treatment, expert opinion based on limited data recommends lifelong monitoring of childhood cancer survivors [9]. As discussed below, planned transitional care is considered to be appropriate for survivors of childhood cancer. The need for more systematic and effective approaches to their care has become acute because of the sheer number of young adult survivors, who currently account for almost 1 in 500 Americans aged 20 to 29 years [1].

29.3.1 Transition of Care: Background and Principles

To date, most of the literature dealing with transition of care has focused on adolescents and young adults with special healthcare needs [10–16]. According to the United States Maternal-Child Health Bureau, the "special needs" population has been defined as, "those who have or are at increased risk for chronic physical, developmental, behavioral, or emotional conditions, and who also require health and related services of a type or amount beyond that required by children generally" [10, 17]. The number of noninstitutionalized children with a chronic condition in the United States alone is estimated to be 4.4 million, or 6.5% of those less than 18 years old [18]. When considering all adolescents with a condition requiring follow-up or surveillance, that figure may be as high as 30%. This population includes those with developmental delay, congenital cardiac anomalies, asthma, cystic fibrosis, diabetes, sickle cell disease, spina bifida, and many with other acquired or congenital disabilities requiring ongoing medical attention. It is estimated that the overall survival of children with special healthcare needs exceeds 80% with current medical care [16]. Because of their similarly high survival rates, risk for developing late effects of treatment and consequent need for lifelong monitoring, childhood cancer survivors are felt to be encompassed by the definition of "special needs" patients cited above. Therefore, many considerations about transition of care for traditional "special needs" population are applicable to this group of patients.

The fundamental challenge is to assist this population in making a successful transition from a child-oriented to an adult-oriented healthcare system. Whereas the general orientation in the former is typically nurturing and directed, the world of adult healthcare requires skills of independence and self-advocacy [14]. Individuals with chronic conditions may need medical care or surveillance, psychosocial support, help with vocational issues if cognitive skills are impaired, consultation regarding fertility if it is impaired by an ongoing condition or previous therapy, and advice regarding insurance coverage. In the United States, it is estimated that one in five young adults (19- to 29-year-olds) with a disability lacks health insurance [19].

From the mid 1980s, medical providers, policy makers, and survivors in the United States have advocated for a standard insuring the seamless, coordinated and comprehensive transition of healthcare for children with special healthcare needs [20]. As a result, pediatric studies have been conducted to identify barriers to successful transition. Although each diagnostic group of young adults may have certain disease-specific issues, themes common to all individuals with special healthcare concerns have emerged.

First, transition is a process rather than a discrete event. Ideally, it should begin in early adolescence with conversation directed to the young person in order to educate the young adolescent about his/her condition and to teach advocacy skills [21]. The transition process spans several years and, if the responsibility for medical care is eventually assumed by an adult-oriented provider who is different from the originating pediatric service, eventuates in a transfer of care. There is agreement that successful transitions of care are not "surprise events," but are the result of careful preparation of the youth, parents, and all involved care providers [22]. A positive attitude is important, which views transition as an expected part of normal development and as something to be celebrated rather than dreaded. Prior to formal transfer of care, complex patients may require a nurse case manager to coordinate the switch and a patient advocate to ensure that needed services will actually be available in the new care setting [18].

Second, flexibility is appropriate in choosing the age for transition and transfer of care. Transition is commonly carried out between approximately 18 and 21 years of age, but the exact time needs to be individualized on the basis of physical development and emotional/social maturity. Two key areas of concern for older adolescents that should be addressed at that time are key symptoms that should prompt them to seek medical evaluation and concerns about sexuality and reproductive health [23].

Third, travel distance to a specialized follow-up center has been identified as an important consideration. In a survey of 334 adults with cystic fibrosis, it was found that 71% of patients receiving care at a cystic fibrosis center lived within 50 miles of that center, while 75.5% of those receiving care somewhere other than a cystic fibrosis center reported the nearest center was over 50 miles away. Distance may be a consideration for individuals choosing a specialty-oriented center [13].

Finally, several barriers that impede successful transition have been identified through focus group/survey methodology. Barriers on the part of providers may include time restrictions, lack of knowledge or training, financial reimbursement and letting go of the established relationship with the child [10, 14, 23–26]. Obstacles to transition for the patient may include dependent behavior, immaturity, lack of support systems, lack of trust in the caregiver, and noncompliance. For the family, the need for control, emotional dependency, overprotectiveness, and lack of trust in the prospective adult care providers may also present barriers to transition [25].

The literature regarding transition for children with special healthcare needs has generally identified four models of care: (1) disease/specialty-specific, (2) adolescent health-focused, (3) a primary care model where the family practitioner or internist is the coordinator, and (4) a single-site model where the ancillary services remain constant. The two predominant models in use appear to be the disease/specialty-specific and adolescent health-centered types [23, 25, 27].

29.3.2 Transition of Care: Key Issues for Childhood Cancer Survivors

Because of the multiple physical and psychosocial risk factors imposed by their therapy and previous disease, childhood cancer survivors require lifelong care [9, 14,

21, 28]. They are at increased risk for secondary neoplasms, organ dysfunction, endocrine abnormalities, neurocognitive deficits, and early death [29–34]. Thus, every long-term survivor of childhood cancer will ultimately need to be transitioned from his or her pediatric environment to an adult care setting. How this can take place and various solutions are presented in the next section. A factor complicating this transition is an apparent lack of knowledge and understanding on the part of the survivor and the primary care physicians regarding the increased risk for these various health and psychosocial impairments [35, 36].

In the cancer survivor literature, the most frequently described approach for LTFU is a clinic designed for this purpose at a pediatric cancer center [1, 37]. However, it is likely that multiple models of care are needed to address the heterogeneity in characteristics, location, and resources of this survivor population. There is an ongoing debate within LTFU programs about how to best provide care for childhood cancer survivors who have reached adulthood. Traditionally, many pediatric oncologists and pediatric oncology nurses have continued to see these patients as needed to provide education and screening for late effects. This practice has continued despite concerns that some adult healthcare needs may not be ideally dealt with by pediatric providers (e.g., screening and treatment for hypertension, infertility, dyslipidemias, and type II diabetes). In addition, because there is a need to record and research late-occurring long-term effects, there is reluctance and often an inability to release patients from follow-up at the pediatric oncology center. In 1998, Oeffinger et al. published data from the Children's Cancer Group and the Pediatric Oncology Group indicating that few programs focus on the long-term healthcare needs of adult survivors of childhood cancer. At that time, most treating institutions were beginning to focus on the continued care of their pediatric cancer survivors. A reported 53% of the institutions interviewed had a LTFU program at their institution. In more than 90% of the programs, adult survivors were followed up in a pediatric institution by a pediatric hematologist-oncologist [38]. Only 13% of responding institutions utilized an adult-oriented provider, and <10% involved a primary-care physician.

29.3.3 Transitional Care Concerns Among Nurses in the Children's Oncology Group

To determine their views on what is the most effective method for providing LTFU services to young adult survivors of childhood malignancies, a project was undertaken by the Late Effects Nursing Subcommittee of the Children's Oncology Group (COG). An additional goal of the study was to determine existing barriers to care and concerns the pediatric oncology team members had in caring for adult survivors in their pediatric settings. Practitioners were also asked what they conceived is the "ideal" follow-up program for adult survivors of pediatric cancer. We were interested in identifying existing successful models of care already in place for young adult childhood cancer survivors that may be adapted for use in other institutions.

To accomplish this, a short, open-ended questionnaire was developed. The pilot survey was performed at the March 2003 COG meeting. Questionnaires were distributed to nursing members who attended the Late Effects section of the Clinical Practice Committee. The survey was received positively with affirmation that care of young adult survivors was an issue of concern to many LTFU programs. A revised questionnaire was sent out later to nurses at other institutions via the COG Late Effects e-mail network. The sample of responding institutions was limited (23 out of a total of >240 COG institutions), but did represent a variety of both large and small medical centers in the United States and Canada. Seventy percent had a relationship with an institution that provided adult care and 30% did not. In addition, 87% of the respondents felt that their LTFU clinic would benefit from affiliating with or developing a LTFU program for adult survivors. The most frustrating issues faced by pediatric providers in caring for adult survivors of childhood cancer were identified. Nurses felt that there were needs specific to the adult population not being met (e.g., obtaining higher education and employment, chronic rehabilitation, assisted-living situations for those with more severe cognitive deficits, addressing the emotional issues of transition, providing written information in Spanish, and providing a separate location away from the pediatric institution where follow-up clinics could be held). A major barrier for adult survivors in the United States is inadequate or absent health insurance. Respondents from COG institutions dealt with this issue in a variety of ways, including 39% who provided free visits or used available funding from their institution; another 26% were unable to see any patients without insurance. Another difficult issue is tracking patients who have become "lost to follow-up." None of the nurses surveyed had a formalized way of finding these patients. Two nurses tried to track patients themselves, making phone calls when they had the time. Nine programs had databases to track patients, but most did not have the personnel to do an adequate job. Three programs relied on Certified Research Assistants to track patients who were treated in studies. Two programs had a cancer registrar involved with the program who tracked patients, and three utilized yearly reminders and newsletters.

Interesting information was revealed when the responding nurses were asked to describe their opinion of an "ideal system" for follow-up of adult survivors. All of the answers were different, reflecting a wide variety of beliefs. Some opinions included:

— Developing a close relationship with an adult facility for transition, and sharing a database.
— Transferring care to an adult primary care provider with access to specialists and psychosocial support.
— Developing an adult practitioner model with a direct link to the pediatric oncologist for consultation.
— Providing a setting that combines adult and pediatric care, with family practitioners, pediatric oncologists or other subspecialists, and pediatric nursing practitioners.
— Transitioning within the same institution to the adult setting.
— Yearly contact by phone, mail or e-mail to maintain a database.

At the heart of the transition issue is a feeling of conflict among pediatric providers. There is a clear desire to maintain a relationship with adult survivors in order to collect data about the effects of childhood cancer and its treatment that may occur much later in life. In addition, there is a desire to keep the survivors

informed of any new developments in the management of late effects. There is also a well-founded concern that survivors may not receive the most comprehensive follow-up care from an adult provider who may be unaware of long-term risks of childhood cancer treatments. At the same time, there is the realization that providing care to adults is outside the scope of practice of pediatric providers, as well as the logistics of continuing to provide care to an ever-growing number of survivors in addition to newly diagnosed patients.

In reality, not all pediatric oncology treatment institutions will choose or are able to have a formal LTFU program for their adult survivors. However, pediatric oncologists, advanced practice nurses, and other team members must remain cognizant of the often-complicated healthcare issues adult survivors may face. They also need to advocate for their patients by acting as a bridge to adult primary care physicians and set up referrals to subspecialists who are familiar with childhood cancer late effects. Advocacy can also come in the form of providing information. The COG recently created formal Long-term Follow-up Guidelines and Health Links for guidance in providing care to survivors. These risk-based, exposure-related clinical practice guidelines provide recommendations for screening and management of late effects that may potentially arise from childhood cancer treatment (these can be accessed at www.survivorshipguidelines.org) [39, 40]. This information is valuable for pediatric oncologists and pediatricians, and is especially useful for adult practitioners who are not familiar with potential or actual late effects of childhood cancer.

29.3.4 Models of Transitional Care As Reported By Nurses in the COG

In the COG nursing survey described above, respondents also provided descriptions of their programs. Based upon those descriptions, the authors grouped programs with similar features and were able to discern four basic models used for care delivery to young adult survivors. Some pediatric treating institutions appeared to use a combination of one or more of the model types. Respondents to the questionnaire represented free-standing pediatric treating institutions, major medical centers, and two Canadian hospitals. This is important because different forms of access to adult care providers may influence the quality of the transition of care. It should be noted that the four basic models that were discerned in this study, and are described below, are not exhaustive of valid approaches to transition of care. Some models that are currently less common, such as that where responsibility for survivor follow-up is formally transferred to community-based adult primary care providers, were not represented in the study sample.

29.3.4.1 Model 1: Adult Practitioner Model

The adult practitioner model was identified when a pediatric oncology advanced practice nurse, experienced in LTFU issues works with an adult practitioner (i.e., an internist or family practice doctor) providing follow up of the pediatric cancer survivor while screening for the patient's potential or actual late effects of therapy. Patient education, health promotion, and health maintenance are important parts of this model of care. This takes place in an adult care facility and patients are referred to a special group of subspecialists who are familiar with the common late effects of the cancer treatment. A social worker or psychologist may be part of the team. The advantages of this model are the ability to capture data and potential for research, easy access to subspecialists, and insurance coverage, particularly if the doctor in-plan is the primary care provider. In addition, the physician is trained in general medicine and can see the survivors for non-cancer-related issues. Disadvantages are that the childhood cancer survivor must go to a new facility for care and medical records may be difficult to obtain.

29.3.4.2 Model 2: Resource Model

The resource model was identified when a young adult or adult survivor is referred to a pediatric treating institution on a one-time or annual basis, but also sees a primary care provider. There is a great deal of communication from the pediatric oncologist to the general medicine physicians. Physicians in the adult setting are directed in their care for the survivors in issues related to late effects. Advantages to the patient include maintaining contact with a pediatric cancer center and having their primary care provider being educated by the pediatric oncologist, an arrangement that can help with insurance coverage. Some disadvantages could be the loss of data on out-going survivors and the amount of paperwork for the pediatric oncologist. In addition, if each primary care practitioner has only one or two survivors in their practice, their expertise with this population could be an issue.

29.3.4.3 Model 3: Switch Model

The switch model was identified when pediatric oncology patients are seen in a major medical center with a pediatric oncology department. Once the young adult survivor is "too old" to be seen in the pediatric setting they will be "switched" to an adult provider within the same medical center. Advantages to the patient are that they are familiar with the setting and location of the hospital or clinic. Data and medical records can also be readily shared. The general consensus among pediatric oncologists is that it is not ideal for adult oncologists to be made responsible for follow-up of these patients due to the demands of treating large numbers of newly diagnosed adults. In this model, it may be better for patients to be referred to general practitioners, internal medicine, or family practice physicians. A collaborative relationship needs to be formed between the pediatric oncology department and the group accepting the survivors for follow-up. Will the pediatric oncologists remain "in the loop" and be utilized for questions? If the answer is no, then the transition process may be less than ideal for the patients.

29.3.4.4 Mode 4: Comfort Model

This model is when the pediatric oncology team keeps the patients coming back for follow-up indefinitely, irrespective of their age or time elapsed since diagnosis. Some of these oncology programs do not have defined LTFU programs and may see their survivors in the general oncology clinic. One advantage of this model is that the young adult and adult survivor is familiar with the pediatric oncologist and staff members. In addition, longitudinal research can be performed on these patients. Disadvantages are the pediatric oncology team's lack of expertise with adult care issues as they arise and lack of "well adult" care provided. Referral to competent, knowledgeable, adult subspecialists can also be difficult to make from a pediatric setting. Finally, treating young adults alongside young children may be uncomfortable for both sets of patients.

29.4 Conclusions

Access to appropriate care for young adults following completion of cancer treatment is necessary both for those who were treated as young adults and for those treated as children. Both groups have increased risks for serious treatment-related complications, although the risks appear to be greatest in those treated during childhood before growth and development were complete. Both groups also face similar challenges characteristic of young adulthood that may interfere with obtaining appropriate medical monitoring, including geographical mobility, incomplete education or vocational training, lack of an established career, uncertain health insurance status, and varying degrees of social maturity.

In addition to all of these, a key challenge for young adult survivors of childhood cancer is making a successful transition of care from the pediatric to adult-oriented healthcare system. The ideal of carrying out such a planned, coordinated transition of care for children with chronic illnesses – including cancer survivors – is now well-accepted. Despite important barriers that can impede transition, several successful models of care are in use that facilitate transition of the lifelong follow-up from the exclusive domain of pediatric oncology to the more suitable realm involving adult medicine. The ever-growing number of childhood cancer survivors requires a concerted effort to develop effective mechanisms for caring for young adult survivors, which will ensure risk-based health monitoring, timely intervention in the event of problems, psychosocial support, wellness education and disease prevention practices, vocational and insurance assistance, and collection of outcomes data, which are vital for the completion of important studies of late effects and transitional care.

References

1. Hewitt M, Weiner SL, Simone JV (2003) Childhood Cancer Survivorship. The National Academies Press, Washington DC, pp 90–127
2. Albritton K, Bleyer WA (2003) The management of cancer in the older adolescent. Eur J Cancer 39:2584–2599
3. Garre ML, Gandus S, Cesana B, et al (1994) Health status of long-term survivors after cancer in childhood: results on a uni-institutional study in Italy. Am J Pediatr Hematol Oncol 16:143–152
4. Vonderweid N, Beck D, Caflisch U, et al (1996) Standardized assessment of late effects in long-term survivors of childhood cancer in Switzerland: results of a Swiss Pediatric Oncology Group (SPOG) pilot study. Int J Pediatr Hematol Oncol 3:483–490
5. Stevens MC, Mahler H, Parkes S (1998) The health status of adult survivors of cancer in childhood. Eur J Cancer 34:694–698
6. Sklar CA (1999) Overview of the effects of cancer therapies: the nature, scale and breadth of the problem Acta Paediatr 88:1–4
7. Oeffinger KC, Eshelman DA, Tomlinson GE, et al (2000) Grading of late effects in young adult survivors of childhood cancer followed in an ambulatory adult setting. Cancer 88:1687–1695
8. Oeffinger KC, Mertens AC, Hudson MM, et al. (2004) Health care of young adult survivors of childhood cancer: a report from the Childhood Cancer Survivor Study. Ann Fam Med 2:61–70
9. Lampkin BC (1993) Introduction and executive summary. Cancer 71:3199–3201
10. Scal P, Evans T, Blozis S, et al (1999) Trends in transition from pediatric to adult health care services for young adults with chronic conditions. J Adolesc Health 24:259–264
11. Boyle MP, Farukki Z, Nosky ML (2001) Strategies for improving transition to adult cystic fibrosis care, based on patient and parent views. Pediatr Pulmonol 32:428–436
12. Flume PA, Anderson DL, Hardy KK, Gray S (2001) Transition programs in cystic fibrosis centers: perceptions of pediatric and adult directors. Pediatr Pulmonol 31:443–450
13. Anderson DL, Flume PA, Hardy KK, Gray S (2002) Transition programs in cystic fibrosis centers: perceptions of patients. Pediatr Pulmonol 33:327–331
14. Fleming E, Carter B, Gillibrand W (2002) The transition of adolescents with diabetes from the children's health care service into the adult health care service: a review the literature J Clin Nurs 11:560–567
15. Madge S, Bryon M (2002) A model for transition from pediatric to adult care in cystic fibrosis. J Pediatr Nurs 17:283–288

16. Geenen SJ, Powers LE, Sells W (2003) Understanding the role of health care providers during the transition of adolescents with disabilities and special health care needs. J Adolesc Health 32:225–233

17. McPherson M, Arango P, Fox H, et al (1998) A new definition of children with special health care needs. Pediatrics 102:137–140

18. Wojciechowski EA, Hurtig A, Dorn L (2002) A natural history study of adolescents and young adults with sickle cell disease as they transfer to adult care: a need for case management services. J Pediatr Nurs 17:18–27

19. White PH (2002) Access to health care: health insurance considerations for young adults with special needs/disabilities. Pediatrics 110:1328–1335

20. Blum RW (2002) Improving transition for adolescents with special health care needs from pediatric to adult-centered health care. Pediatrics 110:1301–1303

21. Rosen DS (1993) Transition to adult health care for adolescents and young adults with cancer. Cancer Suppl 71:3411–3414

22. Reiss J, Gibson R (2002) Health care transition: destinations unknown. Pediatrics 110:1307–1314

23. Scal P (2002) Transition for youth with chronic conditions: primary care physicians' approaches. Pediatrics 110:1315–1321

24. Hobbie WL, Ogle S (2001) Transitional care for young adult survivors of childhood cancer. Semin Oncol Nurs 17:268–273

25. Hergenroeder AC (2002) The transition into adulthood for children and youth with special health care needs. Tex Med 98:51–58

26. Zebrack BJ, Eshelman DA, Hudson MM, et al (2004) Health care for childhood cancer survivors Cancer 100:843–850

27. White P (1999) Transition to adulthood. Curr Opin Rheumatol 11:408–411

28. D'Angio G (1975) Pediatric cancer in perspective: cure is not enough Cancer 35:867–870

29. Nicholson HS, Fears TR, Byrne J (1994) Death during adulthood in survivors of childhood and adolescent cancer. Cancer 73:3094–3102

30. Bhatia S, Robison LL, Oberlin O, et al (1996) Breast cancer and other second neoplasms after childhood Hodgkin disease. New Engl J Med 334:745–751

31. Hudson MM, Jones D, Boyett J, et al (1997) Late mortality of long-term survivors of childhood and adolescent cancer. J Clin Oncol 15:2205–2213

32. Oeffinger KC, Eshelman DA, Tomlinson GE, et al (2000) Providing primary care for long-term survivors of childhood acute lymphoblastic leukemia. J Fam Pract 49:1133–1146

33. Mertens AC, Yasui Y, Neglia JP, et al (2001) Late mortality experience in five-year survivors of childhood and adolescent cancer. J Clin Oncol 19:3163–3172

34. Neglia JP, Friedman DL, Yasui Y, et al (2001) Second malignant neoplasms in five-year survivors of childhood cancer: Childhood Cancer Survivor Study. J Natl Cancer Inst 93:618–629

35. Kadan-Lottick NS, Robison LL, Gurney IG, et al (2002) Childhood cancer survivors' knowledge about their past diagnosis and treatment. JAMA 287:1832–1839

36. Vaughn DJ, Meadows AT (2002) Cancer survivor research: the best is yet to come. J Clin Oncol 20:888–890

37. MacLean WE, Foley GV, Ruccione K, Sklar C (1996) Transitions in the care of adolescent and young adult survivors of childhood cancer. Cancer 78:1340–1344

38 Oeffinger KC, Eshelman DA, Tomlinson GE, Buchanan GR (1998) Programs for adult survivors of childhood cancer. J Clin Oncol 16:2864–2868

39. Children's Oncology Group (2004) Long-term follow-up guidelines for survivors of childhood, adolescent and young adult cancers. www.survivorshipguidelines. org (as of August 12, 2004)

40. Eshelman DA, Landier W, Sweeney T, et al (2004) Facilitating care for childhood cancer survivors: Integrating Children's Oncology Group long-term follow-up guidelines and health links in clinical practice J Pediatr Oncol Nurs 21:271–280

Future Health of Survivors of Adolescent and Young Adult Cancer

Melissa M. Hudson • Kevin C. Oeffinger

Contents

30.1 Introduction

As described in Chap. 27 on late effects, survivors of cancer during adolescence and early adulthood face lifetime risks associated with their previous cancer and cancer therapy. It is well understood that the developing and maturing organ systems of an adolescent or young adult are sensitive to radiation therapy, chemotherapy, and surgery that are delivered to cure the cancer [1, 2]. When alterations in the development or aging of normal tissues reach a critical threshold, organ system dysfunction can result. Virtually all organ systems can be affected, depending upon the cancer therapy exposure, leading to a wide array of late effects, including second cancers, cardiovascular and pulmonary disease, cognitive dysfunction, and musculoskeletal problems. Commonly, late effects may not become apparent for years or even decades after the exposure to the cancer therapies. Of concern, is the potential that persistent, often initially subclinical, effects may exacerbate common diseases associated with aging, such as cardiovascular, skeletal, and endocrine disorders.

Illustrating the impact of late effects of cancer therapy are two seminal papers from the Childhood Cancer Survivor Study (CCSS), a 26-institution cohort study tracking the outcomes of about 14,000 survivors of childhood, adolescent, and young adult cancers diagnosed prior to the age of 21 years [3]. Mertens and colleagues reported that cancer survivors had an excess risk for all-cause mortality (deaths due to any cause) that increased with age [4]. This was due primarily to second cancers and cardiac or pulmonary disease. Hudson et al. reported on the health status of 9,435 young adult survivors, age 18 to 48 years, who were diagnosed with their cancer prior to the age of 21 years [5]. Forty-four percent of the population had at least one moderate to severe adverse outcome of their health status. Some degree of mental health impairment was observed in all diagnostic groups studied, with the highest incidence in survivors of Hodgkin lymphoma, sarcomas, and bone tumors, malignancies that commonly present in adolescence and young adulthood. These findings suggest that the cancer experience during this developmental period results in specific adjustment issues for the cancer patient mature enough to appreciate the gravity of the cancer diagnosis and the risks of treatment side effects.

The physical and emotional impact of cancer should be considered when counseling adolescent and young adult survivors about cancer-related health risks. Importantly, the risks of late effects are modified, either positively or negatively, by a variety of host, treatment, cancer, and behavioral factors (Fig. 30.1). This chapter describes the role of two important components in the lifelong or future health of survivors of cancer diagnosed during adolescence and the early adult years. First, the healthcare of survivors, including screening and surveillance for late effects, is described. Following this, the promotion of healthy lifestyle habits is dis-

cussed, focusing on the interaction of lifestyle habits and the expression of late effects.

30.2 Healthcare of Cancer Survivors

From the perspective of health and chronic disease models, cancer survivors represent an interesting population with health needs and healthcare utilization patterns that vacillates between a wellness and an illness model (Fig. 30.2). Prior to the symptomatic onset of the cancer, most individuals are "healthy" and operate in a wellness model, with preventive healthcare needs that are usually addressed by a primary care physician. With the onset of symptoms and the diagnosis of cancer, the individual then assumes the role of "cancer patient" and is treated for the disease, generally in a chronic care model with care focusing on the disease and provision of care provided largely by the oncology team. Upon completion of therapy and some interval thereafter, depending on the cancer, the patient is declared "cured." Some survivors develop a chronic health problem as an early consequence of the cancer or cancer therapy. For instance, a seizure disorder may result from the location of a brain tumor, or the curative surgery or radiotherapy. Such a survivor may con-

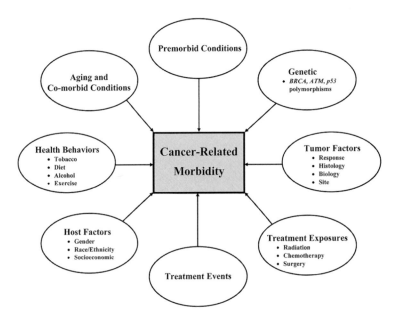

Figure 30.1

Multiple factors contribute to cancer-related morbidity. The risks of late effects may be modified, either positively or negatively, by host (gender, age, race, genetics), cancer (location, histology, biology), or treatment (type, intensity) factors as well as behavioral practices. Practicing healthy lifestyles is the primary method survivors of adolescent and young adult cancers can use to reduce the risk of future health complications. Adapted with permission from Hudson (2005) [1]

tinue in a chronic disease model and be monitored by a neurologist. As another example, an adolescent with an osteosarcoma may require limb-sparing surgery involving a lower extremity. The musculoskeletal system is permanently altered by the tumor and its treatment and long-term monitoring by an orthopedic surgeon would be anticipated. In both of these examples, the survivor would be cared for in a chronic disease model but would also have preventive care needs that would need to be addressed.

Most survivors of adolescent or young adult cancers, however, do not have a chronic health problem upon completion of their cancer therapy, and thus, in a sense, enter back into the wellness model. Importantly, though, they have new long-term health risks, many of which have not been well characterized. Most survivors are not cognizant of their long-term health risks associated with the cancer therapy. Mentally and emotionally, many if not most survivors of adolescent

and young adult cancers figuratively close the door on the cancer chapter of their life. Similarly, most clinicians that provide care for a survivor apart from the cancer center setting are not familiar with the health risks of this relatively small and heterogeneous population. Operating in this mode, most clinicians will note the previous history of the cancer in the medical record, but will usually not consider the survivor as a high-risk individual and will rarely order screening or surveillance studies different than would be warranted in the general population.

A sizeable proportion of survivors, perhaps as much as one-third, will have relatively minimal risk for clinically significant late effects [2]. Receiving healthcare that does not address their previous cancer likely will make little difference in their lives. Most, though, can be stratified into either middle- or high-risk groups. In the traditional wellness model, in which preventive care is delivered to the general population, a similar

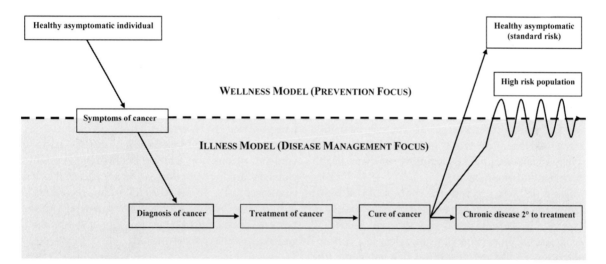

Figure 30.2

Health needs and healthcare utilization of survivors of adolescent and young adult cancer vacillate between a wellness and an illness model. Prior to the symptomatic onset of the cancer, most individuals are "healthy" and operate in a wellness model, with preventive healthcare needs that are usually addressed by a primary care physician. With the onset of symptoms and the diagnosis of cancer, the individual then assumes the role of "cancer patient" and is treated for the disease, generally in a chronic-care model with care focusing on the disease and provision of care provided largely by the oncology team. Upon completion of therapy and some interval thereafter, depending on the cancer, the patient is declared "cured". Some survivors who develop a chronic health problem as an early consequence of the cancer or cancer therapy remain in a chronic-care model

stratification of risk is incorporated. Most screening recommendations are based on genetic predispositions, comorbid health conditions, or lifestyle behaviors.

30.2.1 Risk-Based Healthcare of Survivors

Faced with these risks and challenges, how can the healthcare delivered to survivors be optimized? It is important to recognize that there is a window of opportunity to modify the severity of health outcomes by prevention or early intervention. Early diagnosis and intervention or preventive care targeted at reducing risk for late effects can benefit the health and quality of life of survivors [6]. The outcomes of the following late effects can be influenced by early diagnosis and early intervention: second malignant neoplasms following radiation therapy (breast, thyroid, and skin), altered bone metabolism and osteoporosis, obesity-related health problems (dyslipidemia, hypertension, diabetes mellitus, cardiovascular disease), liver failure secondary to chronic hepatitis C following blood transfusion, and endocrine dysfunction following chest/mantle or cranial radiotherapy. Primary, secondary, and tertiary prevention, including tobacco avoidance/cessation, physical activity, low-fat diet, and adequate calcium intake, can modify risk. Longitudinal care addressing other late effects, such as infertility, musculoskeletal problems, cognitive dysfunction, and psychosocial issues, may also improve survivors' health outcomes and quality of life.

Based on these precepts, the concept of risk-based healthcare of survivors has evolved over the past 10 to 15 years. The term "risk-based healthcare," coined by Meadows, Oeffinger, and Hudson, refers to a conceptualization of lifelong healthcare that integrates the cancer and survivorship experience into the overall lifetime healthcare needs of the individual [2, 6]. We endorse the following basic tenets of risk-based care: (1) longitudinal care that is considered a continuum from cancer diagnosis to eventual death, regardless of age; (2) continuity of care consisting of a partnership between the survivor and a single healthcare provider who can coordinate necessary services; (3) comprehensive, anticipatory, proactive care that includes a systematic plan of prevention and surveillance – a

multidisciplinary team approach with communication between the primary healthcare provider, specialists of pediatric and adult medicine, and allied/ancillary service providers; (4) healthcare of the whole person, not a specific disease or organ system, that includes the individual's family and his cultural and spiritual values; and (5) a sensitivity to the issues of the cancer experience, including expressed and unexpressed fears of the survivor and his or her family/spouse. A systematic plan for lifelong screening, surveillance, and prevention that incorporates risks based on the previous cancer, cancer therapy, genetic predispositions, lifestyle behaviors, and comorbid health conditions should be developed for all survivors.

About one-half of cancer centers have a long-term follow-up (LTFU) program for their survivors [7]. These programs provide screening for late effects, including second cancers, education regarding risks, and promotion of healthy lifestyles. As this is resource-intense and generally a low clinical revenue generator, it is not anticipated that the number of centers in the United States with an LTFU program will substantially increase in the near future. Even in cancer centers with an LTFU program, most survivors gradually disconnect from the cancer center as they age or move away and become "lost to follow-up." Apart from cancer centers, few healthcare professionals see more than a handful of survivors, each with different cancers, treatment exposures, and health risks. This has led to an epidemic of survivors who are not being followed by a clinician familiar with their risks and a general lack of risk-based care. To assist the clinician, regardless of setting, who cares for survivors, the following two sections describe briefly the general care of symptomatic and asymptomatic survivors.

30.2.2 Asymptomatic Survivors

As noted above, depending upon risks, survivors may benefit from early intervention or prevention. To assist the clinician in caring for the asymptomatic survivor, the Children's Oncology Group developed the Long-Term Follow-Up Guidelines for Survivors of Childhood, Adolescent, and Young Adult Cancers [8]. These guidelines were produced through a multidisciplinary effort, cochaired by one of the authors (MMH) and

Wendy Landier, RN, MSN, CPNP. The guidelines can be can be downloaded free of charge at website www.survivorshipguidelines.org. A web-based interactive and user-friendly format of these guidelines, targeted for healthcare professionals and survivors, is under development.

The guidelines are a hybrid, based on evidence and consensus. There is abundant evidence linking cancer treatment exposures to late effects; however, because of the relatively small size of the heterogeneous survivor population, there are no studies (nor will there be in the near future) that show a reduction in morbidity or mortality with screening. As with other high-risk populations that are relatively small, limiting the types of studies evaluating the risks and benefits of screening and surveillance, there are two options in assessing the evidence. The first option is to state that, based on these limitations, there are no high-quality studies, thus limiting the strength of recommendation. However, to do so belies the wealth of high-quality studies from standard-risk populations that are applicable. Evidence gathered from studies in standard-risk populations can be extrapolated and used in the scientific basis of guideline development for high-risk populations. As principles from standard-risk populations are applied to high-risk groups, the two primary differences are timing of initiation and frequency of screening. By virtue of a lack of studies capable of answering these two questions, decisions must be founded on the biology in question within the grounded framework of risk and benefits. To do otherwise, in our opinion, would be akin to placing one's head in the sand and avoiding a difficult question.

30.2.3 Symptomatic Survivors

Although many survivors will remain asymptomatic, some will experience symptoms that may or may not be related to their risks and their previous cancer therapies. Clinicians who are not familiar with the population and are faced with uncertainty will often diverge to the extremes in evaluating a new problem. When young adult survivors present with symptoms not typical of their age group, their symptoms may be dismissed as anxiety or similar conditions, or conversely they may be over tested. Following are three recurrent

themes that we have heard through our experience. A survivor who was treated with mantle or chest radiation faces an increase risk of premature coronary artery disease [9–14]. When a survivor of Hodgkin lymphoma presents as a young adult with chest pain, clinicians who are not cognizant of this risk often attribute the pain to anxiety or gastroesophageal reflux disease. A survivor who had a splenectomy as a staging procedure for their Hodgkin lymphoma faces a lifetime risk of overwhelming sepsis of 2 to 4% [15–18]. Clinicians unfamiliar with this population may not be aggressive in evaluating a febrile illness and miss the opportunity of early diagnosis and prompt treatment of sepsis due to pneumococcus or another encapsulated bacterium. Another example is the obstetrician who is not familiar with the risks of late-onset cardiomyopathy following exposure to anthracyclines [19–21]. The increased intravascular volume associated with pregnancy and the increase cardiac workload during labor and delivery may trigger overt congestive heart failure secondary to an underlying, unrecognized cardiomyopathy.

Illustrating these issues from the survivors' perspective are three responses from young adult survivors from a 4-year study that we conducted, supported through the Robert Wood Johnson Foundation, assessing barriers to long-term healthcare:

"Most of the time I feel that my primary care physician thinks that since I have been diagnosed over 20 years ago, that my cancer history is not important, and that they do not need to do extra tests or even a blood test; this makes me feel frustrated and concerned that if there was something wrong they would just want to watch it for awhile …" "Although I got annual check-ups with an internist, gynecologist, and dermatologist (an oncologist is not appropriate at this point), I don't feel these providers have any special knowledge about long-term studies about my cancer (Hodgkin lymphoma)."

"I am treated no differently than any other patient, except that they order more tests and consider everything suspect. I wish I knew what to look out for in the years ahead."

Two methods can help to remedy this situation: educating survivors regarding the potential late effects of therapy and communicating with other healthcare professionals about the risks and needs of this population. First, it is critically important that the cancer center team educate the survivor and his or her family regarding potential late effects and their presenting symptoms. To be effective, education about late effects should be provided over time, beginning during or soon after completion of therapy. A summary of the cancer and cancer therapy should be provided to all cancer survivors. As needed, this summary should be updated and supplemented by exposure-specific educational materials. An excellent source of such survivor-targeted materials can be found in the Health Links that are provided with the guidelines described above (www.survivorshipguidelines.org).

Communicating with other healthcare professionals is a time-intensive, but critically important endeavor. Regardless of whether or not a survivor is followed in an LTFU program, he will inevitably interface with other healthcare professionals away from the cancer center. Cancer centers should provide contact information and easy accessibility for questions from survivors or their other healthcare providers. Assisting other healthcare professionals in the interpretation of a survivor's presenting symptoms or problems can be life altering.

30.3 Promoting Healthy Lifestyles

30.3.1 Health Behavior Counseling of the Adolescent/Young Adult Cancer Survivor

Cancer and its treatment render adolescent and young adult cancer survivors at greater risk for morbidity from health-risk behaviors than their peers without cancer [4, 5, 22–24]. Chronic or subclinical changes persisting after treatment recovery may result in premature onset of common diseases associated with aging such as obesity, diabetes mellitus, cardiovascular disease, hypertension, and second cancers [22, 24–28]. In young people who are already vulnerable to these conditions, the addition of health-risking behaviors, such as smoking, poor nutrition, and inactivity may increase this risk further. Consequently, health professionals caring for adolescent and young adult survivors have the responsibility and challenge of motivat-

ing the practice of healthy lifestyles in this vulnerable group. Education about cancer-related health risks and risk-modifying measures for the adolescent and young adult cancer survivor can be readily integrated into routine follow-up evaluations. Health education in the oncology setting has several advantages. Childhood cancer survivors have a close, long-term relationship with their oncology staff and generally respect them as credible medical experts. This relationship provides a strong foundation on which to introduce discussions about cancer-related health risks and risk-modifying behaviors. Survivors' enhanced perceptions of vulnerability during the check-up may also create a "teachable moment" that facilitates reception of health promotion messages [29]. In particular, evaluations after completion of therapy in long-term survivors that focus on health surveillance, rather than disease eradication, provide an atmosphere favorable for health promotion discussions.

The optimal components of health promotion counseling of survivors described in detail by Tyc et al. are summarized in Table 30.1 [29]. To be truly informed about potential health risks, survivors need accurate information about their cancer diagnosis, treatment modalities, and cancer-related health risks. This is critical information that many survivors lack [30]. Health counseling should be personalized to consider the unique educational needs related to the individual survivor's cancer experience. The content of traditional adolescent health programs can be modified to include information that enhances the survivor's perception of increased vulnerability. Health behavior discussions should avoid characterizing the survivor as being different from healthy peers. An approach that starts first with a discussion of the adverse effects of health-risking behaviors followed by an explanation of the additional risks predisposed by cancer should reduce the survivor's anxiety and permit identification with peers. The knowledge that certain behaviors are riskier for them than for others may provide some teens with a welcome excuse to resist peer pressure.

Healthcare professionals should also be prepared to address the increased vulnerability of individual patients to specific cancer-related health risks that may be related to sociodemographic factors, cancer treatment modalities, familial or genetic predisposition, and maladaptive health behaviors. Following this discussion, survivors should also be reminded that cancer treatment may accelerate the presentation of common health conditions associated with aging, including organ dysfunction and malignancy. Incorporating personal risk information may increase the significance of the discussion, heighten the survivor's perception of vulnerability, and enhance their reception to health counseling.

In health promotion counseling, clinicians should encourage survivors to establish priority health goals. Behavioral goal setting should include an extensive discussion of the personal benefits of practicing healthy behaviors. Fear of future illness does not provide strong motivation to change for many teens, therefore, the clinician must think broadly when discussing the personal benefits with teens – including financial, cosmetic, and social reasons to choose healthier behaviors. For example, teens may chose not to smoke because of the cost, the effect on yellowing of teeth and nails, the smell, and the conflict it creates with parents and, hopefully, with friends. Deterring an adolescent girl from excessive drinking might include a discussion of avoidance of situations where she can't defend herself from unwanted sexual advances. Potential barriers to and personal costs associated with behavioral change should be explored in detail to identify potential solutions. In these discussions, role playing regarding alternative health actions and problem-solving may be beneficial. Importantly, providers should inquire about the progress of health goals and provide follow-up counseling at subsequent evaluations.

30.3.2 Lifestyle Recommendations for the Adolescent/Young Adult Cancer Survivors

Multiple factors contribute to the risk of cancer-related morbidity in the long-term survivor (Fig. 30.1). Among these, health behaviors represent an important means of risk-reduction that can be readily pursued by survivors. Six common health practices – diet and physical activity, tobacco use, alcohol consumption, sun protection, and dental care – are reviewed below to provide the clinician with fundamental information to facilitate health promotion counseling efforts. The clinician is also referred to the aforementioned Health Links (www.survivorshipguidelines.org).

30.3.3 Diet and Physical Activity

Diet and physical activity are the most important health behaviors that affect cancer and cardiovascular disease risk. Tobacco use may be more problematic in causing second cancers and heart disease (see 30.3.4 Tobacco Use), but obesity is overtaking tobacco use as the greatest health problem faced by cancer survivors. The trend for tobacco use by cancer survivors is favorable, as noted below, but the trend in increasing body weight among cancer survivors is not.

Investigations of dietary practices in childhood cancer survivors have been largely limited to small cohort studies evaluating the relationship of caloric intake with energy expenditure [31–33], nutrient intake with bone mineral density [34–36], or choles-

Table 30.1 Components of health promotion interventions with adolescent cancer patients. Reprinted with permission from Tyc et al. (1999) [29]

Inform of potential health risks.
Address increased vulnerability to health risks relative to healthy peers.
Provide personalized risk information relative to treatment history.
Establish priority health goals.
Discuss benefits of health protective behaviors.
Discuss barriers to/personal costs of engaging in self-protective behaviors.
Provide follow-up counseling.

terol intake with cardiovascular disease risk factors [37]. Results show concerning trends, with energy intake exceeding energy expenditure, suboptimal dietary calcium correlating with osteopenia, and dietary fat intake in levels that will not reduce cholesterol. These findings suggest that childhood cancer survivors would benefit from dietary interventions that match caloric intake with physical activity, optimize calcium and other nutrients needed for bone accretion, and reduce dietary fat.

Likewise, relatively little information is available regarding physical activity in adolescent and young adult cancer survivors [32, 33, 37, 38]. Several studies noted reduced total daily energy expenditure resulting from relative physical inactivity in survivors of childhood acute lymphoblastic leukemia (ALL) and craniopharyngioma [31–33]. In ALL survivors, reduced energy expenditure was correlated with increased percentage of body fat [32, 33]. Similarly, Reilly et al. demonstrated significantly lower energy expenditure in preobese children treated for ALL compared to healthy controls that was related primarily to reduced energy expended on habitual physical activity [38]. In another

study, Oeffinger et al. observed cardiovascular disease risk factors such as obesity, dyslipidemia, hypertension, and insulin resistance in 62% of a cohort of young adult survivors treated for ALL in association with sedentary activity levels [37]. The higher prevalence of obesity in survivors treated with cranial radiation has been attributed to lower physical activity and resting metabolic rate, and hormonal insufficiency [32]. In particular, hypothalamic insult may predispose to obesity through leptin insensitivity [39] and adult growth hormone deficiency, which is associated with higher rates of dyslipidemia, insulin resistance, and cardiovascular mortality [40, 41].

In contrast to the dearth of information about physical activity after treatment for childhood cancer, abundant literature is available documenting an increased incidence of health concerns that are influenced directly by these health behaviors, including overweight/obesity [27, 28, 39, 42, 43], cardiovascular disease [20, 44–48], and osteopenia/osteoporosis [34, 49–53]. In studies of healthy populations, physical inactivity is associated with an increase in all-cause and cardiovascular-related mortality [54–58], coro-

Table 30.2 American Cancer Society (ACS) individual guidelines on nutrition and physical activity for cancer prevention. Adapted from Byers et al. (2002) [76]

1	Eat a variety of healthy foods, with an emphasis on plant sources.
	• Eat five or more servings of a variety of vegetables and fruits each day.
	• Choose whole grains in preference to processed (refined) grains and sugars.
	• Limit consumption of red meats, especially those high in fat and processed.
	• Choose foods that help maintain a healthful weight.
2.	Adopt a physically active lifestyle.
	Adults: engage in at least moderate activity for ≥30 min on ≥5 days of the week (≥45 min of moderate-to-vigorous activity ≥5 days per week may further enhance reductions in the risk of breast and colon cancer.)
3.	Maintain a healthy weight throughout life.
	• Balance caloric intake with physical activity
	• Lose weight if currently overweight or obese.
4.	If you drink alcoholic beverages, limit consumption.

nary heart disease [59–62]. strokes [63]. and osteoporosis [64–66]. Conversely, physical activity has been shown to be protective and reduce risk for coronary heart disease [67], hypertension [68], non-insulin-dependent diabetes mellitus [69, 70], and osteoporosis [71–73]. Therefore, adolescent and young adult cancer survivors, particularly those treated with potentially cardiotoxic cancer therapies, should be routinely counseled regarding the benefits of physical activity in reducing cancer-related morbidity in adulthood.

Adherence to a healthful diet and regular physical activity has been shown to reduce the risk of cancer, cardiovascular disease, and other chronic illnesses [74, 75]. The American Cancer Society outlined nutrition and physical activity guidelines that aim to reduce cancer and cardiovascular disease risk [76]; similar recommendations have been endorsed by the American Heart Association and the Department of Health and Human Services [77, 78]. Briefly summarized in Table 30.2, these guidelines promote balancing fat, protein, and carbohydrate intake to assure nutrient adequacy and maintain health. The benefits of healthful dietary practices should be emphasized during counseling sessions with survivors: higher consumption of vegetables and fruits may be associated with a lower incidence of lung, colorectal, and other gastrointestinal cancers. Eating foods rich in monounsaturated and omega-3 fatty acids (e.g., fish, walnuts) is associated with a lower risk for cardiovascular diseases. Ingestion of healthful carbohydrates like whole grains provides many vitamins and minerals, such as folate, vitamin E, and selenium, which have been associated with a lower risk of colon cancer [79]. Similarly, misperceptions regarding micro- and macronutrients should be corrected: ingestion of specific nutrients in pharmacologic doses does not provide the same benefit of eating a variety of fruits and vegetables, which provide vitamins, minerals, and phytochemicals that work synergistically to reduce cancer risk. The consequences of health-risking dietary practices should be explored in the context of the risks conferred by survivor's cancer treatment and family history: consumption of a high-fat diet may increase the risk of coronary artery disease in a survivor predisposed to cardiac dysfunction following anthracycline chemotherapy or chest radiation.

The American Cancer Society guidelines also provide recommendations regarding regular physical activity, which has been associated with reduced risks of breast, colon, and other cancers, as well as well as cardiovascular health risks [80, 81]. Moderate-to-vigorous physical activity produces beneficial effects on metabolism of stored body fat and physiological functions affecting insulin, estrogen, androgen, prostaglandins, and immune function [75, 82]. Participation in moderate-to-vigorous physical activity for at least 45 min on 5 or more days is advised to be optimal for already active adults; children and adolescents should engage in at least 60 min per day of similar activities. Individuals who are sedentary or just beginning an exercise program are advised to gradually increase to 30 min, of moderate activities, a level that should provide cardiovascular benefit and aid in weight control.

30.3.4 Tobacco Use

In contrast to earlier studies describing tobacco use in childhood cancer survivors [83, 84], recent investigations indicate positive trends in reduction of smoking initiation and an increase in cessation in childhood cancer survivors, suggesting an increased awareness about tobacco-related health risks associated with public health education efforts [85–88]. Children's Cancer Group investigators compared the smoking habits of 592 survivors of acute lymphoblastic leukemia diagnosed between 1970 and 1987 to those of 409 sibling controls [88]. Compared to sibling controls, survivors were significantly less likely to have ever smoked (23% vs. 36%) and less likely to be current smokers (14% vs. 20%). Emmons et al. reported similar results in a CCSS investigation examining the smoking behaviors of over 9,000 adult study participants surviving a childhood cancer diagnosed between 1970 and 1986 [85]. Rates of ever smoking (28%) and currently smoking (17%) reported by survivors were significantly lower than population prevalence rates for both male and female survivors. Other positive findings included evidence that male and female survivors who smoked were also significantly more likely to quit.

These trends are encouraging and provide support for the potential benefits of health education that should continue as long as investigations indicate that childhood cancer survivors continue to compromise their health by smoking or using any form of tobacco. Cigarette smoking has been linked to an increased risk of cardiopulmonary disease including hypertension, emphysema, and stroke. In addition, tobacco use is the most important preventable cause of cancer in adulthood and has been linked to 90% of cases of lung cancer, and one-third of all other cancers including cancers of the mouth, larynx, pharynx, liver, colon, rectum, kidneys, urinary tract, prostate, and cervix. Investigations of adult cancer patients demonstrate additive risks of lung cancer when tobacco carcinogens are combined with thoracic radiation and specific chemotherapeutic agents [89–91]. Although the additional risks conferred by tobacco use to the development of cancer and cardiovascular disease in survivors of cancers presenting during adolescence and young adulthood has not been well studied, an excess risk is anticipated in survivors treated with the antineoplastic modalities outlined in Table 30.3. Therefore, survivors at risk should be reminded of their increased vulnerability to tobacco-related health problems. Likewise, counseling regarding secondhand smoke seems prudent, despite the lack of demonstrating excess risk of adverse tobacco-related health outcomes in cancer survivors exposed to environmental tobacco smoke.

30.3.5 Alcohol

Investigations evaluating the practice of health-risking behaviors in adolescent and young adult cancer survivors indicate rates of alcohol consumption comparable to those of their peers without cancer [92–94]. This statistic is concerning, considering the fact that some cancer treatments and complications predispose the long-term survivor to an increased risk of hepatic dysfunction (Table 30.4). Most contemporary hepatotoxic antineoplastic therapies are associated with acute toxicity, from which the majority of patients recover without apparent long-term sequelae [95]. Conditions reported to exacerbate hepatic dysfunction include chronic hepatitis, particularly chronic hepatitis C (HCV), and hepatic graft-versus-host-disease (GVHD). HCV is the most common etiology of chronic hepatitis, cirrhosis, and hepatocellular carcinoma in the United States. The prevalence of chronic HCV ranges from 6.6 to 49% of childhood cancer survivors who were transfused before contemporary screening of blood donors [96–102]. Contrary to earlier reports demonstrating a mild clinical course in childhood cancer survivors with chronic HCV [96, 99, 100, 103], we now recognize that a significant number of these patients are at risk for adverse outcomes including impaired quality of life, cirrhosis, hepatic failure, and hepatocellular carcinoma [97, 104, 105]. Although the transmission of HCV has declined since the development of blood donor screening tests for the virus, there are many patients surviving with chronic transfusion-acquired infection and many childhood cancer survivors untested and likely unaware of their risk of chronic infection and its implications for future liver health. Because of the high incidence of chronic infection in the majority of individuals exposed to HCV, the potential adverse outcomes associated with chronic infection including liver failure, and the availability of antiviral therapy that significantly reduce

Table 30.3 Antineoplastic therapies with cardiopulmonary toxicities potentiated by tobacco use. Adapted with permission from Tyc et al. (1997) [134]

Potential effects	Therapy
Pulmonary toxicity (pneumonitis, fibrosis, restrictive lung disease)	Bleomycin, lomustin, carmustin, busulfan, cyclophosphamide, methotrexate, cytarabine
Cardiac toxicity (cardiomyopathy)	Anthracyclines: doxorubicin, daunorubicin, idarubicin High-dose cyclophosphamide
Cardiopulmonary toxicity	Thoracic radiation therapy (mantle, mediastinal, lungs, spinal, total body radiation)

this risk, the Centers for Disease Control and Prevention recommend that all individuals at risk transfused before implementation of blood donor testing for HCV (July 1992) should be screened for the disease [106]. Survivors with chronic HCV infection confirmed by a polymerase chain reaction test for viral RNA should be counseled regarding transmission and treatment options. It is important to emphasize that chronic hepatic injury associated with chronic GVHD, chronic infection, nodular regenerative hyperplasia from cytoreductive therapy, or drug-related liver injury, may accelerate the course of liver disease in survivors treated with hematopoietic stem-cell transplantation [107–110].

Liver injury related to treatment for childhood cancer is most often subclinical and may develop without a history of prior acute toxicity, thus it is important for clinicians to obtain a baseline screening of serum transaminases (alanine aminotransferase and aspartate aminotransferase) in asymptomatic survivors. In survivors with cancer-related hepatic dysfunction, preservation of residual hepatocyte function is critical since therapy is not available to reverse hepatic fibro-

sis. In addition to referral for antiviral therapy in cases with chronic HCV, standard recommendations to maintain liver health include abstinence from alcohol use and immunization against hepatitis A and B in patients who have not established immunity to these hepatotrophic viruses. Weight reduction in overweight/obese survivors is also prudent to reduce the risk of hepatic injury from fatty liver hepatitis (steatohepatitis) [111].

In addition to its direct hepatotoxic effects, consumption of alcoholic beverages, particularly in combination with tobacco products, increases the risk of cancers involving the oral cavity, larynx, esophagus, and possibly colon [112–115]. Cancer risk increases in direct proportion to alcohol intake and rises with regular consumption of as few as two drinks per day, with a drink defined as 12 fluid ounces (approx. 355 ml) of beer, 5 fluid ounces of wine (approx. 148 ml), and 1.5 fluid ounces (approx. 44 ml) of 80-proof distilled spirits [112–115]. Alcohol consumption has also been associated with a linear increase in breast cancer incidence in women over the range of consumption reported by most women [116–119]. In one study,

Table 30.4 Antineoplastic therapies with hepatic toxicities potentiated by alcohol use.

Therapy	Potential effects
Dactinomycin	Acute venoocclusive disease
Mercaptopurine	Hepatic dysfunction
Thioguanine	Acute venoocclusive disease
Methotrexate	Hepatic dysfunction
	Hepatic fibrosis
Hepatic radiation (hepatic, whole abdomen, total body)	Hepatic fibrosis
	Cirrhosis
	Hepatocellular carcinoma
Hematopoietic stem cell transplantation	Graft-versus-host-disease
	Chronic hepatitis
	Cirrhosis
	Iron overload
Blood product transfusion	Chronic hepatitis
	Cirrhosis
	Hepatic failure
	Hepatocellular carcinoma

daily consumption of one alcoholic drink was associated with an 11% (95% confidence interval, 7–16%) excess risk of breast cancer compared with nondrinkers [117]. Alcohol is hypothesized to enhance the risk of breast cancer through increases in circulating estrogens or other hormones, reduction in folic acid levels, or by a direct effect on breast tissue [116]. To avoid alcohol-related carcinogenesis, people who drink alcohol should limit intake to no more than two drinks per day for men and one drink per day for women. Because population studies indicate that modest alcohol intake of one to two drinks per day is associated with a lower risk for cardiovascular disease [120], the potential hepatotoxic and carcinogenic risks conferred by regular alcohol consumption must be weighed against its potential cardiovascular benefits.

30.3.6 Sun Protection

The use of sun protection measures is another understudied area of adolescent and young adult cancer survivor health behavior. Recreational and lifestyle preferences have resulted in a steady increase in the incidence of skin cancers, such that skin cancer is now the most common type of cancer diagnosed in adults in the general population [121]. Melanoma and nonmelanoma skin cancers (basal cell and squamous cell carcinoma) have also been reported with increased frequency in survivors of childhood malignancy treated with radiation therapy [122–124]. Non melanoma skin cancers are low-grade lesions that typically develop in skin included in radiation treatment fields, which may be in an unusual or non-sun-exposed part of the body. It is not known if sun protection will reduce the risk of radiation-associated non melanoma skin cancer in childhood cancer survivors [125]. However, public education regarding sun protection and self-examination has been associated with earlier diagnosis and treatment of melanoma in the general population [125]. Therefore, it seems prudent to counsel survivors regarding methods of sun protection, the risk factors and symptoms of skin cancer, and the importance of periodic examination of the skin in and around the radiation field. Adherence to the skin cancer prevention measures recommended for healthy populations are especially important for childhood

cancer survivors [126, 127]. These recommendations include: (1) limiting the amount of time in the sun, especially between 10:00 am and 2:00 pm when ultraviolet rays are most intense; (2) regularly using sunscreen with a sun protection factor of 15 or more; (3) wearing protective clothing, especially when planning extended activities in the sun; and (4) not tanning.

30.3.7 Dental Care

Adolescents and young adults surviving cancer are at risk for oral health problems including salivary gland dysfunction, accelerated dental decay, chronic gingivitis, periodontal disease, and a variety of developmental abnormalities adversely affecting enamel and tooth development [128–132]. Consequently, routine dental care is important for early detection and institution of ameliorative interventions. To date, the only study reporting dental utilization practices in long-term childhood cancer survivors was organized through the CCSS [133]. Dental utilization practices in a CCSS cohort of over 9,000 adult survivors of pediatric malignancies were below recommended levels, even in patients at highest risk for dental abnormalities. Minority status, low educational attainment, annual household income below $20,000, and lack of health insurance were positive predictors for lack of dental follow-up, which are demographic factors associated with inadequate dental utilization in the general population [133]. Clinicians should emphasize that annual dental follow-up is important for all survivors to maintain oral health. Survivors treated with head and neck radiation involving oral cavity structures may require more frequent dental monitoring and intervention to preserve dentition.

30.4 Summary

The achievement of long-term survival in the majority of adolescent and young adults diagnosed with cancer has appropriately focused efforts on maintenance of future health in this growing population. Following the cancer experience, a large proportion of these young men and women will experience some adverse effect on their health [5]. Through risk-based care and education about the health risks conferred by the cancer experience, clinicians caring for long-term survivors play a critical role in the prevention, diagnosis, and rehabilitation of cancer-related complications and adjustment to chronic health conditions predisposed or exacerbated by cancer. Consequently, health professionals caring for adolescent and young adult cancer survivors may positively influence the future health of this vulnerable group by correcting knowledge deficits, addressing factors that enhance the survivor's vulnerability to health problems, and providing personalized health counseling that promotes the practice of health-promoting behaviors.

Acknowledgments

Dr. Hudson is supported by a Cancer Center Support (CORE) Grant CA 21765 from the National Cancer Institute and by the American Lebanese Syrian Associated Charities (ALSAC). Dr. Oeffinger is supported through grants CA 100474 and CA 106972 from the National Cancer Institute and through the Lance Armstrong Foundation.

References

1. Hudson MM (2005) A model for care across the cancer continuum. Cancer 104:2638–2642
2. Oeffinger KC, Hudson MM (2004) Long-term complications following childhood and adolescent cancer: foundations for providing risk-based health care for survivors. CA Cancer J Clin 54:208–236
3. Robison LL, et al (2002) Study design and cohort characteristics of the Childhood Cancer Survivor Study: a multi-institutional collaborative project. Med Pediatr Oncol 38:229–239
4. Mertens AC, et al (2001) Late mortality experience in five-year survivors of childhood and adolescent cancer: the Childhood Cancer Survivor Study. J Clin Oncol 19:3163–3172
5. Hudson MM, et al (2003) Health status of adult long-term survivors of childhood cancer: a report from the Childhood Cancer Survivor Study. JAMA 290:1583–1592
6. Oeffinger KC (2003) Longitudinal risk-based health care for adult survivors of childhood cancer. Curr Probl Cancer 27:143–167
7. Oeffinger KC, et al (1998) Programs for adult survivors of childhood cancer. J Clin Oncol 16:2864–2867
8. Landier W, et al (2004) Development of risk-based guidelines for childhood cancer survivors: the Children's Oncology Group Long-term Follow-Up Guidelines from the Children's Oncology Group Late Effects Committee and Nursing Discipline. J Clin Oncol 22:4979–4990
9. King V, et al (1996) Symptomatic coronary artery disease after mantle irradiation for Hodgkin disease. Int J Radiat Oncol Biol Phys 36:881–889
10. Hancock SL, Tucker MA, Hoppe RT (1993) Factors affecting late mortality from heart disease after treatment of Hodgkin disease. JAMA 270:1949–1955
11. Constine LS, et al (1997) Cardiac function, perfusion, and morbidity in irradiated long-term survivors of Hodgkin disease. Int J Radiat Oncol Biol Phys 39:897–906
12. Boivin JF, et al (1992) Coronary artery disease mortality in patients treated for Hodgkin disease. Cancer 69:1241–1247
13. Hull MC, et al (2003) Valvular dysfunction and carotid, subclavian, and coronary artery disease in survivors of Hodgkin lymphoma treated with radiation therapy. JAMA 290:2831–2837
14. Adams MJ, et al (2003) Radiation-associated cardiovascular disease. Crit Rev Oncol Hematol 45:55–75
15. Chilcote RR, Baehner RL, Hammond D (1976) Septicemia and meningitis in children splenectomized for Hodgkin disease. N Engl J Med 295:798–800
16. Holdsworth RJ, Irving AD, Cuschieri A (1991) Postsplenectomy sepsis and its mortality rate: actual versus perceived risks. Br J Surg 78:1031–1038
17. Ejstrud P, et al (2000) Risk and patterns of bacteraemia after splenectomy: a population-based study. Scand J Infect Dis 32:521–525
18. Bisharat N, et al (2001) Risk of infection and death among post-splenectomy patients. J Infect 43:182–186
19. Hinkle AS, et al (2004) Cardiovascular complications: cardiotoxicity caused by chemotherapy. In: Wallace WHB, Green D (eds) Late Effects of Childhood Cancer. Oxford University Press, New York, pp 85–100
20. Kremer LC, et al (2002) Frequency and risk factors of subclinical cardiotoxicity after anthracycline therapy in children: a systematic review. Ann Oncol 13:819–829
21. Lipshultz SE, et al (1995) Female sex and drug dose as risk factors for late cardiotoxic effects of doxorubicin therapy for childhood cancer. N Engl J Med 332:1738–1743
22. Neglia JP, et al (2001) Second malignant neoplasms in five-year survivors of childhood cancer: childhood cancer survivor study. J Natl Cancer Inst 93:618–629
23. Hudson MM, et al (1998) Increased mortality after successful treatment for Hodgkin disease. J Clin Oncol 16:3592–3600
24. Green DM, et al (1999) Cancer and cardiac mortality among 15-year survivors of cancer diagnosed during childhood or adolescence. J Clin Oncol 17:3207–3215

25. Mertens AC, et al (2002) Pulmonary complications in survivors of childhood and adolescent cancer. A report from the Childhood Cancer Survivor Study. Cancer 95:2431–2441

26. Gurney JG, et al (2003) Endocrine and cardiovascular late effects among adult survivors of childhood brain tumors: Childhood Cancer Survivor Study. Cancer 97:663–673

27. Sklar CA, et al (2000) Changes in body mass index and prevalence of overweight in survivors of childhood acute lymphoblastic leukemia: role of cranial irradiation. Med Pediatr Oncol 35:91–95

28. Oeffinger KC, et al (2003) Obesity in adult survivors of childhood acute lymphoblastic leukemia: a report from the Childhood Cancer Survivor Study. J Clin Oncol 21:1359–1365

29. Tyc VL, Hudson MM, Hinds P (1999) Health promotion interventions for adolescent cancer survivors. Cognit Behav Pract 6:128–136

30. Kadan-Lottick NS, et al (2002) Childhood cancer survivors' knowledge about their past diagnosis and treatment: Childhood Cancer Survivor Study. JAMA 287:1832–1839

31. Harz KJ, et al (2003) Obesity in patients with craniopharyngioma: assessment of food intake and movement counts indicating physical activity. J Clin Endocrinol Metab 88:5227–5231

32. Mayer EI, et al (2000) Energy expenditure, energy intake and prevalence of obesity after therapy for acute lymphoblastic leukemia during childhood. Horm Res 53:193–199

33. Warner JT, et al (1998) Daily energy expenditure and physical activity in survivors of childhood malignancy. Pediatr Res 43:607–613

34. Nysom K, et al (1998) Bone mass and body composition after cessation of therapy for childhood cancer. Int J Cancer Suppl 11:40–43

35. Kadan-Lottick N, et al (2001) Normal bone mineral density after treatment for childhood acute lymphoblastic leukemia diagnosed between 1991 and 1998. J Pediatr 138:898–904

36. van der Sluis IM, et al (2002) Altered bone mineral density and body composition, and increased fracture risk in childhood acute lymphoblastic leukemia. J Pediatr 141:204–210

37. Oeffinger KC, et al (2001) Cardiovascular risk factors in young adult survivors of childhood acute lymphoblastic leukemia. J Pediatr Hematol Oncol 23:424–430

38. Reilly JJ, et al (1998) Reduced energy expenditure in preobese children treated for acute lymphoblastic leukemia. Pediatr Res 44:557–562

39. Davies JH, et al (2004) Osteopenia, excess adiposity and hyperleptinaemia during 2 years of treatment for childhood acute lymphoblastic leukaemia without cranial irradiation. Clin Endocrinol (Oxf) 60:358–365

40. Hew FL, et al (1998) Growth hormone deficiency and cardiovascular risk. Baillieres Clin Endocrinol Metab 12:199–216

41. Davidson MB (1987) Effect of growth hormone on carbohydrate and lipid metabolism. Endocr Rev 8:115–131

42. Didi M, et al (1995) High incidence of obesity in young adults after treatment of acute lymphoblastic leukemia in childhood. J Pediatr 127:63–67

43. Reilly JJ, et al (2000) Risk factors for excess weight gain in children treated for acute lymphoblastic leukaemia. Int J Obes Relat Metab Disord 24:1537–1541

44. Constine LS, et al (2003) Radiation-associated risk factors for premature cardiovascular disease in childhood cancer survivors include accelerated atherosclerosis. Int J Radiat Oncol Biol Phys 57:S199–200

45. Adams MJ, et al (2003) Radiation-associated cardiovascular disease: manifestations and management. Semin Radiat Oncol 13:346–356

46. Kremer LC, et al (2002) Frequency and risk factors of anthracycline-induced clinical heart failure in children: a systematic review. Ann Oncol 13:503–512

47. Nysom K, et al (1998) Relationship between cumulative anthracycline dose and late cardiotoxicity in childhood acute lymphoblastic leukemia. J Clin Oncol 16:545–550

48. Poutanen T, et al (2003) Long-term prospective follow-up study of cardiac function after cardiotoxic therapy for malignancy in children. J Clin Oncol 21:2349–2356

49. Aisenberg J, et al (1998) Bone mineral density in young adult survivors of childhood cancer. J Pediatr Hematol Oncol 20:241–245

50. Arikoski P, et al (1998) Reduced bone mineral density in long-term survivors of childhood acute lymphoblastic leukemia. J Pediatr Hematol Oncol 20:234–240

51. Kaste SC, et al (2001) Bone mineral decrements in survivors of childhood acute lymphoblastic leukemia: frequency of occurrence and risk factors for their development. Leukemia 15:728–734

52. Mandel K, et al (2004) Skeletal morbidity in childhood acute lymphoblastic leukemia. J Clin Oncol 22:1215–1221

53. Hesseling PB, et al (1998) Bone mineral density in long-term survivors of childhood cancer. Int J Cancer Suppl 11:44–47

54. Paffenbarger RS Jr, et al (1986) Physical activity, all-cause mortality, and longevity of college alumni. N Engl J Med 314:605–613

55. Wei M, et al (1999) Relationship between low cardiorespiratory fitness and mortality in normal-weight, overweight, and obese men. JAMA 282:1547–1553

56. Blair SN, Brodney S (1999) Effects of physical inactivity and obesity on morbidity and mortality: current evidence and research issues. Med Sci Sports Exerc 31: S646–662

57. Martinson BC, O'Connor PJ, Pronk NP (2001) Physical inactivity and short-term all-cause mortality in adults with chronic disease. Arch Intern Med 161:1173–1180

58. Macera CA, Powell KE (2001) Population attributable risk: implications of physical activity dose. Med Sci Sports Exerc 33:S635–639; discussion 640–641

59. Paffenbarger RS Jr, Wing AL, Hyde RT (1978) Physical activity as an index of heart attack risk in college alumni. Am J Epidemiol 108:161–175

60. Manson JE, et al (1999) A prospective study of walking as compared with vigorous exercise in the prevention of coronary heart disease in women. N Engl J Med 341:650–658

61. Fletcher G (1999) Physical inactivity as a risk factor for cardiovascular disease. Am J Med 107:10S–11S

62. Williams PT (2001) Physical fitness and activity as separate heart disease risk factors: a meta-analysis. Med Sci Sports Exerc 33:754–761

63. Lee IM, Paffenbarger RS Jr (1998) Physical activity and stroke incidence: the Harvard Alumni Health Study. Stroke 29:2049–2054

64. Espallargues M, et al (2001) Identifying bone-mass-related risk factors for fracture to guide bone densitometry measurements: a systematic review of the literature. Osteoporos Int 12:811–822

65. Greg, EW, Pereira MA, Caspersen CJ (2000) Physical activity, falls, and fractures among older adults: a review of the epidemiologic evidence. J Am Geriatr Soc 48:883–893

66. Madsen KL, Adams WC, Van Loan MD (1998) Effects of physical activity, body weight and composition, and muscular strength on bone density in young women. Med Sci Sports Exerc 30:114–120

67. Morris JN, et al (1990) Exercise in leisure time: coronary attack and death rates. Br Heart J 63:325–334

68. Whelton SP, et al (2002) Effect of aerobic exercise on blood pressure: a meta-analysis of randomized, controlled trials. Ann Intern Med 136:493–503

69. Manson JE, et al (1991) Physical activity and incidence of non-insulin-dependent diabetes mellitus in women. Lancet 338:774–778

70. Helmrich SP, et al (1991) Physical activity and reduced occurrence of non-insulin-dependent diabetes mellitus. N Engl J Med 325:147–152

71. Wolff I, et al (1999) The effect of exercise training programs on bone mass: a meta-analysis of published controlled trials in pre- and postmenopausal women. Osteoporos Int 9:1–12

72. Valdimarsson O, et al (1999) Lean mass and physical activity as predictors of bone mineral density in 16–20-year old women. J Intern Med 245:489–496

73. Gutin B, et al (1999) Effect of physical training and its cessation on percent fat and bone density of children with obesity. Obes Res 7:208–214

74. Glade MJ (1997) Food, nutrition and the prevention of cancer: a global perspective. American Institute for Cancer Research/World Cancer Research Fund, American Institute for Cancer Research, 1997. Nutrition 15:523–526

75. Friedenreich CM (2001) Physical activity and cancer prevention: from observational to intervention research. Cancer Epidemiol Biomarkers Prev 10:287–301

76. Byers T, et al (2002) American Cancer Society guidelines on nutrition and physical activity for cancer prevention: reducing the risk of cancer with healthy food choices and physical activity. CA Cancer J Clin 52:92–119

77. Krauss RM, et al (2000) AHA Dietary Guidelines: revision 2000: a statement for healthcare professionals from the Nutrition Committee of the American Heart Association. Circulation 102:2284–2299

78. US Department of Agriculture and US Department of Health and Human Services (2000) Nutrition and your health: dietary guidelines for Americans (5th edn). Home and Garden Bulletin No. 232. US Government Printing Office, Washington, DC

79. Slavin JL (2000) Mechanisms for the impact of whole grain foods on cancer risk. J Am Coll Nutr 19:300S–307S

80. McTiernan A (2000) Physical activity and the prevention of breast cancer. Medscape Womens Health 5:E1

81. Slattery ML, et al (1997) Physical activity and colon cancer: a public health perspective. Ann Epidemiol 7:137–145

82. Verloop J, et al (2000) Physical activity and breast cancer risk in women aged 20–54 years. J Natl Cancer Inst 92:128–135

83. Haupt R, et al (1992) Smoking habits in survivors of childhood and adolescent cancer. Med Pediatr Oncol 20:301–306

84. Troyer H, Holmes GE (1988) Cigarette smoking among childhood cancer survivors. Am J Dis Child 142:123

85. Emmons K, et al (2002) Predictors of smoking initiation and cessation among childhood cancer survivors: a report from the childhood cancer survivor study. J Clin Oncol 20:1608–1616

86. Emmons KM, et al (2003) Smoking among participants in the childhood cancer survivors cohort: the Partnership for Health Study. J Clin Oncol 21:189–196

87. Larcombe I, Mott M, Hunt L (2002) Lifestyle behaviours of young adult survivors of childhood cancer. Br J Cancer 87:1204–1209

88. Tao ML, et al (1998) Smoking in adult survivors of childhood acute lymphoblastic leukemia. J Natl Cancer Inst 90:219–225

89. Boivin JF (1995) Smoking, treatment for Hodgkin disease, and subsequent lung cancer risk. J Natl Cancer Inst 87:1502–1503

90. van Leeuwen FE, et al (1995) Roles of radiotherapy and smoking in lung cancer following Hodgkin disease. J Natl Cancer Inst 87:1530–1537

91. Kaldor JM, et al (1992) Lung cancer following Hodgkin disease: a case-control study. Int J Cancer 52:677–681
92. Mulhern RK, et al (1995) Health-related behaviors of survivors of childhood cancer. Med Pediatr Oncol 25:159–165
93. Hollen PJ, Hobbie WL (1993) Risk taking and decision making of adolescent long-term survivors of cancer. Oncol Nurs Forum 20:769–776
94. Hollen PJ, Hobbie WL (1996) Decision making and risk behaviors of cancer-surviving adolescents and their peers. J Pediatr Oncol Nurs 13:121–133; discussion 135–137
95. Hudson MM (2004) Hepatic complications. In: Wallace H, Green DM (eds) Late Effects of Childhood Cancer. Arnold, London pp 170–175
96. Cesaro S, et al (1997) Chronic hepatitis C virus infection after treatment for pediatric malignancy. Blood 90:1315–1320
97. Castellino S, et al (2003) The epidemiology of chronic hepatitis C infection in survivors of childhood cancer an update of the St. Jude Children's Research Hospital hepatitis C seropositive cohort. Blood 103:2460–2466
98. Fink FM, et al (1993) Association of hepatitis C virus infection with chronic liver disease in paediatric cancer patients. Eur J Pediatr 152:490–492
99. Locasciulli A, et al (1997) Prevalence and natural history of hepatitis C infection in patients cured of childhood leukemia. Blood 90:4628–4633
100. Paul IM, et al (1999) Chronic hepatitis C virus infections in leukemia survivors: prevalence, viral load, and severity of liver disease. Blood 93:3672–3677
101. Neilson JR, et al (1996) Chronic hepatitis C in long term survivors of haematological malignancy treated in a single centre. J Clin Pathol 49:230–232
102. Strickland DK, et al (2000) Hepatitis C infection among survivors of childhood cancer. Blood 95:3065–3070
103. Arico M, et al (1994) Hepatitis C virus infection in children treated for acute lymphoblastic leukemia. Blood 84:2919–2922
104. Strickland DK, Jenkins JJ, Hudson MM (2001) Hepatitis C infection and hepatocellular carcinoma after treatment of childhood cancer. J Pediatr Hematol Oncol 23:527–529
105. Swilley S, et al (2002) Hepatitis C infection during treatment for childhood cancer: pitfalls in diagnosis and management. Med Pediatr Oncol 39:58–59
106. Centers for Disease Control and Prevention (1998) Recommendations for prevention and control of Hepatitis C virus (HCV) infection and HCV-related chronic disease. MMWR Recomm Rep 47:1–39
107. Socie G, et al (1999) Long-term survival and late deaths after allogeneic bone marrow transplantation. Late Effects Working Committee of the International Bone Marrow Transplant Registry. N Engl J Med 341:14–21
108. Strasser SI, et al (1999) Cirrhosis of the liver in long-term marrow transplant survivors. Blood 93:3259–3266
109. Yau JC, et al (1986) Chronic graft-versus-host disease complicated by micronodular cirrhosis and esophageal varices. Transplantation 41:129–130
110. Knapp AB, et al (1987) Cirrhosis as a consequence of graft versus host disease. Gastroenterology 92:513–519
111. Agrawal S, Bonkovsky HL (2002) Management of non-alcoholic steatohepatitis: an analytic review. J Clin Gastroenterol 35:253–261
112. Marshall JR, Boyle P (1996) Nutrition and oral cancer. Cancer Causes Control 71:101–111
113. Cheng KK, Day NE (1996) Nutrition and esophageal cancer. Cancer Causes Control 7:33–40
114. Riboli E, Kaaks R, Esteve J (1996) Nutrition and laryngeal cancer. Cancer Causes Control 71:147–156
115. Riboli E (1996) Nutrition and cancer of the respiratory and digestive tract: results from observational and chemoprevention studies. Eur J Cancer Prev 5:9–17
116. Smith-Warner SA, et al (1998) Alcohol and breast cancer in women: a pooled analysis of cohort studies. JAMA 279:535–540
117. Longnecker MP (1994) Alcoholic beverage consumption in relation to risk of breast cancer: meta-analysis and review. Cancer Causes Control 5:73–82
118. Longnecker MP (1995) Alcohol and breast cancer. J Clin Epidemiol 48:497–500
119. Franceschi S (1999) Alcohol and cancer. Adv Exp Med Biol 472:43–49
120. Rimm E (2000) Alcohol and cardiovascular disease. Curr Atheroscler Rep 2:529–535
121. Jemal A, et al (2003) Cancer statistics, 2003. CA Cancer J Clin 53:5–26
122. Swerdlow AJ, et al (1997) Second malignancy in patients with Hodgkin disease treated at the Royal Marsden Hospital. Br J Cancer 75:116–123
123. Olsen JH, et al (1993) Second malignant neoplasms after cancer in childhood or adolescence. Nordic Society of Paediatric Haematology and Oncology Association of the Nordic Cancer Registries. BMJ 307:1030–1036
124. Meadows AT, et al (1985) Second malignant neoplasms in children: an update from the Late Effects Study Group. J Clin Oncol 3:532–538
125. Rhodes AR (1995) Public education and cancer of the skin. What do people need to know about melanoma and nonmelanoma skin cancer? Cancer 75:613–636
126. Buller MK, Loescher LJ, Buller DB (1994) "Sunshine and skin health": a curriculum for skin cancer prevention education. J Cancer Educ 9:155–162
127. Buller DB, Callister MA, Reichert T (1995) Skin cancer prevention by parents of young children: health information sources, skin cancer knowledge, and sun-protection practices. Oncol Nurs Forum 22:1559–1566

128. Kaste SC, Hopkins KP, Jenkins JP III (1994) Abnormal odontogenesis in children treated with radiation and chemotherapy: imaging findings. AJR Am J Roentgenol 162:1407–1411

129. Kaste SC, et al (1997) Dental abnormalities in children treated for acute lymphoblastic leukemia. Leukemia 11:792–796

130. Kaste SC, et al (1998) Dental abnormalities in children treated for neuroblastoma. Med Pediatr Oncol 30:22–27

131. Alpaslan G, et al (1999) Disturbances in oral and dental structures in patients with pediatric lymphoma after chemotherapy: a preliminary report. Oral Surg Oral Med Oral Pathol Oral Radiol Endod 87:317–321

Chapter 30

132. Dens F, et al (1995) Dental caries, gingival health, and oral hygiene of long term survivors of paediatric malignant diseases. Arch Dis Child 72:129–132

133. Yeazel MW, et al (2004) An examination of the dental utilization practices of adult survivors of childhood cancer: a report from the Childhood Cancer Survivor Study. J Public Health Dent 64:50–54

134. Tyc VL, Hudson MM, Hinds P, et al (1997) Tobacco use among pediatric cancer patients: recommendations for developing clinical smoking interventions. J Clin Oncol 15:2194–2204

Information and Resources for Young Adults and Adolescents with Cancer

David R. Freyer • Leonard J. Mattano

Contents

31.1 Introduction

In the 1970s and 1980s, the popular American educational television series called "School House Rock!" inspired children and teens with its slogan, "Knowledge is Power" [1]. For today's young adult cancer patients and survivors, that aphorism remains as true now as it was when many of them first discovered the value of learning through the program's catchy songs. As elaborated by Ruccione, successful cancer survivorship addresses the concerns of normalization, living with uncertainty, living with compromise, and overcoming stigma [2]. This requires that healthcare professionals work closely with survivors, their families, and support and advocacy organizations to create a "partnership of empowerment" [3]. It would stand to reason that this involves providing survivors with information concerning their underlying disease, potential medical complications, a range of related psychosocial and financial issues, and available resources. Because information represents knowledge acquired in any manner [4], knowledge is indeed power in the realm of cancer survivorship.

31.2 The Value of Sharing Medical Information

Providing information is beneficial to cancer patients. Studies indicate that nearly 90% of adults with cancer desire maximal information across the continuum of their care [4–6]. Chelf and colleagues reviewed empirical studies that demonstrate measurable benefits from providing cancer patients with information in the areas of treatment decision-making, understanding about treatment, and management of pain and fatigue [4]. Obtaining information is a key coping strategy for some cancer patients [7] and may decrease anxiety through an enhanced sense of control [4]. Yet, in a large, recent study of adult cancer survivors conducted by the Office of Cancer Survivorship at the United States National Cancer Institute (US-NCI), Hewitt and colleagues [8] found that only 58% had received patient education materials from their healthcare providers (94% of whom found them to be helpful). Only 10.9% had direct contact with major cancer organizations such as the US-NCI or the American Cancer Society.

31.3 Methods of Sharing Medically Related Information

There are several effective methods for delivering information to cancer patients. Face-to-face verbal contact between patient and healthcare team is widely agreed to be the cornerstone and the "gold standard" for information sharing. Several studies confirm that healthcare providers are the major and preferred sources of information for cancer patients [4, 5, 9, 10]. In addition to allowing for an exchange of information, direct contact achieves the other aims of medical communication, which are to create a good interpersonal relationship and facilitate medical decision-making [11]. At the same time, research indicates that verbal communication is enhanced if supplemented appropriately with effective materials [4, 9, 12]. These may include written materials (booklets, pamphlets, brochures, books, monographs, and photocopied articles), audio-visual aids (video or audio tapes, DVDs), and computer-based approaches (interactive learning modules and utilization of the World-Wide Web, or Internet). Regardless of the modality used, the caveats summarized by Mills and Sullivan [9] concerning written materials are applicable to all of them. Supplemental information should: (1) reinforce rather than introduce critical new ideas; (2) be accurate and current; (3) address the actual concerns of patients; (4) be presented in a style and at an educational level that can be understood by patients; and (5) be of high quality and presented in an appealing way.

31.4 The Expanding Role of Internet-Based Health and Medical Information Resources

The vast repository of information accessible on the Internet has a prominent role for persons seeking health and medical information. According to a recent survey conducted by the Harris poll, 69% of American adults go on-line from home, work, school, the library or elsewhere [13]. The same survey found that 51% (111 million adults) have ever looked for health-related information on-line, and 35% had done so within the previous month [13]. In a previous survey, it was found that young adults aged 18 to 29 years old accounted for the largest proportion of American adults who go on-line [14]. In that survey, Internet users tended to be Caucasian (76%), have some post-high-school education (63%), and be relatively affluent (46% with an annual income of greater than US$50,000).

The Internet is also a major source of health-related information for cancer patients. In two recent studies conducted in the United States [15] and Canada [5], approximately 50% of adult cancer patients obtained information from the Internet. This was supplemented with printed resources by 79% of the Internet users [15]. In a study of Internet use among a cohort of adults with lung cancer, an association was found with educational level and income [10].

A recent study from the United Kingdom by Ziebland and colleagues [16] suggests that Internet use serves several valuable functions for oncology patients, especially for young adults and including those who are post-treatment. One hundred and seventy-five men and women aged 18 to 83 years with cancer of the breast, bowel, cervix, prostate, or testicle were interviewed. Subjects were recruited from all stages of management (from diagnosis through to long-term follow-up). On average, 44% of patients or their friends and family accessed the Internet (range 26 to 59% across the five diagnostic groups). The highest Internet use was noted in the diagnostic groups having the youngest subjects: testicle (59%), breast (51%), and cervix

(48%). Valuable qualitative data were collected indicating why subjects found the Internet helpful. The main reasons given for using the Internet related to privacy, round-the-clock access, and the ability to search for different types and levels of information as and when needed. The main reasons given by those who did not use the Internet related to a lack of home computer access, and technological unfamiliarity. The Internet was used by these cancer patients during all phases of their illness, including short- and long-term follow-up. Immediately posttreatment, information most frequently sought concerned side effects, reassurance about symptoms and advice on finances. In long-term follow-up, survivors desired to share experience and advice, to contact support groups and to become active in cancer advocacy [16].

Despite its clear value for some, direct information seeking on the Internet by cancer patients faces several limitations. As indicated in the Harris poll cited previously, despite enormous growth in recent years, 30% of adults in the United States are still not on-line and the percentage of users may have reached a plateau [13]. While demographic studies indicate that most users are younger (which could imply a greater comfort level with the technology that will persist with age), they also reveal them to be Caucasian, relatively affluent,

and better educated [13, 17]. Finally, studies have documented concerns about the quality of health information contained on the Internet, in terms of difficulty encountered in searching for relevant information; bias and inaccuracy of key clinical elements in some websites; and the relatively high-grade level of reading needed to understand them [18, 19]. Biermann [20] has drawn attention to the fact that consumers tend to judge health information websites by their "net appeal" (attractiveness of the site) rather than their content.

To address the above concerns and assist patients in searching the Internet for medical information, criteria have been developed for judging the quality of health-related websites and the information they contain (summarized in Table 31.1).

31.5 Using This Chapter

This chapter provides the healthcare professional with a selection of websites (and, by extension, other information obtainable through those websites) that may be shared with their young adult and adolescent survivors of childhood cancer, in order to provide them with appropriate medical care, health-related information, and other resources. It should be noted that the

Table 31.1 Criteria for evaluating medical and health information websites

Health on the Net Foundation: Eight principles in code of conduct[a]	National Cancer Institute: "Ten things to know about evaluating medical resources on the Web"[b]
1. Authority Any medical advice is provided only by medically trained and qualified professionals unless a clear statement made to contrary.	1. Who runs the site? *Those responsible for the site should be clearly indicated.*
2. Complementarity *Information is designed to support, not replace, the relationship between the patient and existing physician.*	2. Who pays for the site? *The source of a site's funding should be clearly stated. Does it sell advertising? Is it sponsored by a company with a financial interest in the product or information presented?*
3. Confidentiality *Confidentiality of personal identity and data of patient are fully respected.*	3. What is the purpose of the site? *Related to who runs and pays for the site, the purpose of the site should be clearly stated and will help evaluate the trustworthiness of information. Check the "About This Site" link.*

Table 31.1 *(continued)*

Health on the Net Foundation: Eight principles in code of conduct[a]	National Cancer Institute: "Ten things to know about evaluating medical resources on the Web"[b]
4. Attribution *Information is supported by clear references to source data with direct links where possible.*	4. Where does the information come from? *Many health and medical sites post information from other sites. If the information is not original, this should be clearly indicated.*
5. Justifiability *Any claims relating to benefits of a specific treatment, commercial product or service should be supported by appropriate, balanced data with sources cited.*	5. What is the basis of the information? *In addition to identifying the author, the evidence for material presented should be described. Medical facts and figures should be referenced. Opinions and advice should be clearly distinguished from evidence-based conclusions.*
6. Transparency of authorship *Information should be provided in the clearest possible manner. Contact addresses should be clearly provided if site visitors wish to obtain more information.*	6. How is the information selected? *Is there an editorial board? Is material reviewed by persons with excellent credentials before it is posted?*
7. Transparency of sponsorship *Support for the site should be clearly identified, including all organizations that have contributed funding.*	7. How current is the information? *Health and medical websites should be reviewed for currency and accuracy on a regular, frequent basis indicated by the date.*
8. Honesty in advertising and editorial policy *A clear statement about advertising as a source of funding should be made, if applicable. A brief description of the advertising policy should be displayed on the site. A clear distinction should be made between advertising or promotional material and the original content provided by the organization operating the site.*	8. How does the site choose links to other sites? *Check the site's policy for choosing links. Some may link to any site that asks or pays for a link, whereas others link only to those meeting certain criteria.*
	9. What information about you does the site collect, and why? *Many sites routinely track visits to determine which pages are being used most. Others may ask a visitor to "subscribe" or "become a member." This may require paying a fee or revealing personal information. Any credible site will indicate exactly what will be done with the information. Be certain to understand the privacy policy, which should be stated clearly. Don't sign up for anything that is not fully understood.*
	10. How does the site manage interactions with visitors? *There should always be a way to contact the site operators with problems, feedback and questions. Are chat rooms or discussions moderated by an expert? Spend some time reading the discussion before becoming a participant.*

[a] Available at: http://www.hon.ch/HONcode/Conduct.html
[b] Available at: http://cancer.gov/cancerinfo/ten-things-to-know

information available through these websites is meant to be shared in the context of an educational approach appropriate for each patient's needs, comprehension, learning style, and available resources.

Information available through these websites has been grouped into five categories: resources for obtaining appropriate medical care (Table 31.2; for assistance in locating qualified providers of cancer treatment and follow-up services for young adults and adolescents); resources for medical information (Table 31.3; for finding specific, detailed information related to cancer treatment and its long-term side effects); *Resources for Financial Information and Assistance* (Table 4; for assisting survivors with issues related to employment, health and life insurance, and paying for medical care); Resources for Information on Wellness and Disease Prevention (Table 31.5; for educating survivors on improving personal health and preventing subsequent cancer and other medical problems); and resources for psychosocial issues and survivor advocacy (Table 31.6; for helping survivors cope with the emotional aspects of cancer and become active in promoting survivorship). Although some websites span more than one category, it was felt that this subject-directed approach would make the information most accessible to the reader.

In selecting websites for inclusion, recognized criteria for evaluating health and medical websites were applied (Table 31.1). At the same time, the list of websites is not represented as being exhaustive, for the ongoing explosion of Web-based health and medical information has made it extremely difficult to create an international compendium that is truly comprehensive. Excellent websites not listed directly will be available through links within those websites that are. An emphasis was placed on including websites particularly relevant to the posttreatment survivor in the young adult or adolescent age group. However, in keeping with the US-NCI Office of Cancer Survivorship's definition of survivor (from the time of diagnosis throughout the balance of that person's life; National Cancer Policy Board 2003) [21], many of the websites provide information directed toward the patient recently diagnosed or receiving treatment. All websites were accessed for currency in Dec. 2006.

Given the aforementioned caveats about sharing medically related information, the following points should be considered when utilizing the websites provided in this chapter:

1. What kind of information or resources does the patient need? For most patients – especially soon after diagnosis – the most effective information is that which is carefully chosen by the health professional to supplement verbal communication and address specific needs (as voiced by the patient and/or recognized by the professional). Some experienced patients with on-line skills may wish to explore this list of websites on their own.

2. What modality of information sharing is best for the patient? For some patients, direct access to websites suggested by the health professional may be the most satisfying. For others, written information or telephone numbers obtained by the health professional through these websites may be more appropriate. Treatment centers may wish to maintain an inventory of written materials from organizations represented in this list of websites.

3. Does the patient have computer access and requisite skills? A substantial proportion of patients will continue not to have ready access to a computer, Internet service, and/or essential computer skills, and the comfort level for using them. For them, printed materials may be the most appropriate. In many treatment centers, computers with Internet access are now provided routinely for patient use at no charge. Assistance should be available for using them on-site during hours convenient for patients. Basic Internet training allows some patients to continue their exploration of Web-based resources at home (if they have a computer with Internet access) or in their own communities (through their workplace or a public library).

4. Which team members carry out patient education? The information provided through these websites crosses professional disciplines and should be made available for physicians, mid-level providers, nurses, and medical social workers to review and use in their interactions with patients. Ideally, these professionals should familiarize themselves in advance with these websites and the information contained therein.

Table 31.2 Resources for obtaining appropriate medical care. *NCI* National Cancer Institute

Website name	Website sponsor (if different)	Summary of information or services provided	Website address
BMT *infonet*	Blood and Bone Marrow Transplant Information Network	Locator service for blood and bone marrow transplant centers where long-term follow-up services or referrals will be available.	www.bmtnews.org
Cancer Council Australia		Under "Information About Cancer" tab, information for locating a cancer specialist in Australia.	www.cancer.org.au
Cancer*Index*	Guide to Internet Resources for Cancer	Broad, inclusive website that is uniquely international in scope, providing extensive links to treatment and follow-up centers in many countries around the world.	www.cancerindex.org
Candle-lighters	Candlelighters Childhood Cancer Foundation	Under "Treatment" > "Comprehensive Follow Up Programs" tabs, description of benefits and desirable characteristics of comprehensive long-term follow-up clinics. Tips for arranging for insurance coverage for evaluation in same.	www.candlelighters.org
CTEP (Clinical Trials Evaluation Program)	National Cancer Institute	Links to home pages of all NCI-supported cooperative groups; useful for locating institutions participating in NCI-funded clinical trials and providing follow-up services for young adult and adolescent survivors.	ctep.cancer.gov/resources/coop.html
CureSearch	Children's Oncology Group and National Childhood Cancer Foundation	Under "Resource Directory" tab, a geographical listing of all Children's Oncology Group institutions in the United States, Canada and Australia. The majority of these provide survivor services to adolescents and some young adults. Those that do not can provide referrals for young adult care.	www.curesearch.org
Macmillan *Cancer Relief*		Organization in the United Kingdom for patients and health professionals. Information includes how to become a Macmillan-affiliated oncology health professional; opportunities for professional development; how to provide a healing care environment for cancer patients.	www.cancerlink.org
National Coalition for Cancer Survivorship		Extensive website with broad information and multiple links. Under "Resource Guide" tab, a listing of NCI-designated comprehensive cancer centers and other centers providing long-term follow-up services to young adult survivors.	www.canceradvocacy.org
Patient-Centered Guides	O'Reilly and Associates	Under "Childhood Cancer Survivors" > "Organizations" tabs, list of well-established survivor programs in the United States meeting certain criteria for inclusion; list not necessarily exhaustive.	www.patientcenters.com

Table 31.2 (continued)

Website name	Website sponsor (if different)	Summary of information or services provided	Website address
Pediatric Oncology Resource Center		List of well-established survivor programs in the United States meeting certain criteria for inclusion; list not necessarily exhaustive.	www.acor.org/ped-onc/survivors
uicc-global cancer control	International Union Against Cancer	Under "Collaboration" tab, contact information for an extensive, international list of member institutions categorized by country, which may be useful for locating care providers.	www.uicc.org

Table 31.3 Resources for obtaining medical information

Website name	Website sponsor (if different)	Summary of information or services provided	Website address
American Cancer Society		Under "Survivors" > "Support for Survivors and Patients" > "Support Programs and Services" tabs, access to "Tender Loving Care" magazine-catalog for information and affordable products for women coping with complications of cancer treatment, including wigs, hairpieces, breast forms, prostheses, bras, swimwear, and more.	www.cancer.org
American Dental Association		Under the "Your Oral Health" tab, this official website of the American Dental Association provides an extensive list of topics pertinent to the cancer patient.	www.ada.org
BMT *infonet*	Blood and Bone Marrow Transplant Information Network	Access to multiple resources of importance to blood and bone marrow transplant patients and survivors. Locator service for transplant centers. Database of transplant drugs and information on major side effects.	www.bmtnews.org
Canadian Cancer Society		Information on specific cancers; cancer encyclopedia. On-line directory of over 4,000 cancer-related services throughout Canada.	www.cancer.ca
Cancer Council Australia		Under "Information About Cancer" tab, numerous links addressing cancer and treatment-related issues for Australian patients.	www.cancer.org.au
Cancer Information Service	National Cancer Institute	Cancer-related information and education network sponsored by the NCI. Toll-free numbers for personalized, confidential responses to specific questions about cancer given in English or Spanish. Under "Cancer Resources" tab, links to informative "What You Need to Know About…" series of disease-specific on-line monographs.	cis.nci.nih.gov

Table 31.3 (*continued*)

Website name	Website sponsor (if different)	Summary of information or services provided	Website address
CancerBACUP		Extensive website for patients in the United Kingdom and mainland Europe. Under respective tabs, information about specific cancers and treatments. Under "Treatment" tab, includes detailed discussion of radiation therapy and side effects. Under "Resources and Support" tab, advice on dealing with numerous long-term side effects and also fertility information and recommendations. Currently has link to CancerBACUP-sponsored website for teenagers that is under construction.	www.cancerbacup.org.uk
CancerHelp UK	Cancer Research UK	Detailed information about specific cancers and treatment. Under "Cancer Treatments" tab, informative discussion of long-term side effects of radiation therapy on various body systems. Suggested reading list available.	www.cancerhelp.org.uk
Cancer*Index*	Guide to Internet Resources for Cancer	Broad, inclusive website that is uniquely international in scope (a major strength of site) providing extensive links to information about specific cancers, treatment modalities, and short- and long-term side effects. Information offered in multiple languages for some resources.	www.cancerindex.org
Cancernet.co.uk		Site in the United Kingdom providing extensive information on specific malignancies and conventional treatment; alternative, hormonal, and other treatments; and a range of fertility and sexuality issues for both women and men.	www.cancernet.co.uk
Cancer-SourceKids.com	Association of Pediatric Oncology Nurses	Under "Teens" and "Learn About Cancer" tabs, provides description of malignancies common in teens and children; and articles written for young people describing need for follow-up care and potential long-term problems.	www.cancersourcekids.com
Candle-lighters	Candlelighters Childhood Cancer Foundation	Under "Treatment" tab, information available concerning treatment modalities, numerous late effects important for the older childhood cancer survivor.	www.candlelighters.org
Chemocare.com	Scott Hamilton and The Cleveland Clinic Foundation	Comprehensive and accessible website for information about chemotherapy and related issues, including specific drugs, managing side effects and maintaining nutrition. Thorough summary of complementary therapy options.	www.chemocare.com
Childhood Cancers	National Cancer Institute	In-depth information on types of childhood cancers; also numerous NCI links for topics related to childhood cancer and treatment.	cancer.gov/cancerinfo/types/childhoodcancers

Table 31.3 (*continued*)

Website name	Website sponsor (if different)	Summary of information or services provided	Website address
Coping with Cancer	National Cancer Institute	In-depth information on dealing with a broad range of side effects resulting from cancer treatment.	cancer.gov/cancertopics/coping
CureSearch	Children's Oncology Group and National Childhood Cancer Foundation	Under "After Treatment" tab, concise, informative, understandable, downloadable summaries of numerous important medical problems (late effects) that may affect some survivors. Under "For Health Professionals" > "Late Effects" tabs, comprehensive, evidence-based medical guidelines for long-term follow-up care are downloadable.	www.curesearch.org
Facing Forward Series: Life After Cancer Treatment	National Cancer Institute	Comprehensive discussion of follow-up care after treatment: what to expect, how to make the most of it.	cancer.gov/cancerinfo/life-after-treatment
fertileHOPE		Comprehensive website addressing the challenge of infertility following cancer treatment, including medical information, parenthood options, resource directory, and financial assistance.	www.fertilehope.org
Liddy Shriver Sarcoma Initiative	Liddy Shriver Sarcoma Initiative	Sarcoma information not readily available elsewhere, particularly for soft-tissue sarcomas. A newsletter (http://liddyshriversarcomainitiative.org/Newsletters/esun_newsletter.htm) reports on recent medical literature and clinical trials.	http://liddyshriversarcomainitiative.org/
Livestrong	Lance Armstrong Foundation	Under "Physical Topics" tab, description of several physical issues that may affect survivors, including both male and female infertility and sexual dysfunction. Healthy behaviors and physical rehabilitation discussed.	www.livestrong.org
Macmillan *cancer relief*		Organization in the United Kingdom with information on cancer, detection, diagnosis, and treatment; also complementary treatment approaches. On-line directory of cancer leaflets, booklets, books and videotapes endorsed by Macmillan.	www.cancerlink.org
Medline Plus	National Institutes of Health	Extensive website offering information, directories of providers, links and lists of resources for a wide range of health-related information. Under "Health Topics" tab, provides comprehensive information on specific cancers and related topics.	medlineplus.gov

Table 31.3 (*continued*)

Website name	Website sponsor (if different)	Summary of information or services provided	Website address
National Center for Complementary and Alternative Medicine	National Institutes of Health	Health information and links to resources about complementary and alternative medicines (CAM), specific alerts and advisories, types of treatments, and how to evaluate CAM practitioners.	nccam.nih.gov
National Coalition for Cancer Survivorship		Under "Resource Guide" and "Essential Care" tabs, in-depth information on specific underlying diagnoses; medical management of pain and other major side effects during and after cancer treatment and more. Much of the information is available in non-English language translations.	www.canceradvocacy.org
People Living With Cancer	American Society of Clinical Oncology	Under "Cancer Type" tab, description of malignancies common in young adults. Under "Coping" tab, discussion of fertility following cancer treatment and pregnancy and cancer, with links to additional resources.	www.plwc.org
PubMed	National Library of Medicine	Powerful search engine of biomedical literature for health-related citations dating to the 1950s.	www.ncbi.nlm.nih.gov/PubMed
Quackwatch – Your Guide to Health Fraud, Quackery and Intelligent Decisions	Quackwatch, Inc. (Stephen Barret, MD)	Topical website providing information and perspectives to protect healthcare consumers from fraud, questionable therapies and misleading information. Portions of site have been translated into languages other than English.	www.quackwatch.org
Teens Living With Cancer	Melissa's Living Legacy Foundation and Children's Oncology Group	Friendly site with language and graphics designed for young adults and teens. Under "Cancer Facts" tab, includes description of common malignancies and their treatment in teens and young adults; also medical dictionary with understandable definitions.	www.teenslivingwithcancer.org
Testicular Cancer Resource Center	Association of Cancer Online Resources	Very complete site for medical and related information concerning this specific cancer of teenage and young adult males, including late effects.	tcrc.acor.org
Ulman Cancer Fund for Young Adults		Under "Treatment Decision Tools" tab, a decision-support tool to assist young adults in understanding treatment options and side effects.	www.ulmanfund.org
Young Survival Coalition		Website of international organization devoted to supporting young women under 40 years of age diagnosed with breast cancer. Information provided on current treatment, research, community branches, and advocacy.	www.youngsurvival.org

Table 31.4 Resources for financial information and assistance

Website name	Website sponsor (if different)	Summary of information or services provided	Website address
American Cancer Society		Under "Survivors" > "Support for Survivors and Patients" > "Support Programs and Services" tabs, access to "Taking Charge of Money Matters" workshop for dealing with financial concerns.	www.cancer.org
Cancer Survivors On Line		Information and additional links and references about financial assistance, health insurance, cancer-related disability, and employment issues; includes summary of the Americans with Disability Act as it applies to cancer survivors.	www.cancersurvivors.org
CancerBACUP		Extensive website for patients in the United Kingdom and mainland Europe. Under "Resources and Support" tab, detailed information about financial issues, including practical advice and resources for assistance.	www.cancerbacup.org.uk
Cancer*Care*		Under "Financial Needs" tab, information and links for finding financial assistance, including programs offered by this organization.	www.cancercare.org
Cancernet.co.uk		Information about insurance and legal issues for cancer patients in the United Kingdom.	www.cancernet.co.uk
Candlelighters	Childhood Cancer Foundation Canada	Under "Programs" tab, information on CCFC Bursaries available for survivors in Canada planning to attend college.	www.candlelighters.ca
Chemocare.com	Scott Hamilton and The Cleveland Clinic Foundation	Comprehensive website for information about chemotherapy. Under "Before and After Chemo" tab, discusses and offers links about financial assistance programs to help pay for chemotherapy medications and treatments.	www.chemocare.com
Childhood Cancer Ombudsman Program	Childhood Brain Tumor Foundation	Investigation and resolution of patient-initiated complaints related to employment and insurance.	www.childhoodbraintumor.org/ombuds.html
CureSearch	Children's Oncology Group and National Childhood Cancer Foundation	Under "After Treatment" tab, information about specific insurance programs and for dealing with insurance issues and denials.	www.curesearch.org
fertileHope		Information and links about insurance coverage of infertility and adoption services, and financial assistance programs for fertility preservation.	www.fertilehope.org
Georgetown University Health Policy Institute		Extensive on-line consumer guides for obtaining and keeping health insurance in the United States; information is specific to all states and District of Columbia.	www.healthinsuranceinfo.net

Table 31.4 (*continued*)

Website name	Website sponsor (if different)	Summary of information or services provided	Website address
Henry J. Kaiser Family Foundation		Consumer guide to handling disputes with employer-based or private health plans.	www.kff.org/consumerguide
Leukemia and Lymphoma Society		Under "Patient Services" > "Stay Informed" > "National Education Workshops" > "Survivor Education Series" tabs, offers access to teaching modules of the "Cancer: Keys to Survivorship" program, which provide specific information and suggested resources for addressing employment issues, cancer-based job discrimination, health insurance regulations and how to obtain and collect health insurance benefits.	www.leukemia-lymphoma.org
Livestrong	Lance Armstrong Foundation	Under "Practical Topics" tab, addresses several related issues including employment discrimination, health and life insurance, life expectancy, planning for the future and others.	www.livestrong.org
NeedyMeds		An information source for pharmaceutical company-sponsored free medication programs for qualified patients lacking insurance. Also links to discount pre-scription card programs, state-sponsored programs and Medicaid sites for assistance in obtaining medications.	www.needymeds.com
National Coalition for Cancer Survivorship		Extensive website. Under "Essential Care" tab, wealth of detailed information regarding employment rights, maximizing health insurance benefits, and how to find potential sources of financial help for cancer survivors. Under "Resources" > "Essential Care" tabs, numerous links and contact information for resources on employment rights and insurance/financial assistance. Under "Cancer Survivor Toolbox" tab, access to skill-building module for helping underinsured and uninsured cancer patients pay for care.	www.canceradvocacy.org
National Children's Cancer Society		Under "How We Can Help" > "Cancer Resources" tabs, extensive list of links to obtain information about (1) health insurance and its legal aspects; (2) college scholarships and more. Under "Program Services" tab, information and on-line application for direct financial assistance from the National Children's Cancer Society for paying insurance premiums and for aspects of medical care.	www.nationalchildrenscancersociety.com

Table 31.4 (continued)

Website name	Website sponsor (if different)	Summary of information or services provided	Website address
Outlook-Life Beyond Cancer	University. of Wisconsin Children's Hospital	(1) Information on how to choose a health insurance plan and prepare for coverage and employment; (2) Information and links to federal, state, and community resources that can provide insurance coverage or financial assistance; (3) Discusses how prior treatment may affect job performance, how to confront medical history at work, and survivor rights at work.	www.outlook-life.org
Patient Advocate Foundation		Active assistance on behalf of patients to resolve insurance, job retention, and/or debt crisis matters.	www.patientadvocate.org
Patient-Centered Guides	O'Reilly and Associates	Extensive website with wealth of information for survivors. Site includes excerpts from books and articles concerning job- and insurance-related issues.	www.patientcenters.com/survivors
Pediatric Oncology Resource Center	Association of cancer online Resources	Extensive list of college scholarships available to cancer survivors.	www.acor.org/ped-onc/scholarships/
Surviving and Moving Forward	The SAMFund	The SAMFund is an organization dedicated to providing grants and scholarships to young adult survivors of cancer as a way to assist in the financial transition off treatment into the "real world."	www.thesamfund.org
Ulman Cancer Fund for Young Adults		Under "Scholarship Info" tab, information on college scholarships available for qualified students living with cancer.	www.ulmanfund.org

Table 31.5 Resources for information on wellness and disease prevention

Website name	Website sponsor (if different)	Summary of information or services provided	Website address
2bMe – A Site for Teens with Cancer	CTFA Foundation and American Cancer Sosiety	Colorful, upbeat website that promotes personal empowerment by providing practical information on skin care, nutrition, activity, and dealing with hair loss (with links to finding head-gear that suits one's style).	www.2bme.org

Table 31.5 (continued)

Website name	Website sponsor (if different)	Summary of information or services provided	Website address
American Cancer Society		Under "Health Information Seekers" > "Prevention and Early Detection" tabs, recommendations for maintaining personal health after treatment, including nutritional and physical activity, cancer prevention and early detection. Under "Survivors" > "Support for Survivors and Patients" > "Support Programs and Services" tabs, a list of several American-Cancer-Society-sponsored programs, including a nutritional and activity improvement program for teens, employee wellness, smoking cessation, and various cancer screening programs.	www.cancer.org
American Institute for Cancer Research		Nutritional and exercise guidelines for survivors.	www.aicr.org/survivor
Canadian Cancer Society		Contact information for Smoker's Helpline available in each province for all smokers, whether or not they are ready to quit. Information concerning genetic cancer risks, cancer-specific screening recommendations, environmental contaminants, and staying well through good nutrition and physical activity.	www.cancer.ca
Cancer Council Australia		Under "Cancer Prevention" tab, information about smoking cessation and prevention of various cancers; includes links to Australian prevention and screening programs. Under "Sun Protection Products" tab, information about Council-endorsed sun protection products and where to obtain them.	www.cancer.org.au
CancerBACUP		Extensive website for patients in the United Kingdom and mainland Europe. Under "Resources and Support" tab, detailed and practical discussion of diet for cancer patients, including special dietary considerations for those who have had stomach surgery.	www.cancerbacup.org.uk
CancerHelp UK	Cancer Research UK	Under "Worried About Cancer?" tab, thorough discussion of cancer screening and prevention. Under "Healthy Eating" tab, detailed, sensible information on nutrition and cooking for cancer patients.	www.cancerhelp.org.uk
Cancernet. co.uk		Site in the United Kingdom offering general and contact information on smoking cessation. Detailed information on dietary and exercise issues.	www.cancernet.co.uk
familydoctor. org	American Academy of Family Physicians	Prevention and wellness information under the headings of healthy living, men's and women's health, health tools and more.	familydoctor.org

Table 31.5 (*continued*)

Website name	Website sponsor (if different)	Summary of information or services provided	Website address
Livestrong	Lance Armstrong Foundation	Under "Survivorship Tools" tab, provides templates for keeping track of medical treatment, creating a health journal, and organizing important, practical information. Under "Physical Topics" tab, healthy behaviors to recover and maintain health are discussed in detail with additional resources provided.	www.livestrong.org
National Children's Cancer Society		Under "How We Can Help" > "Cancer Resources" tabs, extensive list of links including several for smoking cessation information and programs.	www.nationalchildrenscancersociety.com
National Coalition of Cancer Survivorship		Under "Essential Care" tab, extensive information on nutrition and exercise. Under "Resources" > "Essential Care" tabs, links for additional information and help concerning wellness, quality of life, sleep issues, fertility and sexuality, exercise and more.	www.canceradvocacy.org
Office of Cancer Survivorship	National Cancer Institute	Links to federal guidelines and related information for nutrition and cancer screening.	dccps.nci.nih.gov/ocs/resources.html
Outlook-Life Beyond Cancer	University of Wisconsin Children's Hospital	Under "Health Issues and Concerns" tab, Wellness Management offers description of the philosophy and benefits of several health practices for prevention and early detection of adult cancers.	www.outlook-life.org
Patient-Centered Guides	O'Reilly and Associates	Extensive website with wealth of information for survivors. Site includes links to excerpts from books and articles dealing with emotional and psychological challenges, achieving successful transition to adulthood and adult-oriented care, the meaning of surviving life-threatening illness, and related topics	www.patientcenters/survivors
Ulman Cancer Fund for Young Adults		Under "Prevention Tips" tab, pointers for preventing and recognizing cancer of the skin, breast, testicle, and colon	www.ulmanfund.org
WebMD		Extensive website providing wealth of general health information useful to survivors. Under "Condition Centers" tab, in-depth discussions of diseases, conditions and health topics, including diet and nutrition, fitness and exercise, mental health, infertility, men's and women's health issues, sexuality , and much more.	www.webmd.com

Table 31.6 Resources for psychosocial issues and survivor advocacy

Website name	Website sponsor (if different)	Summary of information or services provided	Website Address
Canadian Cancer Society		On-line directory of over 4,000 cancer-related services throughout Canada. Opportunities for donating and getting involved in advocacy efforts. Information for those wishing to donate hair for wigs.	www.cancer.ca
Cancer Survivors On Line		Under "Resources" tab, references and links for information on personal relationships, including communication and sexuality for the survivor.	www.cancersurvivors.org
CancerBACUP		Extensive website for patients in the United Kingdom and mainland Europe. Under "Resources and Support" tab, extensive index of information about CancerBACUP services and centers and other support organizations; detailed discussions of coping with emotional effects and sexuality. Under "Get Involved" tab, multiple opportunities for international events and adventures to raise funds and awareness.	www.cancerbacup.org.uk
CancerHelp UK	Cancer Research UK	Under "Help and Support" tab, extensive list of links and other contact information for general and cancer-specific support organizations in the United Kingdom.	www.cancerhelp.org.uk
CanTeen	The Australian Organization for Young People Living with Cancer	CanTeen is an Australian national organization providing support for adolescents and young adults living with cancer. Member participation is encouraged in camps, other outings, and educational meetings.	www.canteen.org.au
Candlelight-ers	Childhood Cancer Foundation Canada	Under "Programs" tab, information on Candlelighters Teens, a Canada-wide network to support, develop and empower teens with cancer. Contact information provided by province.	www.candlelighters.ca
Children's Cause		Under "Policy" > "Quality Cancer Care and Survivorship" tabs, information about policies, issues, Congressional news, and advocacy resources related to ensuring quality of care.	www.childrenscause.org
CureSearch	Children's Oncology Group and National Childhood Cancer Foundation	Ideas and opportunities for assisting both individuals and organizations in the fight against childhood cancer. Links to legislative contacts provided.	www.curesearch.org
Gilda's Club Worldwide		Gilda's Club provides friendly, supportive meeting places to help build emotional and social support for people living with cancer. Website provides contact information for Gilda's Club homes and links to other resources.	www.gildasclub.org

Table 31.6 *(continued)*

Website name	Website sponsor (if different)	Summary of information or services provided	Website Address
Group Loop	Wellness Community	A safe, on-line community for teens dealing with cancer. Includes on-line discussion boards, support groups and other empowering information written specifically for teens to help them cope.	www.grouploop.org
Livestrong	Lance Armstrong Foundation	Under "Emotional Topics" tab, addresses numerous related issues including communication, dating and new relationships, finding meaning, living with uncertainty, sadness, setting priorities, and more.	www.livestrong.org
Macmillan *cancer relief*		Organization in the United Kingdom offering contact information for Macmillan Cancer Information and Support Centers, and an on-line directory of other support and self-help organizations throughout the United Kingdom. Opportunities for cancer advocacy.	www.cancerlink.org
Outlook-Life Beyond Cancer	University of Wisconsin Children's Hospital	Under "Health Issues and Concerns" tab, Emotional Well-Being discusses potential emotional side effects of life-threatening illness and how to build stronger emotional and physical health.	www.outlook-life.org
Patient-Centered Guides	O'Reilly and Associates	Extensive website with wealth of information for survivors. Site includes links to excerpts from books and articles dealing with emotional and psychological challenges, achieving successful transition to adulthood and adult-oriented care, the meaning of surviving life-threatening illness, and related topics.	www.patientcenters.com
People Living With Cancer	American Society of Clinical Oncology	Under "Coping" tab, information about dealing with emotional aspects of cancer, mental health, relationships, support groups, and sexuality. Also includes expanding section on Cancer in Teenagers and Young Adults, with links to several sites.	www.plwc.org
Planet Cancer		Planet Cancer is dedicated to supporting young adults with cancer. The website is a colorful, hip source of humor, support, and some medical information; serves as a networking forum for patients.	www.planetcancer.org
Pregnant With Cancer Network		Support network connecting persons who have experienced the diagnosis of cancer while pregnant. Some links and other information available.	www.pregnantwithcancer.org

Website name	Website sponsor (if different)	Summary of information or services provided	Website Address
Teenage Cancer Trust		Teenage Cancer Trust supports adolescents and young adults with cancer in the United Kingdom by building hospital units, organizing activities, providing information, and advocating politically. The "Teen Zone" is an on-line forum for patients. Links provided to other international organizations.	www.teencancer.org
Teens Living With Cancer	Melissa's Living Legacy Foundation and Children's Oncology Group	Inviting website with language and graphics geared for teens and young adults addressing numerous personal issues, including relationships with family and friends, body image, self esteem, and sexuality.	www.teenslivingwithcancer.org
Ulman Cancer Fund for Young Adults		Under "Guide to Survival" tab, downloadable guidebook for young adults with cancer written by a survivor with a practical, positive approach.	www.ulmanfund.org
Vital Options International		Vital Options provides dedicated support to young adults with cancer around the world. Website information is available in three languages and includes links to many international on-line resources.	www.thewellnesscommunity.org
Wellness Community		Organization providing support and education to persons living with cancer through participation in free, professionally led workshops and support groups in a supportive, home-like setting. Facilities are located across the United States and are appearing internationally.	www.thewellnesscommunity.org
Wellspring		Canadian network of support centers to meet emotional, social, and informational needs of cancer patients and families.	www.wellspring.ca

Acknowledgments

Valuable assistance in assessing websites was provided by research nurses of the Cook Research Department at DeVos Children's Hospital, Michigan, USA.

References

1. Yohe T, Newall G (1996) School House Rock! The Official Guide. Hyperion, New York
2. Ruccione KS (1994) Issues in survivorship. In: Schwartz CL, Hobbie WL, Constine LS, Ruccione KS (eds) Survivors of Childhood Cancer: Assessment and Management. Mosby, St Louis, pp 329–337
3. Monaco GP (1992) The partnership of empowerment: caregivers and survivors. J Psychosocial Oncol 10:121–133

4. Chelf JH, Agre P, Axelrod A, et al (2001) Cancer-related patient-education: an overview of the last decade of evaluation and research. Oncol Nurs Forum 28:1139–1147

5. Chen X, Siu LL (2001) Impact of the media and the internet on oncology: survey of cancer patients and oncologists in Canada. J Clin Oncol 19:4291–4297

6. Jenkins V, Fallowfield L, Saul J (2001) Information needs of patients with cancer: results from a large study in UK cancer centres. Br J Cancer 84:48–51

7. Van Der Molen B (1999) Relating information needs to the cancer experience: 1. Information as a key coping strategy. Eur J Cancer Care 8:238–244

8. Hewitt M, Breen N, Devesa S (1999) Cancer prevalence and survivorship issues: analyses of the 1992 national health interview survey. J Natl Cancer Inst 91:1480–1486

9. Mills ME, Sullivan K (1999) The importance of information giving for patients newly diagnosed with cancer: a review of the literature. J Clin Nurs 8:631–642

10. Peterson MW, Fretz PC (2003) Patient use of the internet for information in a lung cancer clinic. Chest 123:452–457

11. Ong LM, de Haes JC, Hoos AM, Lammes FB (1995) Doctor-patient communication: a review of the literature. Soc Sci Med 40:903–918

12. Jefford M, Tattersall MHN (2002) Informing and involving cancer patients in their own care. Lancet Oncol 3:629–637

13. Taylor H, Leitman R (2004) No significant change in the number of "cyberchondriacs" – those who go online for health care information. Harris Interactive Health Care News 4:1–4. Available at: www.harrisinteractive. com/news/newsletters_healthcare.asp (accessed June 22, 2004)

14. Taylor H (2002) Internet penetration at 66% of adults (137 million) nationwide. The Harris Poll #18, April 17. Available at: www.harrisinteractive.com/harris_poll/index.asp?PID=295 (accessed June 22, 2004)

15. Basch EM, Thaler HT, Shi W, et al (2004) Use of information resources by patients with cancer and their companions. Cancer 100:2476–2483

16. Ziebland S, Chapple A, Dumelow C, et al (2004) How the internet affects patients' experience of cancer: a qualitative study. BMJ 328:1–6

17. Fogel J (2003) Internet use for cancer information among racial/ethnic populations and low literacy groups. Cancer Control 10:45–51

18. Berland GK, Elliot MN, Morales LS, et al (2001) Health information on the internet: accessibility, quality, and readability in English and Spanish. JAMA 285:2612–2621

19. Eysenbach G, Powell J, Kuss O, Sa ER (2002) Empirical studies assessing the quality of health information for consumers on the world wide web: a systematic review. JAMA 287:2691–2700

20. Biermann JS (2003) Cancer websites you can recommend to your patients. Oncology 17:322–329

21. National Cancer Policy Board; Institute of Medicine and National Research Council (2003) In: Weiner SL, Simone JV, Hewitt M (eds) Childhood Cancer Survivorship: Improving Care and Quality of Life. National Academies Press, Washington DC, p 2

Making Ends Meet: Financial Issues from the Perspectives of Patients and Their Healthcare Team

David R. Freyer • Ronald D. Barr

32.1 Introduction

For most healthcare professionals, the financial aspects of clinical practice are considerably less familiar than the care they actually render. At the same time, few clinicians in today's world fail to appreciate that delivery and financing of care are tightly intertwined. An understanding of key economic issues has become essential for successfully providing oncology care.

Which economic issues are most important depends upon the perspective adopted. An economic evaluation of healthcare services has been defined as a comparison of the costs and consequences of relevant treatment alternatives [1]. In this sense, economic evaluations pertain to specific medical conditions and treatments. A truly comprehensive evaluation considers the viewpoints of all stakeholders, including the patients, providers, third-party payers, and society. In that type of evaluation, a determination of the appropriateness of treatments must ultimately integrate both their effectiveness and their true cost. It has been argued that such analyses should be included routinely as part of randomized clinical trials [1].

This chapter will review some of the key financial issues encountered in the management of adolescent and young adult patients with cancer. In contrast to the economic evaluation just described, the focus of this analysis is a specific patient population rather than a treatment intervention. The perspective taken is that of patients and their healthcare team consisting of the physician, nurse, social worker, and others. Of necessity, limiting the discussion to this perspective excludes other vital economic issues raised by this age group, such as reimbursement of care providers or the cost-utility of successful treatment of young adults who survive and enter society's workforce. Nevertheless, the financial issues raised here do represent genuine concerns of patients who strive to overcome the effects of malignant disease, and rely on the knowledgeable assistance of their oncology team to succeed.

Relative to financial issues, cancer statistics in the adolescent and young adult population are informative but must be interpreted in a clinical context. Although the incidence of newly diagnosed invasive cancer is far lower among persons aged 20 to 29 years (approximately 45 per 100,000 persons) than it is in older adults (approximately 730 per 100,000 for adults aged 50 to 59 years) [2], the financial challenges faced by the younger group are disproportionately complex, and for this reason alone are worthy of concern. Numerically speaking, an even more daunting challenge in the adolescent and young adult population may be posed by young adult survivors of childhood cancer, who outnumber newly diagnosed cancer patients by over four to one (1 in 490 persons versus 1 in 2200 persons, respectively) [2, 3]. This fact requires increased awareness of the similarly complex challenges faced by this growing population.

The financial issues examined in this chapter include employment, health and life insurance, out-of-pocket expenses (the direct, nonmedical cost of obtaining treatment), and selected health-related quality of life (HRQL) issues that may influence them (e.g., education and marital status). For purposes of this discussion, the adolescent and young adult population is divided into two groups, the younger adolescent (less than 18 years old) and the older adolescent and young adult (18 to 29 years old). Younger adolescents are nearly always financially dependent on their parents or guardians, and their financial issues are essentially equivalent to those of younger children. These are mostly associated with active therapy and result in increased family financial burden, largely due to out-of-pocket expenses. In contrast, older adolescent and young adult tend to be financially independent. Their

issues relate to preserving income, paying for medical expenses, providing for dependents, and planning for the future.

32.2 Younger Adolescents: the Financially Dependent Patient

32.2.1 Case Example

A 16-year-old boy was diagnosed with localized osteosarcoma of the right distal femur. He was a full-time high-school student living with both working parents and his siblings, aged 4 and 7 years, approximately 2 h driving time from the oncology center. Treatment lasted 1 year and consisted of intensive, multiagent chemotherapy that required frequent hospitalization for several days at a time. He was referred to a different center for a complex limb-salvage procedure. At diagnosis, the patient's mother, who had worked part-time as an elementary teacher's aide, quit her job in order to attend to her son at the hospital and home. The father, who was employed as a food store manager and received health insurance benefits covering his family, was permitted to reduce his hours by 20% to help care for the patient's younger siblings and assist with transportation to and from the hospital. During treatment, the patient qualified for supplemental coverage of medical expenses through a government-sponsored program for children with serious chronic illnesses. The patient is now in active follow-up 2 years off therapy and is in continuous first remission. Both parents have returned to their previous levels of work.

32.2.2 Major Financial Issues

Adolescents like the one above resemble the younger pediatric patient, as both are financially dependent. Depending on the particular healthcare system, the direct costs of medical care for the majority of children and younger adolescents with cancer are largely paid for, especially in Canada, the United Kingdom, Europe, and other countries with national health programs. In the United States, direct medical costs are mostly covered by insurance through a parent's private or (more commonly) employer-derived group plan, with or without support from various public supplemental programs. Therefore, the major financial concerns for dependent patients are those that contribute to the "family economic burden."

The financial impact of childhood cancer treatment on families has been the subject of surprisingly little study, with only seven publications appearing in the past 25 years [4–10]. While these have originated in diverse societies with a wide variety of healthcare systems (United Kingdom, United States, New Zealand, China, and Canada), the common message is clear: the economic burden can be enormous. For example, even in the Canadian system of universal access and "first dollar coverage," the average costs to families amount to one-third of after-tax income [9].

Data on these costs are difficult to collect comprehensively, especially in the early phase of active treatment soon after diagnosis. Retrospective attempts can result in substantial underestimates and other methodological considerations contribute to systematic underreporting [11]. Even the process of collecting such information on costs imposes an added burden to these families.

Out-of-pocket expenses have been defined as the direct, nonmedical costs of care [12]. These include expenses such as those arising from transportation to and from the treatment center, parking, long-distance telephone calls, extra meals in restaurants, lodgings, childcare for siblings left at home, wigs, copayments for medications covered by insurance, and full payment for those that are not covered. For research and/ or clinical purposes, such expenses can be recorded prospectively in suitably structured diaries, with additional questionnaires capturing other infrequent but substantial expenditures. On the other side of the balance sheet, a record may be kept of reimbursements from insurance companies, social service agencies, and charitable organizations. Notably, these expense reports do not include indirect costs such as lost income, cessation of work not normally performed for remuneration (e.g., housekeeping), and the opportunity costs of family labor (the monetary value of time spent caring for the patient rather than generating income) [13]. In the United States, insurance premiums and consumption of limited benefits represent other indirect costs.

Chapter 32

The financial impact on families of adolescents with cancer is particularly burdensome: the period of active therapy is lengthy compared with other illnesses; the patients experience substantial morbidity; the patients are often too young to have developed support mechanisms outside the family unit; and their families often have other considerable, fixed expenses during this phase of life [9]. Unfortunately, the financial burden of out-of-pocket expenses is magnified in the setting of poverty. Out-of-pocket expenses (and even copayments and insurance premiums in the United States) are fixed and therefore "regressive," accounting for even larger percentages of lower incomes [12]. In poverty, these effects are increased further by "nonmedical financial pressures," such as general social disorganization, lack of education, unstable housing arrangements, family violence, crime, and substance abuse [14].

32.3 Older Adolescent and Young Adult: the Financially Independent Patient or Survivor

Older adolescent and young adult face a number of financial challenges related to their developmental stage. Unlike the younger child, where the combination of responsible adults and existing medical insurance programs assure payment for most oncology services, adolescent and young adult patients are largely "on their own." In the United States, the healthcare financing system for financially independent patients greater than 21 years old is a patchwork of private, federal, state, and local funding programs. The application process to gain access to benefits often requires completion of numerous, unfamiliar forms with long waits for processing at a time when patients are dealing with the shock of a new diagnosis, starting difficult therapy, and feeling physically and emotionally unwell. In the United States, many newly diagnosed young adults are treated in busy, community-based adult oncology office settings where it is uncommon to have social work or financial counseling services available. Finally, the personal and family profiles of these patients can be challenging: careers are not well established; employer-derived medical benefits are marginal or simply not available; their children are very young and require considerable care; and often both of the patient's parents are working – if they are together.

32.3.1 Case Example: The Young Adult On Therapy

A 28-year-old married woman was diagnosed with breast cancer. She and her husband had a total of six children from prior marriages, in addition to discovering during her cancer work-up that she was pregnant with their first child as a couple. The patient had been employed as an office assistant but was unable to continue working following diagnosis, which resulted in loss of her income and her family's primary health insurance benefits. Initial treatment included mastectomy followed by dose-limited chemotherapy for 6 months, during which she received high-risk perinatal services that culminated in the delivery of a healthy full-term baby. Subsequently, she underwent dose-intensive chemotherapy and external beam irradiation, followed by breast reconstruction. During treatment, the patient's husband needed to reduce his work hours substantially to care for the other children and his wife (which he could do with the help of coworkers who donated some of their own earned time-off hours). His secondary health insurance program was limited in scope. With the assistance of a medical social worker, the family enrolled in various government-supported financial and social support programs, obtained payment deferrals from their telephone and utility companies, and received meals and cash gifts from their church. Additional funds needed for living expenses were raised through donation collection cans set out at banks and stores in her community. The patient is now off therapy and recovering, with the husband back to work full-time.

32.3.2 Major Financial Issues

32.3.2.1 Health Insurance

The lack of insurance coverage for medical care and/or medications in the United States is a major issue for this age group. This reflects a relatively high rate of uninsured Americans in this age group in general.

According to the United States General Accounting Office, about 30% of Americans aged 19 to 29 years lack health insurance [15]. Many of these are employed at jobs simply offering no group insurance benefit or by small companies not bound by federal laws governing insurance. Because of the costliness of private health insurance, many in this age group try to save money by "playing the odds" of remaining healthy.

Unless they already carry private or group health insurance, patients in the United States must pursue several strategies for assistance. For patients ≥21 years, the major resource is Medicaid-derived programs ("Medicaid" is a catch-all term referring to various state-administered programs that use both state and federal dollars to pay for medical expenses of qualified individuals). Another option is to apply for non-employer-based group insurance soon after the diagnosis of cancer is made.

Because American private and group health plans vary in scope of coverage, some treatment-related expenses exist whether or not the patient has health insurance. For example, not all insurance programs have benefits for prescription medications. Options for addressing this include enrolling in patient assistance programs offered by some pharmaceutical companies; using samples of oral supportive care medications provided by oncology clinics; and exploring the possibility of obtaining a lower price through international suppliers.

A major portion of medical expenses comprises hospital bills. Patients can work with the hospital billing department to qualify for indigent care status, in which case some services will be provided at no charge, or to set up an affordable long-term payment plan.

Many of the strategies described above can be overwhelming. The assistance of an experienced medical social worker or financial counselor can be invaluable in accessing them. If such is not available in the medical oncology office where the patient is receiving care, a referral may be made to a social worker associated with a nearby hospital-based cancer program.

32.3.2.2 Reduced Work and Loss of Income

This major issue for young adults on therapy results chiefly from decreased hours at paid work for the patient and/or the spouse, who may need to care for the patient or rest of the family. In some cases, the patient may be so medically compromised that temporarily it may not be possible to work at all. Options exist to offset this loss of income, although they are inconsistent and must be used in combination. Some government programs exist to provide supplemental income for patients who are medically unable to work. Another option is to apply shortly after diagnosis for short- or long-term disability insurance through the patient's employer. In this case, the patient must already work for an employer who offers disability insurance and must qualify for the plan.

Diagnosis-specific assistance is available for some patients. Funds from organizations supporting patients with certain diagnoses may be granted as available for miscellaneous expenses, such as house payments and other living expenses. For medically necessary travel, several major airlines offer tickets issued on frequent flyer miles donated by other travelers.

Other funds to help offset lost income may be available through a patient's social network. Churches commonly make benevolent funds available to help pay for food, housing, or transportation. Finally, if a patient has a supportive family and community, fund-raisers may be held, although this practice seems to be more common for childhood cancer patients.

32.3.3 Case Example: The Older Adolescent and Young Adult Survivor of Childhood Cancer

A 24 year old male underwent long-term follow-up clinic evaluation that was initiated by the patient for help with health insurance. Seven years had passed since his last visit. He had been diagnosed at age 15 years with a localized Ewing sarcoma of his right proximal radius. He received standard treatment consisting of multiagent chemotherapy for the disease, as well as resection of the proximal radius for local control. The patient sustained significant anatomical and functional disability affecting his right fingers, hand, and wrist. He was right-handed. The function was improved somewhat after fusion of the radius and ulna and tendon transfer procedure completed at age 17 years. In his period of being lost to follow-up, he was

in prison for 3 years, during which he earned his high school equivalency diploma. However, he had recently lost his job, apartment, and car, and was now living with his mother. He was working for a construction crew, but with his anatomically fixed wrist and limited finger extension, he could only hold the "stop-and-go" traffic sign at the job site. He could not swing a hammer but felt he could operate power tools if given the chance. He had no job-related benefits. He had recently seen a psychiatrist for chronic anxiety and depression.

32.3.4 Major Financial Issues

The financial problems encountered by the young adult survivor of childhood cancer seem to be influenced by the age of the survivor. According to Hays [16], survivors older than approximately 30 years have relatively few problems and tend to resemble control groups, except for obtaining life insurance. In contrast, survivors younger than 30 years exhibit more problems and variance from control groups. The reasons for this may relate to life tasks of the different groups. In almost all respects, the younger adult is less established and still in the process of completing an education, settling on a vocation and redefining primary relationships. Thus, representative problems cluster around the interactions of employment, health insurance, and educational level.

32.3.4.1 Employment

As recently summarized by the Institute of Medicine in the United States, prior to recent protective legislation about 10 to 25% of childhood cancer survivors experienced discrimination or difficulties in employment as adults [17]. In accounting for this, some of the concerns voiced by employers relating to childhood cancer survivors have been possible increased costs due to insurance expenses and lost productivity, as well as negative psychological impact on other employees [17]. Other issues may include out-of-date personnel policies and uninformed managers, difficulty interpreting existing legislative requirements, and misconceptions about a survivor's ability to work.

Currently, the employment picture for this group is mixed, perhaps improving, but difficult to assess due

Table 32.1 Selected United States legislation addressing financial issues of young adults and adolescents with cancer

	Family and Medical Leave Act (FMLA)	Americans with Disabilities Act of 1990 (ADA)	Health Insurance Portability and Accountability Act (HIPAA)	Consolidated Omnibus Budget Reconciliation Act of 1986 (COBRA)
Primary function	• Continuation of employment	• Procurement and retention of employment and benefits (including health insurance)	• Retention of health insurance	• Retention of health insurance
Persons covered	• Employee-cancer patients • Employees with spouse, child, or other dependent with cancer	• Cancer patients and survivors • Employees or prospective employees with dependent cancer patient or survivor	• Employees who become cancer patients	• Employee-cancer patients • Dependent children and spouse (regardless of marital status)
Entities regulated	• Employers with ≥ 50 employees	• Employers with ≥ 15 employees • State and local governments • Legislative branch of federal government • Employment agencies • Labor unions	• All employers	• Public and private employers with ≥ 20 employees
Qualifying conditions	• Serious health conditions rendering employee unable to perform job • Childbirth, adoption, family medical emergencies	• Any disability in qualified individual able to perform essential functions of job • Usually includes cancer whether cured, controlled on treatment, or in remission	• Any prior diagnosis, including cancer	• Any prior diagnosis, including cancer

to changes in government protection and workplace attitudes that may be reflected in only the most recent studies. As summarized by Langeveld and colleagues [18] in a review of 30 empirical studies meeting stringent methodological criteria, some studies have detected no significant difference in the rates or types of employment of survivors compared with controls. However, others have detected a difference. Zeltzer and colleagues found that, compared with siblings, adult survivors of acute lymphoblastic leukemia (ALL) who did not complete higher education had higher unemployment rates or worked less than half-time [19]. Green and colleagues found that female survivors

were unemployed at a rate higher than the national average [20]. A Dutch study found a significantly lower employment rate for both male and female survivors compared with population controls (approximately 53% vs 75%) [21].

Employment discrimination refers to unfair hiring practices or treatment in the workplace due to attitudes concerning a person's ability to work. As summarized by Langeveld [18], some studies have found that, as self-reported, approximately 10–30% of survivors experienced job discrimination. A survey conducted by the United States National Center for Health Statistics found that 23.6% of adult cancer survivors

Table 32.1 (*continued*)

	Family and Medical Leave Act (FMLA)	Americans with Disabilities Act of 1990 (ADA)	Health Insurance Portability and Accountability Act (HIPAA)	Consolidated Omnibus Budget Reconciliation Act of 1986 (COBRA)
Major benefits	• 12 weeks unpaid leave during any 12-month period • Employer must continue benefits (including health insurance) during leave • Restoration of employee at same or equivalent position • Employee must be allowed reduced or intermittent work schedule when necessary	• Prohibits discrimination in hiring, firing and providing benefits on basis of disability • Employers may not ask applicants whether they have had cancer – only whether s/he can perform essential job functions • Employees needing extra time or assistance are entitled to "reasonable accommodation" (e.g., adjustment of work hours or duties to accommodate medical appointments or treatment of side effects)	• Allows employees insured for ≥ 12 months to change jobs without losing coverage, even if previously diagnosed with cancer • Reduces "job lock" (inability to change jobs for fear of losing health insurance) • Group plans may not impose exclusion clauses of > 12 months for pre-existing conditions if medical care received for it within previous 6 months • Requires health plans to renew coverage for groups and individuals • Increases tax deduction for health insurance expenses of self-employed persons	• Requires continuation of group medical coverage to employees who would have lost it due to individual circumstances, including a reduction in work hours or termination for any reason except gross misconduct • Coverage must be continued for 18 months and must be equivalent to group plan offered to other employees • Premiums must be paid by employee but cannot exceed group premium by more than 2% • Secures valuable time to shop for replacement coverage after changing jobs • Extends coverage for employee's childhood cancer survivor who becomes independent and must find new coverage
References	[17]	[17, 29–31]	[17, 30]	[17, 30, 31]

who were less than 35 years at diagnosis had experienced a variety of cancer-related employment problems [22]. Interestingly, the problem of unfair bias seems to be of greater magnitude for those seeking to enter the military, where discrimination was felt to affect 30–80% of survivors [18]. Among Israeli survivors, Dolgin and colleagues found that 46% reported job discrimination and 55% had difficulty gaining entry into the military [23]. Once hired,

income levels of survivors, as summarized by Langeveld [18], seem to be comparable with controls in most studies.

Employment of survivors may be influenced by the type of cancer and the treatment administered. While Nicholson and coworkers detected no difference in employment status for bone tumor survivors compared with siblings [24], Felder-Puig and colleagues found that bone tumor survivors encountered more difficulty with changing jobs and job orientation [25]. Neither study found a difference in income levels for survivors. Novakovic and coworkers found that significantly fewer survivors of Ewing sarcoma than sibling controls were employed full-time [26]. In these studies, survivor cohorts included both patients with upper or lower extremity tumors, but it is not reported whether the site correlated with any employment differences. A more recent report by Nagarajan and colleagues for the Childhood Cancer Survivor Study (CCSS) [27] found that of 694 survivors of lower extremity bone tumors, 97% had ever been employed and 83% had worked during the previous year. Work was associated with a higher educational level, and amputation predicted for lower education and employment, as well as more insurance problems. For both male and female survivors of ALL, Pui and colleagues report that unemployment was higher than national averages (35% versus 5.2% for females; 15.1% versus 5.4% for males) [28]. Patients with central nervous system (CNS) tumors have been identified as having major challenges in education and employment [16]. In a recent Dutch study, employment status was not reported separately for CNS tumor survivors, although this subset was noted to have greater difficulties in other HRQL domains [21]. In the same study, low-dose cranial irradiation was associated with an eight-fold risk of lower educational level.

Military service appears to be a problematic area of employment for survivors. In a study of Dutch survivors, Langeveld found that 55% of males were denied entry compared with 27% of the general population [21]. In Israel, only 49% of survivors served compared with 71% of controls [23]. For entering the United States military, Weiner and colleagues report that medical waivers can be obtained, and that the general rule for entry is that patients must be without evidence of disease and at least 5 years off therapy (2 years for Wilms' and testicular germ-cell tumors) [29].

Several strategies and tools exist to assist adolescent and young adult survivors with employment. In general, treatment centers should routinely provide survivors with information concerning their legal rights and advice on obtaining employment, taking into consideration their specific physical or cognitive challenges.

As summarized in Table 32.1, several federal and state laws in the United States work to protect employment and related rights of survivors. The most significant is the Americans with Disability Act (ADA) of 1990, which prohibits covered employers from discriminating on the basis of disability (including cancer) in hiring, firing, and providing benefits [17, 29–31]. Most states in the United States have similar laws, with a few, including California and Vermont, expressly prohibiting discrimination against cancer survivors [17].

Because adolescent and young adult survivors were diagnosed with cancer before their careers were established, specially tailored programs are required for assisting them with employment. These should be oriented toward completion of education and vocational training rather than rehabilitation, reentry, and retraining, as for older adults [12]. In some instances, programs are available to assist in vocational training and placement, requiring a physician's assessment of physical capabilities. Disabilities generally represent consequences of treatments that were necessary to save the patient's life. As such, the oncology team should endeavor to correct or otherwise manage key disabilities in order to maximize function. Because these are often complicated and require the involvement of other surgical or rehabilitation specialists over time, the issue should be anticipated and undertaken early enough to benefit the survivor seeking to enter the workforce. In addressing employment issues, oncology teams should utilize the expertise of the medical social worker, whose knowledge will be most current in the complex and changing world of survivor employment opportunities and rights [14]. In the years of follow-up leading to young adulthood, adolescent survivors should be counseled to think ahead, stay in school, obtain their diplomas, and seek stable living arrangements, as these other HRQL domains seem to influence employment (as discussed further below). In responding to employment problems, Hoffman has pointed out that lawsuits are not the only or optimal approach [30]. Rather, preemptive strategies for survivors should include: (1) keeping their cancer history private unless it directly affects their job qualifications;

(2) asking about benefits packages only after receiving a written job offer; and (3) stressing their current ability to do the job in question. If necessary, other informal and formal responses to perceived discrimination can be pursued before resorting to expensive and time-consuming litigation [30].

32.3.4.2 Health and Life Insurance

For multiple reasons, the adolescent and young adult population is generally vulnerable to health insurance problems [17]. In the United States, which does not have a nationalized system of healthcare, health insurance is closely related to employment – the "terrible twins" of survivorship [32]. The "aging out" of childhood health plans by survivors often results in a loss of coverage or change to that which is less comprehensive. According to recent data from the United States General Accounting Office, 30% of Americans aged 18 to 24 years and 23% of those aged 25 to 34 years lack any health insurance whatsoever [15].

These facts may have negative effects on adolescent and young adult cancer survivors trying to obtain long-term follow-up services, which are recommended to continue for life [33]. There is a popular misconception that people without health insurance still manage to obtain the medical care they need. In fact, these persons are much more likely to go without needed care. According to White, uninsured patients receive fewer preventative services and less regular care for chronic medical conditions [15].

What is the current state of health insurance coverage for adolescent and young adult survivors of childhood cancer? Several studies suggest increased difficulties obtaining insurance compared with controls, especially for the younger adult. Seven studies of health insurance in this population reviewed by Langeveld [18] suggest that approximately 10 to 25% have difficulty obtaining insurance or have exclusion clauses pertaining to a previous diagnosis of cancer, compared with only 1 to 3% of control groups. In a recent study of adolescent and young adult survivors of lower extremity bone tumors by the CCSS, 87% held health insurance but 30% had difficulty obtaining it [27]. In that study, successfully obtaining insurance was associated with being a nonamputee, completing college, and

being married. Among survivors of acute lymphoblastic leukemia, 28.4% had been denied health insurance and 18.6% were faced with prohibitive premiums. Among the uninsured, 27.7% were not receiving needed care [28]. This lack of coverage seems to be an American phenomenon, as multiple international studies of HRQL describe frequent difficulties in domains such as completing education, finding employment, entering military service, and qualifying for a driver's license, but not in obtaining health insurance. Presumably, this is because national health insurance programs in many other developed countries eliminate the "coverage gap" of American young adults.

Similar shortfalls exist for survivors obtaining life insurance. Again, this seems to be more striking for younger than older adults, although this is not always identified by them as a concern until they are in an established career, have dependents, and own property. Five studies that evaluated life insurance were reviewed by Langeveld [18] and indicate that 24 to 44% of survivors have difficulty obtaining affordable life insurance, compared with approximately 2% of controls. According to the United States Institute of Medicine [17], insurance companies take cancer history into account because life insurance is based on actuarial risk of death, and cancer patients have an increased risk of death at an earlier age. Thus, some life insurance companies will not insure survivors at all, or else charge very high premiums to do so.

In assisting the adolescent and young adult cancer survivor in obtaining or keeping health insurance, the treatment center should begin by routinely providing all survivors with information concerning its importance, how the system works, and how to navigate it successfully. As summarized in Table 32.1, three pieces of legislation in the United States are particularly noteworthy for protecting health insurance for some survivors: the ADA [17, 29–31], the Health Insurance Portability and Accountability Act [17, 30], and the Consolidated Omnibus Budget Reconciliation Act of 1986 [17, 30, 31].

Monaco and colleagues [31] have provided several recommendations for assisting adolescent and young adult survivors with their insurance needs. The overall goals should be to find an insurer who will provide any coverage at all to the survivor, either through offering limited coverage at normal premiums until after the preexisting diagnosis period has expired, or through offering full coverage at a higher rate until the policyholder is considered to be at no increased risk. Open enrollment periods for certain insurance companies and employers may provide an opportunity for survivors to apply. Group insurance plans may also be offered through organizations to which the survivor belongs, such as labor unions, business associations, and religious groups. The most effective strategy, according to the authors [31], is to seek affordable group insurance by securing stable employment with a large company (more than 300 employees). Hoffman has provided several practical suggestions for survivors wishing to shop wisely for health insurance [30]. As with employment, it is critical for treatment centers to assist the patient, especially during the adolescent years of initial follow-up, in anticipating the importance of health insurance and planning accordingly, especially with respect to finding gainful employment.

32.3.4.3 Other Factors Threatening Financial Stability: Education and Marital Status

Across multiple countries, studies of childhood cancer survivors have found that a higher level of educational attainment is associated with employment. In the extensive review by Langeveld and coworkers [18], studies suggest that survivors of CNS tumors, especially if they were treated with irradiation, and patients who were given cranial irradiation for ALL, complete higher education less frequently than other patients. The effect is most striking for those who were diagnosed at a young age. In a study of educational attainment by the CCSS group [35], a lower proportion of survivors than siblings completed high school or college, especially among patients treated for CNS tumors. The use of special education services was higher among survivors (23%) than siblings (8%), which helped offset the educational risk. Among lower-extremity bone tumor survivors, the CCSS group discovered that 93% had graduated from high school (a lower rate than the reference group) and 50% had graduated from college [27]. In that study, it was also noted that patients less than 12 years

old at diagnosis and those who had not undergone amputation were somewhat more likely to graduate from college. In addition, education was a positive predictor for both employment and having health insurance [27]. In a Dutch population, survivors who were female or had a history of either CNS tumor or cranial irradiation for ALL were significantly less likely to complete high school or pursue a graduate degree [21]. In a study in the United Kingdom, 25% of survivors compared with 48% of siblings received higher education, although both levels were higher than the national average of 17.3% [36]. In an Israeli study population, no difference was noted between survivors and siblings for high school graduation or attainment of a university degree [23].

Marital status might also be viewed as an indirect indicator of financial risk because unmarried survivors do not enjoy the security of a spouse's income or benefits providing medical and life insurance. The two largest studies of marriage involving more than 12,000 childhood cancer survivors combined found that, compared with controls, there was a lower prevalence of marriage among survivors in general [37, 38], especially male survivors of CNS tumors [37, 38], and women and whites [37]. In the CCSS, 66% of survivors of lower extremity bone tumors were married or living as married; within that study population, no difference was found for amputees [27]. Among survivors of ALL, the only significant difference in marriage rates was noted for the subset of females who had received cranial irradiation (35.2%) compared with the matched general population (48.8%) [28]. In The Netherlands, survivors of cancer compared with a reference group were significantly less likely to be married, especially among males and those with a history of CNS tumor and/or cranial irradiation [21]. As reviewed by Langeveld, most other studies found similar results [18].

The frequency of divorce reported for childhood cancer survivors varies in different studies [reviewed in 18]. The two largest studies of marital status mentioned above [37, 38] found that divorced survivors had similar characteristics to those who never married. Although the CCSS group [37] found that the overall proportion of survivors who were divorced or separated was lower than that of the United States population, males (especially in the 20- to 24-year-old group) had a higher rate. The authors also state that survivors who had a CNS tumor divorced or separated at a rate higher than those with other diagnoses and matched reference populations. Byrne and colleagues [38] found that male survivors of CNS tumors had a substantially higher divorce rate than controls, especially if diagnosed at a young age.

32.4 Conclusions

Attention to financial issues constitutes an important part of caring for the whole adolescent or young adult with cancer. For the younger adolescent who is financially dependent, the major financial challenge is the family economic burden, which is created by substantial out-of-pocket expenses and reduced income of parents. For the older adolescent or young adult who is financially independent and on treatment, the major financial challenges involve payment for care (particularly in societies without national health programs), loss of income while unable to work, and out-of-pocket expenses. For the financially independent young adult survivor of cancer in childhood or adolescence, serious financial challenges may arise due to difficulties obtaining employment and health and life insurance, especially in certain clinical subgroups such as those who had CNS tumors and/or cranial irradiation. Assisting patients at risk begins with an awareness of the substantial financial problems facing these populations and continues with creative efforts to meet their needs using available resources most suitable for each situation. Especially for survivors, strategies for completing education and finding stable employment should be emphasized and implemented as early as possible.

References

1. Barr RD, Feeny D, Furlong W (2004) Economic evaluation of childhood cancer care. Eur J Cancer 40:1335–1345
2. Ries LAG, Eisner MP, Kosary CL, et al (eds) (2004) SEER Cancer Statistics Review, 1975–2000, National Cancer Institute. Bethesda, MD. Available at: http://seer.cancer.gov/csr/1975_2000/results_single/sect_02_table.02.pdf. Accessed February 1, 2004
3. National Cancer Policy Board; Institute of Medicine and National Research Council. Weiner SL, Simone JV, Hewitt M (eds) (2003) Childhood Cancer Survivorship: Improving Care and Quality of Life. National Academies Press, Washington DC, p 34
4. Lansky SB, Chairs NU, Clark GM, et al (1979) Childhood cancer: non-medical costs of the illness. Cancer 43:403–408
5. Bodkin CM, Pigott TJ, Mann JR (1982) Financial burden of childhood cancer. BMJ 284:1542–1544
6. Pentol A (1983) Cost bearing burdens. Health Soc Serv J 93:1088–1089
7. Bloom BS, Knorr RS, Evans AE (1985) The costs of caring for children with cancer. JAMA 253:2393–2397
8. Martinson IM, Su-Xiao Y, Liang YJ (1993) The impact of childhood cancer on 50 Chinese families. J Pediatr Oncol Nurs 10:13–18
9. Barr RD, Furlong W, Horsman JR, et al (1996) The monetary costs of childhood cancer to the families of patients. Int J Oncol 8:933–940
10. Dockerty JD, Skegg DCG, Williams SM (2003) Economic effects of childhood cancer on families. J Paediatr Child Health 39:254–258
11. Jacobs P, Fassbender K (1998) The measurement of indirect costs in the health economics evaluation literature. Int J Technol Assess Health Care 14:799–808
12. Parsons SK (2002) Financial issues in pediatric cancer. In: Pizzo PA, Poplack DG (eds) Principles and Practice of Pediatric Oncology, 4th edn. Lippincott Williams and Wilkins, Philadelphia, pp 1495–1510
13. Stommel M, Given CS, Given BA (1993) The cost of cancer home care to families. Cancer 71:1867–1874
14. Bonnem S, Ross J (1997) Financial issues in pediatric cancer. In: Pizzo PA, Poplack DG (eds) Principles and Practice of Pediatric Oncology, 3rd edn. Lippincott–Raven, Philadelphia, pp 1357–1365
15. White PH (2002) Access to health care: health insurance considerations for young adults with special health care needs/disabilities. Pediatrics 110:1328–1335
16. Hays DM (1993) Adult survivors of childhood cancer: employment and insurance issues in different age groups. Cancer 71:3306–3309
17. National Cancer Policy Board; Institute of Medicine and National Research Council. Weiner SL, Simone JV, Hewitt M (eds) (2003) Childhood Cancer Survivorship: Improving Care and Quality of Life. National Academies Press, Washington DC, pp 140–163
18. Langeveld NE, Stam H, Grootenhuis MA, Last BF (2002) Quality of life in young adult survivors of childhood cancer. Support Care Cancer 10:579–600
19. Zeltzer LK, Chen E, Weiss R, Guo MD, et al (1997) Comparison of psychologic outcome in adult survivors

of childhood acute lymphoblastic leukemia versus sibling controls: a cooperative Children's Cancer Group and National Institutes of Health study. J Clin Oncol 15:547–556

20. Green DM, Zevon MA, Hall B (1991) Achievement of life goals by adult survivors of modern treatment for childhood cancer. Cancer 67:206–213

21. Langeveld NE, Ubbink MC, Last BF, et al (2003) Educational achievement, employment and living situation in long-term young adult survivors of childhood cancer in the Netherlands. Psychooncology 12:213–225

22. Hewitt M, Breen N, Devesa S (1999) Cancer prevalence and survivorship issues: analyses of the 1992 National Health Interview Survey. J Natl Cancer Inst 91:1480–1486

23. Dolgin MJ, Somer E, Buchvald E, Zaizov R (1999) Quality of life in adult survivors of childhood cancer. Soc Work Health Care 28:31–43

24. Nicholson HS, Mulvihill JJ, Byrne J (1992) Late effects of therapy in adult survivors of osteosarcoma and Ewing sarcoma. Med Ped Oncol 20:6–12

25. Felder-Puig R, Formann A, Mildner A, et al (1998) Quality of life and psychosocial adjustment of young patients after treatment of bone cancer. Cancer 83:69–75

26. Novakovic B, Fears TR, Horowitz ME, et al (1997) Late effects of therapy in survivors of Ewing sarcoma family tumors. J Pediatr Hematol/Oncol 19:220–225

27. Nagarajan R, Neglia JP, Clohisy DR, et al (2003) Education, employment, insurance, and marital status among 694 survivors of pediatric lower extremity bone tumors: a report from the Childhood Cancer Survivor Study. Cancer 97:2554–2564

28. Pui C-H, Cheng C, Leung W, et al (2003) Extended follow-up of long-term survivors of childhood acute lymphoblastic leukemia. N Engl J Med 349:640–649

29. Weiner SL, McCabe MS, Smith GP, et al (2002) Pediatric cancer: advocacy, insurance, education, and employment. In: Pizzo PA, Poplack DG (eds) Principles and Practice of Pediatric Oncology, 4th edn. Lippincott Williams and Wilkins, Philadelphia, pp 1511–1526

30. Hoffman B (1999) Cancer survivors' employment and insurance rights: a primer for oncologists. Oncology 13:841–852

31. Monaco GP, Smith G, Fiduccia D (1997) Pediatric cancer: advocacy, legal, insurance, and employment issues. In: Pizzo PA, Poplack DG (eds) Principles and Practice of Pediatric Oncology, 3rd edn. Lippincott-Raven, Philadelphia, pp 1367–1381

32. Moore DM (1999) The Hoffman article reviewed. Oncology 13:846–849

33. Lampkin BC (1993) Introduction and executive summary. Cancer 71:3199–3201

34. Fishman E (2001) Aging out of coverage: young adults with special health care needs. Health Affairs 20:254–266

35. Mittby PA, Robison LL, Whitton JA, et al (2003) Utilization of special education services and educational attainment among long-term survivors of childhood cancer: a report from the Childhood Cancer Survivor Study. Cancer 97:1115–1126

36. Evans SE, Radford R (1995) Current lifestyle of young adults treated for cancer in childhood. Arch Dis Child 72:423–426

37. Rauck AM, Green DM, Yasui Y, et al (1999) Marriage in the survivors of childhood cancer: a preliminary description from the Childhood Cancer Survivor Study. Med Ped Oncol 33:60–63

38. Byrne J, Fears TR, Steinhorn SC, et al (1989) Marriage and divorce after childhood and adolescent cancer. JAMA 262:2693–2699

Challenges and Opportunities – The Way Ahead

Archie Bleyer • Karen Albritton •

Stuart Siegel • Marianne Phillips •

Ronald Barr

Contents

33.1 Introduction

In contrast to the vast medical literature on cancer during the first 15 years of life (infants, children, and young adolescents) and an even greater volume of literature on cancer in older adults, this book represents the first comprehensive treatise on cancer in older adolescents and young adults. With national and international focuses on younger and older patients during the past half-century, despite the fact that cancer patients diagnosed during late adolescence and early adulthood are at the interface of pediatric and adult oncology, young adults and older adolescents have become orphans, lacking the overall progress made in cancer prevention, diagnosis, and treatment for other age groups [1, 2].

The vast majority of cases of cancer diagnosed before age 30 years appear to be spontaneous and unrelated to either carcinogens in the environment or inherited factors, a distinctly different situation to that which occurs in cancer in older adults. There are exceptions, namely melanomas caused by ultraviolet light, cervical carcinoma due to human papillomavirus infection, Kaposi sarcoma and some non-Hodgkin lymphoma related to the human immunodeficiency virus, and Hodgkin and Burkitt lymphomas associated with the Epstein-Barr virus. However, these account for only one-third of the total cancer problem in all young adults and older adolescents.

As is documented in this book, survival improvement trends portend a worse prognosis for young adults diagnosed with cancer today than for younger children, where as the reverse used to be true, with this deficit increasing with longer duration of follow-up. The deficit in survival improvement is not limited to the United States; rather, it appears to be a global problem.

This chapter summarizes the current status of the epidemiology and outcome of cancer in persons between 15 and 29 years of age. It presents reasons for the lack of progress cited above, as they apply to society, the patient, healthcare professionals, the family and community, the health insurance system, and where and by whom the patient is treated. It then suggests how the multiple challenges posed by this age group can be prioritized, and subsequently, practical solutions developed and implemented.

33.2 Current Status

In this age group, cancer is unique in the distribution of the types that occur. Hodgkin lymphoma, melanoma, testis cancer, female genital tract malignancies, thyroid cancer, soft-tissue sarcomas, non-Hodgkin lymphoma, leukemia, brain and spinal cord tumors, breast cancer, bone sarcomas, and nongonadal germ-cell tumors account for 95% of the cancers in 15- to 29-year-olds. Over a span of only 15 years (i.e., from age 15 to 29 years), the frequency distribution of cancer types changes substantively, such that the pattern demonstrated at the youngest age does not resemble that at the oldest.

The incidence of cancer in the 15- to 29-year age group has increased steadily over the past quarter century. However, the rate of increase is slowing and at the older end of the age range the overall incidence appears to be reducing toward the rate of the 1970s. Reasons for these changes remain speculative.

Compared to females, males in the 15- to 29-year age group are at higher risk of developing cancer and have a lower likelihood of survival. The risks are directly proportional to age. Among the races/ethnicities evaluated, the incidence of cancer in this age group is highest among non-Hispanic whites and lowest among Asians, American Indians, and Alaska Natives. Survival has been worse among African Americans/blacks, American Indians, and Alaska Natives than among the other races and ethnicities.

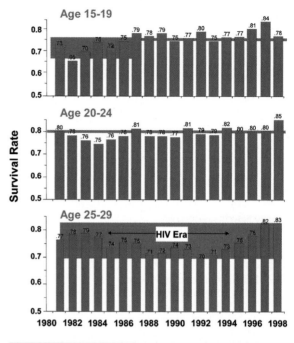

Figure 33.1

Five-year survival for all invasive cancers in patients aged 15 to 19 years (*top panel*), 20 to 24 years (*middle panel*), and 25 to 29 years (*bottom panel*). United States (US) Surveillance and Epidemiology End Results (SEER) database, 1980–1998

At the beginning of the last quarter century, the diagnosis of cancer in 15- to 29-year-olds carried a more favorable prognosis compared to a cancer diagnosis at other ages. Since then, there has been a relative lack of progress in survival improvement among older adolescents and young adults. In the US, the 15- to 19-year age group showed some progress in the early 1980s, but progress has remained relatively static since 1986 (Fig. 33.1, upper panel). In the 20- to 24-year age group, there has been no improvement since 1980 (Fig. 33.1, middle panel). The 25- to 29-year age group actually showed a decline in the overall survival rate in the mid- to late 1980s, probably due to human immunodeficiency virus (HIV)-related cancers, primarily Kaposi sarcoma and non-Hodgkin lymphoma (Fig. 33.1, lower panel). In this age group, the decrease in survival abated as HIV-induced can-

Table 33.1 Factors likely (primary) or unlikely (secondary) to explain the survival deficit

General category	Primary factors[a]	Secondary factors
Personal/patient: older adolescents and young adults	Independence/Autonomy Feelings of Invincibility Under-utilization of Healthcare Services *Awareness* *Delays in Diagnosis* *Health Insurance* Adherence Financial limitations *Participation in clinical trials* *Tumor specimens* *Translational research*	Embarrassment Psychosomatic emphasis Transportation limitations Psychosocial environment during diagnosis and treatment Pharmacokinetic differences
Family/community: family members, colleagues/friends, educators, employers, politicians, legislators, knowledge workers	*Awareness* Lack of education Lack of guidance Inadequate community resources	Constituency influence
Health professional: physicians, nurses, allied health professionals	Awareness *Delays in diagnosis* Healthcare teams Education/training Reimbursement *Health insurance* *Participation in clinical trials* *Tumor specimens* *Translational research* Lack of specialty/discipline	Communication skills Facilities Turf conflicts Lack of dedicated researchers
Societal/Cultural healthcare system	*Awareness* (by employers, school personnel, associates, neighbors, community) *Health insurance* *Delays in diagnosis*	Focus on young and middle age Competing challenges

[a]Items in italics appear in multiple categories

cers were prevented during the 1990s, and there is evidence that a modicum of overall survival improvement has been achieved subsequently (Fig. 33.1, lower panel).

Paramount among other challenges is improving the quality of survival of cancer patients in this age group. This includes enhancing the psychosocial environment during diagnosis and treatment, reducing and preventing acute, chronic and delayed adverse sequelae, and abrogating the financial costs associated with diagnosis, treatment, and long-term follow-up.

33.3 Reasons for Lack of Progress

The relative lack of survival improvement for older adolescent and young adult cancer patients is a complex issue. In this section, probable explanations and contributing factors are specified and potential solutions are suggested. Contributing factors were derived from workshops and discussion groups hosted by the United States National Cancer Institute (NCI) [3], the Children's Oncology Group (COG), the International Society of Pediatric Oncology (SIOP) [4], and from preliminary studies in the United States [5]. Proposed

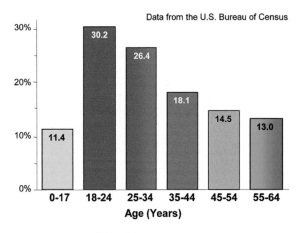

Figure 33.2

Percentage of the US population (aged 18–65 years) without health insurance in 2003. Data are from the US Bureau of Census

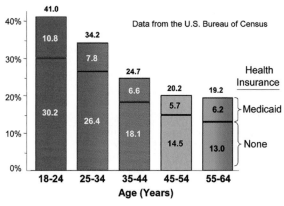

Figure 33.3

Percentage of the US population (aged 18–65 years) with state or no health insurance in 2003. Data are from the US Bureau of Census

explanations were categorized according to whether they applied to individuals (potential patients or patients diagnosed to have cancer), family/community members, the healthcare profession, or society/culture in general. In turn, each category was subdivided into factors that were likely (primary determinants) or unlikely (secondary determinants) to explain the survival deficit (Table 33.1).

33.3.1 Personal/Patient

The personal/patient category includes the individual adolescent and young adult before, during, and after a cancer diagnosis. Importantly, it includes persons before they are diagnosed with cancer because of the importance of early diagnosis in an age group for which prevention is largely ineffective. Factors within this category can be further subdivided into those that are biologic/physical, psychologic/emotional/spiritual, economic/financial, and social. Biologic factors include the unique physiologic and pharmacologic characteristics of adolescent and young adult patients and their array of cancers, many of which are unique to their age.

A primary factor in the personal/patient category is the overarching goal for those in this age group to learn how to become independent and autonomous.

To a large extent, making one's way in the world does not lend itself to concern about the risk of cancer. The individual is much more challenged by tasks of daily living and the immediate future. Another factor is the characteristic, age-specific feeling of immortality and invulnerability, which at no other time in life is more prominent. It is striking how few adolescents and young adults are aware that cancer can and does occur in their age group, or that the risk of developing cancer increases exponentially with age.

Adherence to treatment regimens is another major factor, both in terms of an intrinsic antagonism towards compliance (as a result of the need to become autonomous) and external pressures that mitigate adherence. The former has been well characterized in adolescents, not only with respect to expectations, but also with regard to compliance with chemotherapy [6–9]. Once in college or in the workforce, many young adults face restrictions about taking time for medical concerns. Having to attend class, complete homework, or be on the job make it difficult to adhere to the rigors of diagnosis and treatment, especially when teachers, school administrators and employers are not aware of, or won't accommodate, their student's or employee's needs with respect to cancer management (see 33.3.2 Family/Community below).

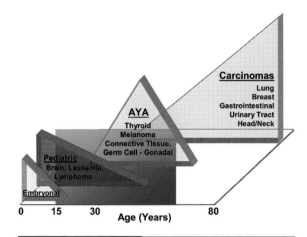

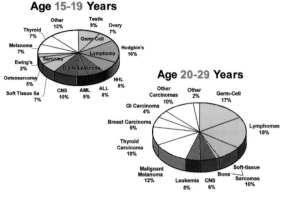

Figure 33.4
Age 15–29 years: the interface of pediatric and adult oncology. *AYA* Adolescents and young adults

Figure 33.5
Cancers in older adolescents and young adults. US SEER, 1975–2001. The segments in color represent "pediatric malignancies". *CNS* Central nervous system, *AML* acute myelogenous leukemia, *ALL* acute lymphoblastic leukemia, *NHL* non-Hodgkin lymphoma, *GI* gastrointestinal

Also important is the frequent lack of, or utilization of, health insurance in adolescents and young adults. As described below and in Chapter 32, Section 3.4.2, this is more problematic in this age group than in any other. In the United States, young adults are the most underinsured age group, falling in the gap between parental coverage and programs designed to provide universal health insurance to children (Medicaid and Children's Health Insurance Programs) on the one hand, and the coverage supplied by a full-time, secure job on the other. Nearly one-third of all 18- to 24-year-olds in the United States are uninsured, and more than 40% are either uninsured (Fig. 33.2) or have Medicaid (state government) assistance (Fig. 33.3) [10]. More than twice the number of 18- to 24-year-olds are uninsured or underinsured as 45- to 54-year-olds (Figs. 33.2 and 33.3).

Young adults and older adolescents also have the lowest rate of primary care use of any age group in the United States [11]. Regardless of health insurance status, adolescents and young adults are more likely than younger children to lack a usual source of care. Without a primary physician with knowledge of the patient's baseline heath status, the symptoms of cancer can be missed.

Cancer patients in the 15- to 29-year age group are at the interface between pediatric and adult oncology (Fig. 33.4). They have cancers that peak in incidence within their age range (Fig. 33.4) and a mix of tumor types (Fig. 33.5) unique to their age. As a result, patients in this specific age group present a special challenge to those trained to care for younger and older persons (see 33.3.3 Health Professional below).

33.3.2 Family/Community

The family/community category includes family members, colleagues/friends, educators, employers, politicians, and knowledge workers, who, in general, also lack awareness of the cancer problem in the adolescent and young adult group. Despite often being the first source of information and guidance for a young person, they almost always lack education and guidance themselves. Patient navigator programs conducted by community volunteers and cancer survivors (e.g., prostate, lung, breast, or colorectal cancer), have been formed in many communities because of this need. However, such programs, when they do exist, are rarely applicable to adolescents or young adults, and community resources that exist at the local level are generally devoted to younger and older patients.

33.3.3 Health Professional

Health professional factors include a lack of awareness about cancer in the adolescent and young adult, in part due to a lack of training and in part to the absence of continuing medical education programs on the topic. Oncology specialists and allied health professionals have less knowledge about treating this age group than of treating children or adults with cancer. Approximately one-half of the cancers in the 20- to 29-year age group constitute those ordinarily treated by adult oncologists (medical, gynecologic, surgical; Fig. 33.5, lower pie diagram); the other half are more familiar to pediatric oncologists and their specialized pediatric diagnostic, therapeutic, and supportive care teams (oncology nurses, radiologists, pathologists, infectious disease specialists, endocrinologists, nephrologists, psychologists, psychiatrists, and social workers). The pediatric approach is favored for 15- to 19-year-olds, because two-thirds to three-quarters of the malignancies that occur in this age group are well known by the pediatric oncology team (Fig. 33.5; upper pie diagram).

In contrast to the breadth of the pediatric oncology team, healthcare teams available to the young adult patient in an adult care program are significantly limited by comparison. It is rare that an adult patient has access to all of the services provided to a patient at a pediatric cancer center (Fig. 33.6). All too often, oncologists and other caregivers on adult services are reluctant to relinquish their young patients to providers who have these services.

In general, specific communication skills are needed to relate to adolescents. Neither adult nor pediatric oncologists are trained with these skills, and difficult topics of conversation, such as sexuality and fertility, are often not addressed.

There is no other patient age group for which the time period to diagnosis is longer, clinical trial participation is lower [12], and fewer tumor specimens are available for translational research (Fig. 33.7). The lack of clinical trial participation is particularly problematic. Only 1 to 2% of all 20- to 29-year-olds with cancer can be identified as participating in a therapeutic clinical trial sometime during their cancer experience. A correlation exists between the level of clinical trial activity and improvement in survival prolongation and

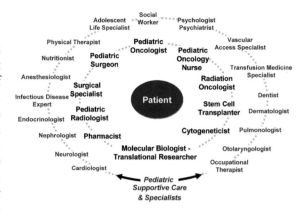

Figure 33.6

Pediatric oncology team

mortality rate reduction [13–15]. These factors explain much of the deficit in translational research and the lack of tumor specimens available for studies assessing molecular and cellular mechanisms of cancer in this age group. There is also a shortage of laboratory-based and clinical researchers dedicated to the study of cancers in the adolescent and young adult age group.

Patterns of care delivered to adolescents and young adults differ from those delivered to younger and older patients. Children are treated almost always in pediatric facilities where the specialists are familiar with their diseases, where they receive age-appropriate therapy, and where they are frequently enrolled in clinical trials [16–18]. By contrast, some adolescents receive care in adult facilities, where certain diagnostic and treatment events take longer to accomplish than in pediatric centers [19]. Adolescents are also more likely to delay contact with the healthcare system; behavior likely related to their increasing autonomy [20–22]. Finally, types of cancer differ between children and adolescents, and the two groups have different tolerances for therapy [23, 24]. Taken together, these factors contribute to delays in diagnosis and treatment for adolescents and young adults with cancer. When their care is managed less efficiently and effectively than that of other age groups, decreased survival is the likely outcome.

As alluded to earlier, few healthcare centers in North America have dedicated units for adolescents and

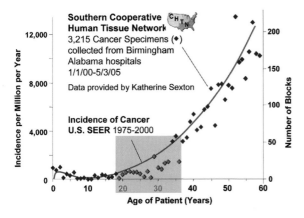

Figure 33.7

Tumor bank specimens (*blue triangles*; data provided by Katherine Sexton) and incidence of cancer (*red triangles*; US SEER, 1975–2000) as a function of age of the patient

young adults. One of the most frequent complaints from patients in this age group is that they have little in common with other patients in the waiting room, out-patient clinic, or hospital environment.

Reimbursement is a factor for both pediatric and adult oncology treatment teams in the United States. The lower rate of health insurance coverage in young adults lowers the reimbursement rate of services rendered and tends to diminish incentives for providers and limit diagnostic evaluation, treatment interventions, and supportive care.

That patients in the adolescent and young adult age group are at the interface between pediatric and adult medicine may lead to uncoordinated care, to uncertainties about who is responsible for their management, and, in worst-case scenarios, to conflicts in management.

33.3.4 Societal/Cultural

The societal/cultural category consists of the challenges societies face in providing for the healthcare needs of older adolescents and young adults. The general public is largely unaware of cancer as a significant healthcare problem among young adults in the United

States. Even healthcare providers at universities and colleges do not have cancer in their curricula. High schools and universities do not have cancer awareness as an essential educational or health evaluation component. It is not surprising, therefore, that the time to diagnosis in older adolescent and young adult patients is not only delayed relative to the time to diagnosis in younger patients, but that it is also correlated with health insurance status, as discussed below.

33.4 Prioritization of Challenges and Potential Solutions

Primary factors (Table 33.1) contributing to the deficit in survival for older adolescents and young adults should be prioritized over secondary factors, and those factors that appear in more than one category are likely to be more important targets for change. Lack of awareness, for example, appears in all of the four major categories. Inadequate health insurance coverage appears in three categories, as does low participation in clinical trials. A deficit in translational research and lack of tumor specimens for research appear in two categories. These four factors – awareness, health insurance, participation in clinical trials, and translational research – may be regarded as paramount and are emphasized in the prioritization review below.

33.4.1 Personal/Patient

Awareness is a primary goal. Older adolescents and young adults not only believe that they are immune to the risks of disease and accident, they do not realize that the risk of cancer is 1:210 for those between 15 and 29 years of age in the United States. Overcoming ideation of invincibility will require local and national educational efforts. The importance of healthcare availability and healthcare insurance coverage will also need more emphasis, while the availability and goals of clinical trials will require particular attention. Moreover, the approaches used to educate and recruit adolescent and young adult cancer patients to clinical trials and translational research efforts will probably need to be quite different from those utilized for older adults.

33.4.2 Family/Community

Those who associate with older adolescents or young adults should be aware that cancer occurs in this age group and be able to advise and encourage a medical evaluation for the symptoms and signs of malignant disease. This applies to family members, friends, neighbors, classmates, teachers, fellow employees, employers, and clergy.

33.4.3 Health Professional

Health professionals must become more aware of cancer occurring during early adulthood, and professional training and continuing education should emphasize the risk of cancer and its common symptoms and signs. Health professionals should become advocates for affordable health insurance. Oncologists should become more cognizant of the gaps in clinical trial activity and translational research in the adolescent and young adult group. They should make available more clinical trials for the adolescent and young adult population and seek ways to increase clinical trial participation specific to this age group.

33.4.4 Societal/Cultural

The lack of awareness of the adolescent and young adult cancer problem should be overcome with public information and education programs. Legislators, health policy administrators, insurance company directors, national medical organization leaders, and leaders of institutions of higher learning should be particularly informed and educated. The role of healthcare insurance should be emphasized, as should the risk of cancer in educational curricula. In the United States, cancer organizations such as the American Society of Clinical Oncology, the American Cancer Society, the National Cancer Institute, the National Comprehensive Cancer Network, C-Change, and the national cancer cooperative groups should make adolescent and young adult oncology a priority (see Appendix 33.1). They should be joined in this effort by private cancer foundations that have a responsibility for young adults or older adolescents, such as Planet Cancer, Fertile Hope, Young Survival Coalition, and The Leukemia and Lymphoma Society (see Appendix 33.1). Ideally, universal healthcare insurance should be available to all persons in the 18- to 29-year age range, until private insurance is provided by an employer or young people can afford or supplement it on their own.

In summary, improving awareness of the cancer problem, providing better healthcare insurance coverage and access to healthcare services, and increasing clinical and translational research on cancer in older adolescents and young adults are challenges that would benefit patients in this age group. This is not to say that challenges such as psychosocial supportive care and dedicated healthcare facilities are not important. On the contrary, they are crucial. However, tackling problems of highest priority is likely to have downstream effects that will alleviate many of the other problems listed in Table 33.1. The solutions will take a coordinated effort at local, regional, national, and international levels. Four additional challenges are discussed in further detail below.

33.5 Longer Time to Diagnosis in Adolescents and Young Adults than in Children

The interval from the onset of the first cancer-specific symptom to the first anti-cancer treatment, known as the waiting time, has been shown to be longer in adolescents than in children [25–28]. Young children (younger than 5 years of age) have been observed to have the shortest waiting times [29]. The waiting time may be influenced by factors related to the individual, to the healthcare system, and/or to the disease. Variation in waiting times among children has been shown to be due primarily to the type of disease, and secondarily to age. The time from onset of symptoms to initial healthcare contact is influenced by individual and healthcare system factors; the time from initial contact to assessment by a treating oncologist or surgeon is most likely affected by healthcare system factors; the time between that assessment and date of first anti-cancer treatment most likely reflects disease-related factors [30–32].

The interval from onset of the first cancer-specific symptom to the day of cancer diagnosis is referred to as the lagtime. Studies in the United States, Canada, Scotland, and Mexico have demonstrated that lagtimes are longer in adolescents than in children [33–37]. In these studies it is unclear whether the longer lagtimes experienced by adolescents – in comparison with younger children – are related to the types of cancers they develop or to other factors related to their age [38].

In the United States, health insurance coverage is a major determinant of lagtimes in patients 15 to 29 years of age [39]. The lagtimes in this age group are correlated more closely with health insurance status than race, ethnicity, gender, marital status, religion, urban versus rural home residence, or median household income of the zipcode of residence [5, 39]. The issue of health insurance coverage is likely a greater factor in 18- to 29-year-olds than in any other age group, since this is the age in the United States at which health insurance coverage is the lowest. Countries with national health insurance are also likely affected by this determinant, since health insurance utilization is lower in the young adult age range than in younger or older persons, despite the universal availability of health insurance.

33.6 Place of Diagnosis and Treatment: Pediatric versus Adult Care Specialists and Facilities

A central, complex issue is the choice of the most appropriate specialist who will manage care for the older adolescent and young adult cancer patient – a pediatric oncologist or an adult oncologist (medical, radiation, surgical, or gynecologic oncologist). For older adolescents, the site of diagnosis and treatment may be problematic since, at least in theory, these patients could be treated at either a pediatric or adult care facility. Leonard and his colleagues in the United Kingdom have pointed out that adult oncologists are "untutored in arranging ancillary medical, psychological, and educational supports that are so important to people who are facing dangerous diseases and taxing treatment at a vulnerable time in their lives" and "unpracticed in managing rare sarcomas." Simultaneously, they have emphasized that pediatric oncologists

"have little to no experience in epithelial tumors or some of the other tumors common in late adolescence" [40]. In 1997, the (admittedly biased) American Academy of Pediatrics issued a consensus statement in which it indicated that referral to a board-eligible or board-certified pediatric hematologist-oncologist and to pediatric subspecialty consultants was the standard of care for all pediatric and adolescent cancer patients [41]. A wider consensus panel that included adult oncologists, the American Federation of Clinical Oncologic Societies, also concluded that "payors must provide ready access to pediatric oncologists, recognizing that childhood cancers are biologically distinct" and that the "likelihood of successful outcome in children is enhanced when treatment is provided by pediatric cancer specialists" [42]. However, neither of these statements defines an age cutoff in the recommendations.

Currently, the choice of specialist is made haphazardly and most often depends upon the decision of the referring physician. Younger children obtain care primarily from pediatricians, who refer to pediatric centers and specialists. Young adult and older adolescent patients are seen by a breadth of specialists for their presenting symptoms of cancer. These include internists, family physicians, gynecologists, emergency room physicians, dermatologists, gastroenterologists, neurologists, and other specialists. These physicians may have very different referral patterns [43], and when the referral of a young adult or adolescent patient is made to an oncologist, it may be to a medical, radiation, surgical, gynecologic, or other oncologic specialist.

The switch from predominantly pediatric to adult medical management tends to occur not at age 21 years or even at age 18 years, as might be expected, but closer to age 15 years. The majority of 15- to 19-year-olds diagnosed with cancer are treated at adult facilities. A cancer registry review in the state of Utah, which has only one pediatric oncology treatment facility, revealed that only 36% of oncology patients 15 to 19 years of age were ever seen at the pediatric hospital [44]. In Canada, only 30% of cancer patients in this age group are managed at pediatric centers [19]. A study of the National Cancer Data Base found that for nearly 20,000 cases of cancer in adolescents aged 15 to 19 years, only

34% were treated at centers that had NCI pediatric cooperative group affiliation [45].

In the end, the healthcare facility decision should be based in large part on which setting will provide the patient with the best outcome. If these are equivalent, "social" or "supportive" factors should next weigh into the decision. For some diseases, data support a particular site or specialist. In North America, a comparison of 16- to 21-year-olds with acute lymphoblastic leukemia (ALL) or acute myeloid leukemia (AML) showed that the outcome was superior for patients treated on cooperative group trials than for those not entered [46]. In France, The Netherlands, and North America, older adolescents with ALL treated on pediatric clinical trials have fared considerably better than those treated on adult leukemia trials [47–49]. In Germany, older adolescents with Ewing sarcoma who were treated at pediatric cancer centers had a better outcome than those treated at other centers [50]. In Italy, young adults with rhabdomyosarcoma fared better if they were treated according to pediatric standards of therapy than when treated ad hoc or on an adult sarcoma regimen [51]. At the University of Texas MD Anderson Cancer Center, the results of treatment for ALL in adults improved substantively after treatment derived from pediatric trials was introduced into the institution's trials [52]. The analysis of data from the United States National Cancer Data Base revealed that adolescents 15 to 19 years of age with non-Hodgkin lymphoma, leukemia, liver cancer, and bone tumors had a survival advantage if treated at an NCI pediatric group institution [45]. Thus, for these pediatric types of cancer, the pediatric specialist/facility is favored.

For other cancers, adult-treating medical/surgical/radiation oncologists are more appropriate providers. Adolescent and young adult patients with melanoma, colorectal carcinoma, breast cancer, or epithelial neoplasm of the ovary may be better served under the care of physicians who are more familiar with these malignancies, such as medical oncologists or gynecologic oncologists. Until pediatric oncologists demonstrate that they have the expertise to treat these relatively nonpediatric cancers, this referral direction should be a first consideration.

The alternative is for adult care specialists/facilities to adopt a pediatric approach, which may be difficult for a variety of historical, sociopolitical, economic, and infrastructure reasons. For example, two adult cooperative groups in the United States (Cancer and Acute Leukemia Group B, and Southwest Oncology Group) are starting a trial of a pediatric regimen taken directly from the COG, which will treat 15- to 29-year-old patients with ALL. Several obstacles have been encountered in planning this approach, including differences in treatment philosophy (e.g., when to resume therapy after myelosuppression relative to the platelet and absolute phagocyte counts, and when to transfuse platelets and red cells), health insurance coverage, adherence of patients to treatment schedules and regimens, and the availability of supportive care and allied health professionals. Nonetheless, these obstacles are expected to be surmounted and the outcomes of young adult patients improved in the process.

Determining which specialist/facility is most appropriate will certainly vary from cancer to cancer and from case to case. Patients at any age who have a "pediatric" tumor, such as rhabdomyosarcoma, Ewing sarcoma, and osteosarcoma, will probably benefit from the expertise of a pediatric oncologist, at least in the form of consultation. Children younger than 18 years of age – and their parents – may benefit from the social and supportive culture of a pediatric hospital regardless of the diagnosis. Individuals between the ages of 16 and 24 years may have varying levels of maturity and independence, and the choice of physician and setting for their care should be determined individually. Pediatric oncologists may be less adept at a nonpaternalistic relationship with the patient (and potentially his or her spouse) and less inclined to consider issues such as sexuality, body image, fertility, and the like. Adult oncologists are more accustomed to dose delays and adjustments, and may be less aggressive with chemotherapy dosing than the pediatric oncologist, whose younger patients can tolerate higher doses. The ultimate challenge would be to develop centers and oncologists devoted solely to the care of this group of patients. Such a dedicated program has been championed in the United Kingdom, at least for older adolescents. Several unique "teenage cancer units" have been established, staffed by physicians and nurses with expertise in adolescent and young adult cancer patient management [53]. This provides the older adolescent

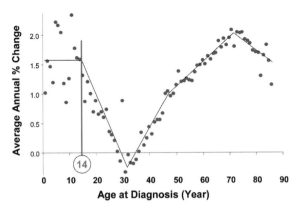

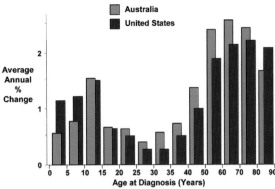

Figure 33.8

Average annual percent change in 5-year survival for all invasive cancers. US SEER, 1975–1997

Figure 33.9

Improvement in 5-year relative survival in Australia and the US as a function of age at diagnosis of invasive cancer: 1982–1997

with age-specific nursing care, recreation therapy, and peer companionship. A similar initiative is underway in Perth, Western Australia with a new building of specific facilities for adolescents up to age 19 years with cancer and plans for a "virtual" multidisciplinary team service to all adolescents regardless of site of care. Eventually, there could be a discipline of adolescent and young adult oncology with its own training programs, science, translational research, clinical trials, and national and international organizations.

33.7 Implications for Other Age Groups

When the average annual percent change in 5-year survival is expressed as a function of specific year of age at diagnosis, the age range affected by adverse trends can be identified more precisely. Such an analysis suggests that progress versus age over the past quarter century in the United States is linear over the 15- to 29-year age span, with inflections at age 14 and 31 years (Fig. 33.8). This suggests that the factors that account for the lack of improvement for the adolescent and young adult group relative to children start at age 15 years, and are increasingly more problematic up to age 30 years. Between 31 and 47 years of age, the trend is reversed with an analogous, nearly mirror-image

linear improvement (Fig. 33.8). This observation indicates that the next oldest 15-year age span (30 to 44 years) should be evaluated in a fashion similar to that undertaken for older adolescents and young adults. This analysis also suggests that the greatest progress in prolonging survival from cancer during the past quarter century in the United States has been in the 60- to 80-year age group, with a peak improvement at age 70 years (Fig. 33.8).

33.8 International Perspectives and Global Challenge

The Surveillance, Epidemiology, and End Results (SEER) data in this monograph are from the United States, and most of the conclusions herein are derived from these SEER data. Nonetheless, most if not all of the observations are applicable to other countries. Certainly, there is a worldwide lack of awareness about cancer in young adults and older adolescents relative to the recognition of cancer in children and older adults. In addition, it is safe to claim that the deficits in clinical trial participation as well as translational research in early adulthood are universal.

The national survival data for Australia show patterns of outcome similar to those observed in the

Table 33.2 Accruals to national cancer treatment trials during the era of national collaboration to augment sarcoma clinical trial development and participation. Clinical trial accrual data were taken from the Cancer Therapy Evaluation Program, National Cancer Institute, courtesy of Michael Montello and Troy Budd

	Age	1998–9	2000–1	2002–3
All cancer	All ages	48,225	57,033	54,717
	<20	9,094	7,791	6,070
	20-39	3,488	3,752	3,411
	40-59	17,403	22,025	22,556
Sarcomas	<40	637	888	929
% of all entries		5.1%	7.7%	9.8%
Other cancers	<40	11,945	10,655	8,552

United States (Fig. 33.9; Australian data kindly provided by C. Stevenson, Australian Institute of Health and Welfare). During the years 1982–1997, 15- to 29-year-old Australians with cancer had the least progress in survival improvement, in comparison with other 15-year groups at younger or older ages. This is consistent with, albeit not as dramatic as, the age pattern in the United States (Fig. 33.9). That Australians enjoy universal health insurance, as do most inhabitants of socioeconomically advantaged countries of the world, suggests that lack of national health insurance in the United States does not alone explain the deficit in America. On the other hand, universal health insurance in Australia does not guarantee access to or use of healthcare services, and is clearly not universally utilized in the young adult age group. Indeed, longer times to a diagnosis of cancer occur in this age group in countries with and without national health insurance, as described above, and in a recent comparison of circumstances in Canada and the United States [54]. Most likely, lack of health insurance and of utilization of healthcare services are global problems in young adults and older adolescents.

There is an obvious need to address the challenges of adolescent and young adult oncology worldwide, perhaps in a manner similar to that described for pediatric oncology [55]. This could be an important opportunity for the International Society of Pediatric Oncology (SIOP) to play a leadership role, as other childhood cancer organizations have exercised nationally. Adoption of a proposed system for the classification of cancers in the 15- to 29-year age group [56] would be a good place to start.

33.9 Future Directions and Interim Solutions

In North America and Australia, the COG has taken a leadership role in meeting the challenges described in this chapter. In conjunction with the NCI and NCI-sponsored adult cooperative groups, four initiatives were identified as priorities for development: (1) improving access to care through understanding barriers to participation, (2) developing a cancer resource network that provides information about clinical trials to patients, families, providers, and the public, (3) enhancing adolescent treatment adherence (compliance with protocol-prescribed therapy), and (4) increasing adolescent and young adult participation in sarcoma trials specifically designed for patients in this age group. The COG Adolescent and Young Adult Committee was formed in 2000 to research the obstacles faced by older adolescents and young adult patients, with the disease focus on sarcomas. The Southwest Oncology Group (for adult patients) subsequently opened the COG trial for metastatic Ewing sarcoma, and thereafter hosted the development of an intergroup sarcoma committee – the Intergroup Con-

Table 33.3 Practical suggestions to enhance early detection of cancer and clinical trial participation in older adolescents and young adults

- Appreciate that cancer occurs in one in every 200 older adolescents and young adults and that everyone is at risk.
- Be aware that young adults often deny symptoms, are too embarrassed to report them, or attribute them to psychosomatic manifestations.
- Encourage and assist young adults to seek care at a comprehensive healthcare center.
- Realize that young adults are least likely to have adequate health insurance, and that they should not allow themselves to "age out" of insurance.
- Know that there are very few known causes of cancer during early adulthood, and that "it just happens", regardless of the health of the person.
- Convey that what is done at the time of the cancer diagnosis is important and that the best outcome is determined by the initial evaluation and therapy. Optimal cancer management means doing it right from the start!
- Once diagnosed with cancer, suggest that young adults ask about clinical trials. If none is available on site, help them find centers that participate in clinical trials suitable for their age.
- Once enrolled on a clinical trial, the adolescent and young adult cancer patient needs understanding and support in order to best adhere to the trial's requisites.

Table 33.4 Recommendation of the Adolescent and Young Adult Oncology Progress Review Group

- Identify the characteristics that distinguish the unique cancer burden in the AYAO patient.
- Provide education, training and communication to improve awareness, prevention, access and quality cancer care for AYAs.
- Create the tools to study the AYA cancer problem.
- Ensure excellence in service delivery across the cancer controll continuum (i.e. prevention, screening, diagnosis, treatment, survivorship, and end of life)..
- Strengthen and promote advocacy and support of the AYA cancer patient.

sortium Against Sarcoma – with formal representation from all the adult cooperative groups as well as the National Cancer Institute of Canada.

Evidence for improvement in the accruals to NCI-sponsored national sarcoma treatment trials is shown in Table 33.2. The proportion of American sarcoma patients younger than age 40 years entered onto the trials has nearly doubled – from 5.1% to 9.8% – during the past 5 years. In contrast, and as a control for this observation, the other cancers that occur in this age group (and that have not yet been addressed) showed a decline in patient accrual.

Another initiative in the United States is the formation of a consortium of all the organizations devoted to assisting adolescents and young adults with cancer. Known as the LiveStrong Young Adult Alliance, this organization is dedicated to improving survival rates and the quality of life of young adults living with cancer by promoting relevant research and the delivery of patient care, generating awareness of the issue, being a voice for young adults with cancer, and advancing helpful community-based programs and services (see Resources). The Alliance will bring together for the first time key voices in the cancer community to improve results for young adults.

In parallel, the United States NCI initiated a Progress Review Group (PRG) to evaluate the national status of young adult cancer outcomes and needs. This

PRG assessed the deficits and scientific issues described in this chapter and addressed others identified by a panel of experts in a 1-year-long process. Specific recommendations for national implementation were presented in late 2006 [57] (Table 33.4). Meanwhile, several practical suggestions should facilitate early detection of cancer in adolescents and young adults and promote referral to a cancer center where clinical trials are a priority (Table 33.3).

In the United Kingdom, initiatives to address the issue of management of adolescents with cancer include national guidelines from the National Institute for Health and Clinical Excellence, which mandates the care for all patients under 19 years of age with cancer to be provided in age-appropriate facilities [58]. In Australia, following a National Senate Inquiry into cancer services and treatment options, specific national recommendations for the management of cancers in the adolescent age groups have been made [59].

33.10 Conclusions

Adolescent and young adult oncology patients belong to a distinct age group and, like pediatric, adult, and geriatric patients, have unique medical and psychosocial needs. Challenges in treating the 15- to 29-year age group include understanding the complex psychosocial environment of this age group, particularly during diagnosis and treatment, managing chronic and delayed adverse sequelae, overcoming a lack of progress in prolonging survival, improving the quality of survival, and addressing the economic costs associated with diagnosis, treatment, and long-term follow-up. The single greatest current challenge in young adults and older adolescents with cancer is to overcome the lack of progress in their survival improvement, a deficit that has spanned nearly a quarter of a century.

There are multiple reasons for the lack of progress. These may be categorized into personal/patient (older adolescents and young adults), family/community (family members, colleagues/friends, educators, employers, politicians, legislators, knowledge workers), health professional (physicians, nurses, allied health professionals), and societal/cultural (healthcare system) factors. The features common to these factors are lack of awareness, inadequate health insurance coverage, lack of clinical trial participation, and a deficit in translational research of the cancers in older adolescents and young adults.

Solutions to the survival deficit include raising awareness about the problem, improving healthcare access and insurance, enhancing understanding of the biology of cancers that occur in this age group, developing national and international organizations to address the deficits, and ultimately, creating a formal discipline of adolescent/young adult oncology.

In particular, resources should be devoted to educating the public, health professionals, insurers, and legislators about cancer during this phase of life and about the special needs of these patients. Specific attention should be paid to the longer delays in diagnosis that occur in older adolescents and young adults relative to younger patients. These are correlated with the quality of health insurance coverage.

Also of special importance is the facility where diagnosis and treatment take place; for several of the pediatric type of malignancies (ALL, AML, Ewing sarcoma, rhabdomyosarcoma), there is evidence that the therapeutic approach taken by pediatric oncologists has led to better survival rates than those applied by medical oncologists and hematologists.

Meanwhile, older adolescents and young adults with cancer should become aware of cancer as a possible illness within their age group, be encouraged to report symptoms without delay, to seek care at a comprehensive healthcare center, to not "age out" of insurance, to understand that what is done at the time of diagnosis is most important, and to ask about and find clinical trials for their age.

Surviving adolescence and young adulthood is difficult enough when all is well and health is robust. Cancer makes this phase of life extraordinarily more challenging and demanding. Medical professionals should pay special attention to the unique transitions faced by these patients; at diagnosis, through the process of informed consent, at initiation of therapy, during school and employment reentrance, at completion of therapy, during posttreatment follow-up, and when switching from pediatric to adult care. Ideally, specialized adolescent and young adult cancer units should be developed with the anticipation that centralization of care and availability of age-targeted clinical trials will lead to improved treatment, survival, and quality of life.

Cancer during adolescence and early adult life is an underestimated challenge that merits specific resources, solutions, and a national focus. Future research should elucidate why survival outcomes for this group have lagged behind those of others and identify the efforts – including better clinical trial accrual – that might remedy the disparity. Finally, more scholarly and focused attention on the unique psychosocial needs of this population will improve the quality of their cancer care and of their survival. At the very least, those at the interface deserve the same attention and progress that has been achieved for younger and older persons.

References

1. Bleyer WA, O'Leary M, Barr R, Ries LAG (eds) (2006) Cancer Epidemiology in Older Adolescents and Young Adults 15 to 29 Years of Age, Including SEER Incidence and Survival, 1975–2000. National Cancer Institute, NIH Pub. No. 06-5767. Bethesda, MD
2. Michelagnoli MP, Pritchard J, Phillips MB (2003) Adolescent oncology – a homeland for the "lost tribe". Eur J Cancer 39:2571–2572
3. Bleyer A, Smith M, Coordinators (1999) Enhancing Accrual of Adolescent and Young Adult Cancer Patients on Clinical Trials. NCI Workshop, 17 June 17, Bethesda, MD
4 Bleyer A (2005) Cancer in older adolescents and young adults: reasons for lack of progress. Pediatr Blood Cancer 45:376
5. Martin S, Ulrich C, Munsell M, et al (2005) Time to cancer diagnosis in young Americans depends on type of cancer and health insurance status. Value Health 8:344
6. Festa RS, Tamaroff MH, Chasalow F, Lanzkowsky (1992) Therapeutic adherence to oral medication regimens by adolescents with cancer. I. Laboratory assessment. J Pediatr 120:807–811
7. Tamaroff MH, Festa RS, Adesman AR, Walco GA (1992) Therapeutic adherence to oral medication regimens by adolescents with cancer. II. Clinical and psychologic correlates. J Pediatr 120:813–817
8. Tebbi CK (1993) Treatment compliance in childhood and adolescence. Cancer 71:3441–3449
9. Kyngas HA, Kroll T, Duffy ME (2000) Compliance in adolescents with chronic diseases: a review. J Adolesc Health 26:379–388
10. DeNavas-Walt C, Proctor BD, Mills RJ (2004) Income, poverty, and health insurance coverage in the United States: 2003. In: US Census Bureau: Current Population Reports. US Government Printing Office, Washington, DC, pp 60–226
11. Ziv A, Boulet JR, Slap GB (1999) Utilization of physician offices by adolescents in the United States. Pediatrics 104:35–42
12. Bleyer A (2005) The adolescent and young adult gap in cancer care and outcome. Curr Probl Pediatr Adolesc Health Care 35:182–217
13. Bleyer A, Montello M, Budd T (2004) Young adults with leukemia in the United States: lack of clinical trial participation and mortality reduction during the last decade. Proc Am Soc Clin Oncol 22:(abstract 586)
14. Bleyer A, Montello M, Budd T, Saxman S (2005) National survival trends of young adults with sarcoma: lack of progress is associated with lack of clinical trial participation. Cancer 103:1891–1897
15. Bleyer A, Budd T, Montello M (2005) Lack of clinical trial participation and of progress in older adolescents and young adults with cancer. Curr Probl Pediatr Adolesc Health Care 35:186–195
16. Huchcroft S, Clarke A, Mao Y, et al (1995) This Battle Which I Must Fight: Cancer in Canada's Children and Teenagers. Supply and Services Canada, Ottawa, Canada
17. Barr RD (1999) On cancer control and the adolescent. Med Pediatr Oncol 32:404–410
18. Greenberg ML, Greenberg CM (1994) A provincial program for childhood cancer control – 1994. Canada: Ministry of Health, Ontario, Toronto
19. Klein-Geltink J, Shaw AK, Morrison HI, et al (2005) Use of paediatric versus adult oncology treatment centres by adolescents 15 to 19 years old: the Canadian Childhood Cancer Surveillance and Control Program. Eur J Cancer 41:404–410
20. Bleyer WA (2002) Cancer in older adolescents and young adults: epidemiology, diagnosis, treatment, survival, and importance of clinical trials. Med Pediatr Oncol 38:1–10
21. White L, Ewing J, Senner AM, et al (2004) Cancer in adolescents and young adults: treatment and outcome in Victoria. Med J Aust 180:653–654
22. Ritchie MA (2001) Sources of support for adolescents with cancer. J Pediatr Oncol Nurs 18:105–110
23. Bleyer A (2002) Older adolescents with cancer in North America deficits in outcome and research. Pediatr Clin North Am 49:1027–1042
24. Albritton K, Bleyer WA (2003) The management of cancer in the older adolescent. Eur J Cancer 39:2584–2599
25. Canadian Childhood Cancer Surveillance and Control Program (2004) Diagnosis and Initial Treatment of Cancer in Canadian Adolescents 15 to 19 Years, 1995–2000. Health Canada, Ottawa, Canada

26. Haimi M, Peretz Nahum M, Ben Arush MW (2004) Delay in diagnosis of children with cancer: a retrospective study of 315 children. Pediatr Hematol Oncol 21:37–48

27. Gibbons L, Mao Y, Levy IG, Miller AB (1994) The Canadian Childhood Cancer Control Program. CMAJ 151:1704–1709

28. Canadian Childhood Cancer Surveillance and Control Program (2003) Diagnosis and Initial Treatment of Cancer in Canadian Children 0 to 14 Years, 1995–2000. Health Canada, Ottawa, Canada

29. Klein-Geltink JE, Pogany LM, Barr RD, et al (2005) Waiting times for cancer care in Canadian children: impact of distance, clinical, and demographic factors. Pediatr Blood Cancer 44:318–327

30. Andersen BL, Cacioppo JT (1995) Delay in seeking a cancer diagnosis: delay stages and psychophysiological comparison processes. Br J Soc Psychol 34:33–52

31. Carvalho AL, Pintos J, Schlecht NF, et al (2002) Predictive factors for diagnosis of advanced-stage squamous cell carcinoma of the head and neck. Arch Otolaryngol Head Neck Surg 128:313–318

32. de Nooijer J, Lechner L, de Vries H (2001) A qualitative study on detecting cancer symptoms and seeking medical help; an application of Andersen's model of total patient delay. Patient Educ Couns 42:145–157

33. Pollock BH, Krischner JP, Vietti TJ (1991) Interval between symptom onset and diagnosis of pediatric solid tumors. J Pediatr 119:725–732

34. Clavarino AM, Lowe JB, Carmont SA, Balanda K (2002) The needs of cancer patients and their families from rural and remote areas of Queensland. Aust J Rural Health 10:188–195

35. Scott-Findlay S, Chalmers K (2001) Rural families' perspectives on having a child with cancer. J Pediatr Oncol Nurs 18:205–216

36. Saha V, Love S, Eden T, et al (1993) Determinants of symptom interval in childhood cancer. Arch Dis Child 68:771–774

37. Fajardo-Gutierrez A, Sandoval-Mex AM, Mejia-Arangure JM, et al (2002) Clinical and social factors that affect the time to diagnosis of Mexican children with cancer. Med Pediatr Oncol 39:25–31

38. Bleyer WA (2003) The scope of the problem of adolescent and young adult cancer. Presented at Proc POGO Symposium on Childhood Cancer, Adolescent and Young Adult Oncology: Walking Two Worlds. 21–22 November 2003, Toronto, Ontario, Canada

39. Bleyer A, Ulrich C, Martin S, et al (2005) Status of health insurance predicts time from symptom onset to cancer diagnosis in young adults. Proc Am Soc Clin Oncol 23:547s

40. Leonard RC, Gregor A, Coleman RE, Lewis I (1995) Strategy needed for adolescent patients with cancer. BMJ 311:387

41. American Academy of Pediatrics Section on Hematology/Oncology (1997) Guidelines for the pediatric cancer center and role of such centers in diagnosis and treatment. Pediatrics 99:139–141

42. American Federation of Clinical Oncologic Societies (1998) Consensus statement on access to quality cancer care. J Pediatr Hematol Oncol 20:279–281

43. Goldman S, Stafford C, Weinthal J, et al (2000) Older adolescents vary greatly from children in their route of referral to the pediatric oncologist and national trials. Proc Am Soc Clin Oncol 18:(abstract 1766)

44. Albritton K, Wiggins CL (2001) Adolescents with cancer are not referred to Utah's pediatric center. Proc Am Soc Clin Oncol 19:(abstract 990)

45. Rauck AM, Fremgen AM, Hutchison CL, et al (1999) Adolescent cancers in the United States: a national cancer data base (NCDB) report. J Pediatr Hematol Oncol 21:310

46. Nachman J, Sather HN, Buckley JD, et al (1993) Young adults 16–21 years of age at diagnosis entered on Children's Cancer Group acute lymphoblastic leukemia and acute myeloblastic leukemia protocols. Results of treatment. Cancer 71:3377–3385

47. Stock W, Sather H, Dodge RK, et al (2000) Outcome of adolescents and young adults with ALL: a comparison of Children's Cancer Group and Cancer and Leukemia Group B Regimens. Blood 96:467a

48. de Bont JM, Holt B, Dekker AW, et al (2004) Significant difference in outcome for adolescents with acute lymphoblastic leukemia treated on pediatric vs adult protocols in the Netherlands. Leukemia 18:2032–2035

49. Boissel N, Auclerc MF, Lheritier V, et al (2003) Should adolescents with acute lymphoblastic leukemia be treated as old children or young adults? Comparison of the French FRALLE-93 and LALA-94 trials. J Clin Oncol (2003)21:760–761

50. Paulussen S, Ahrens S, Juergens HF (2003) Cure rates in Ewing tumor patients aged over 15 years are better in pediatric oncology units. Results of GPOH CESS/EICESS studies. Proc Am Soc Clin Oncol 22:(abstract 816)

51. Ferrari A, Dileo P, Casanova M, et al (2003) Rhabdomyosarcoma in adults. A retrospective analysis of 171 patients treated at a single institution. Cancer 98:571–580

52. Kantarjian HM, O'Brien S, Smith TL, et al (2000) Results of treatment with hyper-CVAD, a dose-intensive regimen, in adult acute lymphocytic leukemia. J Clin Oncol 18:547–561

53. Lewis IJ (1996) Cancer in adolescence. Br Med Bull 52:887–897

54. Barr RD, Greenberg ML (2006) Cancer surveillance and control in adolescents – similarities and contrasts between Canada and the United States. Pediatr Blood Cancer 46:273–277

55. Barr R, Ribeiro R, Agarwal B, Masera G, Hesseling P, Magrath I (2006) Pediatric oncology in countries with limited resources. In: Pizzo PA, Poplack DG (eds) Principles and Practice of Pediatric Oncology, 5th edn. Lippincott Williams and Wilkins, Philadelphia, pp 1604–1616

56. Barr RD, Holowaty EJ, Birch JM (2006) Classification schemes for tumors diagnosed in adolescents and young adults. Cancer 106:1425–1430

57. Closing the Gap: Research and Care Imperatives for Adolescent and Young Adults with Cancer. Report of the Adolescent and Young Adult Oncology Progess. Review Group. US Departement of Health and Human Services and Live Strong™ Young Adult Alliance, 2006

58. National Institute of Clinical Excellence (2005) Improving Outcomes in Children and Young People with Cancer. National Institute of Clinical Excellence, London. www.nice.org.uk

59. Senate Community Affairs References Committee (2005) The Cancer Journey: Informing Choice. Senate Community Affairs References Committee, Commonwealth of Australia; June 2005,www.aph.gov.au/senate.ca

Appendix: Resources

National Cancer Institute Information
http://www.cancer.gov/

The National Cancer Institute (NCI) is a component of the National Institutes of Health (NIH), one of eight agencies that compose the Public Health Service (PHS) in the Department of Health and Human Services (DHHS). The NCI is the Federal Government's principal agency for cancer research and training and coordinates the National Cancer Program, which conducts and supports research, training, health information dissemination, and other programs with respect to the cause, diagnosis, prevention, and treatment of cancer, rehabilitation from cancer, and the continuing care of cancer patients and the families of cancer patients.

The NCI's Web site provides accurate, up-to-date information on many types of cancer, information on clinical trials, resources for people dealing with cancer, and information for researchers and health professionals. Many of the NCI's cancer information resources are accessible through the cancer information page on http://www.cancer.gov/. The NCI's Web site has many resources available in Spanish

NCI publications on adolescent and young adult cancer:

- Childhood Cancers Homepage http://www.cancer. gov/cancerinformation/cancertype/cildhood/ This contains a collection of information sheets about types of childhood cancer, cancer screening and detection, treatment, clinical trials, and cancer literature.
- NCI Research on Childhood Cancers http://cis.nci. nih.gov/fact/6_40.htm. General facts about childhood cancer and research endeavors.
- Young People with Cancer: A Handbook for Parents   http://www.cancer.gov/cancertopics/young-

people. This is an overview of childhood cancer diagnosis, treatment, topics of concern, and additional information for parents.
- Care for Children and Adolescents with Cancer: Questions and Answers http://cis.nci.nih.gov/fact/1_ 21.htm. A fact sheet detailing questions and answers about childhood cancer, childhood cancer centers, and research about treatment for childhood cancers.

SEER: Surveillance, Epidemiology,
and End Results http://seer.cancer.gov/

The Surveillance, Epidemiology, and End Results (SEER) Program of the National Cancer Institute is an authoritative source of information on cancer incidence and survival in the United States. The SEER Program currently collects and publishes cancer incidence and survival data from 14 population-based cancer registries and 3 supplemental registries covering approximately 26% of the United States population. Information on more than 3 million in situ and invasive cancer cases is included in the SEER database, and approximately 170,000 new cases are added each year within the SEER coverage areas. The SEER Registries routinely collect data on patient demographics, primary tumor site, morphology, stage at diagnosis, first course of treatment, and follow-up for vital status. The SEER Program is the only comprehensive source of population-based information in the United States that includes stage of cancer at the time of diagnosis and survival rates within each stage. The mortality data reported by SEER are provided by the National Center for Health Statistics.

The Cancer Statistics Branch (CSB) manages SEER program, and conducts research and developmental activities related to the surveillance of cancer patterns in the United States and monitors progress against cancer. This monograph and other SEER publications/monographs can be viewed at http://seer.cancer.gov/ under Publications.

— Cancer Epidemiology in Older Adolescents and Young Adults 15 to 29 Years of Age, including SEER Incidence and Survival, 1975–2000. Bleyer A, O'Leary M, Barr R, Ries LAG (eds): National Cancer Institute, NIH Pub. No. 06-5767, Bethesda MD, June 2006; also available at www.seer.cancer.gov/publications/aya.

PDQ (Physician Data Query)

http://seer.cancer.gov/cancer_information/doc.aspx?viewid=9D617786-179B-4DB7-8664-885DD33E7D51. NCI's comprehensive cancer database includes summaries on cancer treatment, screening, prevention, genetics, and supportive care, and information on ongoing clinical trials. Some PDQ information is available in Spanish.

NCI Cancer Facts
http://cis.nci.gov/fact/index.htm

A collection of fact sheets that address a variety of cancer topics. Fact sheets are frequently updated and revised in accordance with the latest cancer research.

What You Need to Know About

http://www.cancer.gov/cancer_information/doc.aspx?viewid=920AFA90-5547-4739-8D2D89968F77A87D
A publication series that provides information on many types of cancer. Each publication includes information about symptoms, diagnosis, treatment, emotional issues, and questions to ask your doctor.

International Resources
http://cis.nci.nih.gov/resources/internatinonal.htm

A list of cancer resources that may be particularly helpful to information seekers living outside the United States.

National Institutes of Health Resources
http://cis.nci.nih.gov/resources/nci.htm

A compendium of cancer-related information available from other NIH institutes, offices, and online resources.

MEDLINEplus
http://www.nlm.nih.gov/medlineplus/

The National Library of Medicine's MEDLINEplus Web site includes links to health topics, drug information, a medical encyclopedia, a medical dictionary, health news, directories of doctors, dentists, and hospitals, and other resources and health organizations, including MEDLINE/PubMed. MEDLINE/PubMed is the National Library of Medicine's database of references to more than 14 million articles published in 4,800 biomedical journals.

The National Cancer Institute's Cancer Information Service (CIS)

provides the latest and most accurate cancer information to patients, their families, the public, and health professionals. The CIS is a free public service of the NCI, and serves those in the United States, Puerto Rico, the United States Virgin Islands, and the Pacific Islands. The CIS provides personalized, confidential responses to specific questions about cancer.

— By telephone: United States residents may call the CIS toll free at 1-800-4-CANCER (1-800-422-6237). CIS information specialists answer calls Monday through Friday from 9:00 a.m. to 4:30 p.m. (caller's local time), in English or Spanish. Callers with TTY equipment may call 1-800-332-8615. Callers also have the option of listening to recorded information about cancer 24 h a day, 7 days a week.

— Online: CIS information specialists also offer online assistance in English Monday through Friday from 9:00 a.m. to 11:00 p.m. Eastern Time through the LiveHelp link at http://www.cancer.gov on the Internet.

Information about Clinical Trials
http://clinicaltrials.gov/ClinicalTrials.gov

provides regularly updated information about federally and privately supported clinical research in human volunteers. This site includes information about a trial's purpose, who may participate, locations, and phone numbers for more details.

Office of Cancer Survivorship
http://cancercontrol.cancer.gov/ocs/

The mission of NCI's Office of Cancer Survivorship (OCS) is to enhance the quality and length of survival of all persons diagnosed with cancer and to minimize or stabilize adverse effects experienced during cancer survivorship.
- Develops an agenda for the continuous acquisition of knowledge concerning the problems and challenges facing cancer survivors and their families.
- Supports studies to increase the length of survival for cancer patients and improve the quality of survival of all individuals diagnosed with cancer and their families, including those that involve prevention of subsequent disease and disability.
- Promotes the dissemination of information to professionals who treat cancer patients and to the public concerning the problems and needs of cancer survivors and their families.

Living Beyond Cancer: Finding a New Balance
http://deainfo.nci.nih.gov/ADVISORY/pcp/pcp03-04rpt/Survivorship.pdf

This report of the President's Cancer Panel, a Presidential advisory committee charged with overseeing the development and execution of the National Cancer Program, is the first to take a life span approach to describing cancer survivorship issues, focusing particularly on the posttreatment period. In addition to identifying issues common to people regardless of their age at diagnosis, it enumerates challenges specific to those diagnosed as children (ages 0 to 14 years), adolescents and young adults (ages 15 to 29 years), adults (30 to 59 years of age), and older adults (ages 60 years and older). The findings and 17 recommendations are drawn from testimony received at 5 meetings conducted between May 2003 and January 2004, as well as additional data gathering. The nearly 200 meeting participants included survivors, caregivers, healthcare providers, advocates, and others who candidly described their experiences of life after cancer and the issues of providing care and support. Testimony was provided both in formal hearings and at evening Town Hall meetings.

LIVESTRONG Young Adult Alliance
www.livestrong.org/youngadult

The mission of the LIVESTRONG Young Adult Alliance is to improve survival rates and quality of life for young adults living with cancer by promoting relevant research and the delivery of patient care, generating awareness of the issue, being a voice for young adults with cancer, and advancing helpful community-based programs and services.

Fertile Hope
www.fertilehope.org

Fertile Hope is a national nonprofit organization dedicated to providing reproductive information, support, and hope to cancer patients whose medical treatments present the risk of infertility.

People Living With Cancer
www.peoplelivingwithcance.org

People Living With Cancer, the patient information website of the American Society of Clinical Oncology (ASCO), is designed to help patients and families make informed healthcare decisions. The site has specific sections for adolescents and for young adults, and provides information on more than 85 types of cancer, clinical trials, coping, side effects, a "Find an Oncologist" database, message boards, patient support organizations, and more.

Planet Cancer
www.planetcancer.org

Planet Cancer is a nonprofit organization that supports young adults with cancer in the 18- to 30-year age range. Planet Cancer's dynamic online community uses humor, current news, and interactive forums to help young adults create a network of peer support, as they communicate with other survivors worldwide about issues they face and how to cope with the disease. Planet Cancer also hosts several face-to-face retreats throughout the year, forming strong friendship bonds among young adult cancer patients and survivors.

Ulman Cancer Fund for Young Adults
http://www.ulmanfund/index.asp

The Mission of The Ulman Cancer Fund for Young Adults is to provide support programs, education, and resources – free of charge – to benefit young adults, their families, and friends who are affected by cancer, and to promote awareness and prevention of cancer.

Young Survival Coalition
www.youngsurvival.org/

The Young Survival Coalition (YSC) is the only international, nonprofit network of breast cancer survivors and supporters dedicated to the concerns and issues that are unique to young women and breast cancer. Through action, advocacy, and awareness, the YSC seeks to educate the medical, research, and legislative communities and to persuade them to address breast cancer in women aged 40 years and under. The YSC also serves as a point of contact for young women living with breast cancer.

Vital Options International
www.vitaloptions.org

Vital Options is a communications support and advocacy organization whose mission is to facilitate a global cancer dialogue through communications technology.

Teens Living with Cancer
www.teenslivingwithcancer.org

The original internet resource for 13-to 18-year-olds with cancer, their friends, and families.

Group Loop
www.grouploop.org

Online discussion boards with moderators; only cancer patients are eligible to participate.

Teen Impact
www.teenimpactprogram.com

Children's Hospital of Los Angeles site that has some general resources for teens.

RealTime Cancer
www.realtimecancer.org

Based in eastern Canada but with worldwide application, this site offer personal insights by young adults with cancer.

Leukemia and Lymphoma Society
www.leukemia.org

The Leukemia and Lymphoma Society is the world's largest voluntary health organization dedicated to funding blood cancer research, education, and patient services. The Society's mission: Cure leukemia, lymphoma, Hodgkin lymphoma, and myeloma, and improve the quality of life of patients and their families.

National Comprehensive Cancer Network (NCCN) www.nccn.org

An alliance of 19 of the world's leading cancer centers, is an authoritative source of information to help patients and health professionals make informed decisions about cancer care. Through the collective expertise of its member institutions, the NCCN develops, updates, and disseminates a complete library of clinical practice guidelines. These guidelines are the standard for clinical policy in oncology.

Look Good – Feel Better
www.lookgoodfeelbetter.org

A free, nonmedical, national public service program to help women offset appearance-related changes from cancer treatment. There is also a special program called 2bMe for teenagers.

CancerCare
www.cancercare.org

A nonprofit organization that provides free professional counseling and educational programs for young adults with cancer and their loved ones.

Health Insurance

www.tonikplans.com.
BlueCross & Aetna plans for young adults
in California and Colorado
www.aflac.com/us/en/individuals/cancer.aspx.
Cancer insurance for young adults with cancer.

Information about Specific Cancers
(see also www.cancer.gov)

Sarcoma

The Kristin Ann Carr Sarcoma Fund
www.sarcoma.com
Liddy Shriver Sarcoma Initiative
www.liddyshriversarcomainitiative.com

Breast Cancer

Young Survival Coalition www.youngsurvival.org
See additional information above
Living With It www.livingwithit.org
Another resource for breast cancer support

Cervical Cancer

Papsmear www.papsmear.org

Colon Cancer

Rolling to Recovery www.rollingtorecovery.com

Ovarian Cancer

www.gildasclub.org

Many local Gilda's Clubs offer a group called "Living with cancer in your 20s & 30s."

Educational-Recreational Events/Camps

Camp Make-A-Dream www.campdream.org. Hosts young adults at Camp Make-A-Dream in Gold Creek, Montana for weeklong retreats
First Descents www.firstdescents.com. Free, seven-day kayak camp in Colorado for young adults with cancer.
Tip-of-Toes www.tip-of-toes.org. Expeditions in Canada and points north for teens and young adults with cancer
Teenage Cancer Trust www.teencancer.org International conferences on cancer and the adolescent held every even year in England

Survivorship Guidelines
http://www.survivorshpguidelines.org.

The Children's Oncology Group has posted guidelines for long-term follow-up of pediatric cancer that may help the adolescent and young adult with cancer, including following topics:
Introduction to Long-Term Follow-Up
Emotional Issues
Finding Appropriate Healthcare after Cancer
Health Promotion via Diet and Physical Activity
Educational Issues
Female Health Issues
Male Health Issues
Hearing Problems
Dental Health
Pulmonary Health
Bleomycin Alert
Kidney Health
Liver Health and Hepatitis
Bone Health
Avascular Necrosis
Skin Health
Splenic Precautions
Heart Problems
Eye Problems
Peripheral Neuropathy
Raynaud's Phenomenon

Hypopituitarism
Growth Hormone Deficiency
Hyperprolactinemia
Thyroid Problems
Central Adrenal Insufficiency
Precocious Puberty
Limb Salvage after Bone Cancer
Scoliosis and Kyphosis
Breast Cancer
Reducing the Risk of Second Cancers

Steps for Living
www.StepsForLiving.org

Information about events and resources for survivors of cancer.

Subject Index

C

H

I

T

U

V

W

Y